Cardiac Pacing and Defibrillation:

A Clinical Approach

By

David L. Hayes, M.D.
*Consultant, Division of Cardiovascular Diseases
and Internal Medicine
Mayo Clinic and Mayo Foundation
Professor of Medicine
Mayo Medical School
Rochester, Minnesota*

Margaret A. Lloyd, M.D.
*Consultant, Division of Cardiovascular Diseases
and Internal Medicine
Mayo Clinic and Mayo Foundation
Assistant Professor of Medicine
Mayo Medical School
Rochester, Minnesota*

and

Paul A. Friedman, M.D.
*Senior Associate Consultant
Division of Cardiovascular Diseases
and Internal Medicine
Mayo Clinic and Mayo Foundation
Assistant Professor of Medicine
Mayo Medical School
Rochester, Minnesota*

**Futura Publishing
Company, Inc.**
Armonk, NY

Library of Congress Cataloging-in-Publication Data

Hayes, David L.
    Cardiac pacing and defibrillation : a clinical approach / by David L. Hayes, Margaret A. Lloyd and Paul A. Friedman.
        p. ; cm.
    Includes bibliographical references and index.
    ISBN 13: 978-0-8799-3462-0
    ISBN 10: 0-8799-3462-x
        1. Cardiac pacing. 2. Electric countershock. I. Lloyd, Margaret A. (Margaret Ann), 1942- II. Friedman, Paul A. III. Title.
    [DNLM: 1. Cardiac Pacing, Artificial. 2. Defibrillators, Implantable. 3. Pacemaker, Artificial. WG 168 H417c 2000]
    RC684.P3 H387 2000
    617.4'120645—dc21   00-034098

Blackwell Publishing, Inc., 350 Main Street, Malden, Massachusetts 02148-5018, USA
Blackwell Publishing Ltd, 9600 Garsington Road, Oxford OX4 2DQ, UK
Blackwell Science Asia Pty Ltd, 550 Swanston Street, Carlton South, Victoria 3053, Australia

07 06   8 9

For further information on Blackwell Publishing, visit our website:
www.futuraco.com
www.blackwellpublishing.com

Dedication

DLH: For Sharonne, Sarah, Drew, and my parents.

MAL: For Linda.

PAF: To my wife Vicki, whose love and encouragement make the impossible possible, and to my daughters Lindsay, Hannah, and Maddy.

Preface

Cardiac Pacing and Defibrillation: A Clinical Approach is intended to be a text that is uniformly written with sensible, matter-of-fact methods for understanding and caring for patients with permanent pacemakers and internal cardioverter-defibrillators (ICDs). Our intent was not to create an encyclopedic text. Instead, we meant to provide practical clinical information for those involved in cardiac pacing and defibrillation. Several excellent multiauthored texts provide encyclopedic information. Readers of this text who seek more detailed information about specific subjects are referred to these sources.[1–3]

Cardiac pacing and, more recently, cardiac defibrillation have become fields unto themselves as the technology has proliferated and the devices have rapidly become increasingly more sophisticated. Almost every text that discusses cardiac pacing mentions the first pacemaker implantation in 1958 and the unbelievably rapid advances in technology in the ensuing four decades. Building on the technologic foundation of cardiac pacing, ICD therapy has evolved even more astoundingly. With the first ICD implantation in 1980, who would have imagined the strides made by the turn of the century?

Many experts, myself included, have made the mistake of saying at pivotal developmental points in the past that further advances in pacemaker technology are not possible. Having witnessed the continued improvements in pacemakers and ICDs in recent years, I would not underestimate the potential for future improvements with either device. Clearly, there is still significant opportunity to improve the size, automaticity, and intelligence of future implantable devices.

This text is meant to help the reader understand the technical capabilities of pacemakers and ICDs and how to apply this knowledge clinically. Whether the reader is new to cardiac pacing and defibrillation or is seeing patients with implantable devices every day, we hope that the information we have included will make clinical encounters easier.

One of the inspirations to take on this project was the enjoyment derived from writing *A Practice of Cardiac Pacing* with Dr. Seymour Furman and Dr. David Holmes. They are both outstanding individuals, two of the most respected experts in their fields and valued mentors and friends.

When the decision was made not to pursue another edition of *A Practice of Cardiac Pacing*, I ultimately decided to proceed with a new text and expand the text to include ICD therapy. Again, I was fortunate to recruit the talents of Dr. Paul Friedman and Dr. Margaret Lloyd, both colleagues at the Mayo Clinic. Our institution is favored by a wide breadth of clinical material from which to gain expertise. Working in the same institution with a cohesive approach to patient care made it relatively easy to agree on the "practical approaches" espoused in this text.

I feel strongly that there is merit in a text written by a small number of contributors. Not to detract from the expertise of the contributors or editors of the texts referenced in this book or in others, limiting the number of authors allows a connection from chapter to chapter and a consistent writing style. Our hope is that this choice will make reading and comprehension easier.

The content of this text was determined after a great deal of thought. We have attempted to provide a logical progression from a description of device indications to selection of the most appropriate mode and hardware. From there, we proceed to device implantation and subsequent management with detailed sections on troubleshooting, complications, and follow-up.

We have access to extensive support at the Mayo Clinic, and the preparation of this text has made me appreciate these resources even more. We have leaned heavily on the services of our Section of Scientific Publications and Visual Information Services. Our editorial group is unequaled in their expertise, and although we owe a great deal to the entire section, the book would not have made it to fruition without the help of Roberta Schwartz, John Prickman, Debra Ward, and Renée Van Vleet. Understanding what we wanted to convey in this text, they applied their skills to such details as production, editing, formatting, reference checking, and proofreading.

Our visual information group is equally outstanding. More persons from this area have helped than can be named individually, but those who dealt with our requests, those in the archives section, the medical illustrators, and the graphic artists have all been spectacular.

Many others have influenced this project. All our physician and nursing colleagues in the Pacing and Electrophysiology Group at Mayo Clinic Rochester have had either a direct or an indirect influence on portions of this text. Our intention is not to officially represent our entire practice of pacing and electrophysiology with this text. However, given a significant consistency in the way we practice and how we approach patients, we would expect general agreement with the clinical management strategies put forward in this text.

Dr. Sharonne Hayes, cardiologist and wife, has been immensely helpful by providing expertise and echocardiographic examples in the chapter on hemodynamics. Invaluable assistance has also been obtained in the form of illustrations and hemodynamic expertise from Dr. Rick Nishimura and Dr. Tom Gerber in the hemodynamics chapter.

We also acknowledge Dr. Stephen Hammill, Dr. Robert Rea, Dr. Michael Glikson, Dr. Chuck Swerdlow, and Paul DeGroot, whose careful review and thoughtful comments strengthened the sections on defibrillation and defibrillators. Our work is improved by their input.

David L. Hayes, M.D.

References

1. Ellenbogen KA, Kay GN, Wilkoff BL (editors): Clinical Cardiac Pacing and Defibrillation. Second edition. Philadelphia, WB Saunders Company, 2000
2. Zipes DP, Jalife J (editors): Cardiac Electrophysiology: From Cell to Bedside. Third edition. Philadelphia, WB Saunders Company, 2000
3. Estes NAM III, Manolis AS, Wang PJ (editors): Implantable Cardioverter-Defibrillators: A Comprehensive Textbook. New York, Dekker, 1994

Cardiac Pacing and Defibrillation: A Clinical Approach

1

Clinically Relevant Basics of Pacing and Defibrillation

Margaret A. Lloyd, M.D.,
David L. Hayes, M.D.,
Paul A. Friedman, M.D.

Anatomy and Physiology of the Cardiac Conduction System

The cardiac conduction system consists of specialized tissue involved in the generation and conduction of electrical impulses throughout the heart. In this book, we review how device therapy can be optimally utilized for various forms of conduction system disturbances. An understanding of the normal anatomy and physiology of the cardiac conduction system is key to understanding appropriate utilization of device therapy.

The sinoatrial (SA) node, located at the junction of the right atrium and the superior vena cava, normally is the site of impulse generation (Fig. 1–1). The SA node is composed of a dense collagen matrix containing a variety of cells. The large, centrally located P cells are thought to be the origin of electrical impulses in the SA node, which is surrounded by transitional cells and fiber tracts extending through the perinodal area into the right atrium proper. The SA node is richly innervated

by the autonomic nervous system, which has a key function in rate regulation. Specialized fibers, such as the bundle of Kent, conduct the impulse throughout the right and left atria. The SA node has the highest rate of spontaneous depolarization and under normal circumstances is responsible for generating most impulses.

Atrial conduction fibers converge at the atrioventricular (AV) node, a small subendocardial structure located within the interatrial septum (Fig. 1–1). The AV node likewise receives abundant autonomic innervation, and it is histologically similar to the SA node because it is composed of a loose collagen matrix in which P cells and transitional cells are located. Additionally, Purkinje cells and myocardial contractile fibers may be found. The AV node allows for physiologic delay between atrial and ventricular contraction, resulting in optimal cardiac hemodynamic function. It can also function as a subsidiary "pacemaker" should the SA node fail. Finally, the AV node functions (albeit typically suboptimally) to regulate the number of impulses eventu-

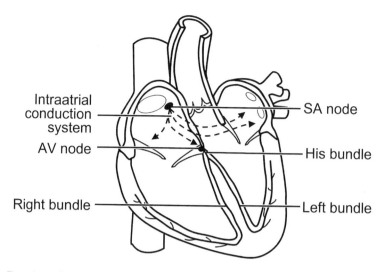

Fig. 1–1. Drawing of the cardiac conduction system. AV, atrioventricular; SA, sinoatrial. See text for details.

ally reaching the ventricle in instances of atrial tachyarrhythmia.

Purkinje fibers emerge from the distal AV node to form the bundle of His, which runs through the membranous septum to the crest of the muscular septum, where it divides into the various bundle branches. The bundle branch system exhibits significant individual variety but is invariably complex. The right bundle is typically a discrete structure running along the right side of the interventricular septum to the anterior papillary muscle, where it divides. The left bundle is usually a large band of fibers fanning out over the left ventricle, sometimes forming functional fascicles. Both bundles eventually terminate in individual Purkinje fibers interdigitating with myocardial contractile fibers. The His-Purkinje system has little in the way of autonomic innervation.

Because of their key function and location, the SA and AV nodes are the most common sites of conduction system failure; it is therefore understandable that the most common indications for pacemaker implantation are SA node dysfunction and high-grade AV block. It should be noted, however, that conduction system disease is frequently diffuse and may involve the specialized conduction system at multiple sites.

Although the earliest pacemakers were designed to treat life-threatening ventricular bradyarrhythmias, current potential indications have drastically expanded to include conditions that do not specifically involve intrinsic conduction system disease. Guidelines have been developed to provide uniform criteria for device implantation, but the importance of the patient's clinical status and any extenuating circumstances should also be considered.

Electrophysiology of Myocardial Stimulation

Stimulation of the myocardium by a pacemaker requires the initiation of a self-propagating wave of depolarization from the site of initial activation, whether from a native "pacemaker" or from an artificial stimulus. Myocardium exhibits a biologic property referred to as "excitability," which is a response to a stimulus out of proportion to the strength of that stimulus.[1] Excitability is maintained by separation of chemical charge, which results in an electrical transmembrane potential. In cardiac myocytes, this electrochemical gradient is created by differing intracellular and extracellular concentrations of sodium (Na^+) and potassium (K^+) ions; Na^+ ions predominate extracellularly and K^+ ions predominate intracellularly. Although this transmembrane gradient is maintained by the high chemical resistance intrinsic to the lipid bilayer of the cellular membrane, passive leakage of these ions occurs across the cellular membrane through ion channels. This passive leakage is offset by two active transport mechanisms, each transporting three positive charges out of the myocyte in exchange for two positive charges that are moved into the myocyte, producing cellular polarization.[2,3] These active transport mechanisms require energy and are susceptible to disruption when energy-generating processes are interrupted.

The chemical gradient has a key role in the generation of the transmembrane action potential (Fig. 1–2). The membrane potential of approximately -90 mV drifts upward to the threshold potential of approximately -70 to -60 mV. At this point, specialized membrane-bound channels modify their conformation from an inactive to an active state, which allows the abrupt influx of extracellular Na^+ ions into the myocyte,[4,5] creating phase 0 of the action potential and rapidly raising the transmembrane potential to approximately $+20$ mV.[6,7] This rapid upstroke creates a short period of overshoot potential (phase 1), which is followed by a plateau period (phase 2) created by the inward calcium (Ca^{++}) and Na^+ currents balanced against outward K^+ currents.[8–10] During phase 3 of the action potential, the transmembrane potential returns to normal, and during phase 4, the gradual upward drift in transmembrane potential repeats. The shape of the transmembrane potential and the relative distribution of the various membrane-bound ion channels differ between the components of the specialized cardiac conduction system.

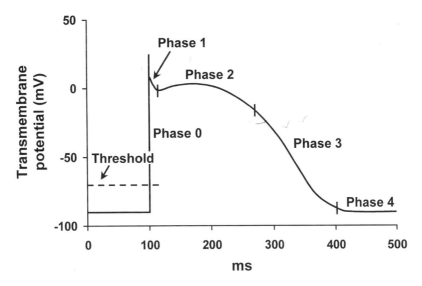

Fig. 1–2. Action potential of a typical Purkinje fiber, with the various phases of depolarization and repolarization (described in the text). (From Stokes KB, Kay GN: Artificial electric cardiac stimulation. *In* Clinical Cardiac Pacing. Edited by KA Ellenbogen, GN Kay, BL Wilkoff. Philadelphia, WB Saunders Company, 1995, pp 3–37. By permission of the publisher.)

Depolarization of neighboring cells occurs as a result of passive conduction via low-resistance intercellular connections called "gap junctions," with active regeneration along cellular membranes.[11,12] The velocity of depolarization throughout the myocardium depends on the speed of depolarization of the various cellular components of the myocardium and on the geometrical arrangement of the myocytes. Factors such as myocardial ischemia, electrolyte imbalance, and drugs may affect the depolarization and depolarization velocity.

Pacing Basics

Stimulation Threshold

Artificial pacing involves delivery of an electrical impulse from an electrode of sufficient strength to cause depolarization of the myocardium in contact with that electrode and propagation of that depolarization to the rest of the myocardium. The minimal amount of energy required to produce this depolarization is called the *stimulation threshold*.[13] The components of the stimulus include the pulse amplitude (measured in volts) and the pulse duration (measured in milliseconds). An exponential relationship exists between the stimulus amplitude and the duration, resulting in a hyperbolic *strength-duration curve*.[14] At short pulse durations, a small change in the pulse duration is associated with a significant change in the pulse amplitude required to achieve myocardial depolarization; conversely, at long pulse durations, a small change in pulse duration has relatively little effect on threshold amplitude (Fig. 1–3). Two points on the strength-duration curve should be noted (Fig. 1–4). The *rheobase* is defined as the smallest amplitude (voltage) that stimulates the myocardium at an infinitely long pulse duration (milliseconds); the *chronaxie* is the

threshold pulse duration at twice the stimulus amplitude, which is twice the rheobase voltage.[15] The chronaxie is important in the clinical practice of pacing because it approximates the point of minimum threshold energy (microjoules) required for myocardial depolarization.[16]

The relationship of voltage, current, and pulse duration to stimulus energy is described by the formula

$$E = V^2/R \times t$$

in which E is the stimulus energy, V is the voltage, R is the total pacing impedance, and t is the pulse duration.[17] This formula demonstrates the relative lack of increase in energy with longer pulse durations.

The strength-duration curve discussed thus far has been that of a constant voltage system, because contemporary permanent pacemakers are constant voltage systems and constant current devices are no longer used (Fig. 1–5). It should be recognized, however, that constant current strength-duration curves can also be constructed.[18] These strength-duration curves, like constant voltage curves, are hyperbolic in shape, but they have a much more gradual decline in current requirements as the pulse width lengthens. Because of this gradual decline, chronaxie of a constant current system is significantly greater than that in a constant voltage system.

Impedance is the term applied to the impediment to current flow in the pacing system. Ohm's law describes the relationship among voltage, current, and resistance as

$$V = IR$$

in which V is the voltage, I is the current, and R is the resistance.[19] Although Ohm's law is used for determining impedance,

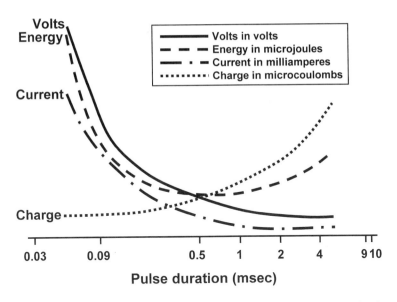

Fig. 1–3. Relationship of charge, energy, voltage, and current to pulse duration. As the pulse duration is shortened, voltage and current requirements increase. Charge decreases as pulse duration shortens. At threshold, energy is lowest at a pulse duration of 0.5 to 1.0 msec and increases at pulse widths of shorter and longer duration. (Modified from Furman S: Basic concepts. *In* A Practice of Cardiac Pacing. Edited by S Furman, DL Hayes, DR Holmes Jr. Mount Kisco, NY, Futura Publishing Company. By permission of the publisher.)

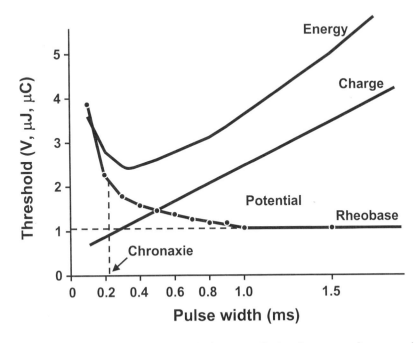

Fig. 1–4. Relationships among chronic ventricular strength-duration curves from a canine, expressed as potential (V), charge (μC), and energy (μJ). Rheobase is the threshold at infinitely long pulse duration. Chronaxie is the pulse duration at twice rheobase. (From Stokes K, Bornzin G: The electrode-biointerface stimulation. *In* Modern Cardiac Pacing. Edited by SS Barold. Mount Kisco, NY, Futura Publishing Company, 1985, pp 33–77. By permission of the publisher.)

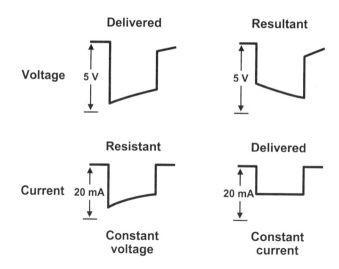

Fig. 1–5. Diagrammatic representation of the delivered voltage and resultant current in a constant-voltage system compared with the delivered current and resultant voltage in a constant-current system. (Modified from Stokes K, Bornzin G: The electrode-biointerface stimulation. *In* Modern Cardiac Pacing. Edited by SS Barold. Mount Kisco, NY, Futura Publishing Company, 1985, pp 33–77. By permission of the publisher.)

technically *impedance* and *resistance* are not interchangeable terms. Impedance implies inclusion of all factors that contribute to current flow impediment, including lead conductor resistance, electrode resistance, and resistance due to electrode polarization. Nevertheless, Ohm's law (substituting impedance for R) is commonly used for calculating impedance. In constant voltage systems, the lower the pacing impedance, the greater the current flow; conversely, the higher the pacing impedance, the lower the current flow. Ideally, the lead conductor material would have a low resistance to minimize the generation of energy-wasting heat as the current flows along the lead, and the electrode would have a high resistance to minimize current flow and negligible electrode polarization. Decreasing the lead radius minimizes current flow by providing greater electrode resistance and increased current density, resulting in greater battery longevity and lower stimulation thresholds.[20]

Polarization refers to layers of oppo-sitely charged ions that surround the electrode during the pulse stimulus.[21] It is related to the movement of positively charged ions (Na^+ and H_3O^+) to the negatively charged electrode; the layer of positively charged ions is then surrounded by a layer of negatively charged ions (Cl^-, HPO_4^-, and OH^-). These layers of charge develop during the pulse stimulus, reaching peak formation at the termination of the pulse stimulus, after which they gradually dissipate. Polarization impedes the movement of charge from the electrode to the myocardium, resulting in a need for increased voltage. Since polarization develops with increasing pulse duration, one way to combat formation of polarization is to shorten the pulse duration. Electrode design has incorporated the use of materials that discourage polarization, such as platinum black, iridium oxide, titanium nitride, and activated carbon.[22–26] Finally, polarization is inversely related to the surface area of the electrode. To maximize the surface area (to reduce polarization) but minimize the radius (to increase electrode impedance), electrode design incorporates a small radius but a porous, irregular surface construction.[27,28] New "high- impedance" leads attempt to maximize the benefits of such design.

Variations in Stimulation Threshold

Myocardial thresholds typically fluctuate, sometimes dramatically, during the first weeks after implantation. After implantation of an endocardial lead, the stimulation threshold typically rises rapidly in the first 24 hours and then gradually increases to a peak at 1 week[29–33] (Fig. 1–6). Over the ensuing 6 to 8 weeks, the stimulation threshold usually declines to a level somewhat higher than that at implantation but less than the peak threshold, known as the "chronic threshold." The magnitude and duration of this early increase in threshold depend in part on lead electrode size, shape, and design; in-

terface between the lead and the myocardium; and individual variation.

Transvenous pacing leads have used passive or active fixation mechanisms to provide a stable electrode-myocardium interface. Active fixation leads typically have higher pacing thresholds at implantation, which frequently decline significantly within the first 15 to 30 minutes after implantation.[34] This effect has been attributed to hyperacute injury due to advancement of the screw into the myocardium. The incorporation of corticosteroid compounds into the electrode design has resulted in significantly lower acute and chronic thresholds.[35–37] Steroid elution was available only in passive fixation leads for many years but has now been available in active fixation leads as well for several years.

On a cellular level, implantation of a transvenous pacing lead results in acute injury to cellular membranes, which is followed by the development of myocar-

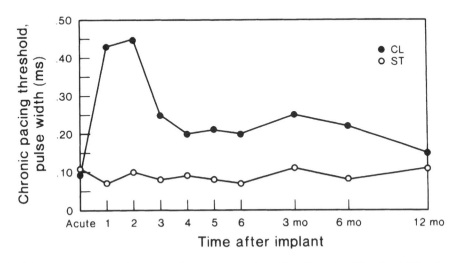

Fig. 1–6. Long-term pacing thresholds from a conventional lead (no steroid elution) (CL; *closed circles*) and a steroid-eluting lead (ST; *open circles*). With the conventional lead, an early increase in threshold decreases to a plateau at approximately 4 weeks. The threshold for the steroid-eluting lead remains relatively flat, with no significant change from short-term threshold measurements. (From Furman S: Basic concepts. *In* A Practice of Cardiac Pacing. Second revised and enlarged edition. Edited by S Furman, DL Hayes, DR Holmes Jr. Mount Kisco, NY, Futura Publishing Company, 1989, pp 23–78. By permission of Mayo Foundation.)

dial edema and coating of the electrode surface with platelets and fibrin. Subsequently, various chemotactic factors are released, and an acute inflammatory reaction consisting of mononuclear cells and polymorphonuclear leukocytes develops. After the acute response, release of proteolytic enzymes and oxygen free radicals by invading macrophages accelerates cellular injury. Finally, fibroblasts in the myocardium begin producing collagen, leading to production of the fibrotic capsule surrounding the electrode. This fibrous capsule ultimately increases the effective radius of the electrode, with a smaller increase in surface area.[38-40]

The stimulation threshold typically has a circadian pattern, generally increasing during sleep and decreasing during the day, probably reflecting changes in autonomic tone. The stimulation threshold may also rise after eating; during hyperglycemia, hypoxemia, or acute viral illnesses; or as a result of electrolyte fluctuations. Many drugs used in patients with cardiac disease likewise increase pacing thresholds (see Chapter 9).

A phenomenon that sometimes develops is *exit block*.[34,41,42] Exit block is a progressive rise in thresholds over time. It occurs despite initial satisfactory lead placement and implantation thresholds, tends to occur in parallel in the atrium and ventricle, and recurs with placement of subsequent leads. Steroid-eluting leads prevent exit block in most, but not all, patients (Fig. 1–7).

Sensing

The first pacemakers functioned as fixed-rate, VOO devices. All current devices offer demand-mode pacing, which is pacing when the intrinsic rate is below the programmed rate. For such devices to function as programmed, accurate and consistent sensing of the native rhythm is essential.

Intrinsic cardiac electrical signals are produced by the wave of electrical current through the myocardium (Fig. 1–8). As the wave front of electrical energy approaches an endocardial electrode, the

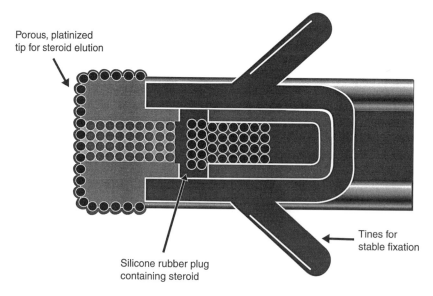

Fig. 1–7. Diagram of a steroid-eluting passive fixation lead. The electrode has a porous, platinized tip. A silicone rubber plug is impregnated with 1 mg of dexamethasone sodium.

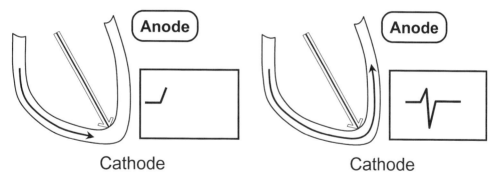

Fig. 1–8. Schema of the relationship of the pacing lead to the recorded electrogram with unipolar sensing. *Left,* As the electrical impulse moves toward the cathode (lead tip), a positive deflection is created in the electrogram. *Right,* As the electrical impulse passes the cathode, the deflection suddenly becomes downward, and as the impulse moves away from the cathode, a negative deflection occurs. (From Kay GN, Ellenbogen KA: Sensing. *In* Clinical Cardiac Pacing. Edited by KA Ellenbogen, GN Kay, BL Wilkoff. Philadelphia, WB Saunders Company, 1995, pp 38–68. By permission of the publisher.)

electrode becomes positively charged relative to the depolarized region, recorded as a positive deflection in the intracardiac electrogram. As the wave front passes directly under the electrode, the outside of the cell abruptly becomes negatively charged, and a sharp negative deflection is recorded, which is referred to as the *intrinsic deflection.*[43,44] It is considered to occur at the moment the advancing wave front passes directly underneath the electrode. Smaller positive and negative deflections preceding and following the intrinsic deflection represent activation of surrounding myocardium. Ventricular electrograms typically are much larger than atrial electrograms because ventricular mass is greater. Fourier transformation has been used to determine the maximum frequency density of atrial and ventricular electrograms, which have generally been found to be in the range of 80 to 100 Hz in the atrium and 10 to 30 Hz in the ventricle. This information has been used to incorporate filtering systems into pulse generators that attenuate signals outside these ranges. Filtering and use of blanking and refractory periods have markedly reduced unwanted sensing, although myopotential frequencies (ranging from 10 to 200 Hz)

considerably overlap with those generated by atrial and ventricular depolarization and are difficult to filter out, especially during sensing in the unipolar mode.[45–47]

Another component of the intracardiac electrogram is the *slew rate,* that is, the peak slope of the developing electrogram[48] (Fig. 1–9). The slew rate represents the maximal rate of change of the electrical potential between the sensing electrodes and is the first derivative of the electrogram (dV/dt). An acceptable slew rate should be at least 0.5 V/sec in both the atrium and the ventricle. In general, the higher the slew rate, the higher the frequency content and the more likely the signal will be sensed. Slow, broad signals, such as those generated by the T wave, are much less likely to be sensed because of a low slew rate and lower frequency density.

Polarization was described previously in this chapter as part of the discussion on stimulation thresholds. Similarly, polarization affects sensing function. After termination of the pulse stimulus, an excess of positive charge surrounds the cathode, which then decays until electrically neutral. Afterpotentials can be sensed with inappropriate inhibition or delay of the subsequent pacing pulse (Fig. 1–10).

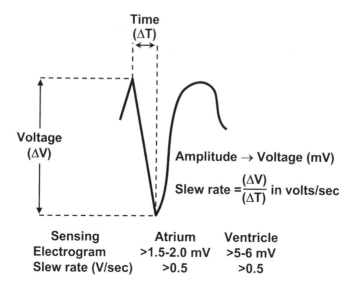

Fig. 1–9. In the intracardiac electrogram, the difference in voltage recorded between two electrodes is the amplitude, which is measured in millivolts. The slew rate is volts per second and should be at least 0.5. (From Kay GN, Ellenbogen KA: Sensing. *In* Clinical Cardiac Pacing. Edited by KA Ellenbogen, GN Kay, BL Wilkoff. Philadelphia, WB Saunders Company, 1995, pp 38–68. By permission of the publisher.)

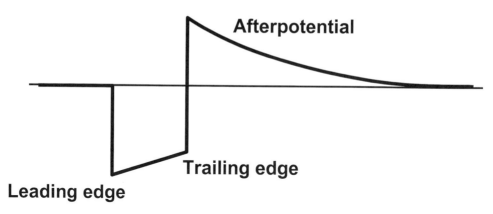

Fig. 1–10. Diagram of a pacing pulse, constant-voltage, with leading edge and trailing edge voltage and an afterpotential with opposite polarity. As described in the text, afterpotentials may result in sensing abnormalities. (From Kay GN, Ellenbogen KA: Sensing. *In* Clinical Cardiac Pacing. Edited by KA Ellenbogen, GN Kay, BL Wilkoff. Philadelphia, WB Saunders Company, 1995, pp 38–68. By permission of the publisher.)

The amplitude of afterpotentials is directly related to both the amplitude and the duration of the pacing pulse; thus, they are most likely to be sensed when the pacemaker is programmed to high voltage and long pulse duration in combination with maximal sensitivity.[49] The use of programmable sensing refractory and blanking periods has helped to prevent the pacemaker from reacting to afterpotentials, although in dual-chamber systems, atrial afterpotentials of sufficient strength and duration to be sensed by the ventricular channel may result in inappropriate ventricular inhibition (*crosstalk*, see below), especially in unipolar systems.[50] Afterpotentials may especially cause problems in devices with automatic threshold measurement and capture detection; the use of leads designed to minimize afterpotentials may increase the effectiveness of such devices.[51]

Similar to pacing thresholds, the amplitude and slew rate of the intracardiac electrogram may demonstrate an abrupt decline during the first week after lead implantation. After 6 to 8 weeks, these values approach implantation values. Acute fixation leads additionally demonstrate a marked decrease in values immediately after lead placement, with increases during the first 20 to 30 minutes after implantation. Corticosteroid-eluting leads typically cause little deterioration in electrogram measurements after implantation.

Source impedance is a term used to describe the voltage drop that occurs from the origin of the intracardiac electrogram to the proximal portion of the lead.[52] Components include the resistance between the electrode and the myocardium, the resistance of the lead conductor material, and the effects of polarization. The resistance between the electrode and the myocardium, as well as polarization, is inversely related to the surface area of the electrode; thus, the effects of both can be minimized by a large electrode surface area. The electrogram actually seen by the pulse generator is determined by the ratio between the sensing amplifier (input impedance) and the lead (source impedance). The greater the ratio of input impedance to source impedance, the less attenuation of the signal from the myocardium. Clinically, impedance mismatch is seen with insulation or conductor failure, which results in sensing abnormalities or failure.

Lead Design

Pacing leads are perhaps the "weak link" in the system, as most pacing system problems are due to failure of some component of the lead. These compo-

nents include the electrode, the conductor, the insulation, and the connector pin (Fig. 1–11 and 1–12). Leads function in a harsh environment in vivo: They must be constructed of materials that provide both mechanical stability and flexibility; they must have satisfactory electrical conductive and resistive properties; the insulating material must be durable but ideally have a low friction coefficient to facilitate implantation; and the electrode must provide good mechanical and electrical contact with the myocardium. Industry continues to modify and improve lead design, but the "ideal" lead has yet to be produced.

As previously discussed, optimal stimulation and sensing thresholds favor an electrode with a small radius and a large surface area. Electrode shape and surface composition have evolved over time. Early models utilized a round helical shape with a smooth metal surface. Electrodes with an irregular, textured surface allow for increased surface area without an increase in electrode radius.[22,23,27,53,54] To achieve increased electrode surface area, manufacturers have used a variety of designs, including microscopic pores, coatings of microspheres, and wire filament mesh.

Unfortunately, relatively few conductive materials have proven to be satisfactory for use in pacing electrodes. Ideally, electrodes are biologically inert, resist degradation over time, and do not elicit a marked tissue reaction at the myocardium-electrode interface. Certain metals, such as zinc, copper, mercury, nickel, lead, and silver, are associated with toxic reactions with the myocardium. Stainless steel alloys are susceptible to corrosion. Titanium and tantalium acquire a surface coating of oxides that impedes current transfer. Materials currently in use are platinum-iridium, Elgiloy (an alloy of cobalt, nickel, chromium, molybdenum, iron, and manganese), platinized titanium-coated platinum, pyrolytic carbon coating a titanium or

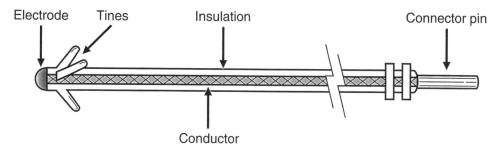

Fig. 1–11. Basic components of a passive fixation pacing lead with tines.

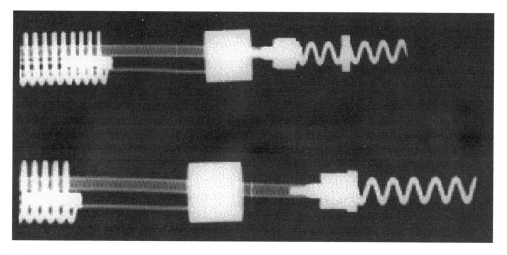

Fig. 1–12. Radiographic example of an active fixation screw-in lead with a retractable screw rather than a screw that is always extended. The screw is extended in the lower image but not in the upper image.

graphite core, iridium oxide, and platinum (Fig. 1–13). Carbon electrodes seem to be least susceptible to corrosion; they have also been improved by a process known as *activation*, which roughens the surface to increase the surface area and allow for tissue ingrowth.[25]

Lead fixation may be active or passive. Passive fixation leads usually incorporate tines or fins at the tip that become ensnared in trabeculated tissue in the right atrium or ventricle, providing lead stability. Active fixation leads have utilized various barbs and screws embedded in the myocardium to provide lead stability. Most active fixation leads now have some type of screw mechanism, either

fixed or retractable, to attach the lead to the myocardium. Although some screws are inactive, most active fixation leads now have screws that are electrically active. There are advantages and disadvantages to each design, and the clinical situation and preference of the operator are important considerations when a lead is chosen. Until recently, corticosteroid elution was available only in passive fixation leads; the introduction of active fixation leads with corticosteroid elution has made this less of a discriminating factor. Considerable myocardial and fibrous tissue enveloping the tip typically develops with passive fixation leads, making future extraction of the lead difficult. Ac-

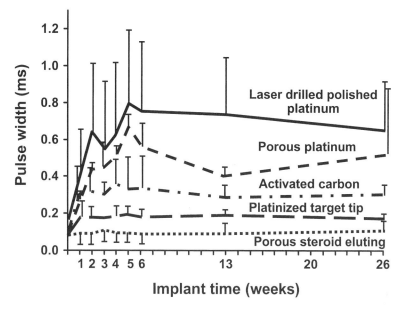

Fig. 1–13. Capture thresholds from implantation to 26 weeks from a variety of unipolar leads with similar geometric surface area electrodes. From top to bottom, the curves represent laser-drilled polished platinum; porous-surface platinum; activated carbon, platinized target tip; and porous steroid-eluting leads. (From Stokes KB, Kay GN: Artificial electric cardiac stimulation. *In* Clinical Cardiac Pacing. Edited by KA Ellenbogen, GN Kay, BL Wilkoff. Philadelphia, WB Saunders Company, 1995, pp 3–37. By permission of the publisher.)

tive fixation leads are sometimes preferable in patients with distorted anatomy, such as those with congenital cardiac defects or those with surgically amputated atrial appendages. Active fixation leads are also preferable in patients with high right-sided pressures and for patients in whom placement of the ventricular lead higher on the septum rather than in the right ventricular apex is desirable. On the other hand, the retraction mechanism of some retractable screws can fail during implantation, especially if multiple attempts are made at positioning, requiring replacement of the lead. Leads with fixed-extended screws can be difficult to advance through the vascular system and past the tricuspid valve and be difficult to rotate to attach the electrode to the myocardium. Like passive fixation leads, active fixation leads can be affected by significant myocardial ingrowth and at-

tachment, making lead extraction difficult should it become necessary.

Conductors are commonly of a multifilament design to facilitate tensile strength and reduce resistance to metal fatigue (Fig. 1–14). Alloys such as MP35N (cobalt, nickel, chromium, and molybdenum), Elgiloy, and nickel-silver are typically used in modern pacing leads. Bipolar leads may be of coaxial design, with an inner coil extending to the distal electrode and an outer coil terminating at the proximal electrode (Fig. 1–15). This design requires that the conductor coils be separated by a layer of inner insulation. Coaxial design remains the most commonly used. Some bipolar leads are coradial, or "parallel-wound"; that is, two insulated coils are wound next to each other. Leads may also be constructed with the conductor coils parallel to each other (multiluminal), again separated by insulating material (Fig. 1–15). Additionally,

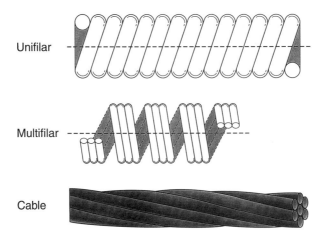

Fig. 1–14. Conductor coils may be of unifilar, multifilar, or cable design. The multifilar and cable designs allow the conductor to be more flexible and more resistant to fracture.

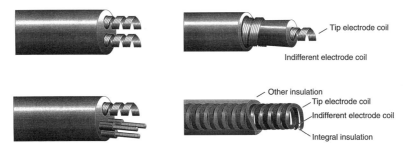

Fig. 1–15. Varieties of conductor construction. *Upper left,* Parallel multifilar coils. *Lower left,* Parallel multifilar coil and three single cables. *Upper right,* Bipolar coaxial design with an inner multifilar coil surrounded by insulation (inner), an outer multifilar coil, and outer insulation. *Lower right,* Individually coated wires wound together in a single multifilar coil for bipolar pacing.

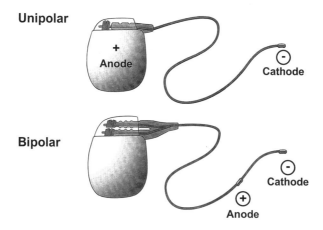

Fig. 1–16. In a unipolar configuration, the pacemaker case serves as the anode, or (+), and the electrode lead tip as the cathode, or (−). In a bipolar configuration, the anode is located on the ring, often referred to as the "ring electrode," proximal to the tip, or cathode. The distance between tip and ring electrode varies among manufacturers and models. (From Mond HG, Helland JR: Engineering and clinical aspects of pacing leads. *In* Clinical Cardiac Pacing. Edited by KA Ellenbogen, GN Kay, BL Wilkoff. Philadelphia, WB Saunders Company, 1995, pp 69–90. By permission of the publisher.)

leads may use a combination of coils and cables. The coil facilitates the passage of a stylet for lead implantation, and the cable allows a smaller lead body.

Two materials have predominated in lead insulation: silicone and polyurethane. Each has its respective advantages and disadvantages, but the overall performance of both materials has been excellent.[55] Table 4–4 in Chapter 4 compares the advantages and disadvantages of these two insulating materials.

The two polymers of polyurethane that have had the widest use are Pellathane 80A and Pellathane 55D. Early after the introduction of polyurethane as an insulating material, it became clear that clinical failure rates with specific leads were higher than acceptable; further investigation revealed that the failures were occurring primarily in leads insulated with the P80A polymer.[53,54] Microscopic cracks developed in the P80A polymer, initially occurring as the heated polymer cooled during manufacturing; with additional environmental stress, these cracks propagated deeper into the insulation, resulting in failure of the lead insulation.

Polyurethane may also undergo oxidative stress in contact with conductors containing silver chloride, resulting in degradation of the lead from the inside and subsequent lead failure. Some current leads use silicone with a polyurethane coating, incorporating the strength and durability of silicone with the ease of handling of polyurethane while maintaining a satisfactory external lead diameter. Laboratory testing and premarketing clinical trials have been inadequate to predict the long-term performance of leads, so that clinicians implanting the devices or performing follow-up in patients with pacing systems must vigilantly monitor lead status.

Contemporary leads and connectors are standardized to conform to international guidelines, which mandate that leads have a 3.2-mm diameter in-line bipolar connector pin.[56] These standards were established because some leads and connector blocks were incompatible, requiring the development of multiple adaptors. Some patients who have functioning leads of the older 5- or 6-mm diameter design require lead adaptors when the pulse generator is replaced.

Bipolar Versus Unipolar Pacing and Sensing

Since the introduction of bipolar leads early in development of pacing systems, the implanting physician has had the option of selecting bipolar or unipolar pacing and sensing. In unipolar systems, the lead tip functions as the cathode and the pulse generator functions as the anode (Fig. 1–16). In bipolar systems, the lead tip functions as the cathode and the lead ring functions as the anode (Fig. 1–16). Unipolar leads are of simpler design, have a smaller external diameter, and may have increased durability. However, they do not offer the option of bipolar function. Bipolar leads may function in the unipolar mode if the pacemaker is so programmed. They are available in several designs, generally coaxial or multiluminal. Regardless of design, the external diameter is usually greater than that of unipolar leads because each coil must be electrically separated by insulating material. Bipolar pacing and sensing are generally preferred over unipolar because bipolar pacing is less likely to result in extracardiac stimulation, which may occur with unipolar pacing. Also, bipolar sensing is less likely to detect myopotentials, far-field signals, and electromagnetic interference.

There are long-standing controversies on the superiority of unipolar over bipolar pacing and sensing configuration. Advocates of unipolar configuration argue that improvements in sensing circuitry and pacemaker filtering capabilities have minimized unipolar oversensing of extracardiac signals. They also argue that bipolar leads have a historically higher failure rate than unipolar leads. Although this is true, if the specific failures of Pellathane 80A and 55D are removed from the analysis, the failure rate between unipolar and bipolar lead designs does not differ significantly.

Unipolar pacing and sensing configuration may be advantageous when a lead is failing because of conductor fracture or insulation break. A lead that is malfunctioning in the bipolar mode may function satisfactorily when programmed to the unipolar configuration (see Chapter 9).

Most current pulse generators offer independently programmable pacing and sensing in each channel; however, bipolar programming of a device attached to a unipolar lead results in no output. Bipolar leads can function in the unipolar mode; the converse is not true.

Pulse Generators

All pulse generators include a power source, an output circuit, a sensing circuit, a timing circuit, and a header with a standardized connector (or connectors) to attach a lead (or leads) to the pulse generator.[57] Most pacemakers of the current generation also include some type of rate-adaptive sensor, telemetry, and microprocessors to allow the device to store diagnostic information that can later be retrieved. Despite increasing complexity, the size of devices has continued to decrease, and the potential longevity of most devices has increased greatly.

Many power sources have been used for pulse generators over the years: nuclear, photoelectric cell, rechargeable nickel-cadmium cell, and biogalvanic energy, to name a few. Lithium iodine cells now power almost all current pulse generators. Lithium is the anodal element and provides the supply of electrons; iodine is the cathodal element and accepts the electrons. The cathodal and anodal elements are separated by electrolyte, which serves as a conductor of ionic movement but a barrier to the transfer of electrons. The circuit is completed by the external load, that is, the leads and myocardium. The battery voltage of the cell depends on the chemical composition of the cell; at the beginning of life for the lithium iodine battery, the cell generates approximately 2.8 V, which decreases to 2.4 V when approximately 90% of the useable battery life has been reached. The voltage then exponentially declines to 1.8 V as the battery reaches end-of-life. At end-of-life, most devices lose telemetry and programming capabilities, frequently reverting to a fixed high output mode to attempt to maintain patient safety. This predictable depletion characteristic has made lithium-based power cells common in current devices.

The battery voltage can be telemetered from the pulse generator; some devices also provide battery impedance (which increases with battery depletion) for additional information about battery life. The battery life can also be estimated by the magnet rate of the device, which changes with a decline in battery voltage. Unfortunately, the magnet rates are not standardized, and rate change characteristics vary tremendously among manufacturers and even among devices produced by the same manufacturer. Therefore, it is important to know the magnet rate characteristics of a given device before using this feature to determine battery status.

The longevity of any battery is determined by several factors, including chemical composition of the battery, size of the battery, external load (pulse duration and amplitude, stimulation frequency, total pacing lead impedance, and amount of current required to operate device circuitry and store diagnostic information), amount of internal discharge, and voltage decay characteristics of the cell. The introduction of high-performance leads and automatic capture algorithms will further enhance device longevity.[51] The basic formula for longevity determination is ampere-hours/current drain $\times$ 114 = longevity in years.

The pacing pulse is generated first by charging of an output capacitor and discharge of the capacitor to the pacing cathode and anode. Since the voltage of a lithium iodine cell is 2.8 V, any pulse amplitude requires the use of a voltage amplifier between the battery and the output capacitor. Current pulse generators are constant-voltage (rather than constant-current) devices, implying delivery of a constant-voltage pulse throughout the pulse duration. In reality, some voltage drop occurs between the leading and the trailing edges of the impulse; the size of this decrease depends on the pacing impedance and pulse duration. The lower the impedance, the greater the current flow from the fixed quantity of charge on the capacitor and the greater the voltage drop throughout the pulse duration.[58] The longer the pulse duration, the more time for current to flow.

The output waveform is followed by a low amplitude wave of opposite polarity, the *afterpotential*. The afterpotential is due to polarization of the electrode at the electrode-tissue interface; formation is due to electrode characteristics as well as to pulse amplitude and duration. The sensing circuit may sense afterpotentials of sufficient amplitude, especially if the sensitivity threshold is low. Newer pacemakers use the output circuit to discharge the afterpotential quickly, thus lowering the incidence of afterpotential sensing.

The intracardiac electrogram is conducted from the myocardium to the sensing circuit via the pacing leads, where it is then amplified and filtered. As mentioned earlier in this chapter, the input impedance must be significantly larger than the sensing impedance to minimize attenuation of the electrogram. A band-pass filter attenuates signals on either side of a center frequency, which varies

among manufacturers (generally ranging from 20 to 40 Hz).[59,60] After filtering, the electrogram signal is compared with a reference voltage, the sensitivity setting; signals with an amplitude of this reference voltage or higher are sensed as true intracardiac events and are forwarded to the timing circuitry, whereas signals with an amplitude below the reference amplitude are categorized as noise, extracardiac or cardiac repolarizations, that is, T waves.

Sensing circuitry also incorporates noise reversion circuits that cause the pacemaker to revert to a noise reversion mode (asynchronous pacing) whenever the rate of signal received by the sensing circuit exceeds the noise reversion rate. This feature is incorporated to prevent inhibition of pacing when the device is exposed to electromagnetic interference. Pulse generators also use Zener diodes designed to protect the circuitry from high external voltages, which may occur, for example, with defibrillation. When the input voltage presented to the pacemaker exceeds the Zener voltage, the excess voltage is shunted back through the leads to the myocardium.

The timing circuit of the pacemaker is a crystal oscillator that regulates the pacing cycle length, refractory periods, blanking periods, and AV intervals with extreme accuracy. The output from the oscillator (as well as signals from the sensing circuitry) is sent to a timing and logic control board that operates the internal clocks, which in turn regulate all the various timing cycles of the pulse generator. The timing and logic control circuitry also contains an absolute maximal upper rate cutoff to prevent "runaway pacing" in the event of random component failure.

Each new generation of pacemakers contains more microprocessor capability. The circuitry contains a combination of ROM (read-only memory) and RAM (random-access memory). ROM is used to operate the sensing and output functions of the device, and RAM is used in diagnostic functions. Larger RAM capability has allowed devices to store increased amounts of retrievable diagnostic information, with the potential to allow downloading of new features externally into an implanted device.

External telemetry is included in all current pacing devices. The pulse generator can receive information from the programmer and send information back by radiofrequency signals. Each manufacturer's programmer and pulse generator operate on an exclusive radiofrequency, preventing the use of one manufacturer's programmer with a pacemaker from another manufacturer. Through telemetry, the programmer can retrieve both diagnostic information and real-time information on battery status, lead impedance, current, pulse amplitude, and pulse duration. Real-time electrograms and marker channels can also be obtained with many devices. The device can also be directed to operate within certain limits and to store specific types of diagnostic information via the programmer.

Pacemaker Nomenclature

A lettered code to describe the basic function of pacing devices, initially developed by the American Heart Association and the American College of Cardiology, has since been modified and updated by the members of the North American Society of Pacing and Electrophysiology and the British Pacing and Electrophysiology Group.[61] This code has five positions to describe basic pacemaker function, although it obviously cannot incorporate all of the various special features available on modern devices (Table 1–1).

The first position describes the chamber or chambers in which electrical stimulation occurs. A reflects pacing in the atrium, V implies pacing in the ventricle, D signifies pacing in both the atrium and the ventricle, and O is used when the device has antitachycardia pacing or cardioversion-defibrillation capability but no bradycardia pacing capability.

The second position describes the chamber or chambers in which sensing occurs. The letter code is the same as that in the first position, except that an O in this position represents lack of sensing in any chamber, that is, fixed-rate pacing. Some devices use an S in both the first and the second positions to indicate single-chamber capability that can be used in either the atrium or the ventricle.

The third position designates the mode of sensing, that is, how the device responds to a sensed event. I indicates that the device inhibits output when an

I	II	III	IV
Table 1–1. NBG* Code			
Chamber(s) paced	Chamber(s) sensed	Response to sensing	Programmability, rate modulation
O = None	O = None	O = None	O = None
A = Atrium	A = Atrium	T = Triggered	P = Simple programmable
V = Ventricle	V = Ventricle	I = Inhibited	M = Multiprogrammable
D =Dual (A + V)	D =Dual (A + V)	D =Dual (T + I)	C = Communicating
			R =Rate modulation

*The North American Society of Pacing and Electrophysiology and the British Pacing and Electrophysiology Group.

Modified from Bernstein et al.[61] By permission of Futura Publishing Company.

intrinsic event is sensed and starts a new timing interval. **T** implies that an output pulse is triggered in response to a sensed event. **D** indicates that the device is capable of dual modes of response (applicable only in dual-chamber systems).

The fourth position reflects both programmability and rate modulation. **O** indicates that none of the pacemaker settings can be changed by noninvasive programming, **P** suggests "simple" programmability (that is, one or two variables can be modified), **M** indicates multiprogrammability (three or more variables can be modified), and **C** indicates that the device has telemetry capability and can communicate noninvasively with the programmer (which also implies multiprogrammability). Finally, an **R** in the fourth position designates rate-responsive capability. This means that the pacemaker has some type of sensor to modulate the heart rate independent of the intrinsic heart rate. All modern devices are multiprogrammable and have telemetry capability; therefore, the **R** to designate rate-responsive capability is the most commonly used currently.

The fifth position is restricted to describing antitachycardia treatment functions. A **P** in this position implies that some pacing algorithm (e.g., scanning, burst, ramp) is capable, and an **S** indicates shocking (cardioversion or defibrillation) capability. A **D** indicates both pacing and shocking capabilities.

All pacemaker functions (whether single- or dual-chamber) are based on timing cycles. Even the function of the most complex devices can be readily understood by applying the principles of pacemaker timing intervals. This understanding is critical to accurate interpretation of pacemaker electrocardiograms, especially during troubleshooting. Pacemaker timing cycles are described in detail in Chapter 6.

Defibrillation Basics

In 1899, Prevost and Battelli[62] noted that the "fibrillatory tremulations produced in the dog" could be arrested with the reestablishment of the normal heartbeat if one submitted the animal "to passages of current of high voltage." Despite these early observations, decades elapsed before broad clinical applicability fueled interest in more widespread investigation of the mechanism underlying defibrillation. With the development of internal defibrillators in the late 1970s came a greater need to quantify defibrillation effectiveness, to understand the factors governing waveform and lead design, and to determine the effect of pharmacologic agents on defibrillation. Remarkably, much of this work was done without a complete understanding of the fundamental mechanism of defibrillation.

This section reviews the emerging insights to the electrophysiologic effects of shocks and how they are related to defibrillation. It also reviews the means of assessing the efficacy of defibrillation (the "defibrillation threshold") and the important effects of waveform, lead design and placement, and pharmacologic agents on defibrillation, with an emphasis on those principles pertaining to clinical practice.

Electrophysiologic Effects of Defibrillation Shocks; Antitachycardia Pacing

Despite the great strides made in understanding the technology required for defibrillation (e.g., lead design and position, waveform selection), the basic mechanism has not been definitively determined. Three contemporary theories accounting for how an electric shock terminates fibrillation coexist with some overlapping: critical mass, upper limit of vulnerability, and progressive depolarization. These are discussed below.

A brief review of the cardiac action potential is useful to facilitate discussion of the effects of defibrillation. The surface electrocardiogram and intracardiac electrogram, common in clinical practice, are the result of extracellular potentials generated by myocardial action potential propagation. An action potential is the transmembrane voltage in a single myocyte over time (Fig. 1–17). The action potential upstroke (phase 0, or depolarization) is mediated by sodium ion flow through voltage-sensitive selective channels, and during ventricular activation it is registered on the surface electrocardiogram as the QRS complex (Fig. 1–18). Repolarization (phase 3) of ventricular myocardium generates the surface electrocardiographic T wave. In its resting state, the myocardium is excitable, and a pacing stimulus, or current injected by the depolarization of a neighboring myocyte, can bring the membrane potential to a threshold value, above which a new action potential ensues. The ability of the action potential of a myocyte to depolarize adjacent myocardium results in propagation of electrical activity through cardiac tissue. Importantly, immediately after depolarization, the myocardium is refractory and cannot be stimulated to produce another action potential until it has recovered excitability (Fig. 1–19). The interval immediately after an action potential during which another action potential cannot be elicited by a pacing stimulus is referred to as the "refractory period."

Ventricular fibrillation is characterized by multiple wandering and colliding wavelets of electrical activation, which propagate into regions in which excitable tissue is encountered. Activation fronts are extinguished when they do not find excitable tissue to enter; conversely, a wave front may split to give off daughter wavelets. These wandering wavelets are self-sustaining once initiated.[63] In the 1940s, Gurvich and Yuniev[64] predicted that electric shocks led to premature tissue stimulation in advance of propagating wave fronts, preventing continued progression of the wave front. This concept of defibrillation as large-scale stimulation remains a central tenet of the currently held theories of defibrillation: the "critical mass" theory, the upper limit of vulnerability theory, and the progressive depolarization (refractory period extension) theory.

Critical Mass

The first theory, the now popular "critical mass theory," proposed that shocks need only eliminate fibrillatory wavelets in a critical amount of myocardium to extinguish the arrhythmia. Experiments in canine models found that injection of potassium chloride (which depolarizes myocardium, rendering it unavailable for fibrillation) into the right coronary artery or the left circumflex artery failed to terminate ventricular fibrillation as often as injection into both the left circumflex and the left anterior descending arteries together. Similarly, electrical shocks of equal magnitude terminated fibrillation most frequently when the electrodes were positioned at the right ventricular apex and the posterior left ventricle, as opposed to two right ventricular electrodes. Thus, it was concluded that if a "critical mass" of myocardium was rendered unavailable for ventricular fibrillation either by potassium injection or by defibrillatory shock, the remaining excitable tissue was insufficient to support the wandering wavelets, and the arrhythmia terminated.[65] However, it was not critical to depolarize every ventricular cell to terminate fibrillation.

Upper Limit of Vulnerability

Studies mapping electrical activation after failed shocks led to several observations not accounted for by the critical mass hypothesis, giving rise to the upper

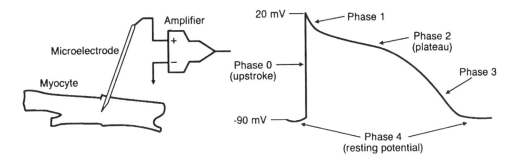

Fig. 1–17. The cardiac action potential. *Left,* Impalement of a single myocyte by a microelectrode. This permits recording of the change in voltage potential over time in a single cell. *Right,* On the graph, voltage (in millivolts) is on the ordinate, time on the abscissa. The action potential in ventricular myocytes begins with a rapid upstroke (phase 0), which is followed by transient early repolarization (phase 1), a plateau (phase 2), and terminal repolarization (phase 3), which returns the membrane potential back to the resting value.

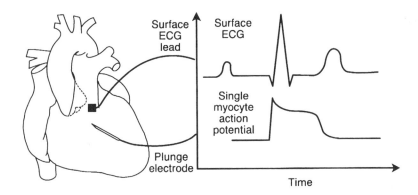

Fig. 1–18. Correlation of cellular and clinical electrical activity. The QRS complex of the surface electrocardiogram (ECG) is generated by the action potential upstroke (phase 0) of ventricular myocytes and the propagation of the upstroke through the ventricular myocardium. Similarly, the T wave is the result of ventricular repolarization (phase 3).

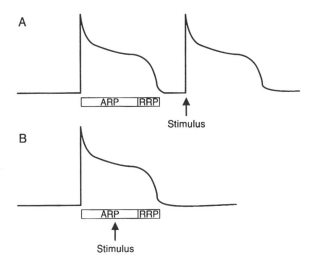

Fig. 1–19. Refractory periods. Myocytes can be stimulated to generate new action potentials, except in their absolute refractory period (ARP). In *A,* a stimulus occurs after the myocyte has fully recovered from the preceding action potential, and a new action potential ensues. In contrast, in *B,* the same stimulus is delivered earlier, the myocyte remains in its absolute refractory period because of the preceding action potential, and no new action potential is elicited. RRP, relative refractory period.

limit of vulnerability theory. First, an iso-electric interval (an electrical pause) was seen after failed shocks before resumption of fibrillation. The relatively long pause suggested that ventricular fibrillation was terminated by the shock and then secondarily regenerated by it[66] (Fig. 1–20). The concept that failed shocks are unsuccessful because they give rise to a new focus of fibrillation rather than because they fail to halt continuing wavelets was further buttressed by a second observation—that postshock conduction patterns were not the continuation of preshock wave fronts.[67] If a failed shock resulted from the inability to halt continuing fibrillation, the assumption was that the postshock wave fronts should be a continuation of the propagating wave fronts present before shock delivery and

that new wave fronts at sites remote from the preshock wave fronts would not be expected. Furthermore, ventricular fibrillation was frequently reinitiated in the regions of lowest shock intensity, suggesting that these low-intensity regions were responsible for reinitiating fibrillation.

Elegant mapping studies demonstrated that shocks with potential gradients less than a minimum critical value—termed the *upper limit of vulnerability* (ULV) (6 V/cm for monophasic shocks, 4 V/cm for biphasic shocks)—could induce fibrillation when applied to myocardium during its vulnerable period. Low-energy shocks did so by creating regions of functional block in vulnerable myocardium at "critical points" that initiated reentry and subsequent fibrillation.[68] Figure 1–21 depicts the vulnerable zone

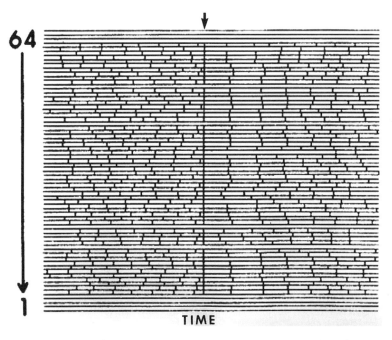

Fig. 1–20. Isoelectric interval after failed shock. Tracings show recordings from 64 electrodes evenly distributed over the epicardial surfaces of both ventricles. At the *arrow*, an unsuccessful 1-J defibrillation shock is delivered. Note that an isoelectric interval (i.e., flat line without activations) immediately follows the shock, that temporal clustering of the first activation follows the failed shock, and that rapid degeneration back to fibrillation then occurs. (Modified from Chen et al.[66] By permission of American Society for Clinical Investigation.)

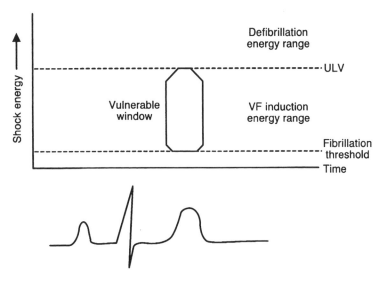

Fig. 1–21. Window of vulnerability during sinus rhythm. During sinus rhythm, the ventricles are vulnerable to ventricular fibrillation (VF) when a shock is delivered on the T wave, in the vulnerable window. To induce fibrillation, the shock energy must be greater than the fibrillation threshold and below the upper limit of vulnerability (ULV). Shocks with energy above the upper limit of vulnerability do not induce fibrillation. Since during VF there is dysynchrony of activation, at any given instant a number of regions are repolarizing (equivalent to the T wave in sinus rhythm), so that a shock with a gradient that is less than the ULV can reinduce fibrillation in these regions. In contrast, shocks with energy above the ULV throughout the myocardium cannot reinitiate VF and are successful. The ULV is correlated with the defibrillation threshold. Further details appear in the text.

during normal sinus rhythm. In sinus rhythm, low-energy shocks delivered during the T wave induce ventricular fibrillation; higher energy shocks—with energy above the ULV—do not. Since at any given time during fibrillation a number of myocardial regions are repolarizing and thus vulnerable, a shock with a potential gradient below the ULV may create a critical point and reinitiate fibrillation. Conversely, a shock with a gradient above the ULV across the entire myocardium does not reinduce ventricular fibrillation and should therefore succeed. During defibrillator testing, shocks are intentionally delivered in the vulnerable zone to induce fibrillation (Fig. 1–22), and the zone of vulnerability has been defined in humans.[69] The fact that the vulnerable zone exists and that the ULV has been correlated with the defibrillation threshold

supports the ULV hypothesis as a mechanism of defibrillation.[70]

Progressive Depolarization

The third theory of defibrillation, the progressive depolarization theory (also referred to as the "refractory period extension theory") incorporates some elements of both critical mass and ULV theories. Using voltage-sensitive optical dyes, Dillon and Kwaku[71] demonstrated that shocks of sufficient strength were able to elicit active responses, even from supposedly refractory myocardium. Thus, as seen in Figure 1–23 *A*, the duration of an action potential can be prolonged (and the refractory period extended) despite refractory myocardium when a sufficiently strong shock is applied.[72] This phenomenon may result from sodium

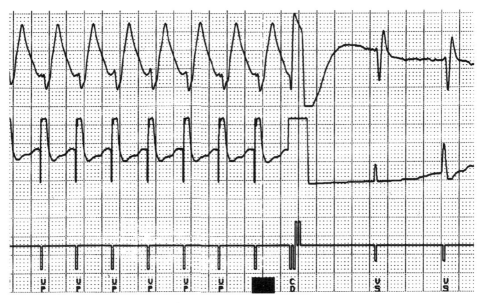

A

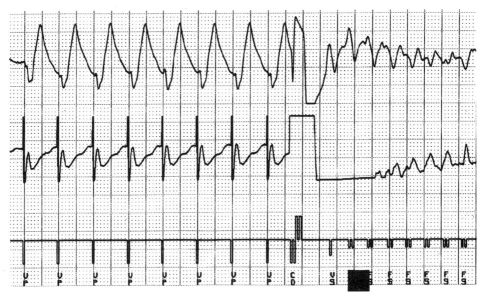

B

Fig. 1–22. Induction of ventricular fibrillation by a T-wave shock during testing of an implantable defibrillator. In *A,* a 1-J shock is delivered 380 msec after the last paced beat. Fibrillation is not induced, because this shock is delivered outside the window of vulnerability. In *B,* the timing of the shock is adjusted to 300 msec after the last paced complex, so that it is delivered more squarely on the T wave, in the window of vulnerability, and fibrillation is induced. The window of vulnerability is defined by both shock energy and timing. CD, charge delivered; FS, fibrillation sense; VP, ventricular pacing; VS, ventricular sensing.

channel reactivation by the shock. The degree of additional depolarization time is a function of both shock intensity and shock timing.[73] Since the shock stimulates new action potentials in myocardium that is late in repolarization and produces additional depolarization time when the myocardium is already depolarized, myocardial resynchronization occurs. This is manifested by myocardial repolarization at a constant time after the shock (second dashed line in Figure 1–23, labeled "constant repolarization time"). Thus, the shock that defibrillates extends overall ventricular refractoriness, limiting the excitable tissue available for fibrillation. It thus extinguishes continuing wavelets and resynchronizes repolarization, so that distant regions of myocardium become excitable simultaneously, preventing dispersion of refractoriness and renewed reentry. Experimental evidence has demonstrated that shocks with a potential gradient above the ULV result in time-dependent extension of the refractory period. In contrast, lower energy shocks may result in a graded response that could create transient block and a critical point, reinducing fibrillation.[73]

To summarize and to put defibrillation theory into clinical perspective, the effects of the application of a voltage gradient across myocardium are a function of field strength and timing. Although the biologic effects of shocks may overlap, this

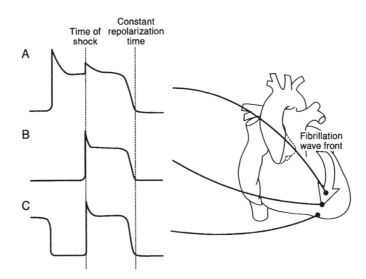

Fig. 1–23. Progressive depolarization. A fibrillatory wave front is depicted by the arrow, and the action potential response to a defibrillatory shock is demonstrated at several points surrounding the wave front. The fibrillatory wave front has just passed through a myocyte at point A when the shock is delivered. The myocyte is in its plateau (phase 2), when it would ordinarily be refractory to additional stimulation. However, when a sufficiently strong shock is delivered, the myocyte can generate an active response with prolongation of the action potential and of the refractory period. The response is referred to as "additional depolarization time." The tissue at point B is at the leading edge of the fibrillatory wave front. The shock strikes this myocardium at the time of the upstroke (phase 0) and has little effect on the action potential. The tissue at point C is excitable (it is the excitable gap that the fibrillatory wave front was about to enter) when the shock is delivered. The shock elicits a new action potential in this excitable tissue. Despite the different temporal and anatomical locations of the three action potentials depicted, after the shock there is resynchronization by the "constant repolarization time." This resynchronization helps prevent continuation of fibrillation.

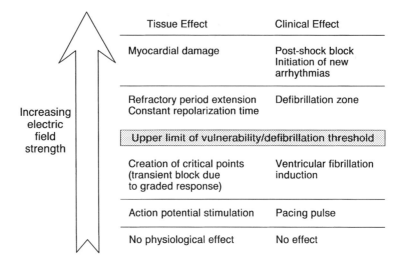

	Tissue Effect	Clinical Effect
	Myocardial damage	Post-shock block Initiation of new arrhythmias
Increasing electric field strength	Refractory period extension Constant repolarization time	Defibrillation zone
	Upper limit of vulnerability/defibrillation threshold	
	Creation of critical points (transient block due to graded response)	Ventricular fibrillation induction
	Action potential stimulation	Pacing pulse
	No physiological effect	No effect

Fig. 1–24. Effects of increasing shock (electrical field) strength on myocardial tissue.

concept is summarized in Figure 1–24. Extremely low energy pulses may have no effect on the myocardium. Stronger pulses (in the microjoule range), such as those used for cardiac pacing, result in action potential generation in nonrefractory myocardium, which leads to a propagating impulse. With increasing electric field strength (to the 1-J area), ventricular fibrillation can be induced with shocks delivered during the vulnerable period. Increasing the shock strength above the ULV (and above the defibrillation threshold) puts the shock in the defibrillation zone. Very high energy shocks can lead to toxic effects, including disruption of cell membranes, postshock block, mechanical dysfunction, and new tachyarrythmias.[73,74]

Antitachycardia Pacing

The concepts of basic myocardial function also explain the mechanism of arrhythmia termination with antitachycardia pacing. As an example, in monomorphic ventricular tachycardia late after myocardial infarction, a reentrant circuit utilizing abnormal tissue adjacent to an infarct is responsible for the arrhythmia (Fig. 1–25). In contrast to ventricular fibrillation, which is composed of multiple wavelets, monomorphic reentrant arrhythmias typically utilize a stable reentrant circuit. For the circuit ventricular tachycardia to perpetuate itself, the tissue immediately in front of the leading edge of the wave front must have recovered excitability so that it can be depolarized (Fig. 1–25). Thus, an excitable gap of tissue must be present in advance of the leading tachycardia wave front or the arrhythmia will terminate. Antitachycardia pacing—delivered as a short burst of pacing impulses at a rate slightly greater than the tachycardia rate—can terminate ventricular tachycardia by depolarizing the tissue in the excitable gap, so that the tissue in front of the advancing ventricular tachycardia wave front becomes refractory, preventing further arrhythmia propagation (Fig. 1–25 B). The ability of a train of impulses to travel to the site of the reentrant circuit and interrupt ventricular tachycardia depends on several factors, including the site of pacing (the

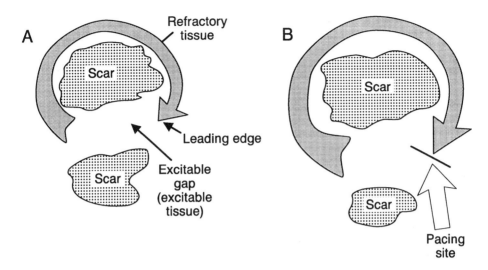

Fig. 1–25. Reentrant ventricular tachycardia circuit. In *A*, a circuit around a fixed scar is depicted by the arrow. The head of the arrow depicts the leading edge of the wave front, and the body of the arrow back to the tail (colored gray) consists of tissue that is still refractory (since the wave front has just propagated through it). The tissue between the tip and the tail of the arrow is excitable and is called the "excitable gap." For the arrow head to continue its course around the scar, an excitable gap must be present; if the wave front encounters refractory tissue, it cannot proceed. In *B*, a wave front generated by an antitachycardia pacing impulse enters the excitable gap and terminates tachycardia. Tachycardias with a small excitable gap (i.e., the head of the arrow follows the tail very closely, so that only a small "moving rim" of excitable tissue is in the circuit) are more difficult to terminate with antitachycardia pacing.

closer to the circuit entrance, the greater the likelihood of circuit penetration and termination), the length of the tachycardia cycle, and the size of the excitable gap. With delivery of antitachycardia pacing, faster and more remote circuits with smaller excitable gaps are generally more difficult to terminate and have a greater risk of degeneration to less organized tachyarrhythmias, including fibrillation. A more detailed discussion of tachycardia resetting, entrainment, and termination via stimulus introduction is available elsewhere.[75] Discussion on use of antitachycardia pacing in implantable devices appears in Chapter 3.

Measuring the Efficacy of Defibrillation

Threshold and Dose Response Curve

At the time of defibrillator insertion, it is critical to determine whether the system implanted can successfully terminate fibrillation. The measure most frequently used to assess the ability of a system to terminate ventricular fibrillation is the *defibrillation threshold* (DFT). The term "threshold" suggests that there is a threshold energy above which defibrillation is uniformly successful and below which shocks fail (Fig. 1–26 *A*). Experimental data and clinical practice, however, invariably demonstrate that a shock of a given strength may terminate fibrillation on one occasion and fail in another episode shortly thereafter without any discernable change in clinical status. The multitude of factors that can affect whether a shock will succeed—patient characteristics, fibrillation duration, degree of ischemia and potassium accumulation, distribution of electrical activation at the time of the shock, circulating pharmacologic agents, and others—result in defibrillation behavior that is best modeled as a random variable, with a calculable probability of success for any given shock strength. Thus, defibrillation is more accurately described by a dose response curve, with an increasing probability of success as the defibrillation energy increases (Fig. 1–26 B). The curve can be characterized by its slope and intercept, and specific points on the curve can be identified, such as ED_{50}, the energy dose with a 50% likelihood of success. Factors adversely affecting defibrillation shift the curve to the right, so that a higher dose of energy is required to achieve a 50% likelihood of success, and improvements in defibrillation (such as superior lead position and improved waveforms or lead design) shift the curve to the left (Fig. 1–27). Because of the large number of fibrillation episodes required to define a curve (30 to 40 inductions), the dose-response curve is not determined in clinical practice, but it remains a useful research tool and conceptual framework.

Relationship Between Defibrillation Threshold and Dose Response Curve

If defibrillation is best described as a dose response curve, where on the curve does the DFT exist (i.e., what is the probability of successful defibrillation at the clinically used DFT energy)? The probability of successful defibrillation at the DFT energy depends entirely on the steps taken to define the threshold. Consider a step-down to failure DFT, in which shocks are delivered beginning at a relatively high energy (e.g., energy with a 99% success rate) and decremented by several joules with each ventricular fibrillation induction until a shock fails (at which point a rescue shock is delivered). The DFT in this protocol is defined as the low-

est energy shock that succeeds (Fig. 1–28). Since the initial energies tested are at the upper end of the dose response curve, successive shocks may have a 98%, 95%, 88%, 85% (and so on) likelihood of success, depending on the starting energy and size of the steps taken. Despite the fairly high likelihood of success for each shock individually, the sheer number of shocks delivered in this range on average result in a shock failing (thus defining the DFT) at a relatively high point on the curve. If this process is repeated many times, a population of DFTs is created, with a mean and expected range. In humans, step-down to failure algorithms have a mean DFT with likelihood of success near 70% but with a standard deviation near 25%.[76,77] Thus, the likelihood of success of a shock delivered at the energy defined as the DFT at a single determination ranges from 25% to 88%, with an average of 71%.[76] In other words, if a defibrillator is programmed to the step-down to failure DFT energy for its first shock, the likelihood that that first shock will succeed can range from 25% to 88% but on average will be 71%.

In contrast to the step-down to failure DFT, in a step-up to success DFT, low-energy shocks are delivered during ventricular fibrillation with incremental doses of energy until a first success occurs, which defines the DFT. In this case, despite the fairly low likelihood of success at each low-energy shock, if enough shocks are delivered, one is likely to succeed, defining the DFT. With this protocol, the mean DFT has a likelihood of success near 30%. Iterative increment-decrement DFT or binary search algorithms that begin in the middle zone of the curve have been shown to approximate the ED_{50}, the energy with a 50% probability of success. In this type of protocol, if the first shock defibrillates the heart, the first shock of the next fibrillation episode uses a lower energy. If the first shock does not defibrillate

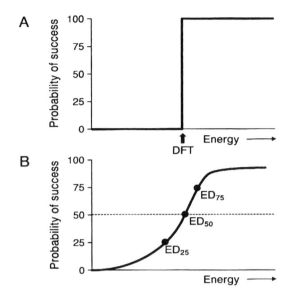

Fig. 1–26. Defibrillation "threshold." *A,* The expected response to shock if a true threshold value existed. In reality, the likelihood of success is a sigmoidal dose response curve, as shown in *B.* The ED_{50} is the energy dose with a 50% likelihood of success, and so on.

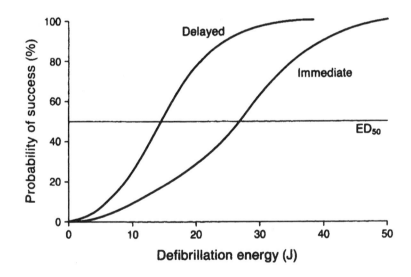

Fig. 1–27. Use of dose response curve to measure effects of an intervention on defibrillation efficacy. The graph shows the effect of thoracotomy on defibrillation in a canine model. The "immediate" group had defibrillation threshold testing done immediately after thoracotomy. Note that the curve is shifted to the right and that the energy with a 50% probability of success is 27 J, compared with 15 J for the "delayed" group, which was allowed 48 to 72 hours of recovery before defibrillation testing. Defibrillation is more effective in the "delayed" group because the probability of success at a given energy is higher in this group. Thus, the curves graphically display diminished defibrillation efficacy immediately after thoracotomy. (From Friedman PA, Stanton MS: Thoracotomy elevates the defibrillation threshold and modifies the defibrillation dose-response curve. J Cardiovasc Electrophysiol 8:68–73, 1997. By permission of Futura Publishing Company.)

Fig. 1–28. Step-down to failure defibrillation threshold (DFT) testing. In this hypothetical example (A), four shocks are required to define the DFT. The first shock is delivered at 20 J and is successful (S). The next shock, delivered at 15 J, also succeeds. A 10-J shock succeeds, and a 5-J shock fails (F), defining the DFT as 10 J (the lowest successful energy). Note from the curve that the likelihood of success at the DFT energy (10 J) is 70%. Now, if the DFT process were repeated, it is possible that the second shock might fail on one occasion (defining the DFT as 20 J) or that all four shocks might succeed on another occasion (and that a lower energy shock would fail to define the DFT), and so on. Thus, repeating the DFT determinations may result in different values for the DFT with each determination. However, if enough repetitions were performed, a population of DFTs, as shown in B, would be created. The most commonly observed DFT in this example would be 10 J, which has a 70% likelihood of success. Further details in text.

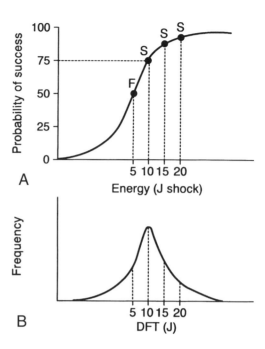

the heart, a second shock at a higher energy is delivered.

Regardless of the DFT protocol, a DFT determination is best conceptualized as a means of approximating a point on the dose response curve, with the specific point estimated being a function of the DFT algorithm chosen. DFT determinations can be very useful tools for assessing defibrillation efficacy. Triplicate DFT measurements, which can be performed with fewer than 10 fibrillation episodes, have been demonstrated to be as reproducible as the true logistic regression model of the dose response curve and to have less variability than other models used to estimate dose response curves. Thus, determination of a DFT before and after an intervention (such as initiation of a drug or movement of a lead to a new position) can determine whether defibrillation efficacy is enhanced or impaired by the intervention.

Defining an Implantation Safety Margin

Given that a DFT determination is an estimated point on the dose response curve and that the probability of successful defibrillation at the DFT is approximately 70% with the commonly used step-down protocol, a safety margin must be added to the DFT energy to increase the odds of success. Although all device shocks could be programmed to deliver the maximum available energy, using a lower energy that can consistently terminate fibrillation has advantages. These include faster charge time and more prompt delivery of therapy (with reduced chance of syncope), battery preservation, diminished risk of AV block, decreased myocardial damage in the regions with the highest voltage gradient, and diminished risk of impaired postshock sensing.[74,78] Thus, the energy programmed should be a value high enough above the DFT to ensure that the shock is on the "plateau" of the dose response curve, where success rates exceed 90%, but not necessarily at maximum output. In humans, adding 10 J to the DFT has been shown to result in first-shock success rates of 99.5% ± 4.3%.[79,80]

In some situations, inducing the absolute fewest fibrillation episodes possible while still ensuring adequate device function is desirable. Defibrillator implantation criteria based on the probability of successful defibrillation of a maximal output first shock have been derived from data obtained in a population of patients with previous implantation. If it is assumed that the defibrillation dose response curves for the population to receive devices are similar to the curves for patients who have had devices implanted in clinical trials (which are used to create the model), defibrillation tests are required only to ensure that the system configuration under evaluation does not have an "undesirable" dose response curve from among the population of available curves. Even a small number of successful shocks makes the probability that the patient undergoing implantation has such an "undesirable" dose response curve low. But before it can be determined that an "undesirable" dose response curve is present, standards of acceptable device function must be defined. For example, if the goal of obtaining a population annual sudden death rate of less than 1% is chosen, the fact that devices can deliver at least four shocks (most deliver six) and that on average a patient will need the device to terminate ventricular fibrillation 1.71 times per year can be used to calculate that the maximal output first-shock efficacy must be at least 86.8% to achieve that low rate of sudden death.[81] Then, with the data from the representative population of patients who had previous implantation, it can be shown that 2 of 2 successful shocks at an energy 10 J less than the maximum device output will achieve the annual sudden death rate desired if all shocks are programmed to the highest output. Thus, the minimum number of shocks required for implantation of an ICD is two. If one shock fails, 2 of 3 successful shocks at a 10-J safety margin have also been shown to predict an annual rate of sudden death of less than 1%.[81]

Defibrillation Testing at Implantation

With the information known about the human defibrillation dose response curve and defibrillation models, a practical approach to implantation testing can be used. Step-down to failure DFT testing can be done with three or four episodes of fibrillation. All patients should have external defibrillation pads placed before the surgical implantation procedure begins, as described in Chapter 5. Testing is done with the device in the surgical pocket and with leads connected. A low-energy shock (generally around 1 J) is delivered to test the lead connections. (In systems that measure high-voltage lead impedance, a test shock is not necessary, because a high-voltage lead impedance value in the normal range confirms the electrical integrity of the connections.) The first-shock energy is programmed to 10 J less than the maximum output of the device, and fibrillation is induced. If the test shock is successful, the first-shock energy is lowered by 5 or 6 J, and after a delay of 3 to 5 minutes, fibrillation is reinduced and the new energy tested. This iterative decremental process is continued until the first shock fails or until an energy of 5 or 6 J succeeds (at which point the DFT is often defined as ≤ 5 or 6 J). The lowest successful energy is taken as the DFT, and the first shock of the device is chronically programmed to the DFT energy plus 10 J. Often during testing, the second defibrillator shock is programmed to an energy equal to the last successful shock energy plus 10 J, and rescue is performed by the defibrillator (rather than externally). Thus, after a 15-J shock is successful, the first shock is programmed to 10 J for the next induction, and the second device shock is programmed to 25 J (which is the current lower boundary for the

DFT [15 J] plus a 10-J safety margin). Occasionally, in patients who have borderline blood pressure after induction of anesthesia or who have other clinical reasons for receiving an absolute minimum number of shocks, two inductions are performed, and a shock with energy that is 10 J less than the maximum output of the device is delivered at each. If both succeed, implantation criteria are met. This approach has the disadvantage of requiring that all shocks be programmed at maximum output chronically.

If an adequate safety margin is not demonstrated (i.e., if fewer than two of three shocks are successful at an energy of 10 J less than the device maximum), a common next step is to reverse the shock polarity (waveform and polarity are discussed in greater detail below). If implantation criteria are still not met, leads are repositioned if it is thought that lead position can be improved, or an additional endovascular lead is added in systems that permit it (optimal lead position is also discussed below). If these approaches fail, a subcutaneous lead is added (see Chapter 5 for implantation technique). Using biphasic waveforms, we have found that subcutaneous leads are required in only 3.7% of devices implanted.[82]

Upper Limit of Vulnerability to Assess Safety Margin

The ULV is the lowest energy above which shocks delivered during the vulnerable period do not induce fibrillation. Since the DFT and ULV are correlated, some investigators have suggested that ULV determinations could be performed to assess defibrillation efficacy with one or no fibrillation episode.[83] During sinus rhythm, test shocks are delivered at the peak of the T wave at initially high energies, with the energy level subsequently decreased in steps until fibrillation is induced, defining a shock that is below the

ULV. Since the ULV may be dependent on the coupling interval, energies are also delivered at various intervals before the T-wave peak to "scan" repolarization. For conventional biphasic waveforms, the ULV corresponds to a 90% successful energy level, and it has been used to provide adequate safety margins at cardioverter-defibrillator implantations and for long-term follow-up in clinical protocols.[84,85] However, since ULV assessment is an indirect measure of defibrillation efficacy, the relationship between the ULV and the DFT may be affected by numerous factors, including electrode configuration, pharmacologic agents, and the protocol used to determine the ULV. In some situations, the changes in ULV may not accurately reflect defibrillation efficacy. Because of the indirect nature of the ULV-DFT relationship, the large body of clinical and experimental data based on DFTs, and the findings of increased myocardial irritability and postshock arrhythmias with repeated high-energy shocks, ULV testing has not yet achieved broad clinical acceptance.

The Importance of Waveform

The shape of a defibrillating waveform can dramatically affect its defibrillation efficacy. In the canine model, for example, Schuder et al.[86] demonstrated that for transthoracic defibrillation, an ascending ramp waveform has a much higher success rate with the same delivered current than does a descending ramp (Fig. 1–29). However, because of the importance of using physically small circuits for implantable devices, a capacitor discharge, which more closely resembles the descending ramp, is employed in devices.

Creating the Defibrillation Waveform

As in pacing, the battery serves as

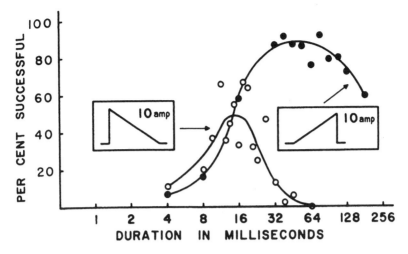

Fig. 1–29. Effect of waveform on defibrillation. The ordinate shows the percentage of successful transthoracic canine defibrillation; on the abscissa is the duration of 10-A triangular shock. The success rate is greater for the ascending ramp than it is for the descending ramp. (From Schuder JC, Rahmoeller GA, Stoeckle H: Transthoracic ventricular defibrillation with triangular and trapezoidal waveforms. Circ Res 19:689–694, 1966. By permission of the American Heart Association.)

the source of electrical charge for cardiac stimulation in defibrillation. Before a high-energy shock can be delivered, the electrical charge must be accumulated in a capacitor, because a battery cannot deliver the amount of required charge in the short time of a defibrillation shock. A capacitor stores charge by means of two large surface area conductors separated by a dielectric (poorly conducting) material, and capacitor size is an important determinant of implantable defibrillator volume, typically accounting for approximately 30% of device size. If fluid analogies are used for electricity—voltage as water pressure and current as water flow (i.e., liters per minute)—the capacitor is analogous to a water balloon, which has a compliance defined by the ratio of volume to pressure. To increase the amount of water put into the balloon, one can increase the pressure or, alternatively, use a balloon with a greater compliance (more stretch for a given amount of pressure). Similarly, the charge stored can be increased by increasing capacitance or by applying greater voltage. The trend in implantable devices has been toward smaller capacitors to create smaller devices.

The charge stored by a capacitor is defined by

$$Charge = capacitance \times voltage$$

The voltage waveform of a capacitor discharged into a fixed resistance load (Fig. 1–30 A) is determined by

$$V(t) = V_i \cdot e^{-t/RC}$$

and the energy associated with the waveform is given by

$$Energy = 0.5 \, CV^2$$

Since the "tail" of the waveform in longer pulses ($\geq$ 10 msec) refibrillates the ventricle (most likely accounting for the

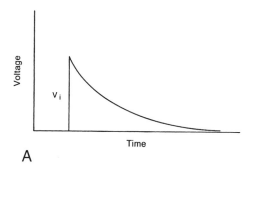

A

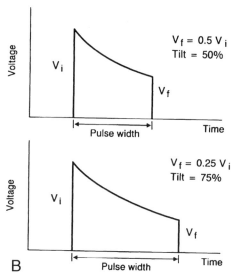

B

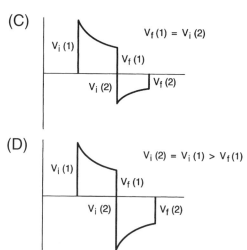

(C)

(D)

Fig. 1–30. Defibrillation waveforms. *A*, Standard capacitor discharge. *B*, Monophasic truncated waveform with initial voltage (V_i), final voltage (V_f), and pulse width labeled. Top waveform has 50% tilt, and bottom waveform has 75% tilt. *C*, Biphasic waveform with leading edge of the first pulse ($V_i(1)$), trailing edge of the first pulse ($V_f(1)$), leading edge of the second pulse ($V_i(2)$), and trailing edge of the second pulse ($V_f(2)$) labeled. Since $V_i(2)$ equals $V_f(1)$, this waveform can be generated by reversing the polarity of a single capacitor after the first pulse is completed. *D*, In contrast, $V_i(2)$ is greater than $V_f(1)$, so that a second capacitor is needed to create this waveform.

superiority of the ascending ramp seen by Schuder et al.[86]), truncated waveforms have been used clinically. The classic monophasic truncated waveform is shown in Figure 1–30 B. The waveform is characterized by the initial voltage (Vi), the final voltage (Vf), and the pulse width or tilt. Tilt is an expression of the percentage decay of the initial voltage. The tilt of a waveform is a function of the size of the capacitor used, the resistance of the leads and tissues through which current passes, and the duration of the pulse. Tilt is defined by the percentage decrease of the initial voltage:

$$\text{Tilt} = (Vi - Vf)/Vi \times 100\%$$

As shown in Figure 1–31, tilt can have an important effect on defibrillation efficacy, with progressive improvement in defibrillation efficacy with decreasing tilt, for a trapezoidal waveform of constant duration. For monophasic wave-

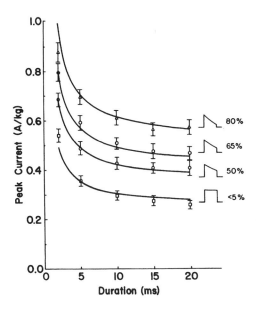

Fig. 1–31. Internal canine defibrillation threshold (peak current) plotted against waveform duration and tilt. Note important effect of tilt on threshold with this waveform. (From Wessale JL, Bourland JD, Tacker WA, Geddes LA: Bipolar catheter defibrillation in dogs using trapezoidal waveforms of various tilts. J Electrocardiol 13:359–365, 1980. By permission of Churchill Livingstone.)

forms formerly used clinically, the optimal tilt was 50% to 80%.

Biphasic Waveforms

Appropriately characterized biphasic shocks can result in significant improvement in defibrillation efficacy, with reductions in DFTs of 30% to 50%.[87] All currently available commercial defibrillators use biphasic waveforms; a typical biphasic waveform is shown in Figure 1–30 C. Biphasic waveforms have numerous clinical advantages, all stemming from their improved defibrillation efficacy. Biphasic waveforms have been shown to result in higher implantation success rates due to their lower DFTs, which are associated

with higher safety margins.[88] Since safety margins are increased, most patients do not require high-energy shocks, and smaller devices can be designed.[89] The improved efficacy of biphasic waveforms permits a greater tolerance in electrode positioning than that required for monophasic waveforms, facilitating the implanting procedure. Additionally, biphasic shocks have been shown to result in faster post-shock recurrence of sinus rhythm and to have greater efficacy than monophasic shocks at terminating ventricular fibrillation of long duration.[90,91]

The mechanism of improved efficacy of biphasic waveforms is not well understood, limiting the ability to determine the ideal biphasic waveform a priori. A large body of evidence, composed predominantly of empirical comparisons of the effects of different modifications to the waveform on the DFT, has shown the importance of tilt, phase duration, and voltage-reversal efficiency on biphasic defibrillation efficacy. However, no single definitive waveform remains; the most efficient waveform for defibrillation in a given system is a function of the leads placed, the capacitance, and possibly individual patient characteristics. Additionally, the interdependence of waveform characteristics (for example, changing the tilt affects pulse width for a given capacitor and resistance) makes the independent effects of each modification difficult to determine. Nonetheless, the general waveform features that tend to result in the lowest DFT with circuit elements similar to those in currently available defibrillators are discussed below. Importantly, biphasic waveforms in which the leading edge voltage of the second pulse is less than or equal to the trailing edge voltage can be created with a single capacitor by reversing the polarity during the shock pulse. Waveforms with a leading edge voltage of the second waveform larger than the trailing edge voltage of the first pulse require a second capacitor and are currently not used by any available implantable device (Fig. 1–30 D).

Phase Duration

Biphasic waveforms have a greater efficacy if more charge is delivered during the first phase. Thus, when a small second phase is added to a monophasic waveform, the defibrillation efficacy improves. With the capacitance values of present defibrillators, if the total pulse duration is kept constant as the duration of the second phase is made longer (and the first shorter), the DFT is progressively reduced to a minimum value. Additional prolongation of the second phase increases the DFT, which ultimately becomes higher than it would be if the first phase were delivered alone as a monophasic shock[92–94] (Fig. 1–32). Thus, commercially available defibrillators have a first-phase duration greater than or equal to the second phase (Fig. 1–33). There are exceptions to this phase duration rule, discussed below in the voltage reversal section. Additionally, these phase duration data were acquired by large capacitors (150 µF) and epicardial leads; data for transvenous systems are less complete. More recent data with transvenous leads and smaller capacitors suggest that there may be two phase durations that minimize the DFT, and that one has a longer second phase than first phase.[95]

Tilt

For monophasic waveforms, optimal tilt is in the 50% to 80% range. For biphasic waveforms, the optimal tilt per phase for single capacitor waveforms with equal tilt for phase 1 and phase 2 is in the 40% to 65% range.[96,97] Optimal tilt depends on capacitance and resistance, and in many commercially available implantable defibrillators, the user cannot program it.

Additionally, because of individual variation, optimal tilt for all patients probably does not exist.

Voltage Reversal

The degree of voltage reversal—the magnitude of change in voltage from the trailing edge of the first pulse to the leading edge of the second pulse—is important for biphasic defibrillation.[98] Greater voltage reversal is associated with improved defibrillation efficacy. Of the commercial waveforms analyzed by Tomassoni et al.,[98] the small voltage reversal Ventritex waveform—in which the leading edge voltage of phase 2 was only one-half the trailing edge voltage of phase 1—was significantly less effective than the CPI waveform, which used equal leading edge phase 2 and trailing edge phase 1 voltages (Fig. 1–33). The Medtronic waveform, which had the same voltage reversal as the CPI waveform, also had a DFT similar to the CPI waveform[98] (Fig. 1–33). Ventritex (St. Jude) no longer uses the small voltage reversal waveform, most likely because of its lower efficacy.

Additional support for the importance of voltage reversal comes from studies using parallel-to-series capacitor switching to create new, experimental waveforms. With this technique, two capacitors are initially connected in parallel, providing greater capacitance. At the time of the phase change during the shock, the capacitors are electronically switched to a series connection, decreasing capacitance and increasing voltage in an additive manner, so that a large voltage reversal is achieved (Fig. 1–34). Parallel-series mode-switched waveforms (60/15 µF) have lower DFTs than single capacitor biphasic waveforms, which have smaller voltage reversals (135/135 µF and 90/90 µF).[99] Interestingly, the second phase of the parallel-series waveform is longer than the first phase but shows im-

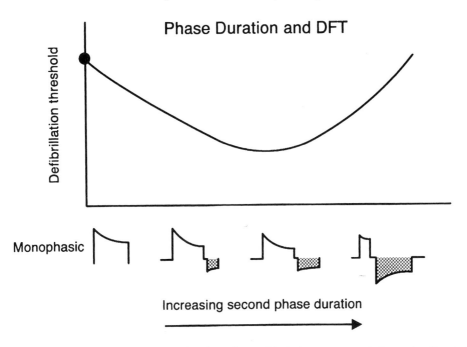

Fig. 1–32. Idealized curve demonstrating the relationship between second phase duration and defibrillation threshold (DFT). Details are in the text.

Manu-facturer	Wave form	Capacitor	Tilt (%)	Pulse width	Voltage reversal	Defibrillation threshold (J)
Guidant	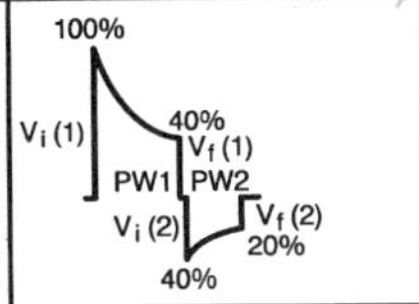 100% $V_i(1)$ 40% $V_f(1)$ PW1 PW2 $V_i(2)$ $V_f(2)$ 20% 40%	140 µf	60/50	PW1 = 60% total PW PW2 = 40% total PW	$V_i(2)=$ $V_f(1)$	9.1 ± 5.5
Medtronic	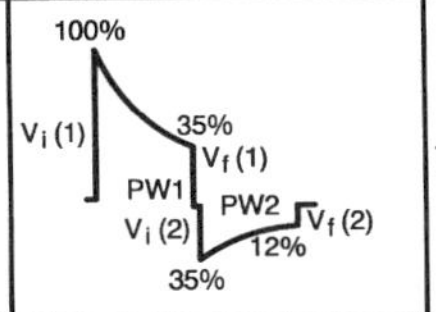 100% $V_i(1)$ 35% $V_f(1)$ PW1 PW2 $V_f(2)$ $V_i(2)$ 12% 35%	120 µf	65/65	PW1 = PW2	$V_i(2)=$ $V_f(1)$	10.2 ± 5.6
Ventritex (St Jude)	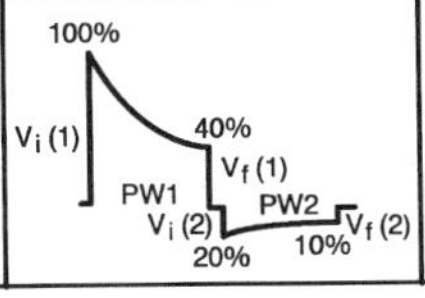 100% $V_i(1)$ 40% $V_f(1)$ PW1 PW2 $V_f(2)$ $V_i(2)$ 20% 10%	150 µf	65/40-50	PW1 = PW2	$V_i(2)=$ ½ $V_f(1)$	13.6 ± 5.5

$P < 0.05$, Guidant (CPI) vs. Ventritex

Fig. 1–33. Characteristics of commercially available waveforms. Because of the important influence of voltage reversal on defibrillation, Ventritex (St. Jude) now uses a different waveform, which has $V_i(2) = V_f(1)$. PW, pulse width; V_f, final voltage; $V_f(1)$, trailing edge of first pulse; $V_f(2)$, trailing edge of second pulse; V_i, initial voltage; $V_i(1)$, leading edge of first pulse; $V_i(2)$, leading edge of second pulse. (Modified from Tomassoni et al.[98] By permission of the American Heart Association.)

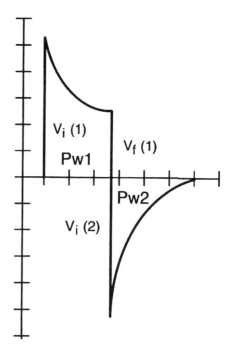

Fig. 1–34. A waveform created with parallel-series capacitor mode switch. Note that the leading edge of the second pulse (V_i (2)) is greater than the trailing edge of the first pulse (V_f (1)), resulting in a large voltage reversal. The second pulse is not truncated, and it is longer than the first pulse (Pw2 > Pw1). This waveform requires two capacitors. Further details are in the text.

proved efficiency, contrary to what might be expected. However, because the capacitance of the second phase is very small, the voltage drops very quickly, so that the duration of the effective voltage may be less in the second phase than in the first. This rapid drop and short pulse width may also explain why this waveform does not refibrillate the ventricle, as hypothesized for waveforms of longer duration, despite not being truncated.

Polarity and Biphasic Waveforms

Polarity is an important determinant of monophasic defibrillation, with lower DFTs found for transvenous systems when the right ventricular electrode is the anode (+).[100,101] The results of studies of biphasic polarity are less uniform, with some reports showing an effect of biphasic polarity and others indicating no effect.[102–104] However, all studies demonstrating a polarity effect have found that waveforms with a first phase in which

the right ventricular electrode is the anode (+) are more effective. Additionally, biphasic polarity has the greatest effect on patients with elevated DFTs. In a study of 60 patients, use of biphasic waveforms with a right ventricular anodal first phase resulted in a 31% reduction in DFT in patients with DFT ≥ 15 J, whereas polarity made no difference in patients with DFTs less than 15 J.[105] Despite the fairly uniform population improvement in DFT with a ventricular anodal first phase polarity among studies in which an effect was seen, there is clearly individual variability, so that if an adequate safety margin cannot be found in a patient, a trial of the opposite polarity is reasonable, regardless of the initial polarity tested.

Mechanism of Improved Efficacy With Biphasic Waveforms

Several theories have been proposed to explain the observed superiority of biphasic over monophasic waveforms.

None provides a complete explanation for the benefits seen, and the fundamental mechanism remains to be determined. However, important basic observations have been made.

First Phase as "Conditioning" Pulse

Successful defibrillation requires sodium channel activation at a time when cells are ordinarily not receptive to physiologic stimulation. The first phase of a pulse may serve to hyperpolarize tissue near the anode, thereby reactivating otherwise inactive sodium channels. This conditioning pulse facilitates excitation by the following pulse.[106]

Refractory Period Shortening

The first phase of a biphasic pulse may shorten the refractory period of myocardial cells. This transient shortening may then facilitate the effective recruitment of sodium channels by the second phase of the pulse. This ultimately extends the duration of the action potential and the refractory period, important putative mechanisms for defibrillation.[94]

Membrane Stabilization

In addition to being more effective and requiring a lower potential gradient for defibrillation, biphasic waveforms are less toxic than monophasic waveforms. In higher voltage gradient regions, membrane disruption and myocardial damage may result from the shock. However, higher voltage gradients are required to produce these toxic effects with biphasic waveforms than with monophasic waveforms. Deleterious postshock effects may be due to membrane microlesions, which permit indiscriminate exchange of ions. The reversal of polarity during the shock may expedite membrane reorientation and repair, decreasing postshock dysfunction.[107]

Measuring Shock Dose

All the discussion to this point has described the shock dose in terms of energy (joules). As noted above, the shape of the waveform is a function of the initial voltage, the size of the capacitor, and the resistance of the load. If a smaller capacitor is used to diminish device size, a larger initial voltage may be needed to deliver an equivalent amount of charge into the fibrillating tissue. Thus, two waveforms may have different leading edge voltages but the same energy if there are differences in capacitance (Fig. 1–35). Therefore, the question of how to determine the "dose" of a shock arises. It is clearly important, because shocks of insufficient dose fail to terminate fibrillation and excessively strong shocks can lead to proarrhythmia or myocardial injury. The "dose" of defibrillation is usually given in units of energy (joules) on the basis of tradition and ease of measurement. Physiologically, however, energy has little bearing on defibrillation; the voltage gradient is the factor that affects membrane channel conductance, and at the tissue level, several decades of animal and human research have shown current to be the most important factor for generating action potentials and for defibrillation.[73] To add to the complexity, energy can be described as the stored energy—the amount of energy stored in the capacitor before shock delivery—or the energy delivered. Since the waveforms are truncated, usually around 10% of the stored energy is not delivered. Additionally, although the term is used clinically, "delivered energy" is highly variable, depending on where the delivery is recorded; energy delivered at the lead surface is not the same as energy delivered

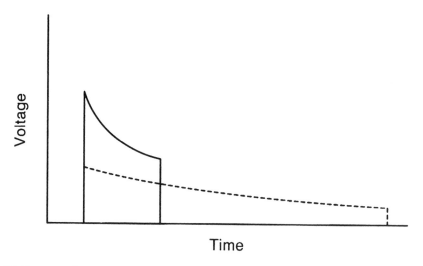

Fig. 1–35. Two waveforms with different voltages but the same energy. The solid waveform has a higher initial voltage but a smaller capacitance and, consequently, a shorter pulse width. The dashed waveform starts with a lower voltage but has a greater capacitance and pulse width, resulting in the same energy delivery despite the marked differences in the voltages. Further details in the text.

only a few millimeters into the tissue. Some device manufacturers, in fact, simply report an arbitrary percentage of the stored energy as the delivered energy. Stored energy, although not a direct indicator of the factors responsible for biologic defibrillation, indicates the size of the device necessary to generate a given energy shock. Over the range of clinically utilized capacitor size and biologic tissue resistance in a given system, a change in energy up or down is reflected by a similar change in voltage and current. In practice, "energy" is the most commonly used term to indicate shock dose.

Use of Waveform Theory in Clinical Practice

The optimal biphasic waveform is specific to device, lead, and patient. In many commercially available devices, the only programmable option is the polarity. Therefore, if a patient undergoing im-plantable defibrillator insertion does not have an adequate defibrillation safety margin, a logical next step is reversal of polarity. If an adequate safety margin is still not met, a lead is often added (discussed below). Tilt or duration could be modified as an alternative next step in systems that offer this feature, although this is infrequently done because predicting optimal tilt for a given patient is difficult.

Lead System and Defibrillation

The most efficient lead system is one that evenly distributes the shock over the myocardium and minimizes the difference in potential between high-gradient and low-gradient zones. This is best accomplished with large contoured epicardial patches positioned so that an imaginary line connecting the centers of the electrodes passes through the ventricular center of mass.[108] However, since epicardial leads require thoracotomy for placement, they are now only rarely used.

Although intrinsically less efficient, transvenous lead systems can now be used almost universally because of the adoption of biphasic waveforms (discussed above) and the introduction of defibrillators in which the pulse generator shell is an active electrode. Because the surface area of the pulse generator is large, the addition of the generator shell as an active electrode reduces the biphasic endocardial DFT by 30% compared with that of a dual-coil defibrillation lead alone.[109] When an active can system with a single distal defibrillation coil is used, addition of a proximal coil has further lowered the DFT in some, but not all, studies.[109,110] Nonetheless, if implantation safety margins cannot be achieved despite waveform modification (reversal of polarity and, rarely, adjustment of tilt and duration), adding a second lead with the elec-

trode positioned near the junction of the right atrium and superior vena cava is a logical next step. If adequate safety margins cannot be achieved despite optimal deployment of endovascular leads, subcutaneous patches or arrays, which further significantly increase defibrillation electrode surface area and can favorably direct greater current through the ventricles, can lead to successful implantation. With biphasic active-electrode pulse generators, subcutaneous leads, which although effective increase system complexity and morbidity, are required in only 3.7% of patients[82] (Fig. 1–36). When they are required, arrays may be more effective than patches, though we found that this benefit was blunted in biphasic systems.[82]

As noted above, defibrillation efficacy is improved with optimal lead positions, although the effectiveness of biphasic waveforms and large surface area of

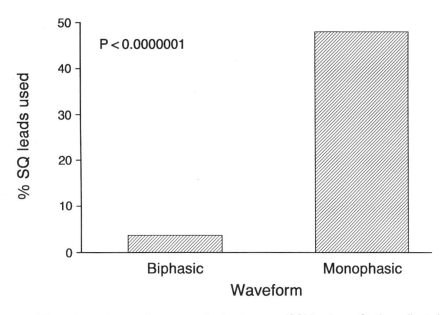

Fig. 1–36. Effect of waveform on frequency of subcutaneous (SQ) lead use. On the ordinate is the frequency of subcutaneous lead usage, and on the abscissa are the subgroups analyzed. In 45 of 94 (48%) patients with monophasic systems, subcutaneous leads were required to meet implantation criteria. In contrast, only 17 of 460 (3.7%) biphasic systems required subcutaneous leads to meet implantation criteria. (From Trusty et al.[82] By permission of Futura Publishing Company.)

the pulse generator has permitted tolerance of less than perfect positions. Generally, defibrillation effectiveness diminishes as the right ventricular electrode is placed in a progressively proximal position, toward the tricuspid valve. Therefore, this lead should be placed as apically as possible. Additionally, a septal location, to direct as much of the electrical field over the left ventricular mass as possible, is desirable.[111] In systems with an active pulse generator shell that permit independent positioning of a proximal defibrillation coil, the proximal lead position can be near the superior vena cava, near its junction with the right atrium, or in the left subclavian vein[112] (Fig. 1–37).

Since in nearly all commercially available defibrillators the pulse generator shell serves as an electrode, its position can also affect defibrillation efficacy. Implantable defibrillators are most commonly placed in the left pectoral region, typically in the prepectoral (subcutaneous) plane. How-

ever, the site of pulse generator placement and vascular access is influenced by multiple factors, including patient and physician preference, anatomical anomalies, previous operations, integrity of the vascular system, and whether a preexisting permanent pacing system is present. In addition to factors specific to the patient, choice of the implantation site can affect ease of technical insertion, defibrillation effectiveness, and long-term rates of lead failure.

Right pectoral implantation may be considered in left-handed persons, hunters who place the rifle butt on the left shoulder, and patients with previous mastectomy, other surgical procedures, or anatomy that precludes left-sided insertion. In systems with both distal and proximal defibrillation coils, the proximal coil is either shifted toward the right hemithorax (if both coils are on the same lead) or, often, advanced to a lower superior vena cava position for greater cardiac proximity (in two-lead systems) with

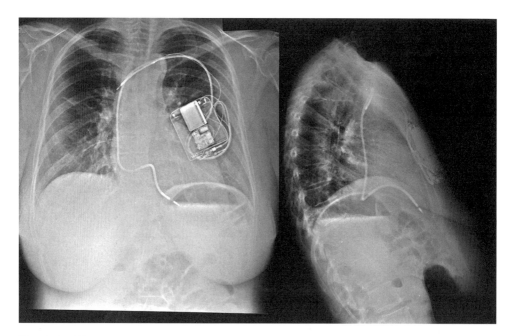

Fig. 1–37. Chest radiographs depict active pulse generator shell system with an added proximal defibrillation coil to optimize defibrillation threshold.

right-sided placement. With active can pulse generators, the largest defibrillation lead surface, the device shell, is shifted away from the ventricular myocardium (Fig. 1–38). These unfavorable restrictions on lead position decrease defibrillation effectiveness.[113,114] With biphasic waveforms, we found that right-sided implantation results in a 6-J increase in DFT compared with left-sided placement (11.3 ± 5.3 J, left-sided; 17.0 ± 4.9 J, right-sided; $P < 0.0001$).[114] Even with the increase, right-sided devices were successfully placed in 19 of 20 patients; in one patient, an acceptable right-sided threshold could not be achieved and that ap-

proach was abandoned. Despite the concern that a right-sided active can might be detrimental by diverting a significant portion of the electrical field away from the ventricles, the large surface area of the shell compensates for this, so that when right-sided implantation is required, active can devices are preferable[114] (Fig. 1–39). In general, however, left-sided insertion is superior to right-sided placement and is used if there are no compelling factors against it.

An alternative site for device placement is the abdomen, but this site is only rarely used. Although not as effective for defibrillation as the left pectoral position,

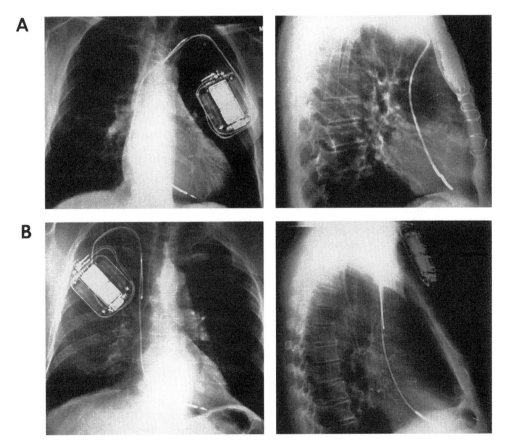

Fig. 1–38. *A,* Posteroanterior and lateral chest radiographs from a patient with a left-sided defibrillator. Note that the proximal defibrillation lead is in the left subclavian vein. *B,* Posteroanterior and lateral chest radiographs from a patient with right-sided defibrillator placement. Note that the proximal defibrillation lead is in the superior vena cava.

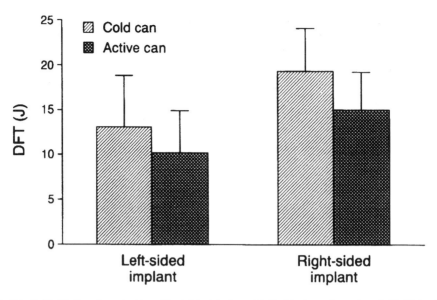

Fig. 1–39. Defibrillation thresholds with right-sided and left-sided cardioverter-defibrillator implantation of active can and cold can devices. Defibrillation threshold (DFT) is on ordinate, and side of placement and can type are on abscissa. (From Friedman et al.[114] By permission of Futura Publishing Company.)

the abdomen appears superior to the right pectoral location for active can placement.[115] However, abdominal insertion is technically more challenging, requiring two incisions, lead tunneling, abdominal dissection (often necessitating surgical assistance), and general anesthesia. Additionally, because of the greater risk of infection, threat of peritoneal erosion, and increased risk of lead fracture, even with totally transvenous systems,[116–118] this position is used only in rare circumstances.

Drugs and Defibrillators

Antiarrhythmic agents are frequently used in patients with implantable defibrillators to treat supraventricular arrhythmias (particularly atrial fibrillation), suppress ventricular tachyarrhythmias, and slow ventricular tachycardia to increase the responsiveness of antitachycardia pacing. In recent implantable defibrillator trials, concomitant use of membrane-active agents (Vaughn-Williams class I or class III

drugs) has ranged from 12% to 31%.[119,120] Several important device-drug interactions must be considered.[121]

1. Detection. Most drugs slow ventricular tachycardia. If slowed below the detection cutoff rate, ventricular tachycardia is not detected by the device and remains untreated. Initiation of antiarrhythmic drugs in patients with ventricular tachycardia is usually followed by device testing to assess detection of ventricular tachycardia.
2. Pacing thresholds. Bradycardia and antitachycardia pacing thresholds may be affected by pharmacologic agents, as discussed in Chapter 13.
3. Pacing requirements. Drugs may exacerbate conduction defects or slow the sinus rate, necessitating pacing for bradycardia.
4. Drug-induced proarrhythmia.
5. Changes in DFT. Although it is well known that pharmacologic agents can modulate defibrillation effective-

Table 1–2.
Effects of Drugs on Defibrillation

Drug	Class*	Effect on defibrillation threshold†
Quinidine	IA	Increase
Procainamide	IA	No change
N-acetylprocainamide	IA	Decrease
Disopyramide	IA	No change
Flecainide	IC	Increase
Moricizine	IC	Increase
Propafenone	IC	No change
Propranolol	II	Increase
Atenolol	II	No change
Isoproterenol	—	Decrease
Sotalol	III	Decrease
Ibutilide	III	Decrease
Dofetilide	III	Decrease
Amiodarone	III	
Oral		Increase
Intravenous		No change or decrease
Diltiazem	IV	Increase
Verapamil	IV	Increase

*Vaughn-Williams classification.
†If study results conflict, the most frequently reported effect is noted.
Modified from Carnes et al.[121] By permission of Pharmacotherapy Publications.

Table 1–3.
Membrane-Active Drugs*

Vaughn-Williams classification	Medication
IA	Quinidine, procainamide, disopyramide
IB	Lidocaine, tocainide, phenytoin
IC	Flecainide, propafenone, encainide, moricizine
III	Sotalol, ibutilide, dofetilide, amiodarone

*These agents may significantly affect defibrillator function, often mandating device testing on initiation.

ness, drug-defibrillation interactions are complex. Moreover, assessment of the influence of drugs on defibrillation is confounded by the effects of anesthetic agents, variability in lead systems and waveforms across studies, and heterogeneity in study subjects (i.e., human, canine, and porcine). In general, however, agents that impede the fast inward sodium current (such as lidocaine) or calcium channel function (such as verapamil) increase the DFT, whereas agents that block repolarizing potassium currents (such as sotalol) lower the DFT. The effects of amiodarone are legion; clinically, long-term administration of amiodarone increases DFTs, whereas intravenous administration has little immediate effect. DFT testing should be performed when administration of drugs that can increase the threshold (especially amiodarone) is initiated, particularly in patients with borderline DFTs. Drug effects on defibrillation are summarized in Table 1–2. As a general rule, ICD evaluation should be considered whenever administration of Vaughn-Williams class I or class III drugs is initiated or their dosage significantly increased. These drugs are listed in Table 1–3. Drug and defibrillator interactions are also discussed in Chapter 13.

References

1. Hodgkin AL, Huxley AF: Quantitative description of membrane current and its application to conduction and excitation in nerve. J Physiol (Lond) 117:500–544, 1952
2. Glitsch HG: Electrogenic Na pumping in the heart. Annu Rev Physiol 44:389–400, 1982
3. Gadsby DC: The Na/K pump of cardiac cells. Annu Rev Biophys Bioeng 13:373–398, 1984
4. Grant AO: Evolving concepts of cardiac sodium channel function. J Cardiovasc Electrophysiol 1:53–67, 1990
5. Makielski JC, Sheets MF, Hanck DA, January CT, Fozzard HA: Sodium current in voltage clamped internally perfused canine cardiac Purkinje cells. Biophys J 52: 1–11, 1987
6. Cohen CJ, Bean BP, Tsien RW: Maximal upstroke velocity as an index of available sodium conductance. Comparison of maximal upstroke velocity and voltage clamp measurements of sodium current in rabbit Purkinje fibers. Circ Res 54:636–651, 1984
7. Kunze DL, Lacerda AE, Wilson DL, Brown AM: Cardiac Na currents and the inactivating, reopening, and waiting properties of single cardiac Na channels. J Gen Physiol 86:691–719, 1985
8. Reuter H: Divalent cations as charge carriers in excitable membranes. Prog Biophys Mol Biol 26:1–43, 1973
9. Hume JR, Giles W: Ionic currents in single isolated bullfrog atrial cells. J Gen Physiol 81:153–194, 1983
10. Hume JR, Giles W, Robinson K, Shibata EF, Nathan RD, Kanai K, Rasmusson R: A time- and voltage-dependent K+ current in single cardiac cells from bullfrog atrium. J Gen Physiol 88:777–798, 1986
11. De Mello WC: Intercellular communication in cardiac muscle. Circ Res 51:1–9, 1982
12. Barr L, Dewey MM, Berger W: Propagation of action potentials and the structure of the nexus in cardiac muscle. J Gen Physiol 48:797–823, 1965
13. Irnich W: The fundamental law of electrostimulation and its application to defibrillation. Pacing Clin Electrophysiol 13: 1433–1447, 1990
14. Blair HA: Time-intensity relations for stimulation of tissue by electric currents. Proc Soc Exp Biol Med 29:615–618, 1932
15. Lapicque L: Définition experimentale de excitabilité. Compt rend Soc Biol 67:280–283, 1909
16. Irnich W: The chronaxie time and its practical importance. Pacing Clin Electrophysiol 3:292–301, 1980
17. Furman S: Basic concepts. In A Practice of Cardiac Pacing. Third edition. Edited by S Furman, DL Hayes, DR Holmes Jr. Mount Kisco, NY, Futura Publishing Company, 1993, pp 34–35
18. Barold SS, Ong LS, Heinle RA: Stimulation and sensing thresholds for cardiac pacing: electrophysiologic and technical aspects. Prog Cardiovasc Dis 24:1–24, 1981
19. Furman S: Basic concepts. In A Practice of Cardiac Pacing. Third edition. Edited by S Furman, DL Hayes, DR Holmes Jr. Mount Kisco, NY, Futura Publishing Company, 1993, p 29
20. Lindemans FW, Denier Van der Gon JJ: Current thresholds and liminal size in excitation of heart muscle. Cardiovasc Res 12:477–485, 1978
21. Moore WJ: Physical Chemistry. Fourth edition. Englewood Cliffs, NJ, Prentice-Hall, 1972, p 510
22. Thuesen L, Jensen PJ, Vejby-Christensen H, Mortensen PT, Thomsen PE: Lower chronic stimulation threshold in the carbon-tip than in the platinum-tip endocardial electrode: a randomized study. Pacing Clin Electrophysiol 12:1592–1595, 1989
23. Walton C, Gergely S, Economides AP: Platinum pacemaker electrodes: origins and effects of the electrode-tissue interface impedance. Pacing Clin Electrophysiol 10:87–99, 1987
24. Garberoglio B, Inguaggiato B, Chinaglia B, Cerise O: Initial results with an activated pyrolytic carbon tip electrode. Pacing Clin Electrophysiol 6:440–448, 1983
25. Bornzin GA, Stokes KB, Wiebusch WA:

A low threshold, low polarization platinized endocardial electrode (abstract). Pacing Clin Electrophysiol 6:A-70, 1983

26. Wiegand UK, Zhdanov A, Stammwitz E, Crozier I, Claessens RJ II, Meier J, Bos RJ, Bode F, Potratz J: Electrophysiological performance of a bipolar membrane-coated titanium nitride electrode: a randomized comparison of steroid and nonsteroid lead designs. Pacing Clin Electrophysiol 22:935–941, 1999

27. Amundson DC, McArthur W, Mosharrafa M: The porous endocardial electrode. Pacing Clin Electrophysiol 2:40–50, 1979

28. Timmis GC, Helland J, Westveer DC: The evolution of low threshold leads. Clin Prog Pacing Electrophysiol 1:313–334, 1983

29. Albert HM, Glass BA, Pittman B, et al: Cardiac stimulation threshold: chronic study. Ann NY Acad Sci 111:889–892, 1964

30. Contini C, Strata G, Pauletti M, Garberoglio B: Measurement of the myocardial stimulation threshold in chronic and acute patients with pacemaker implanted [Italian]. G Ital Cardiol 8 Suppl 1:273–276, 1978

31. Luceri RM, Furman S, Hurzeler P, Escher DJ: Threshold behavior of electrodes in long-term ventricular pacing. Am J Cardiol 40:184–188, 1977

32. Chaptal AP, Ribot A: Statistical survey of strength-duration threshold curves with endocardial electrodes and long-term behavior of these electrodes, Proceedings of the Fifth World Symposium on Cardiac Pacing. Montreal, Canada, Pacesymp, 1979, pp 21–22

33. de Buitleir M, Kou WH, Schmaltz S, Morady F: Acute changes in pacing threshold and R- or P-wave amplitude during permanent pacemaker implantation. Am J Cardiol 65:999–1003, 1990

34. Kay GN, Anderson K, Epstein AE, Plumb VJ: Active fixation atrial leads: randomized comparison of two lead designs. Pacing Clin Electrophysiol 12:1355–1361, 1989

35. Beanlands DS, Akyurekli T, Keon WJ: Prednisone in the management of exit block, Proceedings of the Fifth World Symposium on Cardiac Pacing. Montreal, Canada, Pacesymp, 1979, pp 18–23

36. Mond H, Stokes K, Helland J, Grigg L, Kertes P, Pate B, Hunt D: The porous titanium steroid eluting electrode: a double blind study assessing the stimulation threshold effects of steroid. Pacing Clin Electrophysiol 11:214–219, 1988

37. Kruse IM, Terpstra B: Acute and long-term atrial and ventricular stimulation thresholds with a steroid-eluting electrode. Pacing Clin Electrophysiol 8:45–49, 1985

38. Beyersdorf F, Schneider M, Kreuzer J, Falk S, Zegelman M, Satter P: Studies of the tissue reaction induced by transvenous pacemaker electrodes. I. Microscopic examination of the extent of connective tissue around the electrode tip in the human right ventricle. Pacing Clin Electrophysiol 11:1753–1759, 1988

39. Guarda F, Galloni M, Assone F, Pasteris V, Luboz MP: Histological reactions of porous tip endocardial electrodes implanted in sheep. Int J Artif Organs 5:267–273, 1982

40. Szabo Z, Solti F: The significance of the tissue reaction around the electrode on the late myocardial threshold. *In* Advances in Pacemaker Technology. Edited by M Schaldach, S Furman. New York, Springer-Verlag, 1975, p 273

41. Nagatomo Y, Ogawa T, Kumagae H, Koiwaya Y, Tanaka K: Pacing failure due to markedly increased stimulation threshold 2 years after implantation: successful management with oral prednisolone: a case report. Pacing Clin Electrophysiol 12:1034–1037, 1989

42. King DH, Gillette PC, Shannon C, Cuddy TE: Steroid-eluting endocardial pacing lead for treatment of exit block. Am Heart J 106:1438–1440, 1983

43. Lewis T: The Mechanism and Graphic Registration of the Heart Beat. London, Shaw & Sons, 1925

44. Furman S, Hurzeler P, DeCaprio V: The ventricular endocardial electrogram and pacemaker sensing. J Thorac Cardiovasc Surg 73:258–266, 1977

45. Watson WS: Myopotential sensing in cardiac pacemakers. *In* Modern Cardiac Pacing. Edited by SS Barold. Mount Kisco, NY, Futura Publishing Company, 1985, pp 813–837

46. Parsonnet V, Myers GH, Kresh YM: Characteristics of intracardiac electrograms II: atrial endocardial electrograms. Pacing Clin Electrophysiol 3:406–417, 1980

47. Kleinert M, Elmqvist H, Strandberg H: Spectral properties of atrial and ventricular endocardial signals. Pacing Clin Electrophysiol 2:11–19, 1979

48. Hurzeler P, DeCaprio V, Furman S: Endocardial electrograms and pacer sensing. *In* Advances in Pacemaker Technology. Edited by M Schaldach, S Furman. New York, Springer-Verlag, 1975, p 307

49. Hauser RG, Susmano A: After-potential oversensing by a programmable pulse

generator. Pacing Clin Electrophysiol 4: 391–395, 1981

50. Potential cross-talk in early Gemini 415A pacers with dual anodal rings. Product Safety Alert, Cordis Corporation, 1989

51. Clarke M, Liu B, Schuller H, Binner L, Kennergren C, Guerola M, Weinmann P, Ohm OJ: Automatic adjustment of pacemaker stimulation output correlated with continuously monitored capture thresholds: a multicenter study. European Microny Study Group. Pacing Clin Electrophysiol 21:1567–1575, 1998

52. Kay GN: Basic aspects of cardiac pacing. In Cardiac Pacing. Edited by KA Ellenbogen. Boston, Blackwell Scientific Publications, 1992, pp 32–119

53. Hanson JS: Sixteen failures in a single model of bipolar polyurethane-insulated ventricular pacing lead: a 44-month experience. Pacing Clin Electrophysiol 7:389–394, 1984

54. Raymond RD, Nanian KB: Insulation failure with bipolar polyurethane pacing leads. Pacing Clin Electrophysiol 7:378–380, 1984

55. Kertes P, Mond H, Sloman G, Vohra J, Hunt D: Comparison of lead complications with polyurethane tined, silicone rubber tined, and wedge tip leads: clinical experience with 822 ventricular endocardial leads. Pacing Clin Electrophysiol 6: 957–962, 1983

56. Calfee RV, Saulson SH: A voluntary standard for 3.2 mm unipolar and bipolar pacemaker leads and connectors. Pacing Clin Electrophysiol 9:1181–1185, 1986

57. Furman S: Basic concepts. In A Practice of Cardiac Pacing. Third edition. Edited by S Furman, DL Hayes, DR Holmes Jr. Mount Kisco, NY, Futura Publishing Company, 1993, pp 29–88

58. Tyers GF, Brownlee RR: Power pulse generators, electrodes, and longevity. Prog Cardiovasc Dis 23:421–434, 1981

59. Bicik V, Kristan L: Sine2/triangle/square wave generator for pacemaker testing. Pacing Clin Electrophysiol 8:484–493, 1985

60. Irnich W: Muscle noise and interference behavior in pacemakers: a comparative study. Pacing Clin Electrophysiol 10:125–132, 1987

61. Bernstein AD, Camm AJ, Fletcher RD, Gold RD, Rickards AF, Smyth NP, Spielman SR, Sutton R: The NASPE/BPEG generic pacemaker code for antibradyarrhythmia and adaptive-rate pacing and antitachyarrhythmia devices. Pacing Clin Electrophysiol 10:794–799, 1987

62. Prevost J, Battelli F: Some effects of electrical discharge on the hearts of mammals. Comptes Rendus Acad Sci 129:1267–1268, 1899

63. Moe G: Computer simulation of atrial fibrillation. Comp Biomed Res 2:217–238, 1965

64. Gurvich NL, Yuniev GS: Restoration of regular rhythm in mammalian fibrillating heart. Am Rev Soviet Med 3:236–239, 1946

65. Zipes DP, Fischer J, King RM, Nicoll AdeB, Jolly WW: Termination of ventricular fibrillation in dogs by depolarizing a critical amount of myocardium. Am J Cardiol 36:37–44, 1975

66. Chen PS, Shibata N, Dixon EG, Wolf PD, Danieley ND, Sweeney MB, Smith WM, Ideker RE: Activation during ventricular defibrillation in open-chest dogs. Evidence of complete cessation and regeneration of ventricular fibrillation after unsuccessful shocks. J Clin Invest 77:810–823, 1986

67. Chen PS, Wolf PD, Melnick SD, Danieley ND, Smith WM, Ideker RE: Comparison of activation during ventricular fibrillation and following unsuccessful defibrillation shocks in open-chest dogs. Circ Res 66:1544–1560, 1990

68. Frazier DW, Wolf PD, Wharton JM, Tang AS, Smith WM, Ideker RE: Stimulus-induced critical point. Mechanism for electrical initiation of reentry in normal canine myocardium. J Clin Invest 83:1039–1052, 1989

69. Swerdlow CD, Martin DJ, Kass RM, Davie S, Mandel WJ, Gang ES, Chen PS: The zone of vulnerability to T wave shocks in humans. J Cardiovasc Electrophysiol 8: 145–154, 1997

70. Chen PS, Feld GK, Kriett JM, Mower MM, Tarazi RY, Fleck RP, Swerdlow CD, Gang ES, Kass RM: Relation between upper limit of vulnerability and defibrillation threshold in humans. Circulation 88:186–192, 1993

71. Dillon SM, Kwaku KF: Progressive depolarization: a unified hypothesis for defibrillation and fibrillation induction by shocks. J Cardiovasc Electrophysiol 9:529–552, 1998

72. Sweeney RJ, Gill RM, Steinberg MI, Reid PR: Ventricular refractory period extension caused by defibrillation shocks. Circulation 82:965–972, 1990

73. Dillon SM: The electrophysiological effects of defibrillation shocks. In Implantable Cardioverter Defibrillator Therapy: The Engineering-Clinical Interface. Edited by MW Kroll, MH Lehmann. Norwell, MA, Kluwer Academic Publishers, 1996, pp 31–61

74. Ideker RE, Hillsley RE, Wharton JM: Shock strength for the implantable defibrillator: can you have too much of a good thing? (editorial). Pacing Clin Electrophysiol 15: 841–844, 1992

75. Frazier DW, Stanton MS: Resetting and transient entrainment of ventricular tachycardia. Pacing Clin Electrophysiol 18: 1919–1946, 1995

76. Davy JM, Fain ES, Dorian P, Winkle RA: The relationship between successful defibrillation and delivered energy in open-chest dogs: reappraisal of the "defibrillation threshold" concept. Am Heart J 113: 77–84, 1987

77. Strickberger SA, Daoud EG, Davidson T, Weiss R, Bogun F, Knight BP, Bahu M, Goyal R, Man KC, Morady F: Probability of successful defibrillation at multiples of the defibrillation energy requirement in patients with an implantable defibrillator. Circulation 96:1217–1223, 1997

78. Brady PA, Friedman PA, Stanton MS: Effect of failed defibrillation shocks on electrogram amplitude in a nonintegrated transvenous defibrillation lead system. Am J Cardiol 76:580–584, 1995

79. Strickberger SA, Man KC, Souza J, Zivin A, Weiss R, Knight BP, Goyal R, Daoud EG, Morady F: A prospective evaluation of two defibrillation safety margin techniques in patients with low defibrillation energy requirements. J Cardiovasc Electrophysiol 9:41–46, 1998

80. Marchlinski FE, Flores B, Miller JM, Gottlieb CD, Hargrove WC III: Relation of the intraoperative defibrillation threshold to successful postoperative defibrillation with an automatic implantable cardioverter defibrillator. Am J Cardiol 62:393–398, 1988

81. Degroot PJ, Church TR, Mehra R, Martinson MS, Schaber DE: Derivation of a defibrillator implant criterion based on probability of successful defibrillation. Pacing Clin Electrophysiol 20:1924–1935, 1997

82. Trusty JM, Hayes DL, Stanton MS, Friedman PA: Factors affecting the frequency of subcutaneous lead usage in implantable defibrillators. Pacing Clin Electrophysiol 23:842–846, 2000

83. Swerdlow CD, Kass RM, O'Connor ME, Chen PS: Effect of shock waveform on relationship between upper limit of vulnerability and defibrillation threshold. J Cardiovasc Electrophysiol 9:339–349, 1998

84. Swerdlow CD, Ahern T, Kass RM, Davie S, Mandel WJ, Chen PS: Upper limit of vulnerability is a good estimator of shock strength associated with 90% probability of successful defibrillation in humans with transvenous implantable cardioverter-defibrillators. J Am Coll Cardiol 27:1112–1118, 1996

85. Swerdlow CD, Peter CT, Kass RM, Gang ES, Mandel WJ, Hwang C, Martin DJ, Chen PS: Programming of implantable cardioverter-defibrillators on the basis of the upper limit of vulnerability. Circulation 95:1497–1504, 1997

86. Schuder JC, Gold JH, Stoeckle H, Granberg TA, Dettmer JC, Larwill MH: Transthoracic ventricular defibrillation in the 100 kg calf with untruncated and truncated exponential stimuli. IEEE Trans Biomed Eng 27:37–43, 1980

87. Olsovsky MR, Hodgson DM, Shorofsky SR, Kavesh NG, Gold MR: Effect of biphasic waveforms on transvenous defibrillation thresholds in patients with coronary artery disease. Am J Cardiol 80:1098–1100, 1997

88. Wyse DG, Kavanagh KM, Gillis AM, Mitchell LB, Duff HJ, Sheldon RS, Kieser TM, Maitland A, Flanagan P, Rothschild J, Mehra R: Comparison of biphasic and monophasic shocks for defibrillation using a nonthoracotomy system. Am J Cardiol 71:197–202, 1993

89. Bardy GH, Ivey TD, Allen MD, Johnson G, Mehra R, Greene HL: A prospective randomized evaluation of biphasic versus monophasic waveform pulses on defibrillation efficacy in humans. J Am Coll Cardiol 14:728–733, 1989

90. Schuder JC, McDaniel WC, Stoeckle H: Defibrillation of 100 kg calves with asymmetrical, bidirectional, rectangular pulses. Cardiovasc Res 18:419–426, 1984

91. Jones JL, Swartz JF, Jones RE, Fletcher R: Increasing fibrillation duration enhances relative asymmetrical biphasic versus monophasic defibrillator waveform efficacy. Circ Res 67:376–384, 1990

92. Dixon EG, Tang AS, Wolf PD, Meador JT, Fine MJ, Calfee RV, Ideker RE: Improved defibrillation thresholds with large contoured epicardial electrodes and biphasic waveforms. Circulation 76:1176–1184, 1987

93. Feeser SA, Tang AS, Kavanagh KM, Rollins DL, Smith WM, Wolf PD, Ideker RE: Strength-duration and probability of success curves for defibrillation with biphasic waveforms. Circulation 82:2128–2141, 1990

94. Tang AS, Yabe S, Wharton JM, Dolker M, Smith WM, Ideker RE: Ventricular defibrillation using biphasic waveforms: the importance of phasic duration. J Am Coll Cardiol 13:207–214, 1989

95. Schauerte P, Schondube FA, Grossmann M, Dorge H, Stein F, Dohmen B, Moumen A, Erena K, Messmer BJ, Hanrath P, Stellbrink C: Influence of phase duration of biphasic waveforms on defibrillation energy requirements with a 70-microF capacitance. Circulation 97:2073–2078, 1998

96. Swerdlow CD, Kass RM, Davie S, Chen PS, Hwang C: Short biphasic pulses from 90 microfarad capacitors lower defibrillation threshold. Pacing Clin Electrophysiol 19:1053–1060, 1996

97. Natale A, Sra J, Krum D, Dhala A, Deshpande S, Jazayeri M, Newby K, Wase A, Axtell K, VanHout WL, Akhtar M: Relative efficacy of different tilts with biphasic defibrillation in humans. Pacing Clin Electrophysiol 19:197–206, 1996

98. Tomassoni G, Newby K, Deshpande S, Axtell K, Sra J, Akhtar M, Natale A: Defibrillation efficacy of commercially available biphasic impulses in humans. Importance of negative-phase peak voltage. Circulation 95:1822–1826, 1997

99. Yamanouchi Y, Mowrey KA, Nadzam GR, Hills DG, Kroll MW, Brewer JE, Donohoo AM, Wilkoff BL, Tchou PJ: Large change in voltage at phase reversal improves biphasic defibrillation thresholds. Parallel-series mode switching. Circulation 94:1768–1773, 1996

100. Bardy GH, Ivey TD, Allen MD, Johnson G, Greene HL: Evaluation of electrode polarity on defibrillation efficacy. Am J Cardiol 63:433–437, 1989

101. Strickberger SA, Hummel JD, Horwood LE, Jentzer J, Daoud E, Niebauer M, Bakr O, Man KC, Williamson BD, Kou W, Morady F: Effect of shock polarity on ventricular defibrillation threshold using a transvenous lead system. J Am Coll Cardiol 24:1069–1072, 1994

102. Strickberger SA, Man KC, Daoud E, Neary MP, Horwood LE, Niebauer M, Hummel JD, Morady F: Effect of first-phase polarity of biphasic shocks on defibrillation threshold with a single transvenous lead system. J Am Coll Cardiol 25:1605–1608, 1995

103. Natale A, Sra J, Dhala A, Jazayeri M, Deshpande S, Axtell K, Akhtar M: Effects of initial polarity on defibrillation threshold with biphasic pulses. Pacing Clin Electrophysiol 18:1889–1893, 1995

104. Shorofsky SR, Gold MR: Effects of waveform and polarity on defibrillation thresholds in humans using a transvenous lead system. Am J Cardiol 78: 313–316, 1996

105. Olsovsky MR, Shorofsky SR, Gold MR: Effect of shock polarity on biphasic defibrillation thresholds using an active pectoral lead system. J Cardiovasc Electrophysiol 9:350–354, 1998

106. Zhou X, Smith WM, Justice RK, Wayland JL, Ideker RE: Transmembrane potential changes caused by monophasic and biphasic shocks. Am J Physiol 275: H1798–1807, 1998

107. Jones JL, Jones RE: Decreased defibrillator-induced dysfunction with biphasic rectangular waveforms. Am J Physiol 247:H792–H796, 1984

108. Ideker RE, Wolf PD, Alferness C, Krassowska W, Smith WM: Current concepts for selecting the location, size and shape of defibrillation electrodes. Pacing Clin Electrophysiol 14:227–240, 1991

109. Gold MR, Foster AH, Shorofsky SR: Lead system optimization for transvenous defibrillation. Am J Cardiol 80:1163–1167, 1997

110. Bardy GH, Dolack GL, Kudenchuk PJ, Poole JE, Mehra R, Johnson G: Prospective, randomized comparison in humans of a unipolar defibrillation system with that using an additional superior vena cava electrode. Circulation 89:1090–1093, 1994

111. Winter J, Heil JE, Schumann C, Lin Y, Schannwell CM, Michel U, Schipke JD, Schulte HD, Gams E: Effect of implantable cardioverter/defibrillator lead placement in the right ventricle on defibrillation energy requirements. A combined experimental and clinical study. Eur J Cardiothorac Surg 14:419–425, 1998

112. Gold MR, Olsovsky MR, DeGroot PJ, Cuello C, Shorofsky SR: The effect of superior vena cava coil position on active can defibrillation thresholds (abstract). Pacing Clin Electrophysiol 22: A22, 1999

113. Epstein AE, Kay GN, Plumb VJ, Voshage-Stahl L, Hull ML, for the Endotak Investigators: Elevated defibrillation threshold when right-sided venous access is used for nonthoracotomy implantable defibrillator lead implantation. J Cardiovasc Electrophysiol 6:979–986, 1995

114. Friedman PA, Rasmussen MJ, Grice S, Trusty J, Glikson M, Stanton MS: Defibrillation thresholds are increased by right-sided implantation of totally transvenous implantable cardioverter defib-

rillators. Pacing Clin Electrophysiol 22:1186–1192, 1999

115. Heil JE, Lin Y, Derfus DL, Lang DJ: Impact of ICD electrode position on transvenous defibrillation thresholds (abstract). Pacing Clin Electrophysiol 18:873, 1995

116. Reddy RK, Gleva MJ, Gliner BE, Dolack GL, Kudenchuk PJ, Poole JE, Bardy GH: Biphasic transthoracic defibrillation causes fewer ECG ST-segment changes after shock. Ann Emerg Med 30:127–134, 1997

117. Luria D, Rasmussen MJ, Hammill SC, Friedman PA: Frequency and mode of detection of nonthoracotomy implantable defibrillator lead failure (abstract). Pacing Clin Electrophysiol 22:705, 1999

118. Brady PA, Friedman PA, Trusty JM, Grice S, Hammill SC, Stanton MS: High failure rate for an epicardial implantable cardioverter-defibrillator lead: implications for long-term follow-up of patients with an implantable cardioverter-defibrillator. J Am Coll Cardiol 31:616–622, 1998

119. Moss AJ, Hall WJ, Cannom DS, Daubert JP, Higgins SL, Klein H, Levine JH, Saksena S, Waldo AL, Wilber D, Brown MW, Heo M, for the Multicenter Automatic Defibrillator Implantation Trial Investigators: Improved survival with an implanted defibrillator in patients with coronary disease at high risk for ventricular arrhythmia. N Engl J Med 335:1933–1940, 1996

120. The Antiarrhythmics Versus Implantable Defibrillators (AVID) Investigators: A comparison of antiarrhythmic-drug therapy with implantable defibrillators in patients resuscitated from near-fatal ventricular arrhythmias. N Engl J Med 337:1576–1583, 1997

121. Carnes CA, Mehdirad AA, Nelson SD: Drug and defibrillator interactions. Pharmacotherapy 18:516–525, 1998

2

Hemodynamics of Pacing

Margaret A. Lloyd, M.D., David L. Hayes, M.D.

Our understanding of the hemodynamic consequences of cardiac pacing has paralleled the rapid technologic advances in cardiac pacing we have witnessed over the past 5 decades.[1-3] Dual-chamber pacing, rate responsiveness, programmable and rate-responsive atrioventricular (AV) intervals, alternative-site pacing, and new multichamber (biatrial or biventricular, or both) pacing devices are all attempts to mimic normal cardiac conduction and physiology as much as technologically feasible.

Application of the appropriate pacing therapy first requires understanding of normal physiology, the various interrelated components contributing to the normally functioning cardiovascular system, and the effects of various cardiac and noncardiac diseases on these individual components as well as on function of the whole. Given that our understanding of cardiac function in normal and abnormal conditions is incomplete and that current technology is imperfect, the goal to perfectly mimic the normal cardiovascular system under all conditions has yet to be met. Nevertheless, hemodynamic pacing continues to attract intense interest as technologic advances bring us closer to that goal.

Cardiovascular Physiology

Challenge to the cardiovascular system, such as exercise or emotion, usually results in an increase in cardiac output, which is determined by heart rate and stroke volume. The relative contribution of each is variable and in part determined by age, the type and intensity of activity, baseline cardiovascular conditioning, and whether there is underlying cardiac or noncardiac disease (Fig. 2–1).

The cardiovascular demands incurred with exercise are usually met primarily by an increase in heart rate and secondarily by increases in stroke volume. Aerobically trained athletes can increase stroke volume proportionally more, thus enabling them to reach the same cardiac output with a relatively smaller increase in heart rate. Stroke volume is defined as the amount of blood ejected with each ventricular contraction, that is, end-diastolic volume minus end-systolic volume. In the normal heart, end-diastolic volume depends on diastolic filling pressure, total blood volume, distribution of that blood volume, and atrial systole (preload). End-systolic volume depends on myocardial contractility and afterload. The Frank-Starling law relates the degree

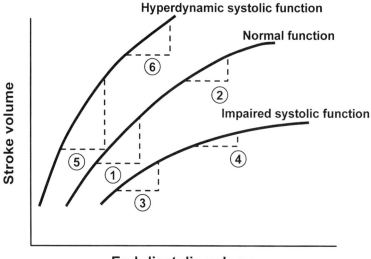

End-diastolic volume

Fig. 2–1. Left ventricular (LV) function curve indicating the relationship between LV end-diastolic volume and stroke volume. Normal LV function is represented by the middle curve. If LV systolic function is on the ascending limb of the curve, an increase in end-diastolic volume results in a significant increase in stroke volume (1). This increase is even greater for patients with hyperdynamic systolic function (5) and less for patients with impaired systolic function (3). At greater end-diastolic volumes, that is, higher LV filling pressures, further increasing the end-diastolic volume results in smaller increments in stroke volume. Even though patients with normal (2) or hyperdynamic (6) LV function may have a greater absolute increase in stroke volume, any increase in stroke volume for patients with LV dysfunction may be critically important (4). (Modified from Greenberg B, Chatterjee K, Parmley WW, Werner JA, Holly AN: The influence of left ventricular filling pressure on atrial contribution to cardiac output. Am Heart J 98:742–751, 1979. By permission of Mosby.)

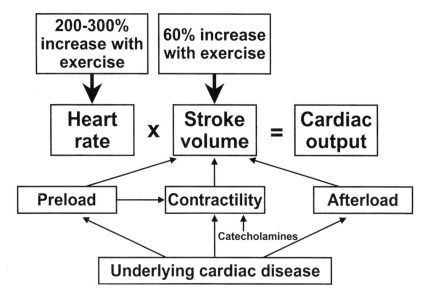

Fig. 2–2. Determinants of cardiac output during exercise. (Modified from Janosik and Labovitz.[1] By permission of WB Saunders Company.)

of left ventricular (LV) filling pressure to cardiac output at various degrees of contractility (Fig. 2–2).

All these relationships can be modulated by metabolic alterations, changes in autonomic tone or neurohormonal milieu, pharmacologic agents, and changes in the cardiac rhythm. For example, the increase in sympathetic tone associated with an increase in heart rate decreases the AV interval. Antiarrhythmic drugs can increase or decrease the heart rate at rest and in response to exercise, either by a direct effect on the sinus node or by effects on the autonomic nervous system.

Abnormal Physiology

A large segment of the pacing population has cardiac or noncardiac disease (or both types) that affects cardiac performance. Again, these conditions can be characterized as those affecting heart rate, those affecting stroke volume, and those affecting both.

Chronotropic incompetence may be due to isolated sinus node dysfunction, autonomic dysfunction, or the effects of drugs that blunt the chronotropic response to physiologic stress. Persons with normal LV function may be asymptomatic at rest but experience various degrees of symptoms with activity, depending on activity level, concurrent conditions, such as pulmonary disease, and severity of chronotropic incompetence. Persons with LV dysfunction may be less tolerant because of impaired stroke volume and have a relatively greater dependence on heart rate to maintain cardiac output. Patients may be unaware of how symptomatic they are unless objectively evaluated.

Myocardial contractility may be impaired by coronary artery disease, myocardial infarction, nonischemic cardiomyopathy, chronic valvular disease, or pericardial disease. Patients with LV dysfunction regardless of cause are more dependent on factors such as preload and afterload to maintain optimal stroke volume. Many of these patients have associated conduction system disease, such as various degrees of sinus node dysfunction, AV nodal disease, or His-Purkinje disease. AV or interventricular dyssynchrony can worsen already impaired myocardial performance. Metabolic abnormalities, such as chronic acidosis, hypoxia, and hypercarbia, depress cardiac performance. Many patients with severe LV dysfunction also have autonomic dysfunction that further limits the ability of the heart to increase heart rate and stroke volume with physiologic stress.

Many persons with LV dysfunction have concomitant renal failure, diabetes mellitus, and hypertension, all of which may affect indices of preload, afterload, and autonomic function as well as directly impair myocardial contractility. Drugs used in the treatment of these conditions, atrial fibrillation, and coronary artery disease may further affect these functions and directly suppress intrinsic conduction. Understandably, determining which patients will benefit from hemodynamic pacing techniques and which pacing technique will most benefit any individual patient is complex and incompletely understood at this time.

Basics of Hemodynamic Pacing

Atrioventricular Dissociation and Ventriculoatrial Conduction

The earliest indication for pacing was complete heart block, and ventricular pacing was the only pacing mode available. Establishing a stable ventricular rhythm was lifesaving and overshadowed the fact that normal cardiac function was not reestablished. Additionally, some patients experienced hemodynamic decline with this mode of pacing. Later it was established that the hemodynamic impairment

Table 2–1.
Pacemaker Syndrome

Potential symptoms
- Weakness
- Chest pain
- Syncope or near-syncope
- Dyspnea
- Cough
- Neck pulsations
- Apprehension
- Abdominal pulsations

Potential physical findings
- Hypotension
- Congestive heart failure
- Cannon "a" waves
- Blood pressure decline during ventricular pacing
- Decrease in cardiac output and arterial pressure
- Increase in peripheral vascular resistance during monitoring

is due to ventriculoatrial conduction or contraction (or both) against a closed AV valve and may result in symptoms that constitute pacemaker syndrome.[3,4] Ventriculoatrial conduction can result in activation of mechanical stretch receptors in the walls of the atria and pulmonary veins (Fig. 2–3). Vagal afferents transmit these impulses centrally, and reflex peripheral vasodilatation results. In addition, various neurohormonal agents, such as atrial natriuretic peptide, are activated. Pacemaker syndrome may be manifested by a variety of symptoms and physical signs (Table 2–1 and Fig. 2–4). Pacemaker syndrome was initially identified as a complication of VVI pacing; however, it may occur with any pacing mode when there is AV dissociation. It may also occur in persons with a markedly prolonged AV delay, with atrial systole effectively occurring concurrently with or after ventricular systole.

The prevalence of pacemaker syndrome is difficult to determine and depends in part on how it is identified. Studies evaluating objective clinical impairment with pacing in a nontracking mode suggest that the incidence may be in the range of 7% to 10%.[4] However, in a crossover study by Heldman et al.[5] of patients with pacing in each of the DDD and VVI modes for a week in randomized order, 83% of them experienced some subjective degree of pacemaker syndrome with pacing in the VVI mode. This finding suggests that when patients have some basis for comparison, they are more aware of symptoms of pacemaker syndrome (Fig. 2–5).

Atrioventricular Synchrony

The contribution of AV synchrony to maintaining physiologic cardiac performance has been confirmed by multiple studies over the past 25 years (Fig. 2–6). AV synchrony is estimated to increase stroke volume by as much as 50% and in normal hearts may decrease left atrial pressure and increase cardiac index by as much as 25% to 30%[6] (Fig. 2–3). Although patients with normal ventricular function may have the greatest *absolute* degree of improvement, a greater degree of *relative* improvement is typical in patients with severe left ventricular systolic dysfunction (Table 2–2). In these patients, any improvement derived from appropriately timed atrial systole may be beneficial.

Mitral valve closure and diastolic filling are influenced by the timing of atrial

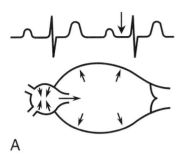

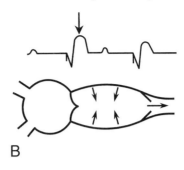

A   B

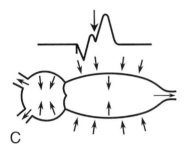

C

Fig. 2–3. *A,* Optimal cardiac filling with atrioventricular (AV) synchrony. *B,* With VVI pacing, the ventricle is not optimally filled and there is contraction against a closed AV valve. *C,* As a result of the loss of AV synchrony, venous pressure is increased, and multiple symptoms may ensue. (From Levine PA, Mace RC: Pacing Therapy: A Guide to Cardiac Pacing for Optimum Hemodynamic Benefit. Mount Kisco, NY, Futura Publishing Company, 1983, pp 29, 36. By permission of the publisher.)

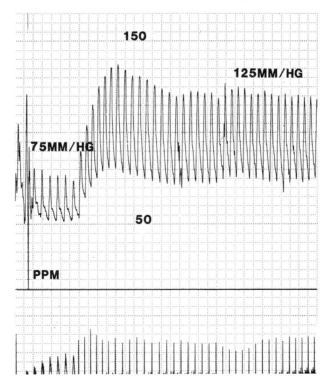

Fig. 2–4. Hemodynamic tracing from a patient with a VVI pacemaker. The arterial blood pressure increases with the transition from VVI pacing to normal sinus rhythm. (From Hayes DL, Holmes DR Jr: Hemodynamics of cardiac pacing. *In* A Practice of Cardiac Pacing. Third edition. Edited by S Furman, DL Hayes, DR Holmes Jr. Mount Kisco, NY, Futura Publishing Company, 1993, pp 195–218. By permission of Mayo Foundation.)

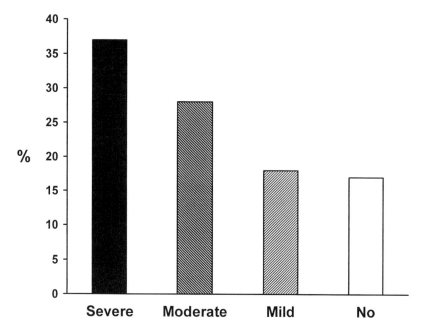

Fig. 2–5. Degree of symptoms detected in patients randomized to DDD and VVI pacing modes. Overall, 83% of patients had some symptoms consistent with pacemaker syndrome. (Modified from Heldman et al.[5] By permission of Futura Publishing Company.)

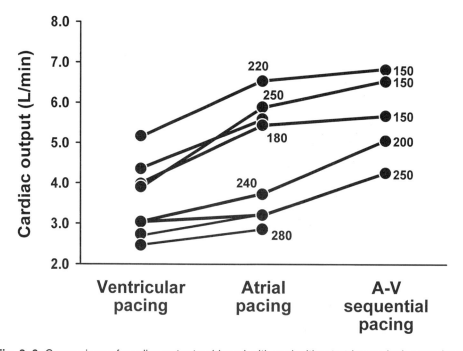

Fig. 2–6. Comparison of cardiac output achieved with and without atrioventricular synchrony. (Modified from Hartzler GO, Maloney JD, Curtis JJ, Barnhorst DA: Hemodynamic benefits of atrioventricular sequential pacing after cardiac surgery. Am J Cardiol 40:232–236, 1977. By permission of Excerpta Medica.)

Table 2–2.
Maintenance of Atrioventricular (AV) Synchrony

Resting state
  Normal ventricular filling and normal ventricle
  • Maintains optimal preload
  • Contributes up to 20% of cardiac output compared with ventricular-based pacing
  • Prevents increase of venous pressure (occurring with atrial systole against a closed
    AV valve or with ventricular systole and an open AV valve)
  • Prevents AV valve regurgitation (occurring with ventricular systole against an open
    AV valve)
  Left ventricular impairment and increased filling pressure
  • Has diminishing effect on cardiac output inversely proportional to the degree of left
    ventricular impairment
  • Prevents AV valve regurgitation (occurring with ventricular systole against an open
    AV valve)
Moderate to maximal exercise
  Normal ventricular filling and normal ventricle
  • Maintains optimally timed preload
  • Contributes only a small amount of increased cardiac output (<10%) compared with
    rate-matched asynchronous pacing
  • Prevents AV valve regurgitation (occurring with ventricular systole against an open
    AV valve)
  Left ventricular impairment and increased filling pressure
  • Has little effect on cardiac output
  • Prevents AV valve regurgitation (occurring with ventricular systole against an open
    AV valve)

and ventricular contraction. If the AV interval is too long, mitral valve closure may occur early and impair diastolic filling time. If the AV interval is too short, atrial contribution to ventricular filling may be impaired because the mitral valve fails to close before left ventricular systole. Patients with severe diastolic dysfunction benefit even more with appropriately timed atrial systole, because dependence on optimal preload is even greater to maintain satisfactory cardiac output.

The influence of pacing mode on factors indirectly but importantly related to cardiovascular performance has also been studied. P-synchronous pacing has been shown to result not only in significantly higher cardiac outputs than those with VVI pacing but also in lower systemic vascular resistance, lower serum lactate levels, smaller AV oxygen gradients, and lower levels of circulating vasoactive peptides and norepinephrine.[7]

Conversely, a comparison of long-term ventricular and P-synchronous pacing in patients with complete heart block did not show a significant difference in systemic or pulmonary vascular resistance and myocardial oxygen consumption either at rest or during exercise.[8]

Mechanical AV delay varies between paced and sensed atrial beats because of the intrinsic delay in atrial activation after atrial pacing, that is, intra-atrial conduction.[9] The absolute intra-atrial conduction delay varies significantly among patients and also depends on underlying conduction or myocardial disease (Fig. 2–7). One study found the mean intra-atrial delay to be 27 msec,[10] and another demonstrated an 8% improvement in resting cardiac output when independently programmable AV delays were used for paced and sensed beats.[11] Different AV intervals are standard on most dual-chamber pacemakers.

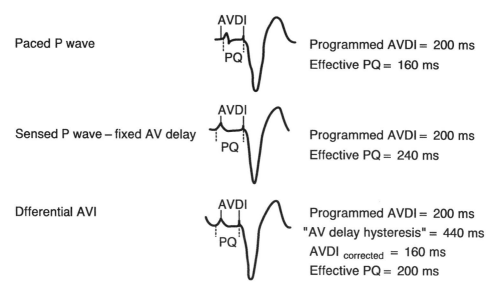

Fig. 2–7. A differential atrioventricular interval (AVDI) attempts to correct for the timing differences between a paced and a sensed atrial event. When the atrium is paced, the atrioventricular interval (AVI) begins with delivery of the pacing artifact. However, there is latency between delivery of the pacing artifact and actual depolarization. Depending on interatrial conduction time, the paced-sensed difference can be great. In this diagram, the AVI is programmed to 200 msec for each event, but the effective AVI is 160 msec after the sensed atrial event and 240 msec after the paced atrial event. (From Janosik et al.[11] By permission of the American College of Cardiology.)

Most current pacing devices offer not only independently programmable paced and sensed AV intervals but also a rate-responsive AV interval. Conduction through the AV node normally accelerates through the action of the sympathetic nervous system with physiologic increases in heart rate, resulting in shorter AV intervals at higher heart rates. Any variation in heart rate has been well demonstrated to result in an immediate, precise, and inversely proportional variation in the AV interval in normal hearts.[12] A linear relationship exists between heart rate and the AV interval, with a decrease of 4 msec in the AV delay for each heart rate increase of 10 msec, independent of age or baseline PR interval[13] (Fig. 2–8). In patients with conduction system disease or autonomic dysfunction, the AV delay may not shorten with heart rate increase. Rate-adaptive AV interval attempts to

mirror normal physiology and allow a higher maximal tracking rate (Fig. 2–9). Multiple studies have reported improved hemodynamic indices during exercise with a rate-adaptive AV interval compared with those with a fixed AV interval[12,14] (see Chapter 6).

Optimization of the AV interval has been a source of frustration for many years. When dual-chamber pacemakers were first introduced and only a fixed AV interval was possible, very simple programming guidelines were followed. In general, if the patient had intact AV conduction, the AV interval was programmed long enough to allow intrinsic conduction. If the patient had AV block, the AV interval was programmed to mimic what was considered to be a normal PR interval, that is, 150 to 200 msec. However, this guideline failed to consider either the previously described mechanical intra-

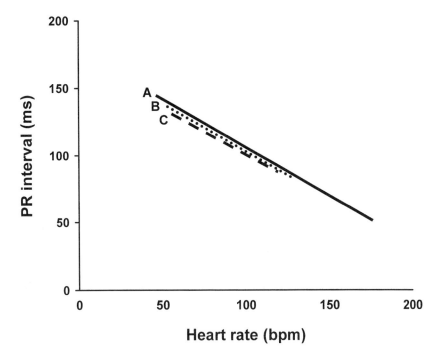

Fig. 2–8. Linear regression of PR interval (msec) and heart rate (bpm) from electrocardiograms of young healthy subjects (A), older healthy subjects (B), and patients after myocardial infarction (C). Linear shortening of the interval occurs as exercise intensity increases. (From Rees et al.[13] By permission of Pulsus Group.)

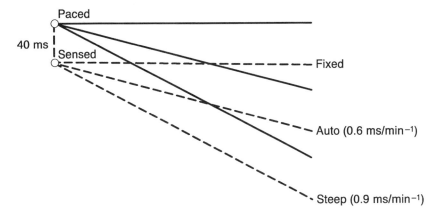

Fig. 2–9. Schematic representation of the atrioventricular (AV) interval response when both differential AV interval and rate-adaptive AV interval are activated. The solid lines represent paced atrial events and the dashed lines sensed atrial events.

atrial delay from atrial pacing to atrial depolarization or the effect of any interatrial conduction delay.[9]

Doppler echocardiographic measurements have been the most definitive means to optimize AV interval (Fig. 2–10, 2–11, and 2–12). Even though Doppler studies are time consuming and highly operator-dependent, the techniques are better validated than any others. The

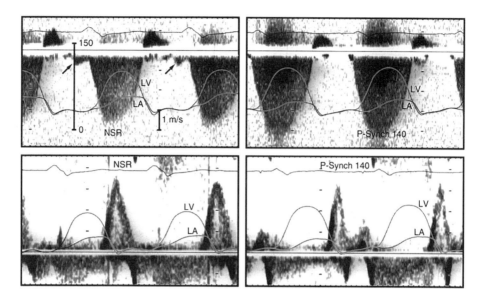

Fig. 2–10. Upper frames are continuous wave Doppler tracings of mitral regurgitation signals in normal sinus rhythm (NSR) (*left*) and P-synchronous (P-Synch) pacing at an atrioventricular interval of 140 msec (*right*). There are corresponding pulsed-wave mitral inflow signals in the lower frames. In sinus rhythm, there is evidence of diastolic mitral regurgitation (*arrows*), and left atrial (LA) pressure is increased. The mitral inflow signal, *lower panel,* demonstrates fusion of the E and A waves and a short diastolic filling period. P-synchronous pacing demonstrates lower left atrial pressure, higher left ventricular (LV) peak systolic pressure, which corresponds with the disappearance of diastolic mitral regurgitation, and marked improvement in left ventricular filling characteristics. There are distinct E and A waves, and the diastolic filling period is improved. (From Symanski and Nishimura.[46] By permission of Mosby.)

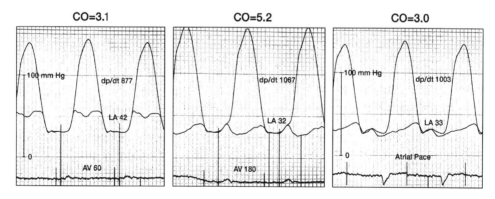

Fig. 2–11. Simultaneous electrocardiographic, aortic pressure, and left ventricular pressure tracings from a patient with dilated cardiomyopathy show that an atrioventricular (AV) interval that is too short compromises left ventricular diastolic filling, causing an increase in left ventricular filling pressures and reduced cardiac output (CO). When the AV interval is too long, the diastolic filling time is diminished, and there is inefficient coordination between early and atrial diastolic filling. On pulsed-wave Doppler mitral inflow tracings, this would be seen as E and A wave fusion. LA, left atrium. (From Nishimura RA, Symanski JD, Hurrell DG, Trusty JM, Hayes DL, Tajik AJ: Dual-chamber pacing for cardiomyopathies: a 1996 clinical perspective. Mayo Clin Proc 71:1077–1087, 1996. By permission of Mayo Foundation.)

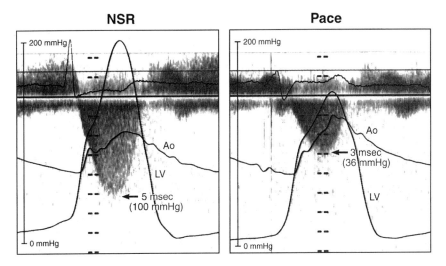

Fig. 2–12. Continuous wave Doppler tracings of left ventricular (LV) outflow tract signals with simultaneous aortic (Ao) and LV pressure tracings in sinus rhythm (NSR) (*left*) and with P-synchronous pacing (*right*). Both the Doppler signal and the corresponding pressure tracings demonstrate a significant reduction in the LV outflow tract gradient with pacing. (From Symanski and Nishimura.[46] By permission of Mosby.)

ultimate goal of Doppler-directed AV interval optimization is to optimize cardiac output without compromising filling pressures.

A detailed description of Doppler techniques is beyond the scope of this text. The basic procedure for optimizing the AV interval in patients with systolic dysfunction involves measuring hemodynamics, stroke volume, and diastolic function at various AV intervals (Table 2–3). (We do at least three intervals, typically 50, 100, and 150 msec. Additional AV intervals may be used in an effort to further optimize hemodynamics.) The optimal AV interval is determined by integrating the various measurements and determining a balance between optimal diastolic filling and cardiac output.

When the AV interval is optimized for patients with hypertrophic cardiomyopathy, the same measurements are done, but in addition the LV outflow tract gradient is measured (Fig. 2–13). A balance is found between minimizing the outflow tract gradient and maintaining cardiac

output and adequate diastolic filling, ensuring that the AV interval is short enough for ventricular capture.

Plethysmographic techniques have also been used to optimize the AV interval and to maximize cardiac output. Although less well validated than Doppler studies, early results with these techniques are promising.[15,16] Plethysmography would provide a significantly less expensive alternative to Doppler techniques.

A major weakness that remains is the inability to optimize the AV interval during exercise. Optimization at rest is not necessarily the same as optimization during exercise. Studies are necessary to define a technique for AV interval optimization that is applicable to exercise.

Chronotropic Response

Multiple studies have demonstrated that chronotropic competence is the most important contributor to cardiac output, especially at moderate or extreme degrees

Table 2–3.
Worksheet Used for Optimization of the Atrioventricular Interval

1. LVOT diameter ____ cm*	Atrioventricular delay, msec†		
	50	100	150
2. HR, bpm			
3. BP, mm Hg			
4. LVOT velocity, m/sec			
5. LVOT TVI, cm			
6. Mitral E wave, m/sec			
7. Mitral A wave, m/sec			
8. DT, msec			
9. DFT, msec			
10. SV, mL			
11. CO, L/min			

SV = 0.785 × LVOT diameter² × LVOT TVI.

BP, blood pressure; CO, cardiac output; DFT, defibrillation threshold; DT, deceleration time; HR, heart rate; LVOT, left ventricular outflow tract; SV, stroke volume; TVI, time velocity integral.

*LVOT is measured only once per study.

†Indicate if different atrioventricular interval due to programmable options.

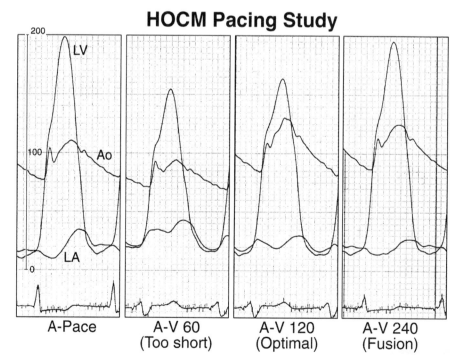

HOCM Pacing Study

A-Pace

A-V 60 (Too short)

A-V 120 (Optimal)

A-V 240 (Fusion)

Fig. 2–13. Tracings from an invasive study of atrioventricular interval optimization in a patient with hypertrophic obstructive cardiomyopathy (HOCM). In this example, the optimal atrioventricular interval was 120 msec. Ao, aorta; LA, left atrium; LV, left ventricle. (From Symanski and Nishimura.[46] By permission of Mosby.)

of exercise[17–19] (Fig. 2–14). At rest and at lower levels of activity, AV synchronization has a greater role in maintaining an appropriate cardiac output (Fig. 2–15 and 2–16). Because most of the pacing population is at the lower end of the activity curve most of the time and a significant proportion of these patients are also dependent on adequate preload because of decreased ventricular compliance, AV synchrony is perhaps just as important as rate responsiveness for achieving optimal

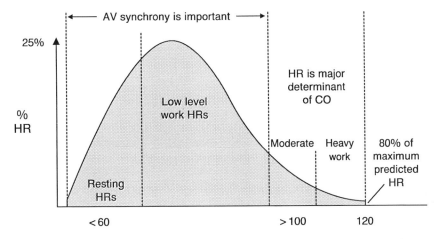

Fig. 2–14. Schematic representation of the contribution of atrioventricular synchrony and rate response to cardiac output (CO) at various levels of activity. At rest and low levels of activity, maintenance of atrioventricular synchrony makes a proportionately greater contribution to cardiac output. At higher exercise levels, cardiac rate (HR) clearly contributes more to cardiac output.

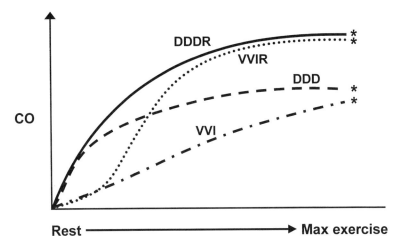

Fig. 2–15. Schematic representation of expected cardiac output (CO) response to exercise with various pacing modes in a patient with chronotropic incompetence (*). In this representation, the patient is presumed to be chronotropically incompetent. (If the patient had the ability to mount a normal rate response, greater cardiac output could be obtained with the non-rate-adaptive pacing modes [i.e., VVI and DDD] than that depicted in this diagram.) Whether any measurable difference would occur between VVIR and DDDR at peak exercise would depend on many factors, including sensor programming, underlying cardiac disease, and type of conduction system disease. (From Hayes DL, Holmes DR Jr: Hemodynamics of cardiac pacing. *In* A Practice of Cardiac Pacing. Third edition. Edited by S Furman, DL Hayes, DR Holmes Jr. Mount Kisco, NY, Futura Publishing Company, 1993, pp 195–218. By permission of Mayo Foundation.)

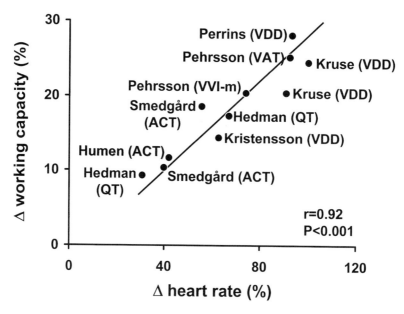

Fig. 2–16. Representation of multiple studies comparing the relative contribution of heart rate and atrioventricular synchrony to work capacity. All studies agree that heart rate is the greatest contributor during exercise. (From Nordlander et al.[17] By permission of Futura Publishing Company.)

cardiovascular hemodynamics in the typical patient. Restoration of both rate responsiveness and AV synchrony should be the goal of physiologic pacing and should be viewed as a complementary achievement.

Optimal Right Ventricular Pacing Site

Significant discussion, controversy, and investigation have taken place on the hemodynamic advantages of alternative sites of right ventricular (RV) pacing, that is, pacing from other than the apex. Although several studies have now been published, many of the series are small, some involving long-term pacing and others short-term observation only.

In a study of 89 patients, RV outflow tract pacing improved cardiac output more than did "traditional" apical pacing.[20] The authors hypothesized that the increase in cardiac output was due to normalization of the QRS axis, resulting in less anisotropic conduction and more efficient contraction of the left ventricle. On the basis of observations in a small number of patients, they raised the question of whether the decrease in blood pressure noted with temporary apical ventricular pacing during coronary angiography and angioplasty is due to loss of atrial "kick" or simply to less efficient ventricular depolarization with apical pacing or to both. Other studies[21] also demonstrated comparable hemodynamics with atrial pacing and single-chamber ventricular pacing from the septum. Single-chamber apical pacing, however, was associated with a significant decrease in mean aortic pressure. Of the 89 patients studied,[20] 5 were restudied 6 months after implantation and were found to have continued improvement in cardiac output with RV outflow tract pacing in comparison with apex pacing, suggesting that the increase in cardiac output was not simply a short-term phenomenon.

In a study of 14 patients, Buckingham et al.[22] compared three pacing site combinations: RV apex, RV outflow tract, and both. Their outcomes suggested that in patients with poor LV function, there may be subtle improvements in diastolic and systolic function with pacing in the RV outflow tract and at combined sites in the right ventricle compared with traditional RV apex pacing. In a study of 13 patients with normal left ventricular function, DDD pacing from the RV outflow tract or proximal septum did not improve cardiac function in relation to apical pacing.[23]

In a temporary pacing study in 17 patients, RV outflow tract pacing resulted in higher cardiac indices than those with apex pacing. The authors concluded that stimulation of the RV outflow tract offered a significant hemodynamic benefit during single-chamber pacing over that with conventional apex pacing, particularly in patients without significant coronary artery disease or left ventricular dysfunction.[24]

Having introduced the discrepancies in the literature on whether the benefit of RV outflow tract pacing was limited to patients with abnormal cardiac function, Ishikawa et al.[25] found that cardiac function was improved by RV outflow pacing compared with RV apex pacing regardless of the pacing mode (11 patients with DDD and 2 with VVI pacemakers because of chronic atrial fibrillation) or cardiac function.

At this time, the literature is confusing because of the anatomical terms used to describe alternative RV pacing sites. The difficulty in comparing different ventricular pacing sites has led to proposed nomenclature to describe alternative RV pacing sites, that is, other than the apical pacing site.[26] The proposed sites are as follows (Fig. 2–17):

- RV inlet septal pacing. Pacing above, on, or beneath the annulus of the septal-anterior tricuspid valve leaflets, yielding relatively normal QRS morphology and axis (A).
- RV infundibular septal pacing. Pacing proximal to the pulmonic valve distal to, or near, the crista supraventricularis, yielding left bundle branch block and a vertical axis (B).

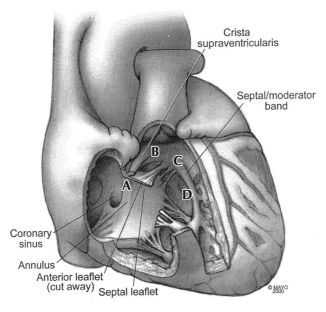

Fig. 2–17. Schematic representation of alternative right ventricular pacing sites proposed by Giudici and Karpawich[26] (see text). (By permission of Mayo Foundation.)

- RV outflow septal pacing. Pacing most commonly referred to as RV outflow tract pacing near the septal-moderator band insertion at a mid-position on the RV septum, yielding left bundle branch block and a vertical axis (C).
- RV apical septal pacing. Pacing proximal to the septal-moderator band continuity that does not typically produce a vertical QRS axis (D).

Effect of Pacing Mode on Morbidity and Mortality

An early study by Rosenqvist et al.[27] paved the way for intense clinical interest in and subsequent clinical trials on the effect of pacing mode on morbidity and mortality and on the potential adverse effects of VVI pacing (Fig. 2–18). At 4 years of follow-up, atrial fibrillation had occurred in 47% of the patients receiving VVI pacing but in only 7% of those receiving AAI pacing ($P < 0.0005$); congestive heart failure occurred in 37% of the VVI group

and in 15% of the AAI group ($P < 0.005$); and mortality was 23% in the VVI group and 8% in the AAI group ($P < 0.025$).

Many other investigators performed retrospective reviews to assess the effect of pacing mode on mortality (Fig. 2–19). Despite the inherent weaknesses of retrospective analyses, it is difficult to dismiss the similar finding among all the studies of significantly lower mortality with DDD or AAI pacing than with VVI pacing and significantly lower incidences of atrial fibrillation.[28]

Lamas et al.[29] reported survival in a large population of patients (20,948) with sinus node dysfunction. The population was a random sample of the complete United States cohort of Medicare patients receiving pacing for sinus node dysfunction in 1988 through 1990. The DDD/DDDR pacing mode was an independent correlate of survival.

A number of prospective trials now completed or under way are summarized in Table 4–2 (Chapter 4). Andersen et al.[30] published the first prospective data on pacing mode and survival. Among 225

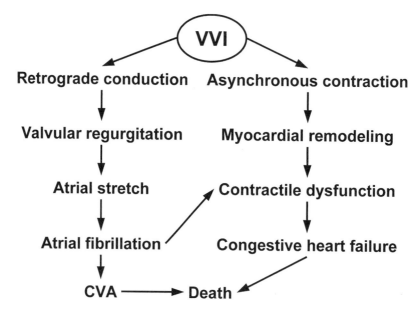

Fig. 2–18. Potential adverse clinical outcomes from VVI pacing. CVA, cerebrovascular accident. (Modified from Gillis AM: Pacing to prevent atrial fibrillation. Cardiol Clin 18:25–36, 2000. By permission of WB Saunders Company.)

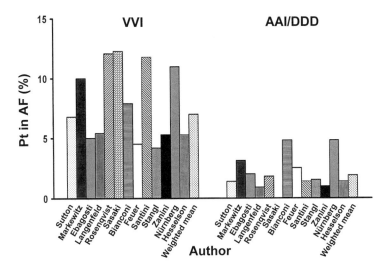

Fig. 2–19. Representation of various retrospective studies comparing morbidity and mortality between VVI and DDD or other atrial-based pacing modes. There is a definite trend to a lower incidence of atrial fibrillation with DDD or other atrial-based pacing modes. AF, atrial fibrillation; AF (%), percentage of patients in whom atrial fibrillation developed per year of follow-up. (Data from Barlow M, Kerr CR, Connolly SJ: Survival, quality-of-life, and clinical trials in pacemaker patients. *In* Clinical Cardiac Pacing and Defibrillation. Second edition. Edited by KA Ellenbogen, GN Kay, BL Wilkoff. Philadelphia, WB Saunders Company, 2000, pp 383–404.)

patients (mean age, 76 years) with sinus node dysfunction randomized to AAI or VVI pacing, the incidence of atrial fibrillation was higher in the VVI group (AAI group, 14%; VVI group, 23%; $P = 0.12$) and the incidence of thromboembolism was also higher in the VVI group than in the AAI group ($P = 0.0083$). Although no difference in mortality could be detected at the initial analysis at 3.3 years, subsequent analysis at 5.5 years showed improved survival and less heart failure in the AAI group.[31] In addition, there was a persistent reduction in the incidences of atrial fibrillation and thromboembolic events (Fig. 2–20).

Lamas et al.[32] subsequently developed a prospective, randomized, single-blind trial, Pacemaker Selection in the Elderly (PASE), to compare DDDR and VVIR pacing modes. There was no statistically significant difference in quality of life between DDDR and VVIR pacing modes, but there was a trend toward improved quality of life in patients with

sinus node dysfunction randomized to dual-chamber pacing. Perhaps more significant was a crossover of 26% of patients from ventricular pacing to dual-chamber pacing because of pacemaker syndrome.

The PASE study was the template for the subsequent MOST (Mode Selection Trial) study. In this study of 2,000 patients with sinus node dysfunction randomized to either VVI or DDD pacing, primary end points are all causes of mortality and cerebrovascular accidents. Results are expected in 2000.

The Canadian Trial of Physiologic Pacing (CTOPP)[33] compared VVIR with DDDR or AAIR and had primary end points of overall mortality and cerebrovascular accidents and secondary end points of atrial fibrillation, hospitalizations for congestive heart failure, and death due to a cardiac cause. CTOPP demonstrated that physiologic pacing (DDD/AAI) was associated with a reduced rate in the development of chronic atrial fibrillation, from 3.78% to 2.87% per year, at the 3-year

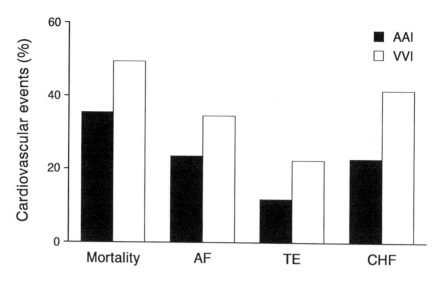

Fig. 2–20. Outcomes from the Danish pacemaker (Andersen et al.[30]) trial. See text. AF, atrial fibrillation; CHF, congestive heart failure; TE, thromboembolism. (From Solomon AJ, Gersh BJ: Effect of recent randomized trials on current pacing practice. Cardiology in Review 7:9–16, 1999. By permission of Lippincott Williams & Wilkins.)

analysis. No significant improvement in quality of life or mortality was demonstrated with dual-chamber pacing. However, there was a slight divergence of the mortality curves favoring dual-chamber pacing. In addition, quality of life was improved in subsets of patients. These included patients who were pacemaker-dependent and patients with severe diastolic or systolic dysfunction (Gillis A, personal communication, October 1999).

In a smaller trial by Schrepf et al.,[34] paroxysmal atrial fibrillation occurred more frequently with VVI pacing than with DDD pacing. However, the Pac-A-Tach trial[35] found no significant difference in recurrence of atrial tachyarrhythmias by intention to treat at 1 year—48% in DDDR and 43% in VVI.

A prospective, randomized British trial, UKPACE (United Kingdom Pacing and Cardiovascular Events), has been started to compare DDD with VVI pacing modes in 2,000 patients 70 years of age and older requiring permanent pacing for second- or third-degree AV block.[36]

The prospective data to date lack consistency, but we believe that subsequent analyses may minimize the inconsisten-cies. Specifically, it is difficult to ignore the similarity between the mortality data from the initial CTOPP analysis and the early Andersen et al. analysis. Also, longer term follow-up of the CTOPP population will determine whether patient preference parallels that in the PASE trial.

Pacing in Hypertrophic Obstructive Cardiomyopathy

The many subtypes and multiple clinical presentations of hypertrophic obstructive cardiomyopathy (HCM) have made it difficult to compare and identify optimal diagnostic and treatment modalities. Patients with HCM have various degrees of septal hypertrophy and outflow tract obstruction, and they may experience exertional dyspnea, angina, syncope, or sudden cardiac death. Symptoms may be due to massive hypertrophy and myocardial microischemia, mitral regurgitation from displacement of the mitral valve apparatus, outflow tract obstruction severe enough to cause hemodynamic embarrassment, or impaired diastolic function. Treatment has traditionally been with β-adrenergic and calcium blocking agents and, in medically refractory cases, surgical septal myectomy (sometimes with concurrent mitral valve repair or replacement). Some patients have required postoperative pacing because of damage to the conduction system at the time of myectomy or pacing therapy for the severe bradycardia produced in some by medical therapy.

McDonald et al.[37] described the use of dual-chamber pacing as a primary treatment for outflow tract obstruction in 1988. Subsequent investigators have evaluated both invasive and noninvasive hemodynamic values in both short-term and long-term pacing therapy.

Fananapazir et al.[38] reported on 84 patients with HCM and drug-resistant symptoms who were treated by dual-chamber pacemakers programmed to the DDD mode with AV intervals short enough to fully activate the ventricle from the pacing site at the RV apex (according to electrocardiographic criteria). After a mean of 2.3 years, symptoms resolved (28 patients) or decreased (47 patients) in 89% of the patients. This outcome was associated with a significant improvement in mean New York Heart Association functional class, from 3.2 to 1.6, and a reduction in the LV outflow tract gradient from 96 to 27 mm Hg in patients with significant outflow obstruction. These benefits persisted after cessation of pacing during normal sinus rhythm, as did some changes on the surface electrocardiogram (T-wave morphology) and the signal-averaged electrocardiogram.

The most widely accepted hypothesis to explain the improvement in hemodynamics that may occur during pacing in patients with HCM is that the altered septal activation caused by RV apical pacing may result in less narrowing of the LV outflow tract and a subsequent decrease in the Venturi effect, respon-sible for systolic anterior motion of the mitral valve[39] (Fig. 2–21). However, the persistence of improvement after cessation of pacing in some series and the observation that subjective and objective improvement may also be seen in some patients with left bundle branch block suggest that the effect of long-term pacing cannot be attributed solely to alteration of the septal activation sequence by ventricular pacing. There are hypotheses that permanent pacing in patients with HCM may result in long-term remodeling of the left ventricle,[40] but this possibility is not well established.

Pacing in HCM has been the subject of several randomized single-center and multicenter trials (Table 2–4). A single-center, randomized, crossover trial de-monstrated symptomatic improvement in 63% of patients with pacing in the DDD mode[43] (Fig. 2–22). However, 42% of patients had improvement with

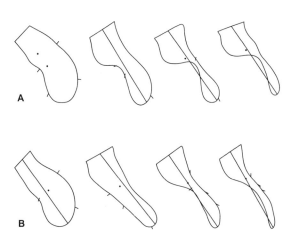

Fig. 2–21. Schematic representation of ventriculograms from a patient with hypertrophic obstructive cardiomyopathy. The *row A diagrams* represent septal motion during intrinsic ventricular depolarization and reflect marked left ventricular outflow obstruction. With atrioventricular sequential pacing (*row B diagrams*) the ventricular depolarization pattern is altered and left ventricular outflow obstruction decreased. (From Jeanrenaud et al.[39] By permission of the journal.)

Table 2–4.
Trials Assessing the Effect of Pacing Mode on Morbidity and Mortality

Study	Patient inclusion criteria	End points	Treatment arms	Key results
Danish study[31]	• Sick sinus syndrome requiring pacing	• Mortality • CV death • AF • TE events • Heart failure • AV block	• AAI pacing (n = 110) vs. • VVI pacing (n = 115)	• Cumulative incidence of CV death, PAF, chronic AF, and TE events lower with AAI pacing • Less severe heart failure with AAI • Multivariate analysis: AAI associated with freedom from TE events, survival from CV death
PASE[32]	• Age ≥ 65 yr • Need for PPM to prevent or treat bradycardia	• QOL • All-cause mortality • First nonfatal CVA or death • First hospitalization for CHF • AF • PM syndrome	• Single-blind, randomized, controlled comparison; VVIR pacing vs. • DDDR pacing	• QOL improved significantly, but no difference between pacing modes • 26% of pt with VVIR crossover to DDDR due to PM syndrome • Trends of borderline statistical significance in end points favoring DDDR in pt with SND
CTOPP[33]	• Initial PM • Life expectancy > 1 yr • Not in chronic AF	• Cardiovascular mortality or stroke • Paroxysmal or chronic AF • Hospitalization for CHF • QOL • 6-min walk	• DDD/R or AAI/R pacing vs. • VVI/R pacing	• No difference in QOL, VVI vs. DDD/AAI • No statistically significant difference in mortality or stroke • No difference in hospitalizations • 24% decrease in incidence of chronic or paroxysmal AF with DDD/AAI
MOST[41]	• SND requiring PM • NSR or atrial standstill at time of implantation	• Stroke • Health status • Cost-effectiveness • Total mortality • CV mortality • AF • Heart failure score • PM syndrome	• DDDR vs. • VVIR	• In progress

continues

Table 2–4. (*Continued*)

Study	Patient inclusion criteria	End points	Treatment arms	Key results
UKPACE[36]	• Age ≥ 70 yr • High-grade AV block requiring PPM	• All-cause mortality	• DDDR (50%) vs. • VVIR (25%) vs • VVI (25%)	• In progress
DANPACE[42]	• Tachycardia-bradycardia syndrome with normal AV conduction	• All-cause mortality • CV mortality • Incidence of AF and TE events • QOL • Cost-effectiveness	• AAIR vs. • DDDR	• In progress

AF, atrial fibrillation; AV, atrioventricular; CHF, congestive heart failure; CTOPP, Canadian Trial of Physiologic Pacing; CV, cardiovascular; CVA, cardiovascular accident; DANPACE, Danish Pacing Trial; MOST, Mode Selection Trial; NSR, normal sinus rhythm; PAF, paroxysmal atrial fibrillation; PASE, Pacemaker Selection in the Elderly; PM, pacemaker; PPM, permanent pacemaker; QOL, quality of life; SND, sinus node dysfunction; TE, thromboembolic; UKPACE, United Kingdom Pacing and Cardiovascular Events.

programming to a low pacing rate in the AAI mode, that is, effectively no pacing, suggesting a significant placebo effect.

In the PIC (Pacing in Cardiomyopathy) study, a multicenter, randomized, crossover study,[44] dual-chamber pacing resulted in a 50% reduction of the LV outflow tract gradient, a 21% increase in exercise duration, and improvement in New York Heart Association functional class compared with baseline status (Fig. 2–23). When clinical features, including chest pain, dyspnea, and subjective health status, were compared between DDD and back-up AAI pacing, there was no significant difference, again suggesting a significant placebo effect.

In another randomized, double-blind, crossover study, the M-PATHY (Multicenter Study of Pacing Therapy for Hypertrophic Cardiomyopathy) trial, patients were randomized to 3 months each of DDD or AAI pacing (rate, 30) in a crossover design. No significant differences were evident between pacing and no pacing, either subjectively or objectively, when exercise capacity, quality-of-life score, treadmill exercise time, and peak oxygen consumption were compared.[45] Patients reported symptomatic improvement with pacing, a result suggesting a substantial placebo effect, and a small subset of patients older than 65 had significant objective improvement, a suggestion that DDD pacing might be a viable option in these patients. The investigators concluded that pacing should not be considered a primary treatment for HCM and that subjective benefit without objective evidence of improvement should be interpreted cautiously.

When pacing is used for the patient with HCM, AV interval programming is crucial to achieve optimal hemodynamic improvement. Ventricular depolarization must occur as a result of pacing. Therefore, the AV interval must be short enough to result in depolarization by the paced event. However, the shortest AV interval is not necessarily the best[46] (Fig. 2–13). Some experts have advocated AV nodal ablation to assure paced ventricular depolarization if rapid intrinsic AV nodal conduction prevents total ventricular depolarization by the pacing stimulus.[39]

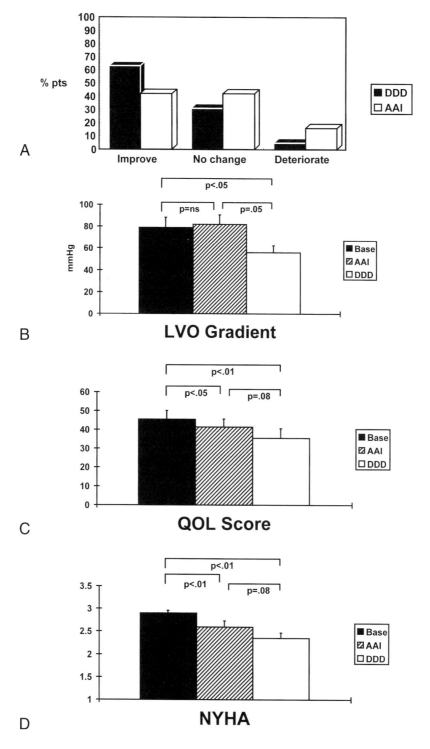

Fig. 2–22. Subjective response to pacing in a single-center, controlled, double-blind, randomized study in which patients received DDD pacing with optimized atrioventricular interval or no pacing (AAI at 30 bpm). Shown from the same study are (*B*) changes in left ventricular outflow (LVO) gradient, (*C*) quality of life (QOL) score, and (*D*) change in functional New York Heart Association (NYHA) class. There was statistically significant improvement in functional class in the patients who were not paced, that is, AAI at 30 bpm, indicating a significant placebo effect. (Courtesy of Dr. R.A. Nishimura, Mayo Clinic.)

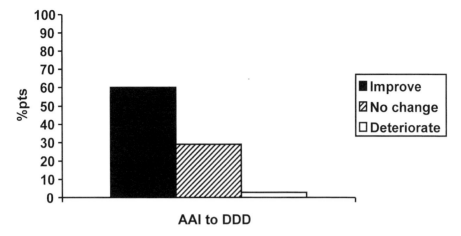

Fig. 2–23. Subjective response to pacing in the Pacing in Cardiomyopathy (PIC) trial, a multi-center, controlled, double-blind, randomized study in which patients received DDD pacing or no pacing (AAI backup pacing). This study also demonstrated a significant placebo effect from implantation of the pacemaker.

Septal myotomy-myectomy remains the definitive therapy for outflow tract obstruction in HCM, and dual-chamber pacing exclusively for the treatment of the gradient should still be considered secondarily. However, in patients who have a strong desire to avoid surgery, dual-chamber pacing can be considered if short-term studies suggest benefit with RV apical pacing, total ventricular preexcitation can be achieved without an unduly short AV delay, and the patient clearly understands that long-term benefit is unknown at this time and that surgical intervention may still be required.

Finally, it should be understood that symptoms associated with HCM are frequently multifactorial and that the cause may be something other than dynamic outflow tract obstruction.

Atrial fibrillation is poorly tolerated in HCM because of diastolic dysfunction, and there is a higher than expected prevalence of functional accessory pathways that facilitate rapid ventricular rates, resulting in symptoms that may be indistinguishable from hemodynamic obstruction. Rapid atrial fibrillation may degenerate into malignant ventricular ar-

rhythmias, and patients may be at risk for primary ventricular arrhythmias.

Pacing in Congestive Heart Failure

Congestive heart failure (CHF) affects 1% to 2% of the United States population and is the most common diagnosis at hospital dismissal.[47,48] Although medical therapy has been shown to improve survival and functional status in these patients, many remain symptomatic despite maximally tolerated doses.[49,50] Patients who remain symptomatic with medical therapy have an observed annual mortality of 12% to 40%.[49–51] Therefore, many efforts have been made to improve hemodynamics in such patients by nonpharmacologic means, including cardiac pacing.

Dual-Chamber Pacing

In the early 1990s, right-sided AV sequential (dual-chamber) pacing with short AV delays was proposed as empirical therapy to relieve CHF symptoms in patients with severe LV dysfunction.[52,53] In 1990, Hochleitner et al.[53] reported improvement in LV ejection fraction and functional class with pacing at a short AV delay in patients with dilated cardiomyopathy. The 16 patients studied were critically ill and refractory to maximal medical management. The baseline PR interval was 200 msec (range, 140 to 320 msec); patients received empirical pacing at an AV delay of 100 msec.

In subsequent investigations, hemodynamic improvement by dual-chamber pacing was shown to be related to optimal synchronization of atrial and ventricular contractions.[54] However, only patients with CHF who have prolonged PR intervals, in which atrial contraction occurs so prematurely that the atrial "kick" to ventricular contraction is lost, appear to derive benefit from dual-chamber pacing. Conversely, in patients with normal or short AV conduction, the diastolic filling period does not change and cardiac output decreases by 23%, most likely because of the systolic and diastolic dyssynergy induced by RV pacing.[54] Consequently, clinical trials showed that dual-chamber pacing had limited long-term efficacy as an adjunct to medical therapy in relieving CHF symptoms.[55,56]

Left Ventricular and Biventricular Pacing

Progressive QRS widening develops during the course of disease in 68% of patients with cardiomyopathy and baseline intraventricular conduction abnormality. Complete LBBB is present in more than 80% of patients with end-stage cardiomyopathy within 6 weeks before death.[57] Similar to the hemodynamic effects of isolated LBBB, LBBB in cardiomyopathy increases isovolumic contraction and relaxation times, thereby increasing the duration of mitral regurgitation and shortening LV filling time, with the net effect of decreasing preload (Fig. 2–24). The duration of mitral regurgitation is more sensitive to heart rate in patients with LBBB than in those without.[58] The magnitude of these effects is proportional to the QRS duration. Regionally diminished myocardial function or disturbed temporal sequence of contraction secondary to abnormal electrical activation disproportionately worsens systolic dysfunction in cardiomyopathy, since the remaining myocardium cannot provide the compensatory increase in fiber shortening necessary to maintain stroke volume.[59] Therefore, LV pacing and simultaneous biventricular RV and LV (multisite) pacing have recently been used to alter the ventricular electrical and mechanical activation sequence in patients with severe, symptomatic LV dysfunction and intraventricular conduction delay or LBBB.[60–68]

Influence of Pacing Site

The site of latest LV activation during RV apical pacing is the posterior or posteroinferior base.[69] Since the electrical activation sequence in LBBB is very similar to that in RV pacing, LV pacing at the posterior or posteroinferior base should have a normalizing effect on ventricular activation. Consequently, monoventricular LV pacing in patients with severe LV dysfunction and LBBB yields a hemodynamic response similar to that of biventricular pacing and significantly higher than that of RV pacing[62,70] (Fig. 2–25). Moreover, pacing of the midlateral area or posterior area of the left ventricle in this situation leads to greater improvement in pulse pressure and dP/dt than pacing of anterior or apical LV sites.[70]

Monoventricular LV pacing in LBBB does not cause premature contraction of the left ventricle relative to the right ventricle, most likely because of the slow conduction associated with pacing of myocardium compared with intrinsic

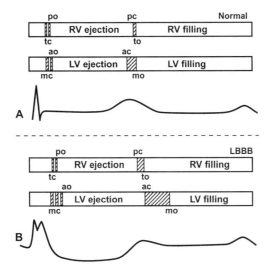

Fig. 2–24. Relationship between right ventricular (RV) and left ventricular (LV) events in normal subjects (*A*) and in patients with left bundle branch block (LBBB) (*B*). In the normal group, LV events either precede or occur simultaneously with RV events. In LBBB, the sequence is reversed, with RV events preceding those of the left ventricle. po, to, ao, mo: time of pulmonic, tricuspid, aortic, and mitral valve openings; pc, tc, ac, mc: time of respective valve closures. (Modified from Grines CL, Bashore TM, Boudoulas H, Olson S, Shafer P, Wooley CF: Functional abnormalities in isolated left bundle branch block. The effect of interventricular asynchrony. Circulation 79:845–853, 1989. By permission of the American Heart Association.)

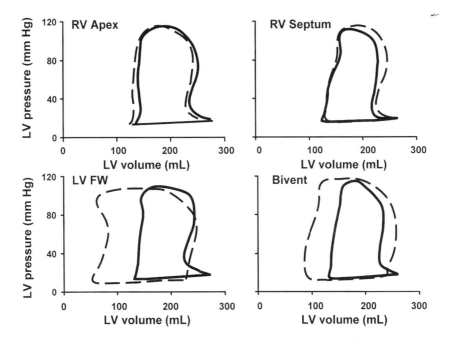

Fig. 2–25. Left ventricular (LV) pressure and volume loops demonstrating change in stroke volume and stroke work during intrinsic rhythm with standard dual-chamber *P*-synchronous pacing, biventricular pacing, and left ventricular pacing. FW, free wall; RV, right ventricular. (From Kass et al.[62] By permission of the American Heart Association.)

conduction by the right bundle. Therefore, mechanical ventricular synchrony is achieved despite early activation of the left ventricle.[62] The reduced hemodynamic effects of simultaneous biventricular compared with monoventricular LV pacing[62,64,65] suggest that some delay between RV and LV stimulation may be beneficial given the degree of LV hypertrophy frequently present in patients with cardiomyopathy. The functional status of the myocardium in the paced segment also affects the hemodynamic results: In patients with coronary artery disease, pacing of ischemic myocardium is not as effective as pacing of myocardium with normal regional function[71] and adversely affects the relationship of LV dP/dt to end-diastolic volume.

Mechanisms Underlying the Benefits of Left Ventricular and Biventricular Pacing

The mechanisms by which LV and biventricular pacing improve mechanical LV function in patients with CHF and LBBB are not entirely understood. Electrical resynchronization between the right ventricle and the left ventricle should eliminate the adverse effects of LBBB-induced mechanical ventricular dyssynchrony on regional LV systolic function. However, biventricular pacing in the absence of conduction system disease is hemodynamically superior to RV pacing despite similarly paced QRS duration.[66] Also, hemodynamic improvement with LV pacing in LBBB is equivalent to if not better than that with biventricular pacing even though it does not shorten the QRS complex.[62,64] Preliminary studies have shown that the improvement in systolic dP/dt by LV pacing in LBBB is proportional to the reduction of the electromechanical delay within the left ventricle.[67] This finding implies that synchronization of LV wall motion is important in the improvement of systolic function. Therefore, for achieving benefit from pacing therapy, electrical resynchronization evidenced by QRS narrowing may be less important than the LV pacing site and the associated change in LV contraction efficiency.[62,68,70] The hemodynamic improvements in systolic LV function with pacing may not be due to mechanical factors alone. Systemic or intramyocardial release of catecholamines, reflex-mediated baroreceptor and autonomic nervous system activation, and release of vasodilatory substances, such as atrial natriuretic peptides, have all been demonstrated for dual-chamber pacing and may well have a role in biventricular and LV pacing.[19,72]

Hemodynamic Benefits of Pacing in Neurocardiogenic Syndromes

Hemodynamic considerations are important during pacing for neurocardiogenic syncope.[73–76] Understanding the physiology involved is crucial to understanding the hemodynamics.[77] The carotid sinus reflex is the physiologic response to pressure exerted on the carotid sinus. Stimulation results in activation of baroreceptors within the wall of the carotid sinus, and they initiate an afferent response. Discharge from vagal efferents then results in cardiac slowing. Although this reflex is physiologic, some persons have an exaggerated or even pathologic response. This reflex has two components, cardioinhibitory and vasodepressor. A cardioinhibitory response results from increased parasympathetic tone and may be manifested by sinus arrest, sinus bradycardia, PR prolongation, or advanced AV block. The vasodepressor response is due to sympathetic withdrawal and secondary hypotension. Although a pure cardioinhibitory or pure vasodepressor response can occur, a mixed response is most common.

Tilt-table testing can provide the physiologic environment to reproduce vasovagal syncope (Fig. 2–26). With head-up tilt, susceptible patients have decreased venous return and subsequent decrease in LV filling. This response triggers stimulation of baroreceptors and adrenergic discharge, which can result in efferent vagal discharge and sympathetic withdrawal. Vasodilatation and hypotension as well as cardiac slowing may result. It is important to document whether the predominant cause of symptoms is cardioinhibitory or vasodepressor, because therapy differs. Tilt-table testing is often helpful in determining the predominant cause.

Drugs such as β-blockers are commonly used as first-line therapy. Although significant controversy persists, vasovagal syncope can be aborted or blunted by dual-chamber pacing, and even if syncope does occur, pacing can prolong consciousness to avoid injury.[73]

VVI pacing usually fails to ameliorate symptoms even if a bradycardiac response prevails,[78] because the absence of AV synchrony aggravates the peripheral vasodilatation that generally accompanies this condition. However, existing data suggest that dual-chamber AV synchronous pacing provides a beneficial effect. In one study, tilt-table testing was performed on 3 successive days in 10 patients with predominantly cardioinhibitory neurally mediated syncope. The first and second studies served as controls and as proof of reproducibility of syncope. On the third day, tilt testing was repeated with a temporary pacemaker programmed to dual-chamber pacing mode. Syncope was prevented in five of six patients. The mean time that tilt-up was tolerated was prolonged from less than 1 minute to more than 3 minutes, along with a significant increase in cardiac output and arterial blood pressure.[73] After permanent pacemaker implanta-tion, symptoms were abolished in 21 of 40 patients during a mean follow-up period of 24 months.[74] At a mean follow-up of 39 months, symptomatic improvement was documented in 84% of 37 patients, with complete resolution of symptoms in 35% and a marked reduction in the total number of episodes.[76] The authors concluded that most cases of vasovagal syncope can be aborted by pacing, and even if syncope occurs, pacing can prolong consciousness to avoid serious injury.

Conversely, the beneficial effect of pacing was challenged in a series of 22 patients with bradycardia during neurocardiogenic syncope in whom pacing failed to prevent a significant drop in blood pressure during a repeat tilt test.[78] Nonetheless, pacing significantly altered symptoms. Of 21 patients with an abnormal response to the initial tilt test, 18 had syncope and 3 had presyncope. During repeat tilt testing, 5 patients experienced syncope, 15 presyncope, and 1 no symptoms. Although presyncope was not prevented in most patients, the shift from syncope in 18 patients to syncope in only 5 patients represented significant clinical improvement.

In the North American Vasovagal Pacemaker Study (VPS-1), 46 patients with recurrent syncope and a positive tilt test result were randomized to dual-chamber pacemaker therapy with a special feature known as Rate Drop or to no pacemaker therapy.[79] (The Rate Drop algorithm allows the pacemaker to pace at a faster rate if bradycardia suddenly occurs.) Stopped prematurely because of the benefit observed with pacemaker therapy, the study revealed that only 17% of patients with pacing had recurrent syncope compared with 59% of patients without pacing.

Brignole et al.[80] randomized 60 patients with carotid sinus hypersensitivity to pacing or no pacing. At a mean follow-up of 36 months, syncope recurred in 9% of patients with pacing but in 57% of patients without pacing.

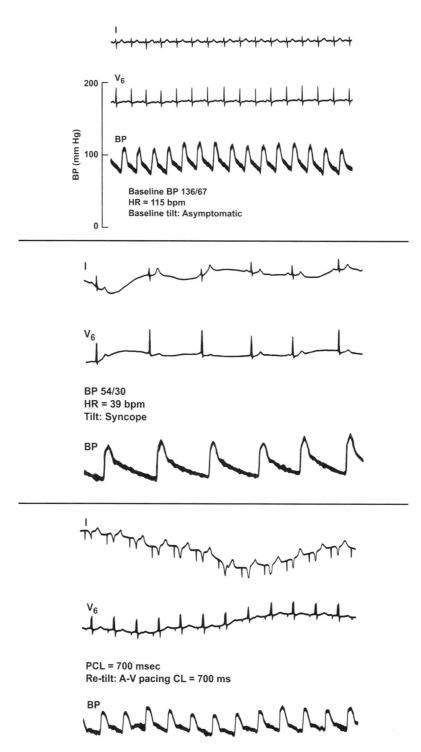

Fig. 2–26. Electrocardiographic and arterial blood pressure recordings obtained during tilt testing. *Top panel,* Tilt with the patient asymptomatic demonstrates normal sinus rhythm at a heart rate (HR) of 115 bpm and baseline blood pressure (BP) of 136/67. *Middle panel,* Tilt during syncope; the heart rate is 39 bpm and the blood pressure 54/30. *Bottom panel,* Subsequent tilt with atrioventricular (A-V) sequential pacing at a cycle length (PCL) of 700 msec (86 bpm). Significant vasodepression remains, but with the heart rate maintained, the patient experienced only presyncope. (Courtesy of Dr. W.-K. Shen, Mayo Clinic.)

Additional trials are under way to assess pacing therapy in both neurocardiogenic syncope and carotid sinus hypersensitivity.

Hemodynamic Benefits of Pacing in First-Degree Atrioventricular Block

Hemodynamic compromise due to marked first-degree AV block is well documented.[81,82] It is unfortunate that the symptoms have been described as those of pacemaker syndrome.[82] The hemodynamic compromise and symptoms in these patients are due to loss of optimal AV relationships. Although loss of AV synchrony is a factor in pacemaker syndrome, as previously discussed, other adverse hemodynamic conditions, such as atrial stretch, contribute as well. Pacing therapy should not be limited to first-degree AV block. Patients with type I second-degree AV block, traditionally a nonindication for pacing, who have hemodynamic compromise due to AV dyssynchrony and not necessarily bradycardia should also probably be considered for permanent pacing.

Conclusions

The goal of physiologic pacing should be to restore normal physiology as much as possible. This would include restoration of rate responsiveness in all patients and restoration of AV synchrony in all patients with the exception of those with chronic atrial fibrillation.

The hemodynamic importance of optimizing the AV interval is well established, and different AV intervals and rate-adaptive AV intervals are probably appropriate in most patients receiving pacing.

Retrospective work performed over the past several decades and more recent prospective studies have demonstrated the superiority of atrial-based pacing. Although the results of the prospective studies are not entirely consistent, we believe that longer follow-up of prospective study patients and additional prospective studies will minimize these current inconsistencies.

There is no uniform agreement on the indications for and efficacy of pacing in patients with HCM or dilated cardiomyopathy who do not have a traditional indication for pacing. The current experience is less than enthusiastic for pacing in patients with HCM, although a small subset of patients clearly does benefit from dual-chamber pacing.

In patients with CHF, trials under way will further our understanding of the pathophysiology of CHF and the optimal role of pacing in treatment. These trials will provide better insight into the most favorable site for biventricular pacing or whether LV pacing alone may be superior. Similarly, continuing studies are needed before definitive statements can be made about the optimal RV pacing site, regardless of LV function.

References

1. Janosik DL, Labovitz AJ: Basic physiology of cardiac pacing. *In* Clinical Cardiac Pacing. Edited by KA Ellenbogen, GN Kay, BL Wilkoff. Philadelphia, WB Saunders Company, 1995, pp 367–398
2. Kyriakides ZS, Kolettis TM, Kremastinos D: Cardiac pacing and coronary hemodynamics. Prog Cardiovasc Dis 41:471–480, 1999
3. Buckingham TA, Janosik DL, Pearson AC: Pacemaker hemodynamics: clinical implications. Prog Cardiovasc Dis 34:347–366, 1992
4. Ausubel K, Furman S: The pacemaker syndrome. Ann Intern Med 103:420–429, 1985
5. Heldman D, Mulvihill D, Nguyen H, Messenger JC, Rylaarsdam A, Evans K, Castellanet MJ: True incidence of pacemaker syndrome. Pacing Clin Electrophysiol 13:1742–1750, 1990
6. Barold SS, Zipes DP: Cardiac pacemakers

and antiarrhythmic devices. *In* Heart Disease: A Textbook of Cardiovascular Medicine. Fourth edition. Edited by E Braunwald. Philadelphia, WB Saunders Company, 1992, pp 726–755

7. Kruse I, Arnman K, Conradson TB, Ryden L: A comparison of the acute and long-term hemodynamic effects of ventricular inhibited and atrial synchronous ventricular inhibited pacing. Circulation 65: 846–855, 1982

8. Nordlander R, Pehrsson SK, Astrom H, Karlsson J: Myocardial demands of atrial-triggered versus fixed-rate ventricular pacing in patients with complete heart block. Pacing Clin Electrophysiol 10:1154–1159, 1987

9. Wish M, Fletcher RD, Gottdiener JS, Cohen AI: Importance of left atrial timing in the programming of dual-chamber pacemakers. Am J Cardiol 60:566–571, 1987

10. Ausubel K, Klementowicz P, Furman S: Interatrial conduction during cardiac pacing. Pacing Clin Electrophysiol 9:1026–1031, 1986

11. Janosik DL, Pearson AC, Buckingham TA, Labovitz AJ, Redd RM: The hemodynamic benefit of differential atrioventricular delay intervals for sensed and paced atrial events during physiologic pacing. J Am Coll Cardiol 14:499–507, 1989

12. Ritter P, Daubert C, Mabo P, Descaves C, Gouffault J: Haemodynamic benefit of a rate-adapted A-V delay in dual chamber pacing. Eur Heart J 10:637–646, 1989

13. Rees M, Haennel RG, Black WR, Kappagoda T: Effect of rate-adapting atrioventricular delay on stroke volume and cardiac output during atrial synchronous pacing. Can J Cardiol 6:445–452, 1990

14. Mehta D, Gilmour S, Ward DE, Camm AJ: Optimal atrioventricular delay at rest and during exercise in patients with dual chamber pacemakers: a non-invasive assessment by continuous wave Doppler. Br Heart J 61:161–166, 1989

15. Hayes DL, Hayes SN, Hyberger LK, Friedman PA: Atrioventricular interval optimization technique: impedance measurement vs echo/Doppler (abstract). Pacing Clin Electrophysiol 21:969, 1998

16. Raisinghani A, Diaco NV, Sageman SW, Spiess BD, Williams BR, Belott P, Ohmori K, DeMaria AN: The COST Study: a multicenter trial comparing measurements of cardiac output by thoracic electrical bioimpedance with thermodilution (abstract). J Am Coll Cardiol 31 Suppl A:430A, 1998

17. Nordlander R, Hedman A, Pehrsson SK: Rate responsive pacing and exercise capacity—a comment (editorial). Pacing Clin Electrophysiol 12:749–751, 1989

18. Fananapazir L, Srinivas V, Bennett DH: Comparison of resting hemodynamic indices and exercise performance during atrial synchronized and asynchronous ventricular pacing. Pacing Clin Electrophysiol 6:202–209, 1983

19. Kruse I, Arnman K, Conradson TB, Ryden L: A comparison of the acute and long-term hemodynamic effects of ventricular inhibited and atrial synchronous ventricular inhibited pacing. Circulation 65:846–855, 1982

20. Giudici MC, Thornburg GA, Buck DL, Coyne EP, Walton MC, Paul DL, Sutton J: Comparison of right ventricular outflow tract and apical lead permanent pacing on cardiac output. Am J Cardiol 79:209–212, 1997

21. Karpawich PP, Mital S: Comparative left ventricular function following atrial, septal, and apical single chamber heart pacing in the young (abstract). Pacing Clin Electrophysiol 20:1983–1988, 1997

22. Buckingham TA, Candinas R, Attenhofer C, Van Hoeven H, Hug R, Hess O, Jenni R, Amann FW: Systolic and diastolic function with alternate and combined site pacing in the right ventricle. Pacing Clin Electrophysiol 21:1077–1084, 1998

23. Alboni P, Scarfo S, Fuca G, Mele D, Dinelli M, Paparella N: Short-term hemodynamic effects of DDD pacing from ventricular apex, right ventricular outflow tract and proximal septum. G Ital Cardiol 28:237–241, 1998

24. de Cock CC, Meyer A, Kamp O, Visser CA: Hemodynamic benefits of right ventricular outflow tract pacing: comparison with right ventricular apex pacing. Pacing Clin Electrophysiol 21:536–541, 1998

25. Ishikawa T, Sumita S, Kikuchi M, Kosuge M, Sugano T, Shigemasa T, Endo T, Kuji N, Kimura K, Tochikubo O, Ishii M: Hemodynamic effects of right ventricular outflow pacing [Japanese]. J Cardiol 30:125–130, 1997

26. Giudici MC, Karpawich PP: Alternative site pacing: it's time to define terms (editorial). Pacing Clin Electrophysiol 22:551–553, 1999

27. Rosenqvist M, Brandt J, Schuller H: Long-term pacing in sinus node disease: effects of stimulation mode on cardiovascular morbidity and mortality. Am Heart J 116:16–22, 1988

28. Barold SS, Santini M: Natural history of

sick sinus syndrome after pacemaker implantation. *In* New Perspectives in Cardiac Pacing, 3. Edited by SS Barold, J Mugica. Mount Kisco, NY, Futura Publishing Company, 1993, pp 169–211

29. Lamas GA, Pashos CL, Normand SL, McNeil B: Permanent pacemaker selection and subsequent survival in elderly Medicare pacemaker recipients. Circulation 91:1063–1069, 1995

30. Andersen HR, Thuesen L, Bagger JP, Vesterlund T, Thomsen PE: Prospective randomised trial of atrial versus ventricular pacing in sick-sinus syndrome. Lancet 344:1523–1528, 1994

31. Andersen HR, Nielsen JC, Thomsen PE, Thuesen L, Mortensen PT, Vesterlund T, Pedersen AK: Long-term follow-up of patients from a randomised trial of atrial versus ventricular pacing for sick-sinus syndrome. Lancet 350:1210–1216, 1997

32. Lamas GA, Orav EJ, Stambler BS, Ellenbogen KA, Sgarbossa EB, Huang SK, Marinchak RA, Estes NA III, Mitchell GF, Lieberman EH, Mangione CM, Goldman L: Quality of life and clinical outcomes in elderly patients treated with ventricular pacing as compared with dual-chamber pacing. Pacemaker Selection in the Elderly Investigators. N Engl J Med 338:1097–1104, 1998

33. Gillis AM, Kerr CD, Connolly SJ, Gent M, Roberts R, for the CTOPP Investigators: Identification of patients most likely to benefit from physiologic pacing in the Canadian Trial of Physiologic Pacing (abstract). Pacing Clin Electrophysiol 22:728, 1999

34. Schrepf R, Koller B, Pache J, Hofmann M, Goedel-Meinen L, Schömig A: Results of the randomized prospective DDD vs. VVI trial in patients with paroxysmal atrial fibrillation (abstract). Pacing Clin Electrophysiol 20:1152, 1997

35. Wharton JM, Sorrentino RA, Campbell P, Gonzalez-Zuelgaray J, Keating E, Curtis A, Grill C, Hafley G, Lee K, and the PAC-A-TACH Investigators: Effect of pacing modality on atrial tachyarrhythmia recurrence in the tachycardia-bradycardia syndrome: preliminary results of the Pacemaker Atrial Tachycardia trial (abstract). Circulation 98 Suppl:I-494, 1998

36. Toff WD, Skehan JD, De Bono DP, Camm AJ: The United Kingdom Pacing and Cardiovascular Events (UKPACE) trial. United Kingdom Pacing and Cardiovascular Events. Heart 78:221–223, 1997

37. McDonald K, McWilliams E, O'Keeffe B,

Maurer B: Functional assessment of patients treated with permanent dual chamber pacing as a primary treatment for hypertrophic cardiomyopathy. Eur Heart J 9:893–898, 1988

38. Fananapazir L, Cannon RO III, Tripodi D, Panza JA: Impact of dual-chamber permanent pacing in patients with obstructive hypertrophic cardiomyopathy with symptoms refractory to verapamil and beta-adrenergic blocker therapy. Circulation 85:2149–2161, 1992

39. Jeanrenaud X, Goy JJ, Kappenberger L: Effects of dual-chamber pacing in hypertrophic obstructive cardiomyopathy. Lancet 339:1318–1323, 1992

40. Fananapazir L, Epstein ND, Curiel RV, Panza JA, Tripodi D, McAreavey D: Long-term results of dual-chamber (DDD) pacing in obstructive hypertrophic cardiomyopathy. Evidence for progressive symptomatic and hemodynamic improvement and reduction of left ventricular hypertrophy. Circulation 90:2731–2742, 1994

41. Lamas GA: Pacemaker mode selection and survival: a plea to apply the principles of evidence based medicine to cardiac pacing practice. Heart 78:218–220, 1997

42. Andersen HR, Nielsen JC: Pacing in sick sinus syndrome—need for a prospective, randomized trial comparing atrial with dual chamber pacing. Pacing Clin Electrophysiol 21:1175–1179, 1998

43. Nishimura RA, Hayes DL, Ilstrup DM, Holmes DR Jr, Tajik AJ: Effect of dual-chamber pacing on systolic and diastolic function in patients with hypertrophic cardiomyopathy. Acute Doppler echocardiographic and catheterization hemodynamic study. J Am Coll Cardiol 27:421–430, 1996

44. Kappenberger L, Linde C, Daubert C, McKenna W, Meisel E, Sadoul N, Chojnowska L, Guize L, Gras D, Jeanrenaud X, Ryden L: Pacing in hypertrophic obstructive cardiomyopathy. A randomized crossover study. PIC Study Group. Eur Heart J 18:1249–1256, 1997

45. Maron BJ, Nishimura RA, McKenna WJ, Rakowski H, Josephson ME, Kieval RS: Assessment of permanent dual-chamber pacing as a treatment for drug-refractory symptomatic patients with obstructive hypertrophic cardiomyopathy. A randomized, double-blind, crossover study (M-PATHY). Circulation 99:2927–2933, 1999

46. Symanski JD, Nishimura RA: The use of pacemakers in the treatment of cardiomy-

opathies. Curr Probl Cardiol 21:385–443, 1996

47. Eriksson H: Heart failure: a growing public health problem. J Intern Med 237:135–141, 1995

48. Ho KK, Pinsky JL, Kannel WB, Levy D: The epidemiology of heart failure: the Framingham Study. J Am Coll Cardiol 22 Suppl A:6A–13A, 1993

49. Cohn JN, Johnson G, Ziesche S, Cobb F, Francis G, Tristani F, Smith R, Dunkman WB, Loeb H, Wong M, Bhat G, Goldman S, Fletcher RD, Doherty J, Hughes CV, Carson P, Cintron G, Shabetai R, Haakenson C: A comparison of enalapril with hydralazine-isosorbide dinitrate in the treatment of chronic congestive heart failure. N Engl J Med 325:303–310, 1991

50. Packer M, Bristow MR, Cohn JN, Colucci WS, Fowler MB, Gilbert EM, Shusterman NH: The effect of carvedilol on morbidity and mortality in patients with chronic heart failure. U.S. Carvedilol Heart Failure Study Group. N Engl J Med 334:1349–1355, 1996

51. Doval HC, Nul DR, Grancelli HO, Perrone SV, Bortman GR, Curiel R: Randomised trial of low-dose amiodarone in severe congestive heart failure. Grupo de Estudio de la Sobrevida en la Insuficiencia Cardiaca en Argentina (GESICA). Lancet 344:493–498, 1994

52. Brecker SJ, Xiao HB, Sparrow J, Gibson DG: Effects of dual-chamber pacing with short atrioventricular delay in dilated cardiomyopathy. Lancet 340:1308–1312, 1992

53. Hochleitner M, Hortnagl H, Ng CK, Gschnitzer F, Zechmann W: Usefulness of physiologic dual-chamber pacing in drug-resistant idiopathic dilated cardiomyopathy. Am J Cardiol 66:198–202, 1990

54. Nishimura RA, Hayes DL, Holmes DR Jr, Tajik AJ: Mechanism of hemodynamic improvement by dual-chamber pacing for severe left ventricular dysfunction: an acute Doppler and catheterization hemodynamic study. J Am Coll Cardiol 25:281–288, 1995

55. Gold MR, Feliciano Z, Gottlieb SS, Fisher ML: Dual-chamber pacing with a short atrioventricular delay in congestive heart failure: a randomized study. J Am Coll Cardiol 26:967–973, 1995

56. Linde C, Gadler F, Edner M, Nordlander R, Rosenqvist M, Ryden L: Results of atrioventricular synchronous pacing with optimized delay in patients with severe congestive heart failure. Am J Cardiol 75:919–923, 1995

57. Wilensky RL, Yudelman P, Cohen AI, Fletcher RD, Atkinson J, Virmani R, Roberts WC: Serial electrocardiographic changes in idiopathic dilated cardiomyopathy confirmed at necropsy. Am J Cardiol 62:276–283, 1988

58. Xiao HB, Lee CH, Gibson DG: Effect of left bundle branch block on diastolic function in dilated cardiomyopathy. Br Heart J 66:443–447, 1991

59. Herman MV, Heinle RA, Klein MD, Gorlin R: Localized disorders in myocardial contraction. Asynergy and its role in congestive heart failure. N Engl J Med 277:222–232, 1967

60. Cazeau S, Ritter P, Bakdach S, Lazarus A, Limousin M, Henao L, Mundler O, Daubert JC, Mugica J: Four chamber pacing in dilated cardiomyopathy. Pacing Clin Electrophysiol 17:1974–1979, 1994

61. Cazeau S, Ritter P, Lazarus A, Gras D, Backdach H, Mundler O, Mugica J: Multisite pacing for end-stage heart failure: early experience. Pacing Clin Electrophysiol 19:1748–1757, 1996

62. Kass DA, Chen CH, Curry C, Talbot M, Berger R, Fetics B, Nevo E: Improved left ventricular mechanics from acute VDD pacing in patients with dilated cardiomyopathy and ventricular conduction delay. Circulation 99:1567–1573, 1999

63. Leclercq C, Cazeau S, Le Breton H, Ritter P, Mabo P, Gras D, Pavin D, Lazarus A, Daubert JC: Acute hemodynamic effects of biventricular DDD pacing in patients with end-stage heart failure. J Am Coll Cardiol 32:1825–1831, 1998

64. Blanc JJ, Etienne Y, Gilard M, Mansourati J, Munier S, Boschat J, Benditt DG, Lurie KG: Evaluation of different ventricular pacing sites in patients with severe heart failure: results of an acute hemodynamic study. Circulation 96:3273–3277, 1997

65. Auricchio A, Stellbrink C, Block M, Sack S, Vogt J, Bakker P, Klein H, Kramer A, Ding J, Salo R, Tockman B, Pochet T, Spinelli J: Effect of pacing chamber and atrioventricular delay on acute systolic function of paced patients with congestive heart failure. The Pacing Therapies for Congestive Heart Failure Study Group. The Guidant Congestive Heart Failure Research Group. Circulation 99:2993–3001, 1999

66. Auricchio A, Salo RW: Acute hemodynamic improvement by pacing in patients with severe congestive heart failure. Pacing Clin Electrophysiol 20:313–324, 1997

67. Gras D, Mabo P, Tang T, Luttikuis O, Chatoor R, Pedersen AK, Tscheliessnigg HH,

Deharo JC, Puglisi A, Silvestre J, Kimber S, Ross H, Ravazzi A, Paul V, Skehan D: Multisite pacing as a supplemental treatment of congestive heart failure: preliminary results of the Medtronic Inc. InSync Study. Pacing Clin Electrophysiol 21: 2249–2255, 1998

68. Saxon LA, Kerwin WF, Cahalan MK, Kalman JM, Olgin JE, Foster E, Schiller NB, Shinbane JS, Lesh MD, Merrick SH: Acute effects of intraoperative multisite ventricular pacing on left ventricular function and activation/contraction sequence in patients with depressed ventricular function. J Cardiovasc Electrophysiol 9:13–21, 1998

69. Vassallo JA, Cassidy DM, Miller JM, Buxton AE, Marchlinski FE, Josephson ME: Left ventricular endocardial activation during right ventricular pacing: effect of underlying heart disease. J Am Coll Cardiol 7:1228–1233, 1986

70. Auricchio A, Klein H, Tockman B, Sack S, Stellbrink C, Neuzner J, Kramer A, Ding J, Pochet T, Maarse A, Spinelli J: Transvenous biventricular pacing for heart failure: can the obstacles be overcome? Am J Cardiol 83:136D–142D, 1999

71. Raichlen JS, Campbell FW, Edie RN, Josephson ME, Harken AH: The effect of the site of placement of temporary epicardial pacemakers on ventricular function in patients undergoing cardiac surgery. Circulation 70:I118–I123, 1984

72. Ellenbogen KA, Thames MD, Mohanty PK: New insights into pacemaker syndrome gained from hemodynamic, humoral and vascular responses during ventriculo-atrial pacing. Am J Cardiol 65:53–59, 1990

73. Fitzpatrick A, Theodorakis G, Ahmed R, Williams T, Sutton R: Dual chamber pacing aborts vasovagal syncope induced by head-up 60 degrees tilt. Pacing Clin Electrophysiol 14:13–19, 1991

74. Fitzpatrick A, Sutton R: Tilting towards a diagnosis in recurrent unexplained syncope. Lancet 1:658–660, 1989

75. Morgan JM, Amer AS, Ingram A, Fitzpatrick A, Sutton R: Diagnosis and management of vasovagal syndrome (abstract). Pacing Clin Electrophysiol 14:667, 1991

76. Sutton R: Vasovagal syncope: clinical presentation, classification and management. *In* Cardiac Pacing and Electrophysiology: A Bridge to the 21st Century. Edited by AE Aubert, H Ector, R Stroobandt. The Netherlands, Kluwer Academic Publishers, 1994, pp 15–22

77. Maloney JD, Jaeger FJ, Rizo-Patron C, Zhu DW: The role of pacing for the management of neurally mediated syncope: carotid sinus syndrome and vasovagal syncope. Am Heart J 127:1030–1037, 1994

78. Sra JS, Jazayeri MR, Avitall B, Dhala A, Deshpande S, Blanck Z, Akhtar M: Comparison of cardiac pacing with drug therapy in the treatment of neurocardiogenic (vasovagal) syncope with bradycardia or asystole. N Engl J Med 328:1085–1090, 1993

79. Connolly SJ, Sheldon R, Roberts RS, Gent M: The North American Vasovagal Pacemaker Study (VPS). A randomized trial of permanent cardiac pacing for the prevention of vasovagal syncope. J Am Coll Cardiol 33:16–20, 1999

80. Brignole M, Menozzi C, Lolli G, Bottoni N, Gaggioli G: Long-term outcome of paced and nonpaced patients with severe carotid sinus syndrome. Am J Cardiol 69:1039–1043, 1992

81. Barold SS: Indications for permanent cardiac pacing in first-degree AV block: class I, II, or III? (Editorial.) Pacing Clin Electrophysiol 19:747–751, 1996

82. Kuniyoshi R, Sosa E, Scanavacca M, Martinelli M, Magalhaes L, Hachul D, Lewandowski A, Sarabanda A, Bellotti G, Pileggi F: The pseudo-pacemaker syndrome [Portuguese]. Arq Bras Cardiol 63:111–115, 1994

3

Indications for Pacemakers and ICDs

David L. Hayes, M.D.,
Paul A. Friedman, M.D.

Guidelines for implantation of cardiac pacemakers and defibrillators have been established by a task force formed jointly by the American College of Cardiology (ACC) and the American Heart Association (AHA). The first set of guidelines for pacemaker indications was published in 1984. The guidelines were revised in 1991 and 1998[1] and implantable cardioverter-defibrillator (ICD) criteria added. Although occasional cases cannot be categorized, the ACC/AHA guidelines are, for the most part, all-encompassing and have been widely endorsed. Current guidelines are based on the strength of available data and expert opinion; the indications have been divided into the following three classes:

Class I—Use of pacemakers and ICDs is widely accepted and supported by published studies and the literature.

Class II—Pacemakers and ICDs are frequently used, and supportive data exist, although opinion diverges on the usefulness and efficacy of device therapy.

Class IIa—The preponderance of the evidence favors the use of pacemakers and ICDs. (In the most recent guidelines, there are no class IIa recommendations for ICDs.)

Class IIb—Evidence supporting the clinical use of pacemakers and ICDs exists, but agreement on usefulness and efficacy is less well established.

Class III—Conditions for which pacemakers and ICDs are not useful or effective and in some cases may be harmful; ICDs are contraindicated in these conditions.

Indications for Permanent Pacing

The precise criteria for the implantation of a permanent pacemaker vary from institution to institution. As the ACC/AHA guidelines classification implies, some conduction disturbances generally are accepted as definite indications for permanent pacing and others are generally agreed not to require permanent pacing. In a number of conduction disturbances, the need for permanent pacing is debatable, but pacing probably is necessary and depends on the clinical circumstances. Because of changes in diagnosis and therapy, the absolute indications for permanent pacing are constantly evolving. Difficulties arise when an attempt is made to list rigid indications for implanted pacemaker insertion.

Before concluding that permanent pacing is in the best interest of the patient, the physician must carefully and thoughtfully analyze the patient. This analysis should include the general medical status as well as the specifics of the cardiac rhythm disturbance.

In keeping with the format of the ACC/AHA guidelines, indications for pacing are covered by underlying conduction system disorder or disease process, including

- Acquired atrioventricular (AV) block
- Acute myocardial infarction
- Chronic bifascicular and trifascicular block
- Sinus node dysfunction
- Neurocardiogenic syncope and carotid sinus hypersensitivity
- Prevention and termination of tachyarrhythmias
- Hypertrophic cardiomyopathy
- Dilated cardiomyopathy and congestive heart failure
- After cardiac transplantation

The ACC/AHA guidelines also include a section on pacing indications for pediatric patients. In this chapter, specific pediatric considerations are included within the larger categories; for example, congenital AV block is included in the section on AV block.

Atrioventricular Block

AV block is the impairment of conduction of a cardiac impulse from the atrium to the ventricles. It can occur at different levels, depending on whether it is proximal to the AV node, at the level of the AV node, or at the level of the His-Purkinje conduction system (Table 3–1).

Electrocardiographically, AV block has been divided into first-, second-, and third-degree (complete) heart block. First-degree heart block is a prolonged PR interval without failure of ventricular conduction. The normal PR interval is defined electrocardiographically as a range of 120 to 200 msec. First-degree AV block is usually secondary to a delay of impulse conduction through the AV node or the atrium (Fig. 3–1).

Second-degree heart block occurs when an atrial impulse that should be conducted to the ventricle is not. The nonconducted P waves may be intermittent or frequent, at regular or irregular intervals, and preceded by fixed or lengthening PR intervals. A distinguishing feature is that conducted P waves are related to the QRS complex in a recurrent pattern and are not random. Second-degree AV block has been classified into type I and type II Mobitz block. Typical type I second-degree AV block (Wenckebach block, Mobitz I) is characterized by progressive PR prolongation culminating in a nonconducted P wave (Fig. 3–2). In type II second-degree AV block (Mobitz II), the PR interval remains constant before the blocked P wave (Fig. 3–3). The AV block is intermittent and generally repetitive and may result in several nonconducted P waves in a row. Mobitz I and II are applied to the two types of block, whereas "Wenckebach block" refers to Mobitz I block only.

Type II second-degree AV block often precedes the development of higher grades of AV block, whereas type I second-degree AV block is usually a less severe conduction disturbance and does not consistently progress to more advanced forms of AV block. Type I AV block with a normal QRS complex usually takes place at the level of the AV node, proximal to the bundle of His.

Table 3–1.
Indications for Pacing in Atrioventricular (AV) Block

Class I
1. Third-degree AV block at any anatomical level associated with any one of the following conditions:
   a. Bradycardia with symptoms presumed to be due to AV block. Arrhythmias and other medical conditions that require drugs that result in symptomatic bradycardia.
   b. Documented periods of asystole > 3.0 seconds or any escape rate < 40 bpm in awake, symptom-free patients.
   c. After catheter ablation of the AV junction
   d. Postoperative AV block that is not expected to resolve.
   e. Neuromuscular diseases with AV block, such as myotonic muscular dystrophy, Kearns-Sayre syndrome, Erb's dystrophy (limb-girdle and peroneal muscular atrophy).
2. Second-degree AV block regardless of type or site of block, with associated symptomatic bradycardia.
3. Congenital third-degree AV block in a patient with a wide QRS escape rhythm or ventricular dysfunction or in an infant with a ventricular rate < 50 to 55 bpm or with congenital heart disease and a ventricular rate < 70 bpm.
Class IIa
1. Asymptomatic third-degree AV block at any anatomical site with average awake ventricular rates ≥ 40 bpm.
2. Asymptomatic type II second-degree AV block.
3. Asymptomatic type I second-degree AV block at intra- or infra-His levels found incidentally at electrophysiologic study for other indications.
4. First-degree AV block with symptoms suggestive of pacemaker syndrome and documented alleviation of symptoms with temporary AV pacing.
5. Congenital third-degree AV block beyond the first year of life with an average heart rate < 50 bpm or abrupt pauses in ventricular rate that are two or three times the basic cycle length.
6. Long QT syndrome with 2:1 AV or third-degree AV block.
Class IIb
1. Marked first-degree AV block (> 0.30 second) in patients with LV dysfunction and symptoms of congestive heart failure in whom a shorter AV interval results in hemodynamic improvement, presumably by decreasing left atrial filling pressure.
2. Transient postoperative third-degree AV block that reverts to sinus rhythm with residual bifascicular block in the pediatric patient.
3. Congenital third-degree AV block in the asymptomatic neonate, child, or adolescent with an acceptable rate, narrow QRS complex, and normal ventricular function.
Class III
1. Asymptomatic first-degree AV block.
2. Asymptomatic type I second-degree AV block at the supra-His (AV node) level or not known to be intra- or infra-Hisian.
3. AV block expected to resolve and unlikely to recur (e.g., drug toxicity, Lyme disease).

AV block that is 2:1 may be type I or type II second-degree AV block. If the QRS complex is narrow, the block is more likely to be type I, that is, located within the AV node, and one should search for transition of the 2:1 block to 3:2 block, during which the PR interval lengthens in the second cardiac cycle (Fig. 3–4). If the QRS complex is wide (Fig. 3–5 and 3–6), the level of block is more likely distal to the His bundle and the escape focus is usually less reliable. If preexisting bundle branch block is present, the block may be located either in the AV node or in the His-Purkinje system.

Third-degree (complete) AV block implies that there is no conduction of the atrial impulses to the ventricle (Fig. 3–7).

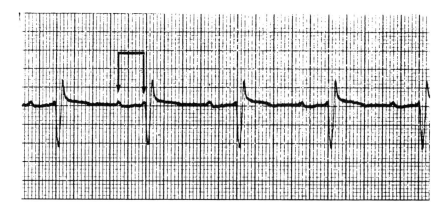

Fig. 3–1. First-degree atrioventricular block in which there is, by definition, prolongation of the PR interval greater than 200 msec. Here, the PR interval, noted by *arrows,* is approximately 300 msec.

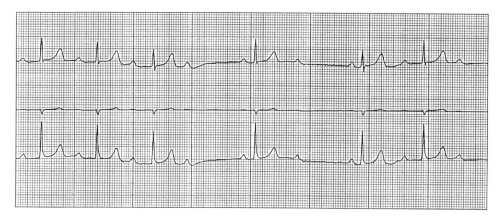

Fig. 3–2. Wenckebach atrioventricular block (Mobitz I) conduction defect allows progressive prolongation of the PR interval until a P wave is blocked. The cycle then recurs.

It is important to separate this from AV dissociation due to a subsidiary pacemaker, usually junctional, that paces more rapidly than the underlying sinus rate. In third-degree AV block, in contrast, the atrial rate is faster than the ventricular escape and there is no AV nodal conduction.

Third-degree (complete) AV block may be congenital or acquired. In the congenital form of complete heart block, there is anatomical discontinuity in the conduction pathway. Pacing for this disorder was controversial for many years because many patients with congenital complete heart block consider themselves asymptomatic, and there was conflicting information on the risk of sudden death. However, subjective improvement is usually noted once rate response is restored with permanent pacing. In addition, data support improved survival with permanent pacing.[2–4] Indications for pacing in pediatric patients are congenital complete heart block with a wide QRS escape rhythm or ventricular dysfunction and, in the infant, a ventricular rate of less than 50 to 55 bpm or associated congenital heart disease with a ventricular rate of less than 70 bpm. In addition, a class IIa indication is congenital complete heart block beyond the first year of life with an average

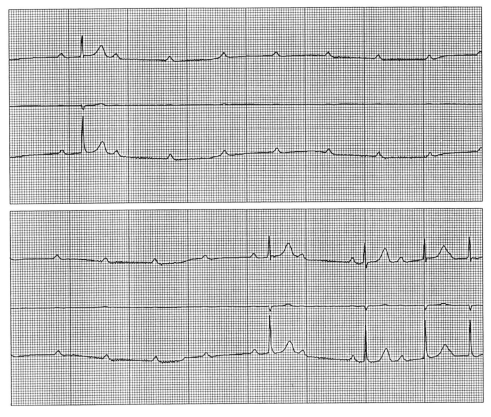

Fig. 3–3. High-grade atrioventricular (AV) block in which there is sporadic failure to conduct from atrium through AV node. In this example, the first and last P waves appear to result in ventricular depolarization, with a PR interval of approximately 220 msec. Between QRS complexes, however, nine P waves are not conducted through the AV node, and the result is a 7.4-second period of ventricular asystole.

heart rate of less than 50 bpm or abrupt pauses in ventricular rate that are two or three times the basic cycle length. Finally, congenital complete heart block in the neonate, child, or adolescent with an acceptable rate, narrow QRS, and normal ventricular function is considered a class IIb indication. In other words, pacing can be justified in any patient with congenital complete heart block.

Acquired complete heart block most commonly is due to aging with or without calcification of the conduction system or is secondary to ischemic disease, for example, previous myocardial infarction with damage extending to involve the conduction system. Complete heart block can also be related to a number of systemic illnesses, many of which have been described in single case reports (Table 3–2). Iatrogenic causes of complete heart block also exist. Postoperative complete heart block has been the most common iatrogenic cause in the past. However, AV nodal ablation for the definitive treatment of supraventricular tachyarrhythmias has become an increasingly more common acquired cause of complete heart block.

Acquired complete heart block can be either intermittent or fixed. Patients with abnormalities of AV conduction may be asymptomatic or experience severe symptoms related to profound brady-

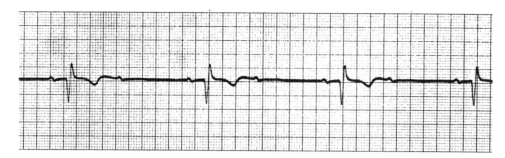

Fig. 3–4. Atrioventricular block, 2:1, in which the QRS complex appears narrow. When the conduction ratio remains in a 2:1 pattern, it is impossible to tell from the electrocardiogram exactly where in the atrioventricular node the conduction disturbance occurs. A narrow QRS complex suggests that the conduction defect is "intra-His" rather than "infra-His," which would result more commonly in a wide QRS complex.

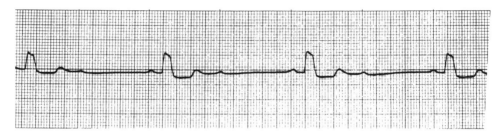

Fig. 3–5. Atrioventricular block, 2:1, with a left intraventricular conduction delay. This pattern suggests an infra-His conduction defect.

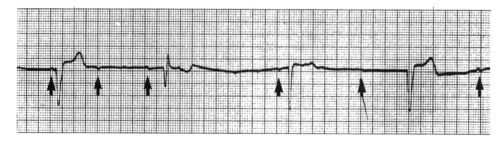

Fig. 3–6. Subsequent electrocardiographic recording from the patient whose recording is shown in Figure 3–3. This tracing shows intermittent complete heart block with junctional escape beats (*arrows* indicate P waves).

cardia or ventricular arrhythmias. Decisions on the need for a pacemaker in the patient with impaired AV conduction, whether complete heart block or second-degree AV block, are influenced by a number of factors, the most important of which is whether or not the patient has symptoms that may be directly attributed to the arrhythmia. It has been well documented that patients with complete heart block and syncope have improved survival with permanent pacing.

Atrial fibrillation with a slow ventricular response should be considered AV block, although it is often categorized as sinus node dysfunction. Patients with this anomaly should receive a pacemaker if the bradycardia is causing symptoms (Fig. 3–8).

Some inconsistencies can be found in the current ACC/AHA guidelines for pacing in AV block.[5]

The designation of asymptomatic complete heart block with ventricular es-

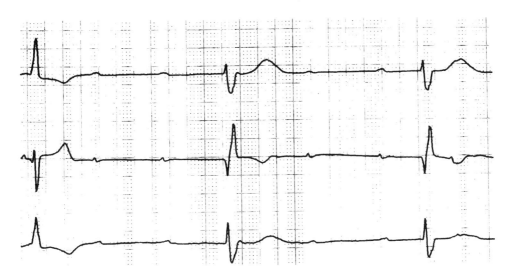

Fig. 3–7. Complete heart block is characterized by dissociation between atrial and ventricular activity. The atrial rate approximates 27 bpm, whereas the ventricular rate is approximately 75 bpm.

Table 3–2.
Causes of Acquired Atrioventricular (AV) Block

Idiopathic (senescent) AV block	Infiltrative
Coronary artery disease	Sarcoidosis
Calcific valvular disease	Amyloidosis
Postoperative or traumatic	Hemochromatosis
AV node ablation	Malignant disease (lymphomatous or solid tumor)
Therapeutic radiation to the chest	Neuromuscular
Infectious	Progressive external ophthalmoplegia,
Syphilis	Kearns-Sayre syndrome
Diphtheria	Myotonic muscular dystrophy
Chagas' disease	Peroneal muscular atrophy, Charcot-Marie-Tooth
Tuberculosis	disease
Toxoplasmosis	Scapuloperoneal syndrome
Lyme disease*	Limb-girdle dystrophy
Viral myocarditis (Epstein-Barr,	Drug effect
varicella, etc.)	Digoxin
Infective endocarditis	Beta-blockers
Collagen-vascular	Calcium-blocking agents
Rheumatoid arthritis	Amiodarone
Scleroderma	Procainamide
Dermatomyositis	Class 1C agents: propafenone, encainide,
Ankylosing spondylitis	flecainide
Polyarteritis nodosa	
Systemic lupus erythematosus	
Marfan's syndrome	

*Should not require permanent pacing; temporary pacing only until infection is treated.

cape rates greater than 40 bpm is a class II indication for pacing. Although the literature does not make the distinction and no clinical trials have been done to provide data in this subset of patients, the arguments for this conduction system abnormality as a class I indication are very practical. Once again, is the patient truly asymptomatic and is the patient or the clinician certain of this? To determine

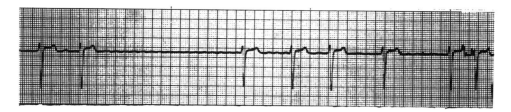

Fig. 3–8. Atrial fibrillation with a variable ventricular response and a period of asystole approximately 3.5 seconds in duration.

whether symptoms do or do not exist, what diagnostic procedures, such as ambulatory monitoring and exercise testing, should be done?

No definitive evidence exists on the focus or long-term stability of the escape rate. The rate definition of greater than 40 bpm is arbitrary and unnecessary. It is not the escape rate per se that is critical to stability but rather the site of origin of the escape rhythm, junctional or ventricular; rate instability may not be predictable or obvious. Irreversible acquired complete heart block should be a class I indication.

The current guidelines[1] include pacing in patients with neuromuscular diseases and AV block, for example, myotonic muscular dystrophy, Kearns-Sayre syndrome, limb-girdle dystrophy of Erb, and peroneal muscular atrophy. However, pacing is advocated only as a class I indication in third-degree AV block. Critical review of the literature[6–9] reveals controversy about the optimal timing for pacing in these patients. The potential for sudden death in this group of patients is well documented, and, certainly, third-degree block warrants pacing;[6–9] however, because of the unpredictable progression to symptomatic bradycardia, pacing probably should be considered much earlier in the disease process. The safest and most rational approach may be to offer pacing once any conduction abnormality is noted and subsequent follow-up reveals any progression. If the patient remains without symptoms and long-term follow-up does not reveal progression of the conduction abnormality, continued observation is rea-sonable. However, to wait for third-degree, or even second-degree, block to appear to satisfy the current guidelines may expose patients to substantial risk of syncope or even sudden death.

The current guidelines[1] do not discuss 2:1 AV block, possibly because of the difficulty in classifying this electrocardiographic finding.[10] Although 2:1 AV block per se cannot be definitively characterized as type I or type II block, it may evolve into either. An attempt to alter the AV conduction ratio, either by exercise or by pharmacologic means, for example, with atropine, may allow diagnostic localization of the conduction abnormality.

Confusion arises when the term "advanced AV block" is used in the current guidelines[1] to describe both second- and third-degree AV block. Higher degrees of block, such as 3:1 and 4:1, should be described as advanced second-degree AV block,[10] and complete heart block should be reserved for AV dissociation when the atrial rate exceeds the junctional or ventricular escape rate.

The indications for pacing in type II second-degree AV block are somewhat confusing.[1] "Asymptomatic type II second-degree AV block" is a class IIa indication under the category "Acquired Atrioventricular Block." However, "type II second-degree AV block" (symptoms not specified) is a class I indication under the category "Chronic Bifascicular and Trifascicular Block."[1] In the section "Acquired Atrioventricular Block," symptoms must be present for a class I specification. Although not clearly stated, it is likely that the difference is justified by the assumption that second-degree AV block that occurs with chronic bifascicular or trifascicular block may imply more significant and diffuse conduction system disease. Regardless of the rationale, because more than 70% of type II second-degree AV block is associated with a wide QRS complex,[11] it should be a class I indication in all cases, whether paroxysmal or chronic.

Type I second-degree AV block at intra-His or infra-His levels found incidentally at electrophysiologic study performed for other indications is a class IIa indication for pacing. Type I second-degree AV block not known to be intra- or infra-Hisian is a class III (nonindication) designation for pacing. Infranodal block, which implies diffuse conduction system disease, should be considered a class I indication for pacing. If an asymptomatic patient has type I second-degree AV block with a narrow QRS, His bundle recordings are generally neither recommended nor necessary. However, type I second-degree AV block with a narrow QRS that is found to be infranodal at an electrophysiologic study performed for other reasons should be considered a class I indication, because the patient is likely to have diffuse conduction system disease.

A previous study[12] indicated that asymptomatic patients in type I second-degree AV block for most of the day should be considered for permanent pacemaker implantation on the basis of survival data that showed that the prognosis for this rhythm disturbance, unrelated to QRS duration and acute myocardial infarction, was as poor as that for type II second-degree block. However, these data have not been reproduced elsewhere. Therefore, in asymptomatic patients who have narrow QRS type I second-degree block, pacing is not currently recommended.[13]

Symptomatic first-degree AV block is now included as a class IIa indication for pacing. The guideline states that pacing should be considered in "first-degree AV block with symptoms suggestive of pacemaker syndrome and documented alleviation of symptoms with temporary AV pacing." Hemodynamic compromise due to marked first-degree AV block is well documented.[14] It is unfortunate that the symptoms are described as those of pacemaker syndrome. The hemodynamic compromise and symptoms in these patients are due to loss of optimal AV relationships. Although loss of AV synchrony is a factor in pacemaker syndrome, other adverse hemodynamic conditions, such as atrial stretch, contribute as well. Pacing therapy should not be limited to first-degree AV block. Patients with type I second-degree AV block, traditionally not an indication for pacing, who have hemodynamic compromise due to AV dyssynchrony and not necessarily bradycardia should also probably be considered for permanent pacing as a class II indication.

The necessity and appropriateness of a temporary AV pacing study are arguable, especially if the PR interval is very long and does not shorten during exercise. In a hemodynamically compromised patient, hemodynamic improvement probably can be demonstrated during a temporary pacing study. During such a resting study, however, it may not be possible to demonstrate relief of symptoms, and exercise studies are difficult to execute with temporary AV sequential pacing in place. Therefore, some patients with marked first-degree or type I second-degree AV block and symptoms compatible with AV dyssynchrony should be considered for permanent pacing and not be subjected to a temporary pacing study, which adds unnecessary additional risk and cost without definite quantifiable outcomes.

The guidelines appropriately discuss potentially reversible causes of AV block for which permanent pacing should not be used. For example, the guidelines list electrolyte abnormalities, Lyme disease, and some instances of perioperative AV block due to hypothermia or inflammation. Potentially reversible causes of AV block or sinus node dysfunction not discussed are sleep apnea and related sleep disorders.[15] Although the literature contains limited information, in patients without seriously symptomatic bradyarrhythmias, any consideration of pacing can reasonably be delayed until the sleep disorder is treated. Similarly, the current guidelines do not include vagally mediated bradyarrhythmias secondary to a reversible medical illness or to physiologic changes in autonomic tone. For example, pauses that occur during emesis and asymptomatic pauses during sleep discovered incidentally by electrocardiographic monitoring do not require permanent pacing.

Acute Myocardial Infarction

Patients with myocardial infarction may experience a variety of conduction disturbances largely related to the site of the infarction and the coronary artery involved.[16] Rigid classification is difficult because of the variations in coronary circulation (Table 3–3).

Pacing, both temporary and permanent, after acute myocardial infarction was required more often in the prethrombolytic era. Since thrombolytic use has become commonplace, data on the need for permanent pacing after myocardial infarction are scarce. It should be stressed that the requirement for temporary pacing in acute myocardial infarction does not constitute an indication for permanent pacing.

Anterior myocardial infarctions are more likely to be accompanied by intraventricular conduction defects or AV block (or both). The long-term prognosis in survivors of acute myocardial infarction who have had AV block is related primarily to the extent of myocardial injury rather than to the AV block per se.

Patients with an inferior myocardial infarction may have a variety of conduction disturbances. Supraventricular arrhythmias associated with an inferior myocardial infarction are sinus bradycardia, sinus arrest, atrial fibrillation, and atrial flutter. AV nodal conduction disturbances, including first-degree AV

Table 3–3.
Indications for Pacing After Acute Myocardial Infarction

Class I
1. Persistent second-degree atrioventricular (AV) block in the His-Purkinje system with bilateral bundle branch block or third-degree AV block within or below the His-Purkinje system after acute myocardial infarction.
2. Transient advanced (second- or third-degree) infranodal AV block and associated bundle branch block. If the site of block is uncertain, an electrophysiologic study may be necessary.
3. Persistent and symptomatic second- or third-degree AV block.
Class IIa
None
Class IIb
1. Persistent second- or third-degree AV block at the AV node level.
Class III
1. Transient AV block without intraventricular conduction defects.
2. Transient AV block with isolated left anterior fascicular block.
3. Acquired left anterior fascicular block without AV block.
4. Persistent first-degree AV block with bundle branch block that is old or of indeterminate duration.

block and Mobitz I (Wenckebach) AV block, may also occur after an acute inferior myocardial infarction, and in a minority of patients, higher grades of AV block (Mobitz II and complete heart block) develop. Patients require temporary pacing if they are hemodynamically unstable. However, few have persistent high-grade AV block or sinus node dysfunction that requires permanent pacing.

"Transient advanced (second- or third-degree) infranodal AV block and associated bundle branch block" after an acute myocardial infarction are considered class I indications.[1] The ACC/AHA guideline states that "if the site of block is uncertain, an electrophysiological study may be necessary." The true value of an electrophysiologic study in this situation of transient AV block is unclear unless it demonstrates relatively uncommon abnormalities, such as a markedly prolonged HV interval, that is, one exceeding 100 msec, or the induction of second- or third-degree AV block with a gradual increase in the rate of atrial pacing. In this context, a simple but reasonable clinical rule of thumb in the patient with transient (second- or third-degree) AV block and associated bundle branch block after an acute myocardial infarction is useful: After an anterior wall myocardial infarction, a pacemaker is indicated if vagal block is excluded, because the block is almost certainly infranodal; after an inferior wall myocardial infarction, no pacemaker is needed. Thus, transient second-degree or complete AV nodal block with bundle branch block is not generally a class I indication for pacing in patients with inferior myocardial infarction, because the prognosis is good and is not adversely affected by the AV block.

Chronic Bifascicular and Trifascicular Block

Permanent pacing in patients with conduction disturbances of two or more fascicles of the ventricular conduction system depends on assessment of the risk of development of complete AV block, either transient or permanent (Table 3–4).[17,18] High mortality and a significant incidence of sudden death are known to be associated with bifascicular or trifascicular block and syncope, which, without pacing, commonly lead to complete heart block. Thus, defining the cause of syncope in patients with bifascicular and trifascicular block is important for documenting whether intermittent complete heart block is present. If this is docu-

---

Table 3–4.
Indications for Pacing in Chronic Bifascicular and Trifascicular Block

Class I
1. Intermittent third-degree atrioventricular (AV) block.
2. Type II second-degree AV block.
Class IIa
1. Syncope not proved to be due to AV block when other likely causes, specifically ventricular tachycardia, have been excluded.
2. Incidental finding at electrophysiologic study of markedly prolonged HV interval (> 100 msec) in asymptomatic patients.
3. Incidental finding at electrophysiologic study of pacing-induced infra-His block that is not physiologic.
Class IIb
None.
Class III
1. Fascicular block without AV block or symptoms.
2. Fascicular block with first-degree AV block without symptoms.

mented, a permanent pacemaker should be implanted. However, the incidence of progression of bifascicular block to complete heart block is low. Furthermore, no clinical or laboratory variables have proved valuable or definitive in identifying patients at a high risk of death from future bradyarrhythmias due to progression of the conduction disease. Specific controversy has arisen about patients with right bundle branch block and left anterior hemiblock. Although these patients have increased cardiovascular mortality, conduction abnormalities and bradycardia are not the causes of death in a sufficiently high proportion to warrant routine prophylactic pacing.

Measurement of the HV interval (a measure of conduction of the His-Purkinje system) at times helps in identifying patients at higher risk for the development of symptomatic high-grade AV block. In patients with a markedly prolonged HV interval, prophylactic pacing may be indicated because of an increased incidence of symptomatic bradycardia. The degree of HV interval lengthening necessary to justify prophylactic pacemaker placement is controversial. Some have advocated pacing for an HV interval of more than 100 msec, and others have considered pacing for an HV interval of more than 70 msec, especially if the patient is to receive cardioactive drugs that have the potential for further impairment of the conduction system. For patients with a normal or less prolonged HV interval, electrophysiologic testing does not reliably differentiate high-risk from low-risk groups. The clinical usefulness of routine electrophysiologic studies is not established in patients with bifascicular block. Therefore, such studies in asymptomatic patients with bifascicular block usually are not necessary.

Sinus Node Dysfunction

Sinus node dysfunction (sick sinus syndrome and tachycardia-bradycardia syndrome) includes a variety of cardiac arrhythmias that have been classified in several ways.[19] Sinoatrial disturbances included are sinus bradycardia (Fig. 3–9), sinus arrest (Fig. 3–10), sinoatrial block, and paroxysmal supraventricular tachycardias alternating with periods of bradycardia or asystole (Table 3–5 and Fig. 3–11).

The definition of bradycardia varies, but it is generally agreed to denote rates of less than 40 bpm during waking hours. There is disagreement about the absolute cycle length of an asystolic period that should require pacing. Sinus pauses of 3 seconds or greater or sustained symptomatic sinus rates below 40 bpm in the awake patient are indications for permanent pacing. Sinus bradycardia during sleep in an otherwise asymptomatic patient should not be considered an indication for pacing. Because of the uncertainty of the definition of bradycardia and the duration of sinus pauses that require treatment, it is important to take the patient's clinical condition into consider-

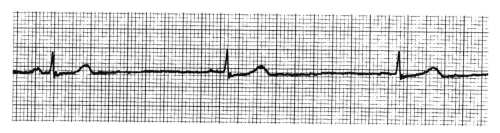

Fig. 3–9. Sinus bradycardia occurs at a rate of 39 bpm. The patient had symptoms at this rate that were alleviated after DDD pacing.

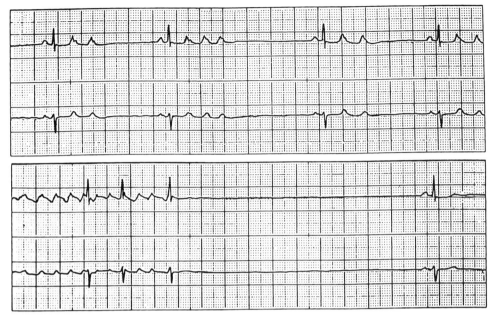

Fig. 3–10. Continuous electrocardiographic tracing from a patient with tachycardia-bradycardia syndrome reveals intermittent sinus rhythm and atrial flutter with sinus arrest and a 4.5-second pause.

Table 3–5.
Indications for Pacing in Sinus Node Dysfunction

Class I
1. Sinus node dysfunction with documented symptomatic bradycardia, including frequent sinus pauses that produce symptoms. In some patients, bradycardia is iatrogenic and occurs as a consequence of essential long-term drug therapy of a type and at a dose for which there are no acceptable alternatives. The definition of bradycardia varies with the patient's age and expected heart rate.
2. Symptomatic chronotropic incompetence.
Class IIa
1. Sinus node dysfunction occurring spontaneously or as a result of necessary drug therapy with heart rate < 40 bpm when a clear association between significant symptoms consistent with bradycardia and the actual presence of bradycardia has not been documented.
2. Asymptomatic sinus bradycardia in a child with complex congenital heart disease who has a resting heart rate < 35 bpm or pauses in ventricular rate > 3 seconds.
Class IIb
1. In minimally symptomatic patients, chronic heart rate < 30 bpm while awake.
2. Asymptomatic sinus bradycardia in an adolescent with congenital heart disease who has a resting heart rate < 35 bpm or pauses in ventricular rate > 3 seconds.
Class III
1. Sinus node dysfunction in asymptomatic patients, including those in whom substantial sinus bradycardia (heart rate < 40 bpm) is a consequence of long-term drug treatment.
2. Sinus node dysfunction in patients with symptoms suggestive of bradycardia that are clearly documented as not associated with a slow heart rate.
3. Sinus node dysfunction with symptomatic bradycardia due to nonessential drug therapy.
4. Asymptomatic sinus bradycardia in the adolescent when the longest RR interval is < 3 seconds and the minimum heart rate is > 40 bpm.

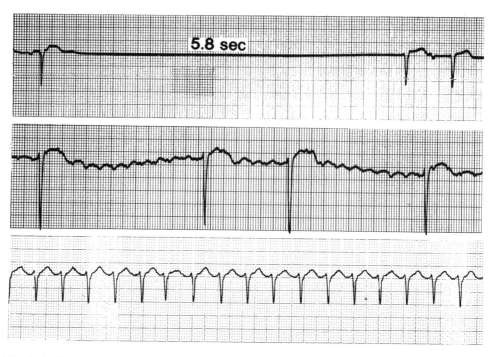

Fig. 3–11. Three electrocardiographic tracings obtained from the same patient over a 12-hour period. The *top tracing* demonstrates sinus arrest with a 5.8-second pause terminated by a junctional escape beat. The *middle tracing* reveals atrial flutter with a slow ventricular response. The *bottom tracing* shows supraventricular tachycardia.

ation, including age, associated disease, medications, and symptoms.

In sinus node dysfunction, correlation of symptoms with the specific arrhythmia is essential. Patients who have episodes of both tachycardia and bradycardia and are asymptomatic may not require therapy. Others become symptomatic when treated for tachycardia because the treatment produces symptomatic bradycardia. Treatment for tachycardia may, therefore, require permanent antibradycardia pacing.

Neurally Mediated Syncope

There are several types of neurally mediated syncope, some of which may be an indication for permanent pacing (Table 3–6). The terminology used for the various disorders is unnecessarily confusing. Disorders include asymptomatic carotid sinus hypersensitivity, carotid sinus syndrome, benign vasovagal syncope, and malignant vasovagal syncope.

Understanding the physiology involved is crucial to understanding the clinical manifestations.[20] The carotid sinus reflex is the physiologic response to pressure exerted on the carotid sinus. Stimulation results in activation of baroreceptors within the wall of the carotid sinus. Vagal efferents then result in cardiac slowing. Although this reflex is physiologic, some persons have an exaggerated or even pathologic response. This reflex has two components, a cardioinhibitory response and a vasodepressor response. A cardioinhibitory response results from increased parasympathetic tone and may be manifested by any or all of the following: sinus bradycardia (Fig. 3–12), PR prolongation, and advanced AV block. The vasodepressor response is due to decreased sympathetic activity and second-

Table 3–6.
Indications for Pacing in Neurocardiogenic Syncope and Carotid Sinus Hypersensitivity

Class I
1. Recurrent syncope caused by carotid sinus stimulation; minimal carotid sinus pressure induces ventricular asystole of > 3 seconds' duration in patients not receiving medication that could depress the sinus node or AV conduction.

Class IIa
1. Recurrent syncope without clear provocative events and with a hypersensitive cardioinhibitory response.
2. Syncope of unexplained origin when major abnormalities of sinus node function or AV conduction are discovered or provoked in electrophysiologic studies.

Class IIb
1. Neurally mediated syncope with significant bradycardia reproduced by a head-up tilt with or without isoproterenol or other provocative maneuvers.

Class III
1. A hyperactive cardioinhibitory response to carotid sinus stimulation in patients without symptoms.
2. A hyperactive cardioinhibitory response to carotid sinus stimulation in patients with vague symptoms, such as dizziness and light-headedness.
3. Recurrent syncope, light-headedness, or dizziness without a hyperactive cardioinhibitory response.
4. Situational vasovagal syncope in which avoidance behavior is effective.

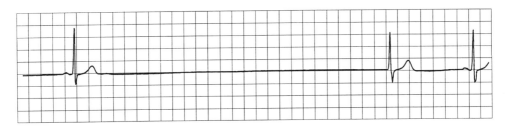

Fig. 3–12. Carotid sinus massage is often effective in demonstrating the basis of syncope or dizziness. Gentle massage of the carotid sinus at the bifurcation of the common carotid artery may produce atrioventricular block or, in this instance, prolonged sinus arrest with junctional escape.

ary hypotension. Although pure cardioinhibitory or pure vasodepressor responses may occur, a mixed response is most common.

The definitions of normal and abnormal responses are somewhat arbitrary. Ventricular asystole of 3 seconds or greater or a substantial decrease in blood pressure (30 to 50 mm Hg) is abnormal. An abnormal response to carotid sinus massage occurs in 25% to 30% of patients older than 50. Although most of these patients are asymptomatic during carotid sinus massage and have no clinical history of syncope, others may have had recurrent syncope. Patients with syncope may have a typical history related to a tight collar or neck extension but more commonly have not identified any definite provocative maneuvers. If carotid sinus massage reproduces the patient's symptoms and is associated with significant cardioinhibition or vasodepression, a diagnosis of carotid sinus syndrome can be made and treatment could be initiated. If carotid sinus massage yields a positive result but does not reproduce the patient's symptoms, a hypersensitive carotid reflex has been demonstrated, but it may not be of clinical significance, and other causes for syncope should be investigated. However, if the result of carotid sinus massage is negative, tilt testing may be indicated.

Tilt testing can provide the physiologic environment to reproduce malignant vasovagal syncope[20,21] (Fig. 3–13). With head-up tilt, susceptible patients have decreased venous return and a subsequent decrease in left ventricular filling, which may result in efferent vagal discharge. Stimulation of baroreceptors and adrenergic discharge may also result in efferent vagal discharge. Vasodilatation and hypotension as well as cardiac slowing may result from efferent vagal discharge. It is important to document whether the predominant cause of symptoms is cardioinhibitory or vasodepressor in origin because therapy

differs. Tilt-table testing is often helpful in determining the predominant cause (Fig. 3–14).

In the patient with significant cardioinhibition, permanent pacing is appropriate and should eliminate most, if not all, of the patient's symptoms. In the patient with pure vasodepression, however, other measures, such as drugs and compressive stockings, are chosen for treatment. In the patient with a mixed response but a significant vasodepressor response, dual-chamber permanent pacing with the capability of hysteresis has been shown to help blunt the vasodepressor-related symptoms. In this situation, the pacemaker is programmed to a hysteresis rate that allows the patient to remain in normal sinus rhythm most of the time, that is, 40 to 50 ppm, and to a pacing rate of 80 to 100 ppm. Therefore, when an episode of cardioinhibition and vasodepression occurs, as the patient's intrinsic heart rate slows to less than

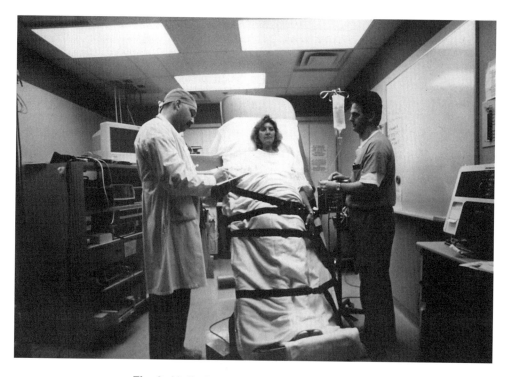

Fig. 3–13. Patient undergoing tilt-table testing.

BP 54/30
HR = 39 bpm

Baseline BP 136/67
HR = 115 bpm

Tilt: syncope

Baseline Tilt: asymptomatic

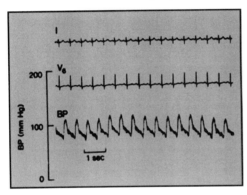

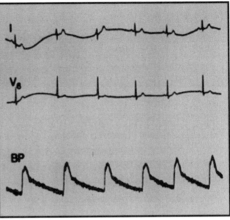

PCL = 700 msec

Re-tilt: A-V pacing CL = 700 ms

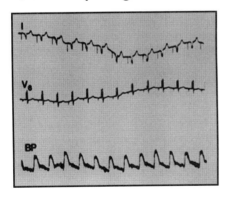

Fig. 3–14. Electrocardiographic and arterial blood pressure recordings obtained during tilt testing. *Top left panel,* Recordings made during tilt with the patient asymptomatic demonstrate normal sinus rhythm at a heart rate (HR) of 115 bpm and baseline blood pressure (BP) of 136/67. *Top right panel,* Recordings during syncope, at which time the heart rate was 39 bpm and the blood pressure 54/30. *Bottom panel,* During a subsequent tilt with atrioventricular (A-V) sequential pacing at a cycle length (CL) of 700 msec (86 bpm), significant vasodepression was still present, but with the heart rate maintained, the patient experienced only presyncope. PCL, pacing cycle length. (Courtesy of Dr. W.-K. Shen, Mayo Clinic.)

the hysteresis rate, the pacemaker begins pacing at the programmed rate of 80 to 100 ppm. Ideally, to allow restoration of the patient's intrinsic rhythm, the pacemaker should be capable of search hysteresis, whereby at programmed intervals, the pacemaker intermittently suspends pacing to determine whether the patient's intrinsic rate is once again greater than the hysteresis rate.

Benign vasovagal syncope, or a "simple faint," usually does not require therapy. Associated rhythms are usually prolonged sinus arrest without nodal or ventricular escape and may be associated with dramatic symptoms, including syncope, often undiagnosed for prolonged periods (Fig. 3–15). Syncope has been reported during many activities, such as swallowing, coitus, cough, micturition,

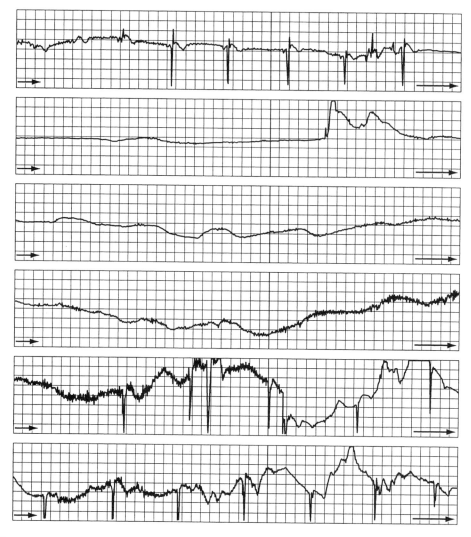

Fig. 3–15. Continuous electrocardiographic recording in a 55-year-old man who has hyper-vagotonia with greater than 30 seconds of asystole. Recovery with sinus bradycardia takes place in the *fifth panel.*

and respiration. Pacemaker implantation may be an effective means of preventing syncope, but there is some controversy about whether the patients should receive permanent pacing.[22–24] The argument against pacing is that such vagally mediated events usually do not significantly increase mortality. However, the situations during which the events occur, such as operation of a motor vehicle or heavy machinery, may predispose the patient or bystanders to danger.

Prevention and Termination of Tachyarrhythmias

The ACC/AHA guidelines include a section on pacing for the prevention and termination of tachyarrhythmias (Tables 3–7 and 3–8). Pertinent guidelines include class I indications of pacing for (1) symptomatic paroxysmal supraventricular tachycardia reproducibly terminated by pacing if drugs and catheter ablation do not control the arrhythmia or produce

Table 3–7.
Indications for Pacemakers That Automatically Detect and Pace to Terminate Tachycardia

Class I
1. Symptomatic recurrent supraventricular tachycardia that is reproducibly terminated by pacing after drugs and catheter ablation fail to control the arrhythmia or produce intolerable side effects.
2. Symptomatic recurrent, sustained ventricular tachycardia as part of an implantable cardioverter-defibrillator system.
Class IIa
None.
Class IIb
1. Recurrent supraventricular tachycardia or atrial flutter that is reproducibly terminated by pacing as an alternative to drug therapy or ablation.
Class III
1. Tachycardias frequently accelerated or converted to fibrillation by pacing.
2. Accessory pathways with the capacity for rapid anterograde conduction whether or not the pathways participate in the mechanism of the tachycardia.

intolerable side effects and (2) symptomatic recurrent sustained ventricular tachycardia (VT) as part of an ICD system. The second indication is discussed in the ICD section of this chapter. As for the first class I indication, pacing is now rarely used for prevention of supraventricular tachycardia because catheter ablation techniques have become widely used. Similarly, for the class IIb indication of supraventricular tachycardia or atrial flutter that is reproducibly terminated by pacing, permanent pacing as an alternative to drug therapy or ablation, although justifiable, is rarely done.

In the "Pacing Indications to Prevent Tachycardia" section of the guidelines, the class IIa indication for pacing in high-risk patients with congenital long QT syndrome should be noted. This is discussed under "Implantable Cardioverter-Defibrillator Indications," below.

Hypertrophic Cardiomyopathy

If the patient with hypertrophic cardiomyopathy (HCM) has any of the previously discussed indications for pacing, HCM is not necessary for justification of

Table 3–8.
Pacing Indications to Prevent Tachycardia

Class I
1. Sustained pause-dependent ventricular tachycardia with or without prolonged QT, in which the efficacy of pacing is thoroughly documented.
Class IIa
1. High-risk patients with congenital long QT syndrome.
Class IIb
1. Atrioventricular reentrant or atrioventricular node reentrant supraventricular tachycardia not responsive to medical or ablative therapy.
2. Prevention of symptomatic, drug-refractory recurrent atrial fibrillation.
Class III
1. Frequent or complex ventricular ectopic activity without sustained VT in patients without long QT syndrome.
2. Long QT syndrome due to reversible causes.

pacing. The current guidelines, however, go beyond conventional indications for pacing and include a class IIb indication for "medically refractory, symptomatic hypertrophic cardiomyopathy with significant resting or provoked [left ventricular] outflow obstruction."

The addition of a hemodynamic indication for pacing in patients with medically refractory HCM is overdue. However, the guidelines are vague in defining what a "significant" resting or provoked left ventricular outflow obstruction gradient should be in patients with obstructive HCM. No firm consensus exists, but gradients "significant" enough to warrant consideration for pacing have been suggested to be a resting gradient of 30 mm Hg or greater and a provoked gradient of 50 mm Hg or greater.[25]

Dilated Cardiomyopathy

A class IIb indication for pacing in dilated cardiomyopathy is now included as "symptomatic, drug-refractory dilated cardiomyopathy with prolonged PR interval when acute hemodynamic studies have demonstrated hemodynamic benefit of pacing."

Although significant potential exists for clinical improvement by pacing in patients with dilated cardiomyopathy and congestive heart failure, there is general agreement that standard dual-chamber pacing, even if the patient has a prolonged PR interval or diastolic mitral regurgitation by echocardiography, will benefit very few. At present, it is not possible to accurately predict who will benefit from standard dual-chamber pacing. Current data suggest that biventricular pacing or possibly single-site left ventricular pacing are the configurations that will result in hemodynamic improvement.[26]

There is no good evidence that a temporary hemodynamic pacing study (part of the ACC/AHA guidelines) will predict the long-term outcome of perma-

nent pacing. It may help optimize the AV interval, but no further claim can be made. Temporary pacing thus adds unnecessary risk and cost without proven objective benefit.

Pacing After Cardiac Transplantation

The incidence of bradyarrhythmias after cardiac transplantation has been reported to be 8% to 23%.[27] Sinus node dysfunction is the usual cause of bradyarrhythmias. Although bradyarrhythmias often are no longer displayed 6 to 12 months after transplantation, pacing is indicated for symptomatic bradyarrhythmias or chronotropic incompetence.

Indications for the Implantable Cardioverter-Defibrillator

Background

Development of the ICD was pioneered by Dr. Michel Mirowski in the late 1960s after the death of a close friend and mentor who had been hospitalized with recurrent ventricular tachyarrhythmias. His frustration with the limitations of available therapies for high-risk persons led to the concept of an implantable device that would continuously monitor cardiac rhythm and deliver defibrillating shocks for ventricular tachyarrhythmias when they occurred. During the 1970s, experimental models were built and refined, leading to the first implantation of an ICD in 1980 in a patient with two previous cardiac arrests. Over the next several years, ICD therapy was limited to patients with documented cardiac arrest due to ventricular fibrillation, and device availability was limited to a few centers.[28,29] In 1985, after a review of the available data, the Food and Drug Administration (FDA) granted approval for commercial use of the device. ICD experience and utilization grew, and evidence of effectiveness in terminating malignant ventricular arrhythmias mounted, so that by 1991, when two expert panels published independent recommendations for ICD use, the indications had broadened to include patients with drug-refractory ventricular fibrillation (VF) or VT, patients with VT or VF in whom arrhythmias could not be induced (so that electrophysiologic study could not assess drug effectiveness), and patients who did not tolerate antiarrhythmic drugs.[30,31] Since that time, further refinements in ICD technology, loss of faith in the universal effectiveness of drug therapy, and accumulating prospective clinical evidence have led to the use of ICDs as the treatment of first choice for patients at high risk for lethal arrhythmias.

Several factors have resulted in the use of ICDs becoming the de facto standard therapy for patients at high risk for sudden cardiac death. First, a series of observational studies demonstrated the uniform effectiveness of implantable devices in treating ventricular tachyarrhythmias and lowering annual rates of sudden cardiac death to 1% to 2%.[32–36] Although it was evident that ICDs reduced arrhythmic death, enthusiasm for use of the device was tempered by concern that total mortality might not be significantly reduced and that arrhythmic deaths were being shifted into heart failure deaths. Subsequently, however, a series of independent prospective, randomized trials comparing ICDs with the best available antiarrhythmic drug therapy demonstrated a significant reduction in all-cause mortality with ICD therapy.[37,38] Perhaps almost as important, advances in device technology have greatly diminished implant morbidity and have led to widespread patient and physician acceptance of the therapy. The adoption of biphasic waveforms (which enhance defibrillation effectiveness) and improved lead design have permitted the use of transvenous systems, eliminating the need for thora-

cotomy.[39,40] Great reduction in the size of the device has permitted pectoral implantation and has improved patient comfort.[41] The addition of tiered therapies, including painless antitachycardia pacing and low-energy synchronized cardioversion, and the development of specificity algorithms to limit inappropriate therapies have further added to the versatility and usability of the device.[34,42] Thus, it has become clear that ICDs are effective; the challenge for the physician is to assess the patient's risk of life-threatening arrhythmia to determine whether ICD therapy is indicated.

Assessing the Patient

The goal of ICD therapy is to prevent premature arrhythmic death in a person who might otherwise enjoy long-term survival free of the risk of imminent death from coexisting cardiac or noncardiac disease. Like the bradycardia indications, the ACC/AHA guidelines are widely accepted; they are referred to in the discussion below. Tables 3–9, 3–10, and 3–11 list the ACC/AHA classes I, II, and III indications for ICD implantation. Although risk stratification remains complex and controversial for many populations, it can be greatly simplified by considering primary and secondary prevention separately. Secondary prevention, which is the use of ICD therapy in patients with significant clinical events—out-of-hospital cardiac arrest, documented VF or VT, or syncope in patients with significant structural heart disease and inducible ventricular arrhythmias—has been well established and is generally accepted. Primary prevention requires assessment of future arrhythmia risk, which is determined by careful history-taking, physical examination, and assessment of cardiovascular function. This is discussed in greater detail below. Studies now under way will further refine ICD indications (Tables 3–12 and 3–13).

Table 3–9.
Implantable Cardioverter-Defibrillator Class I Indications

1. Cardiac arrest due to ventricular fibrillation (VF) or ventricular tachycardia (VT) not due to a transient or reversible cause.
2. Spontaneous sustained VT.
3. Syncope of undetermined origin with clinically relevant, hemodynamically significant sustained VT or VF induced at electrophysiologic study when drug therapy is ineffective, not tolerated, or not preferred.
4. Nonsustained VT with coronary disease, previous myocardial infarction, left ventricular dysfunction, and inducible VF or sustained VT at electrophysiologic study that is not suppressible by a class I antiarrhythmic drug.

Table 3–10.
Implantable Cardioverter-Defibrillator Class II Indications

Class IIa
None.
Class IIb
1. Cardiac arrest presumed to be due to ventricular fibrillation when electrophysiologic testing is precluded by other medical conditions.
2. Severe symptoms attributable to sustained ventricular tachyarrhythmias while the patient awaits cardiac transplantation.
3. Familial or inherited conditions with a high risk for life-threatening ventricular tachyarrhythmias, such as long QT syndrome or hypertrophic cardiomyopathy.
4. Nonsustained ventricular tachycardia with coronary artery disease, previous myocardial infarction, left ventricular dysfunction, and inducible sustained ventricular tachycardia or ventricular fibrillation at electrophysiologic study.
5. Recurrent syncope of undetermined origin with ventricular dysfunction and inducible ventricular arrhythmias at electrophysiologic study when other causes of syncope have been excluded.

Table 3–11.
Implantable Cardioverter-Defibrillator Class III Indications

1. Syncope of undetermined cause in a patient without inducible ventricular tachyarrhythmias.
2. Incessant ventricular tachycardia (VT) or ventricular fibrillation.
3. Ventricular fibrillation or VT resulting from arrhythmias amenable to surgical or catheter ablation; for example, atrial arrhythmias associated with the Wolff-Parkinson-White syndrome, right ventricular outflow tract VT, idiopathic left ventricular tachycardia, or fascicular VT.
4. Ventricular tachyarrhythmias due to a transient or reversible disorder (e.g., acute myocardial infarction, electrolyte imbalance, drugs, trauma).
5. Significant psychiatric illnesses that may be aggravated by device implantation or may preclude systematic follow-up.
6. Terminal illnesses with projected life expectancy ≤ 6 months.
7. Patients with coronary artery disease who have left ventricular dysfunction and prolonged QRS duration without spontaneous or inducible sustained or nonsustained VT and who are undergoing coronary bypass surgery.
8. New York Heart Association class IV drug-refractory congestive heart failure in patients who are not candidates for cardiac transplantation.

Table 3–12.
Secondary Prevention of Sudden Cardiac Death

Study	Patient inclusion criteria	End point(s)	Treatment arms	Key results
AVID[38]	• Survivor of cardiac arrest • VT with syncope • Symptomatic sustained VT with LVEF ≤ 0.40	• Total mortality • Mode of death • Quality of life • Cost benefit	• Amiodarone or sotalol	• Significant improvement in overall survival with ICD
CASH[43]	• Survivor of cardiac arrest	• Total mortality • Recurrences of arrhythmias requiring CPR • Recurrence of unstable VT	• ICD • Amiodarone, propafenone, or metoprolol	• Significant improvement in overall survival with ICD
CIDS	• Survivor of cardiac arrest • Syncope with symptomatic sustained VT with LVEF ≤ 0.35 or syncope with inducible VT	• Total mortality	• Amiodarone	• No significant improvement in survival with ICD
MAVERIC[44]	• Resuscitated VT/VF, SCD • Sustained non-syncopal VT	• All-cause mortality • Event-free survival • Costs • Quality of life	• Empirical amiodarone • EP-guided therapy (drug or nondrug)	• Ongoing
PRIDE	• Sustained VT • VF or aborted sudden death • Dilated nonischemic cardiomyopathy with EF ≤ 0.35, syncope, and NSVT or positive SAECG	• All-cause mortality • Recurrence of VT/VF • Cost-effectiveness	• EP-guided drug or device therapy • Immediate ICD implantation	• Ongoing
ASTRID[45]	• Patients with Ventak AV1810 implanted for current indication • DFT < 600 V and minimum 1 mV atrial, 5 mV ventricular EGM amplitudes at implantation	• Time to first occurrence of inappropriate therapy • Health care utilization • Quality of life	• Standard-features programming • Enhanced-features programming	• Completed; results not published

continues

Table 3–12. (*Continued*)

Study	Patient inclusion criteria	End point(s)	Treatment arms	Key results
VT-MASS	• ICD indication • EF > 20%	• Combined end point of symptomatic arrhythmia, appropriate ICD therapy, or death	• ICD and metoprolol • ICD and sotalol • ICD without AAD or BB	• Ongoing

AAD, antiarrhythmia drugs; ASTRID, Atrial Sensing to Reduce Inappropriate Defibrillation; AVID, Antiarrhythmics Versus Implantable Defibrillators; BB, beta-blockers; CASH, Cardiac Arrest Study-Hamburg; CIDS, Canadian Implantable Defibrillator Study; CPR, cardiopulmonary resuscitation; DFT, defibrillation threshold; EF, ejection fraction; EGM, electrogram; EP, electrophysiologic; ICD, implantable cardioverter-defibrillator; LVEF, left ventricular ejection fraction; MAVERIC, Midlands Trial of Empirical Amiodarone Versus Electrophysiologically Guided Intervention and Cardioverter Implantation in Ventricular Arrhythmias; NSVT, nonsustained ventricular tachycardia; PRIDE, Primary Implantation of Cardioverter-Defibrillator in High-Risk Ventricular Arrhythmias; SAECG, signal-averaged electrocardiography; SCD, sudden cardiac death; VT, ventricular tachycardia; VT-MASS, Metropolol and Sotalol for Sustained Ventricular Tachycardia.

Secondary Prevention

Cardiac arrest due to VF or VT not due to a transient or reversible cause (ACC/AHA guidelines, class I, indication 1). Persons who have a cardiac arrest due to VF or VT without acute myocardial infarction or a clearly reversible cause are at high risk for recurrent sudden cardiac arrest. Early natural history studies demonstrated recurrence rates of life-threatening arrhythmias in these patients that ranged from 30% to 50% at 2 years of follow-up.[1] Randomized prospective trials have shown significant reductions in total mortality and arrhythmic deaths in patients receiving ICDs compared with patients treated with amiodarone given empirically or sotalol guided by electrophysiologic testing, the agents most effective in treating these persons at high risk.[38,54,55]

Defibrillator use in patients with cardiac arrest presumed to be due to VF but in whom electrophysiologic testing is precluded by other medical conditions was rated a class IIb indication (supportive evidence, but less well established) by the ACC/AHA guidelines committee. In our practice, if the concomitant medical conditions are not expected to result in near-

or intermediate-term mortality, patients with VT or VF arrest routinely receive ICDs if they are well enough to tolerate the procedure. Although electrophysiologic study may guide ICD programming[56] and selection (by assessing sinoatrial and AV nodal conduction), can in exceedingly rare cases detect an accessory pathway not otherwise evident, and can ascertain bundle branch reentry VT, in most cases the study does not alter the decision to implant a device in a patient with a fatal or near-fatal arrhythmic event. Thus, the inability to perform an electrophysiologic study does not warrant withholding lifesaving therapy in a patient who may otherwise benefit.

Spontaneous sustained VT (ACC/AHA guidelines, class I, indication 2). Patients with sustained VT and syncope or sustained VT with ejection fraction of 0.40 or less and symptoms suggestive of hemodynamic compromise (near syncope, congestive heart failure, or angina) have significantly improved survival when treated with ICDs compared with antiarrhythmic drugs.[38] These patients are uniformly treated with ICDs if they are appropriate candidates. In contrast, patients with previous myocardial infarction or

Table 3–13.
Primary Prevention of Sudden Cardiac Death

Study	Patient inclusion criteria	End point(s)	Treatment arms	Key results
MADIT[37,46]	• Q-wave MI ≥ 3 weeks • Asymptomatic NSVT • LVEF ≤ 0.35 • Inducible and nonsuppressible VT on EPS with procainamide • NYHA Class I-III	• Overall mortality • Costs and cost-effectiveness	• ICD ($n = 95$) • Conventional therapy ($n = 101$)	• ICDs reduced overall mortality by 54% • ICDs cost $16,900 per life-year saved versus conventional therapy
CABG-PATCH[47]	• Scheduled for elective CABG surgery • LVEF < 0.36 • Abnormal SAECG	• Overall mortality	• ICD ($n = 446$) • Standard treatment ($n = 454$)	• Survival not improved by prophylactic implantation of ICD at time of elective CABG
MUSTT[48]	• CAD • EF ≤ 0.40 • NSVT • Inducible VT or VF	• Sudden arrhythmic death or spontaneous sustained VT	• ICD in nonsuppressible group • Antiarrhythmic drug therapy in suppressible group • No therapy	• Ongoing
Cardiomyopathy Study[49]	• Nonischemic DCM • LVEF ≤ 0.30 • NYHA class II or III	• Total mortality • Sudden death • Serious arrhythmia	• ICD • Standard treatment	• Ongoing
Defibrillat	• Patients with CHF awaiting heart transplant	• Total mortality • Serious arrhythmias	• ICD • Standard treatment	• Ongoing
BEST[50]	• Acute MI • EF ≤ 0.40 • SDRR < 70 msec or ≥ 109 VPCs/hr or abnormal SAECG	• All-cause mortality • Cost-effectiveness	• Conventional and BB therapy • EPS: if inducible, ICD and BB; if noninducible, BB	• Ongoing
DINAMIT	• Acute MI (6–21 days) • LVEF ≤ 0.35 • HR ≥ 80 bpm or SDRR < 70 msec	• All-cause mortality • Quality of life • Cost-effectiveness	• Conventional therapy • ICD	• Ongoing
MADIT-II[51]	• Prior MI • EF ≤ 0.30	• All-cause mortality • Cost-effectiveness	• Conventional therapy • ICD	• Ongoing

continues

Table 3–13. (*Continued*)

Study	Patient inclusion criteria	End point(s)	Treatment arms	Key results
SCD-HeFT*[52]	• Ischemic or nonischemic cardiomyopathy • EF ≤ 0.35 • NYHA class II or III • Appropriate ACE inhibitor • No history of sustained VT/VF	• All-cause mortality • Quality of life • Cost-effectiveness • Morbidity • Incidence of arrhythmias	• Placebo and standard therapy vs. • Amiodarone and standard therapy vs. • ICD and standard therapy	• Ongoing
DEFINITE*	• Symptomatic nonischemic cardiomyopathy • NSVT • Low EF	• All-cause mortality	• ICD, standard drug therapy, and BB vs. • Standard drug therapy and BB only	• Ongoing
DEBUT (SUDS)	• Survivor of sudden cardiac death from resuscitated VT/VF • Probable sudden cardiac arrest with RBBB and ST elevation	• All-cause mortality • Rhythms via stored EGMs that triggered ICD shocks	• ICD vs. • BB	• Ongoing
Ventak-CHF/Contak CD[53]	• Indication for ICD • Symptomatic CHF on stable drugs, including ACE • EF ≤ 0.35 • QRS > 120 msec	• Functional capacity • Qualtiy of life • NYHA class	• Biventricular pacing or no pacing and then crossover	• Ongoing

ACE, angiotensin-converting enzyme; BB, beta-blocker; BEST-ICD, Beta-Blocker Strategy Plus Implantable Cardioverter-Defibrillator; CABG, coronary artery bypass graft; CABG-PATCH, Coronary Artery Bypass Graft Patch Trial; CAD, coronary artery disease; CHF, congestive heart failure; DCM, dilated cardiomyopathy; DEBUT (SUDS), Defibrillator Versus Beta-Blockers for Unexplained Death in Thailand (Sudden Unexplained Death Syndrome); Defibrillat, Defibrillator Implantation as a Bridge to Transplantation; DEFINITE, Defibrillator in Non-Ischemic Cardiomyopathy Treatment Evaluation; DINAMIT, Defibrillator in Acute Myocardial Infarction Trial; EF, ejection fraction; EGM, electrogram; EPS, electrophysiologic study; HR, heart rate; ICD, implantable cardioverter-defibrillator; LVEF, left ventricular ejection fraction; MADIT, Multicenter Automatic Defibrillator Implantation Trial; MI, myocardial infarction; MUSTT, Multicenter Unsustained Tachycardia Trial; NSVT, nonsustained ventricular tachycardia; NYHA, New York Heart Association; RBBB, right bundle branch block; SAECG, signal-averaged electrocardiography; SCD-HeFT, Sudden Cardiac Death-Heart Failure Trial; SDRR, standard deviation of RR interval; Ventak-CHF/Contak CD, Ventak-Congestive Heart Failure/Contak Cardioverter-Defibrillator; VF, ventricular fibrillation; VPC, ventricular premature contraction; VT, ventricular tachycardia.

*Primary prevention in patients with heart failure.

mild cardiomyopathy who have VT that is exceedingly well tolerated and is not associated with hemodynamic compromise and who have normal or near normal ventricular function do not have an established survival benefit with device therapy. Nonetheless, because of the effectiveness of ICDs in terminating ventricular tachyarrhythmias, the high success rate of painless antitachycardia pacing in controlling many of these VTs, and the established capability of ICDs for treating potential concomitant arrhythmias (for example, bradycardia associated with conduction system disease or sinus node dysfunction), device therapy is often appropriately used in these patients. However, patients with preserved ventricular function and well-tolerated VT may also be considered candidates for primary antiarrhythmic drug treatment or catheter ablation, and the choice of therapy is tailored by patient age and preference, concomitant medical illnesses, and physician preference.

Syncope of undetermined origin with clinically relevant, hemodynamically significant sustained VT or VF induced at electrophysiological study when drug therapy is ineffective, not tolerated, or not preferred (ACC/AHA guidelines, class I, indication 3). Patients with syncope and inducible ventricular arrhythmias are at high risk for recurrent events and for sudden cardiac death, particularly if dilated cardiomyopathy or previous myocardial infarction and depressed ventricular function are present. In patients with significant structural heart disease and inducible arrhythmias, syncope is a clinically important event, and ICD use in this situation can loosely be categorized as secondary prevention.

Primary Prevention and Assessment of Specific Disease States

Accurate determination of underlying cardiac disease is paramount for predicting an asymptomatic or minimally symptomatic person's risk of having life-threatening arrhythmias develop and for providing appropriate therapy. For some specific disease states, established methods of risk assessment exist, whereas for many others, predictors of arrhythmic events are poorly defined and the approach remains controversial. Techniques such as signal-averaged electrocardiography, heart rate variability, and T-wave alternans, among others, have been assessed, but none has adequate predictive power to independently guide patient management at present. Nonetheless, it has become increasingly clear that the underlying disease has an important role in prognosis and influences the decision on whether to implant an ICD as part of the treatment protocol.[1] Once again, clinical trials are imperative to determine the clinical benefit of ICD implantation as primary prevention of life-threatening arrhythmias (Table 3–13). The approach to specific disease states is discussed below.

Coronary Artery Disease

Patients with coronary artery disease, previous myocardial infarction, depressed ventricular function (ejection fraction $\leq$ 35%), and nonsustained VT are at increased risk for ventricular tachyarrhythmias despite the lack of arrhythmia symptoms, with a 2-year mortality around 30%.[57] Of this population, patients at electrophysiologic study with inducible VT not suppressible by class I antiarrhythmic drugs had a significant reduction in mortality with ICD therapy compared with conventional therapy (predominantly amiodarone) in a randomized, prospective trial.[37] On the basis of this trial, the ACC/AHA Guidelines Committee recognized ICD use as a class I indication in this population (the only class I indication for primary prevention), and the FDA broadened ICD indications to include this group. If patients with coronary disease, previous myocardial infarction, and left ventricular dysfunction have inducible VT or VF at electrophysiologic study but a class I drug efficacy is not assessed, ICD use is rated class IIb by the ACC/AHA guidelines. Given the demonstrated and consistent superiority of ICD therapy over drug therapy for high-risk patients with left ventricular dysfunction in several published and presented studies,[37,58] in our practice we do not routinely require failure of a class I agent before ICD use if VT is induced at electrophysiologic study. Additionally, we recommend ambulatory monitoring to screen for nonsustained VT in asymptomatic patients with prior myocardial infarction and left ventricular dysfunction who have no indications for revascularization and who have not had a recent (within 3 weeks) infarction, and we offer invasive electrophysiologic study for further risk stratification when nonsustained VT (> 3 beats, > 100 bpm) is found (Table 3–14).

Although this approach toward asymptomatic patients with coronary disease and ventricular dysfunction is supported by the available data, it has several limitations. Since nonsustained VT is episodic, the sensitivity of periodic screening is limited. The requirement of an invasive study for risk stratification exposes patients to a small risk and has practical limitations in broad applicability. More important, although it is clear that patients with inducible ventricular tachyarrhythmias are at high risk for future clinical events, patients with noninducible arrhythmia may also have a somewhat elevated risk.[58] Studies in progress, such as the Sudden Cardiac Death-Heart Failure Trial and Multicenter Automatic Defibrillator Implantation Trial II, which are randomizing patients to device or medical therapy on the basis of noninvasive risk stratification alone, will better define the appropriate management of this population. In the meantime, it is important that all patients with ventricular dysfunction receive pharmacologic therapy with mortality-reducing agents, such as angiotensin-converting enzyme inhibitors and beta-blockers, regardless of device use.

Table 3–14.
Primary Prevention After Myocardial Infarction

Study	Patient inclusion criteria	End point(s)	Treatment arms	Key results
SEDET	• Acute MI (1–3 weeks) • Ineligible for thrombolysis • EF ≥ 0.15 to ≤ 0.40 • Nonsustained VT or ≥ 10 PVCs/hr between 6 and 21 days after MI	• All-cause mortality • Quality of life • Incidence of VT • Sudden and nonsudden death • Cardiac death • Predictive value of BRS and HRV	• ICD vs. • Conventional therapy	• Ongoing
IRIS	• Acute MI • Fast NSVT > 150 bpm • HR > 100 bpm at admission	• All-cause mortality • Resource utilization • Quality of life	• ICD vs. • Conventional therapy	• Ongoing

BRS, baroreceptor sensitivity; EF, ejection fraction; HR, heart rate; HRV, heart rate variability; ICD, implantable cardioverter-defibrillator; IRIS, Immediate Risk Stratification Improves Survival; MI, myocardial infarction; NSVT, nonsustained ventricular tachycardia; PVC, premature ventricular contraction; SEDET, South European Defibrillator Trial; VT, ventricular tachycardia.

Hypertrophic Cardiomyopathy

The natural history of patients with HCM is characterized by slow progression of symptoms such as dyspnea and angina. Without arrhythmia, the prognosis is often relatively good; however, patients with HCM have an increased risk for sudden death, from 3% to 6% annually, and approximately 50% of deaths are sudden.[59,60] HCM is the most common cause of sudden death in otherwise healthy young persons. Symptoms such as palpitations and syncope may be difficult to assess in patients with HCM because of the potential for multiple etiologic factors, including autonomic dysregulation, an outflow gradient, atrial fibrillation, and ventricular tachyarrhythmias. Moreover, these and other factors, such as subendocardial ischemia, enhanced AV nodal conduction of atrial fibrillation, conduction defects, and septal myocyte disarray, have been proposed as triggers for sudden death. Because of the complexity of the pathogenesis of sudden death, risk stratification is difficult. There is no clear consensus in the literature on the predictive power of ambulatory monitoring and electrophysiologic study, and many studies suffer from small patient numbers or limited follow-up.[61,62] Given the known progressive phenotypic expression of HCM over time, assessment of the pathologic substrate at any one point may have limited long-term predictive power. Ultimately, the best prognostic study may be a blood test to determine the specific genetic defect.

Despite the challenges in assessing patients with HCM, there are several areas of broad consensus. The available data suggest that ventricular tachyarrhythmias are the cause of sudden death in most patients, even if initially triggered by one or several mechanisms. Patients fortunate enough to survive an episode of out-of-hospital cardiac arrest or who have sustained ventricular tachyarrhythmias are at highest risk for sudden death and should generally undergo ICD implantation. Patients without a dramatic clinical event but with other risk factors, particularly young age, syncope, malignant family history, and a markedly thickened ventricular septum, are also at increased risk.[60] Because of low implant morbidity and the ensured compliance of ICD therapy, combined with the uncertain effectiveness of antiarrhythmic drugs in this population,[62] we often offer device therapy to these patients, although the approach is highly individualized. Device use in this population may be further supported by our observation of frequent appropriate ICD discharges in high-risk patients without antecedent clinical events, a finding also obtained in a multicenter review.[59,63] Secondary benefits of ICD therapy in this population are the potential for dual-chamber pacing to alleviate symptomatic gradients in a subset of patients and the growing availability of devices that deliver therapy specific for atrial arrhythmias, including atrial defibrillation. These advantages, however, are tempered by the concern of committing patients, often young, to lifelong hardware implantation, the long-term need for system revisions, and the possibility of inappropriate shocks and concomitant anxiety. Thus, although device therapy is often used in patients with risk factors, the approach is tailored after extensive discussion with the patient. The ACC/AHA guidelines committee issued a class IIb indication for patients with "familial or inherited conditions with a high risk for life-threatening ventricular tachyarrhythmias such as long QT syndrome or hypertrophic cardiomyopathy."

Long QT Syndrome

Familial long QT syndrome is a rare disorder of cardiac ion channels resulting in abnormal repolarization, usually manifested as a long QT interval with abnormal T-wave morphology on the surface electrocardiogram[64] (Fig. 3–16). Patients with the syndrome have a propensity for syncope, polymorphic VT (torsades de pointes), and sudden cardiac death.[65] Without treatment, the 1-year mortality approaches 20% and the 15-year mortality surpasses 50%.[65] Since this is primarily an electrical disorder, typically seen in patients without significant heart disease or structural abnormalities, arrhythmia control results in an excellent prognosis. Because a sudden increase in sympathetic activity often acts as the arrhythmia trigger, first-line treatment frequently consists of β-adrenergic receptor blocker therapy. Although this therapy can effectively control symptoms and reduce the risk of sudden death for many patients, the risk is not eliminated. In long QT syndrome registries, 9% of sudden death events occurred during therapy with β-adrenegic blocking agents.[66] Additionally, up to 25% of patients with long QT syndrome remain symptomatic despite high-dose β-adrenergic blocker therapy, and these patients most likely represent a high-risk subgroup. Although antibradycardia pacing (to prevent proarrhythmic pauses and to shorten depolarization) and left cardiac sympathetic denervation can diminish the risk of sudden death, it is not eliminated.

ICD therapy is recommended for patients who present with aborted sudden death, sustained ventricular arrhythmias, or recurrent syncope despite medical therapy. Patients with a strong family history of sudden cardiac death, particularly if other risk factors are present (deafness, syncope, female sex, markedly prolonged QTc interval [> 0.55 to 0.60]), are also frequently offered this therapy, although the approach is individualized. Because missing only 1 or 2 days of beta-blocker therapy can be fatal,[67] the dual-chamber capability of ICDs may diminish tachyarrhythmia frequency, and the implant morbidity of nonthoracotomy ICDs is low, patients who cannot tolerate the drugs or who are noncompliant may also benefit from ICD therapy. In persons with a strong family history and a normal QTc interval, familial genetic evaluation can be an invaluable assessment tool, although it is expensive, time-consuming, labor-intensive, and most often not available. Persons without symptoms who have a normal QT interval are generally observed or treated with β-adrenergic blocking agents, depending on the situation.

Brugada Syndrome, Ventricular Fibrillation, and Arrhythmogenic Right Ventricular Dysplasia

In 1992, Pedro and Josep Brugada described eight patients with right bundle branch block who had ST segment elevation in V_1–V_3 with syncope due to polymorphic VT or sudden death. Since the initial description, the number of patients described worldwide has grown dramatically. The Brugada syndrome, as it has since been named, has been recognized as the cause of sudden death that is endemic in young Asian Pacific men. There are no associated structural cardiac abnormalities. The syndrome is known in Thailand as "Lai Tai," in the Philippines as "Bangungut," and in Japan as "Pokkuru," terms that refer to sudden death at night or during sleep, and the syndrome is the most common cause of natural death in young Thai men. The syndrome is due to sodium channel mutations, distinct from those in long QT syndrome, which result in abnormal repolarization, most prominent in the right ventricular epicardium. A high rise in vagal tone has been reported to occur just before VF episodes. The electrocardiographic abnormalities may not always be present, but they can be unmasked by procainamide or ajmaline challenge. Beta-adrenergic blocking agents and amiodarone have not been effective in

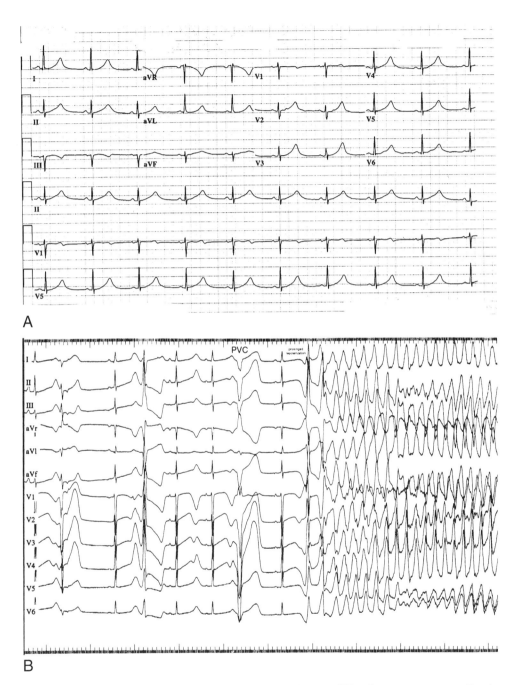

Fig. 3–16. Long QT syndrome. *A,* Electrocardiogram shows a QTc of 575 msec, suggesting in-creased risk of an arrhythmic event. This patient had a confirmed lesion affecting the cardiac potassium channel KVLQT1. *B,* In a rhythm strip from a different patient, torsades de pointes is initiated during a dobutamine challenge. A short interval is terminated by a premature ven-tricular contraction (PVC), which in turn is followed by a long interval. The short-long sequence results in marked additional prolongation of repolarization, and a second PVC on the T wave initiates the arrhythmia.

preventing death; ICDs have. Given the 30% incidence of recurrent arrhythmic events in patients with symptoms at 3 years, defibrillator therapy is warranted. Additionally, because of the similarly high incidence of aborted sudden death in asymptomatic persons with the typical electrocardiographic pattern, electrophysiologic study and an ICD should be strongly considered.[68,69]

Idiopathic VF may be a variant of the Brugada syndrome without abnormalities of the resting electrocardiogram, although this possibility remains unclear. Most patients have a history of syncope caused by bursts of polymorphic VT or VF that terminate spontaneously. VF typically begins with a short-couple extrasystole, which initiates a rapid polymorphic VT that promptly deteriorates to VF. VF is usually inducible at electrophysiologic study. Although some investigators have suggested therapy with class Ia agents guided by electrophysiologic study and report favorable long-term outcomes with this approach, most favor ICD implantation.[70]

Arrhythmogenic right ventricular dysplasia is characterized by fibrous and fatty replacement of the myocardium, preferentially in the right ventricle, although involvement can spread to both chambers. Right ventricular adipose and small bulges (aneurysms) can frequently

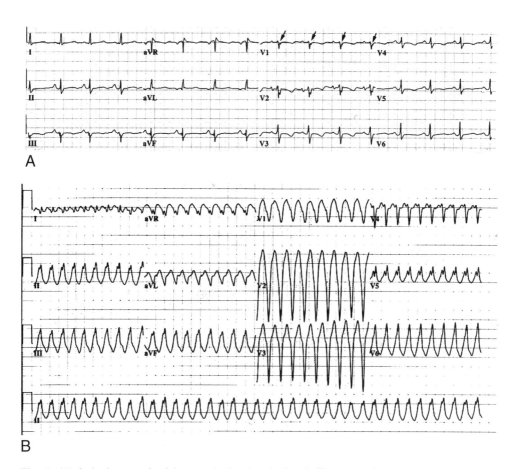

Fig. 3–17. Arrhythmogenic right ventricular dysplasia. *A*, Electrocardiogram shows right precordial T wave inversions and epsilon waves (*arrows*). *B*, Ventricular tachycardia in the same patient. Note the left bundle branch block pattern, which originated in the right ventricle.

be detected by magnetic resonance imaging or ultrafast computed tomography, which may be preferable. The electrocardiogram classically demonstrates inverted T waves in the right precordium, and in approximately 30% of cases, classic epsilon waves are seen (Fig. 3–17). In contrast to the Brugada syndrome or idiopathic VF, in which polymorphic arrhythmias are present, arrhythmogenic right ventricular dysplasia more commonly results in fast monomorphic VT. Since left ventricular function is often preserved, hemodynamic collapse is less frequent, although sudden death has been reported as the first presentation of the disease. Treatment approaches have included medications, catheter ablation, and surgical ventriculotomy or disarticulation to prevent electrical substrate communication with the remainder of the myocardium. For patients with refractory arrhythmias, defibrillator therapy provides prophylaxis against syncope due to rapid and hemodynamically unstable VT. The frequency of appropriate therapy in patients with arrhythmogenic right ventricular dysplasia may be high, supporting the role of ICD therapy in this patient population and necessitating adjuvant medical or catheter therapy to prevent excessive shocks.[71,72]

Contraindications to Implantable Cardioverter-Defibrillator Therapy

Contraindications to ICD therapy are summarized in Table 3–3. Patients who have incessant arrhythmias that cannot be controlled by adjuvant medical, catheter-based, or surgical therapy are not candidates for device implantation. Patients whose arrhythmias are clearly due to a transient or reversible disorder, such as acute myocardial infarction, significant electrolyte imbalance, drug ingestion, or trauma, do not have a greatly increased risk of recurrent arrhythmia and should not receive implantable defibrillator therapy. Patients with significant psychiatric illnesses that may be aggravated by device shocks and patients with terminal ill-

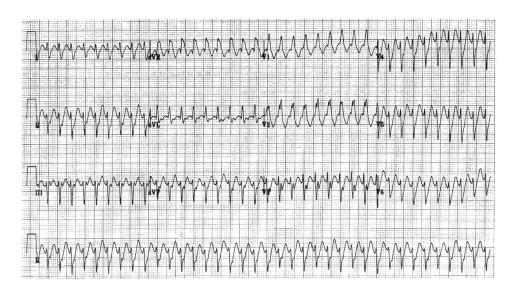

Fig. 3–18. Electrocardiogram showing fascicular ventricular tachycardia. Note the right bundle branch block pattern with far-left axis deviation, consistent with an arrhythmia focus in the left posterior fascicle. Ablation success rates exceed 90% for this arrhythmia, so that defibrillator therapy is not typically indicated.

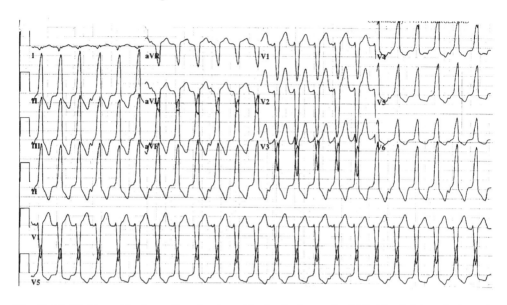

Fig. 3–19. Right ventricular outflow tract ventricular tachycardia (VT). The left bundle branch block with positive QRS complexes in II, III, and aVF is characteristic; because of the high outflow origin of the tachycardia, wave fronts propagate toward the inferior leads. This tracing also demonstrates atrioventricular (A-V) dissociation (best seen in lead II). Because of the rapid rate of the tachycardia, only every third VT complex can conduct retrogradely to the AV node, resulting in 3:1 ventriculoatrial conduction. AV dissociation in this situation is not indicative of AV block; in fact, this patient has normal AV nodal conduction during sinus rhythm. Right ventricular outflow tract VT is best treated with catheter ablation; defibrillator therapy is not indicated.

ness, including New York Heart Association class IV drug-refractory congestive heart failure in patients who are not candidates for transplantation, should also not receive defibrillators. Additionally, patients with VF or VT resulting from arrhythmias amenable to surgical or catheter ablation, such as right ventricular outflow tract VT, idiopathic left ventricular VT, fascicular VT, or Wolff-Parkinson-White syndrome with ventricular tachyarrhythmias secondary to rapid anterograde conduction of atrial fibrillation, should not generally undergo ICD therapy (Fig. 3–18 and 3–19).

The ACC/AHA guidelines also indicate that patients with syncope of undetermined cause in whom there are no inducible arrhythmias should not receive defibrillators. Although this recommendation is well supported for patients without cardiac abnormalities, it may not apply in patients with structural heart disease for which electrophysiologic study is not predictive of arrhythmia. For example, the usefulness of electrophysiologic study in patients with dilated cardiomyopathy remains controversial, and the limited available data suggest that ICD therapy in patients with dilated cardiomyopathy and syncope may be of benefit even with negative findings on electrophysiologic study.[73,74]

Conclusions

Appropriate defibrillator use requires stratification of risk for each patient. This can be simplified by considering secondary and primary prevention separately. Because of demonstrated effectiveness, proven superiority over medical therapy, and low implant morbidity, ICDs have become standard therapy for secondary prevention of life-threatening ventricular tachyarrhythmias. Selecting patients for primary prevention requires careful assessment of patient history, family history, and underlying disease state. Patients at high risk for life-threatening arrhythmias generally benefit from ICD therapy. Great reduction in size, improved specificity of therapy, and availability of dual-chamber pacing and atrial-specific treatments have increased patient and physician acceptance and lowered the threshold of device therapy in primary prevention of sudden death. New insights into the pathophysiology of cardiac disease, improved tools for risk stratification, and additional innovations in ICD design will lead to both further refinements in patient selection and more widespread use of the device for patients at risk of sudden death.

References

1. Gregoratos G, Cheitlin MD, Conill A, Epstein AE, Fellows C, Ferguson TB Jr, Freedman RA, Hlatky MA, Naccarelli GV, Saksena S, Schlant RC, Silka MJ, Ritchie JL, Gibbons RJ, Eagle KA, Gardner TJ, Lewis RP, O'Rourke RA, Ryan TJ, Garson A Jr: ACC/AHA guidelines for implantation of cardiac pacemakers and antiarrhythmia devices: a report of the American College of Cardiology/American Heart Association Task Force on Practice Guidelines (Committee on Pacemaker Implantation). J Am Coll Cardiol 31:1175–1209, 1998

2. Michaelsson M, Jonzon A, Riesenfeld T: Isolated congenital complete atrioventricular block in adult life. A prospective study. Circulation 92:442–449, 1995

3. Dewey RC, Capeless MA, Levy AM: Use of ambulatory electrocardiographic monitoring to identify high-risk patients with congenital complete heart block. N Engl J Med 316:835–839, 1987

4. Sholler GF, Walsh EP: Congenital complete heart block in patients without anatomic cardiac defects. Am Heart J 118:1193–1198, 1989

5. Hayes DL, Barold SS, Camm AJ, Goldschlager NF: Evolving indications for permanent cardiac pacing: an appraisal of the 1998 American College of Cardiology/American Heart Association Guidelines (editorial). Am J Cardiol 82:1082–1086, 1998

6. Fragola PV, Autore C, Magni G, Antonini G, Picelli A, Cannata D: The natural course of cardiac conduction disturbances in myotonic dystrophy. Cardiology 79:93–98, 1991

7. Bialer MG, McDaniel NL, Kelly TE: Progression of cardiac disease in Emery-Dreifuss muscular dystrophy. Clin Cardiol 14:411–416, 1991

8. Polak PE, Zijlstra F, Roelandt JR: Indications for pacemaker implantation in the Kearns-Sayre syndrome. Eur Heart J 10:281–282, 1989

9. Komajda M, Frank R, Vedel J, Fontaine G, Petitot JC, Grosgogeat Y: Intracardiac conduction defects in dystrophia myotonica. Electrophysiological study of 12 cases. Br Heart J 43:315–320, 1980

10. Surawicz B, Uhley H, Borun R, Laks M, Crevasse L, Rosen K, Nelson W, Mandel W, Lawrence P, Jackson L, Flowers N, Clifton J, Greenfield J Jr, De Medina EO: The quest for optimal electrocardiography. Task Force I: standardization of terminology and interpretation. Am J Cardiol 41:130–145, 1978

11. Denes P: Atrioventricular and intraventricular block. Circulation 75 Suppl:III-19-III-25, 1987

12. Shaw DB, Kekwick CA, Veale D, Gowers J, Whistance T: Survival in second degree atrio-ventricular block. Br Heart J 53:587–593, 1985

13. Connelly DT, Steinhaus DM: Mobitz type I atrioventricular block: an indication for permanent pacing? (Editorial.) Pacing Clin Electrophysiol 19:261–264, 1996

14. Barold SS: Indications for permanent cardiac pacing in first-degree AV block: class I, II, or III? (Editorial.) Pacing Clin Electrophysiol 19:747–751, 1996

15. Stegman SS, Burroughs JM, Henthorn RW: Asymptomatic bradyarrhythmias as a marker for sleep apnea: appropriate recognition and treatment may reduce the need for pacemaker therapy. Pacing Clin Electrophysiol 19:899–904, 1996

16. Barold SS, Falkoff MD, Ong LS, Vaughan MJ, Heinle RA: Atrioventricular block in acute myocardial infarction: new developments. *In* New Perspectives in Cardiac Pacing. 2. Edited by SS Barold, J Mugica.

Mount Kisco, NY, Futura Publishing Company, 1991, pp 3–21

17. Englund A, Bergfeldt L, Rehnqvist N, Astrom H, Rosenqvist M: Diagnostic value of programmed ventricular stimulation in patients with bifascicular block: a prospective study of patients with and without syncope. J Am Coll Cardiol 26:1508–1515, 1995

18. Dhingra RC, Denes P, Wu D, Chuquimia R, Amat-y-Leon F, Wyndham C, Rosen KM: Syncope in patients with chronic bifascicular block. Significance, causative mechanisms, and clinical implications. Ann Intern Med 81:302–306, 1974

19. Dreifus LS, Michelson EL, Kaplinsky E: Bradyarrhythmias: clinical significance and management. J Am Coll Cardiol 1: 327–338, 1983

20. Abi-Samra F, Maloney JD, Fouad-Tarazi FM, Castle LW: The usefulness of head-up tilt testing and hemodynamic investigations in the workup of syncope of unknown origin. Pacing Clin Electrophysiol 11:1202–1214, 1988

21. Almquist A, Goldenberg IF, Milstein S, Chen MY, Chen XC, Hansen R, Gornick CC, Benditt DG: Provocation of bradycardia and hypotension by isoproterenol and upright posture in patients with unexplained syncope. N Engl J Med 320: 346–351, 1989

22. Brignole M, Menozzi C, Lolli G, Oddone D, Gianfranchi L, Bertulla A: Pacing for carotid sinus syndrome and sick sinus syndrome. Pacing Clin Electrophysiol 13: 2071–2075, 1990

23. Sutton R: Pacing in sick sinus syndrome and carotid sinus hypersensitivity. *In* New Perspectives in Cardiac Pacing. 2. Edited by SS Barold, J Mugica. Mount Kisco, NY, Futura Publishing Company, 1991, pp 53–58

24. Sra JS, Jazayeri MR, Avitall B, Dhala A, Deshpande S, Blanck Z, Akhtar M: Comparison of cardiac pacing with drug therapy in the treatment of neurocardiogenic (vasovagal) syncope with bradycardia or asystole. N Engl J Med 328:1085–1090, 1993

25. Symanski JD, Nishimura RA: The use of pacemakers in the treatment of cardiomyopathies. Curr Probl Cardiol 21:385–443, 1996

26. Auricchio A, Stellbrink C, Block M, Sack S, Vogt J, Bakker P, Klein H, for the Pacing Therapies for Congestive Heart Failure Study Group, Kramer A, Ding J, Salo R, Tockman B, Pochet T, Spinelli J, for the Guidant Congestive Heart Failure Research Group: Effect of pacing chamber and atrioventricular delay on acute systolic function of paced patients with congestive heart failure. Circulation 99: 2993–3001, 1999

27. DiBiase A, Tse TM, Schnittger I, Wexler L, Stinson EB, Valantine HA: Frequency and mechanism of bradycardia in cardiac transplant recipients and need for pacemakers. Am J Cardiol 67:1385–1389, 1991

28. Mirowski M, Reid PR, Mower MM, Watkins L, Gott VL, Schauble JF, Langer A, Heilman MS, Kolenik SA, Fischell RE, Weisfeldt ML: Termination of malignant ventricular arrhythmias with an implanted automatic defibrillator in human beings. N Engl J Med 303:322–324, 1980

29. Lehmann MH, Steinman RT, Schuger CD, Jackson K: The automatic implantable cardioverter defibrillator as antiarrhythmic treatment modality of choice for survivors of cardiac arrest unrelated to acute myocardial infarction. Am J Cardiol 62: 803–805, 1988

30. Lehmann MH, Saksena S, for the NASPE Policy Conference Committee: Implantable cardioverter defibrillators in cardiovascular practice: report of the Policy Conference of the North American Society of Pacing and Electrophysiology. Pacing Clin Electrophysiol 14: 969–979, 1991

31. Dreifus LS, Fisch C, Griffin JC, Gillette PC, Mason JW, Parsonnet V: Guidelines for implantation of cardiac pacemakers and antiarrhythmia devices. A report of the American College of Cardiology/American Heart Association Task Force on Assessment of Diagnostic and Therapeutic Cardiovascular Procedures (Committee on Pacemaker Implantation). J Am Coll Cardiol 18:1–13, 1991

32. Saksena S, Breithardt G, Dorian P, Greene HL, Madan N, Block M: Nonpharmacological therapy for malignant ventricular arrhythmias: implantable defibrillator trials. Prog Cardiovasc Dis 38: 429–444, 1996

33. The PCD Investigator Group: Clinical outcome of patients with malignant ventricular tachyarrhythmias and a multiprogrammable implantable cardioverter-defibrillator implanted with or without thoracotomy: an international multicenter study. J Am Coll Cardiol 23:1521–1530, 1994

34. Zipes DP, Roberts D, for the Pacemaker-Cardioverter-Defibrillator Investigators: Results of the international study of the implantable pacemaker cardioverter-

defibrillator. A comparison of epicardial and endocardial lead systems. Circulation 92:59–65, 1995

35. Bardy GH, Yee R, Jung W, for the Active Can Investigators: Multicenter experience with a pectoral unipolar implantable cardioverter-defibrillator. J Am Coll Cardiol 28:400–410, 1996

36. Wever EF, Hauer RN, Schrijvers G, van Capelle FJ, Tijssen JG, Crijns HJ, Algra A, Ramanna H, Bakker PF, Robles de Medina EO: Cost-effectiveness of implantable defibrillator as first-choice therapy versus electrophysiologically guided, tiered strategy in postinfarct sudden death survivors. A randomized study. Circulation 93:489–496, 1996

37. Moss AJ, Hall WJ, Cannom DS, Daubert JP, Higgins SL, Klein H, Levine JH, Saksena S, Waldo AL, Wilber D, Brown MW, Heo M, for the Multicenter Automatic Defibrillator Implantation Trial Investigators: Improved survival with an implanted defibrillator in patients with coronary disease at high risk for ventricular arrhythmia. N Engl J Med 335: 1933–1940, 1996

38. The Antiarrhythmia Versus Implantable Defibrillators (AVID) Investigators: A comparison of antiarrhythmic-drug therapy with implantable defibrillators in patients resuscitated from near-fatal ventricular arrhythmias. N Engl J Med 337: 1576–1583, 1997

39. Gold MR, Shorofsky SR: Transvenous defibrillation lead systems. J Cardiovasc Electrophysiol 7:570–580, 1996

40. Friedman PA, Stanton MS: Thoracotomy elevates the defibrillation threshold and modifies the defibrillation dose-response curve. J Cardiovasc Electrophysiol 8: 68–73, 1997

41. Stanton MS, Hayes DL, Munger TM, Trusty JM, Espinosa RE, Shen WK, Osborn MJ, Packer DL, Hammill SC: Consistent subcutaneous prepectoral implantation of a new implantable cardioverter defibrillator. Mayo Clin Proc 69:309–314, 1994

42. Friedman PA, Stanton MS: The pacer-cardioverter-defibrillator: function and clinical experience. J Cardiovasc Electrophysiol 6:48–68, 1995

43. Siebels J, Cappato R, Ruppel R, Schneider MA, Kuck KH: Preliminary results of the Cardiac Arrest Study Hamburg (CASH). Am J Cardiol 72:109F-113F, 1993

44. Pathmanathan RK, Lau EW, Cooper J, Newton L, Skehan JD, Garratt CJ, Griffith MJ: Potential impact of antiarrhythmic drugs versus implantable defibrillators on the management of ventricular arrhythmias: the Midlands trial of empirical amiodarone versus electrophysiologically guided intervention and cardioverter implant registry data. Heart 80:68–70, 1998

45. Dorian P, Newman D, Thibault B, Phillipon F, Kimber S: A randomized clinical trial of a standardized protocol for the prevention of inappropriate therapy using a dual chamber implantable cardioverter defibrillator (abstract). Circulation 100 Suppl:I-786, 1999

46. Moss AJ: Background, outcome, and clinical implications of the Multicenter Automatic Defibrillator Implantation Trial. Am J Cardiol 80:28F–32F, 1997

47. Bigger JT Jr, for the Coronary Artery Bypass Graft (CABG) Patch Trial Investigators: Prophylactic use of implanted cardiac defibrillators in patients at high risk for ventricular arrhythmias after coronary-artery bypass graft surgery. N Engl J Med 337:1569–1575, 1997

48. Buxton AE, Fisher JD, Josephson ME, Lee KL, Pryor DB, Prystowsky EN, Simson MB, Di Carlo L, Echt DS, Packer D, Greer GS, Talajic, and the MUSTT Investigators: Prevention of sudden death in patients with coronary artery disease: the Multicenter Unsustained Tachycardia Trial (MUSTT). Prog Cardiovasc Dis 36:215–226, 1993

49. The German Dilated CardioMyopathy Study Investigators: Prospective studies assessing prophylactic therapy in high risk patients: the German Dilated CardioMyopathy Study (GDCMS)—study design. Pacing Clin Electrophysiol 15: 697–700, 1992

50. Raviele A, Bongiorni MG, Brignole M, Cappato R, Capucci A, Gaita F, Mangiameli S, Montenero A, Pedretti R, Salerno J, Sermasi S: Which strategy is "best" after myocardial infarction? The Beta-blocker Strategy plus Implantable Cardioverter Defibrillator Trial: rationale and study design. Am J Cardiol 83: 104D–111D, 1999

51. Moss AJ, Cannom DS, Daubert JP, Hall WJ, Higgins SL, Klein H, Wilber D, Zareba W, Brown MW: Multicenter Automatic Defibrillator Implantation Trial II (MADIT II): design and clinical protocol. Ann Noninvasive Electrocardiol 4:83–91, 1999

52. Bardy GH, Lee KL, Mark DB, Poole JE, Fishbein DP, Troutman C, Anderson J, Johnson G, Christian V, and the SCD-HeFT Pilot investigators: Sudden Cardiac

Death in Heart Failure Trial: pilot study (abstract). Pacing Clin Electrophysiol 20:1148, 1997

53. Saxon LA, Boehmer JP, Hummel J, Kacet S, De Marco T, Naccarelli G, Daoud E, for the VIGOR CHF and VENTAK CHF Investigators: Biventricular pacing in patients with congestive heart failure: two prospective randomized trials. Am J Cardiol 83:120D–123D, 1999

54. Mason JW, for the Electrophysiologic Study versus Electrocardiographic Monitoring Investigators: A comparison of seven antiarrhythmic drugs in patients with ventricular tachyarrhythmias. N Engl J Med 329:452–458, 1993

55. The CASCADE Investigators: Randomized antiarrhythmic drug therapy in survivors of cardiac arrest (the CASCADE Study). Am J Cardiol 72:280–287, 1993

56. Glikson M, Luria D, Friedman PA, Trusty JM, Benderly M, Hammill SC, Stanton MS: Are routine arrhythmia inductions necessary in patients with pectoral implantable cardioverter defibrillators? J Cardiovasc Electrophysiol 11:127–135, 2000

57. Bigger JT Jr, Fleiss JL, Kleiger R, Miller JP, Rolnitzky LM: The relationships among ventricular arrhythmias, left ventricular dysfunction, and mortality in the 2 years after myocardial infarction. Circulation 69:250–258, 1984

58. Buxton AE, Lee KL, Fisher JD, Josephson ME, Prystowsky EN, Hafley G: A randomized study of the prevention of sudden death in patients with coronary artery disease. Multicenter Unsustained Tachycardia Trial Investigators. N Engl J Med 341:1882–1890, 1999

59. Maron BJ, Shen WK, Link MS, Epstein AE, Almquist AK, Daubert JP, Bardy GH, Favale S, Rea RF, Boriani G, Estes NA, Spirito P, Casey SA, Stanton MS, Betocchi S: Efficacy of implantable cardioverter defibrillators for the prevention of sudden death in patients with hypertrophic cardiomyopathy. N Engl J Med 342:365–373, 2000

60. Spirito P, Seidman CE, McKenna WJ, Maron BJ: The management of hypertrophic cardiomyopathy. N Engl J Med 336:775–785, 1997

61. Borggrefe M, Breithardt G: Is the implantable defibrillator indicated in patients with hypertrophic cardiomyopathy and aborted sudden death? (Editorial.) J Am Coll Cardiol 31:1086–1088, 1998

62. Kuck KH: Arrhythmias in hypertrophic cardiomyopathy. Pacing Clin Electrophysiol 20: 2706–2713, 1997

63. Lobo TJ, Friedman PA, Rea RF, Munger TM, Hammill SC, Osborn MJ, Packer DL, Stanton MS, Shen WK: Clinical outcome following cardioverter defibrillator implantation in patients with hypertrophic cardiomyopathy (abstract). J Am Coll Cardiol 31 Suppl A:435A, 1998

64. Moss AJ: Clinical management of patients with the long QT syndrome: drugs, devices, and gene-specific therapy. Pacing Clin Electrophysiol 20:2058–2060, 1997

65. Schwartz PJ: The long QT syndrome. Curr Probl Cardiol 22:297–351, 1997

66. Moss AJ, Schwartz PJ, Crampton RS, Locati E, Carleen E: The long QT syndrome: a prospective international study. Circulation 71:17–21, 1985

67. Gronefeld G, Holtgen R, Hohnloser SH: Implantable cardioverter defibrillator therapy in a patient with the idiopathic long QT syndrome. Pacing Clin Electrophysiol 19:1260–1263, 1996

68. Brugada P, Brugada R, Brugada J, Geelen P: Use of the prophylactic implantable cardioverter defibrillator for patients with normal hearts. Am J Cardiol 83:98D–100D, 1999

69. Gussak I, Antzelevitch C, Bjerregaard P, Towbin JA, Chaitman BR: The Brugada syndrome: clinical, electrophysiologic and genetic aspects. J Am Coll Cardiol 33:5–15, 1999

70. Viskin S, Belhassen B: Polymorphic ventricular tachyarrhythmias in the absence of organic heart disease: classification, differential diagnosis, and implications for therapy. Prog Cardiovasc Dis 41:17–34, 1998

71. Link MS, Wang PJ, Haugh CJ, Homoud MK, Foote CB, Costeas XB, Estes NA III: Arrhythmogenic right ventricular dysplasia: clinical results with implantable cardioverter defibrillators. J Interventional Card Electrophysiol 1:41–48, 1997

72. Fontaine G: The use of ICD's for the treatment of patients with arrhythmogenic right ventricular dysplasia (ARVD) (letter). J Interventional Card Electrophysiol 1:329–330, 1997

73. Knight BP, Goyal R, Pelosi F, Flemming M, Horwood L, Morady F, Strickberger SA: Outcome of patients with nonischemic dilated cardiomyopathy and unexplained syncope treated with an implantable defibrillator. J Am Coll Cardiol 33:1964–1970, 1999

74. Brilakis E, Shen WK, Hammill SC, Friedman PA: Improved survival with device therapy in patients with idiopathic dilated cardiomyopathy and syncope (abstract). Circulation 100 Suppl:I-643, 1999

4

Generator and Lead Selection

David L. Hayes, M.D., Paul A. Friedman, M.D.

The purpose of this chapter is to provide direction in choosing the most appropriate pulse generator—pacemaker or implantable cardioverter-defibrillator (ICD)—and leads for a given patient. It is not possible to provide guidelines that meet the needs of every patient; indeed, pulse generator selection, both pacemaker and ICD, must be individualized.

Pacemaker Selection

Generalizations can be made about the most appropriate pacing mode and specific programmable parameters for a given underlying rhythm disturbance or other cardiovascular problem that requires permanent pacing[1] (Table 4–1).

In addition, basic hemodynamic issues should be kept in mind during pacemaker selection. These are covered in detail in Chapter 2. In summary, controversy still exists on whether morbidity and mortality are less with an atrial-based pacing mode, that is, AAI or dual-chamber, than with ventricular pacing.[2–6] Emerging findings in prospective studies are not consistent. However, our belief is that dual-chamber pacing has long-term hemodynamic benefits, and longer-term follow-up of

some of the morbidity-mortality prospective trials may yield more consistent results. Table 4–2 summarizes the status of trials to date (for a detailed discussion, see Chapter 2).

Many algorithms have been used for pulse generator and mode selection (Fig. 4–1 and 4–2). Although all rules have exceptions, a very simple approach is appropriate for most patients. For patients with chronic atrial fibrillation and a slow ventricular response in whom pacing is required, VVIR is the mode of choice. This is the only clear-cut indication for single-chamber ventricular pacing. Obviously, other patients may have associated comorbidities or other issues that would favor use of a single-chamber ventricular pacemaker, either VVI or VVIR. For example, in a patient with other irreversible medical problems or dementia in whom longevity or activity level (or both) is markedly limited, a simple device may be the most appropriate. These decisions must be made individually. However, even in the most ill patient in whom a pacemaker is being implanted, one must be certain that a simpler device, that is, VVI, does not make the patient worse by causing pacemaker syndrome.[10,11] Even for a patient with another irreversible and possibly

Table 4–1.
Indications for Various Pacing Modes

Mode	Generally agreed-upon indications	Controversial indications	Contraindications
VVI	AF with symptomatic bradycardia in the CC patient	Symptomatic bradycardia in the patient with associated terminal illness or other medical conditions from which recovery is not anticipated and pacing is life-sustaining only	Patients with known PM syndrome or hemodynamic deterioration with ventricular pacing at the time of implantation CI patient who will benefit from rate response Patients with hemodynamic need for dual-chamber pacing
VVIR	Fixed atrial arrhythmias (AF or atrial flutter) with symptomatic brady-cardia in the CI patient	Same as for VVI	Same as for VVI
AAI	Symptomatic bradycardia as a result of SND in the otherwise CC patient when AV conduction can be proven normal		SND with associated AV block demonstrated either spontaneously or during preimplantation testing In the unlikely event that atrial sensing is inadequate
AAIR	Symptomatic bradycardia as a result of SND in the CI patient when AV conduction can be proven normal		Same as for AAI
VDD	Congenital AV block AV block when sinus node function can be proven normal		SND AV block accompanied by SND When adequate atrial sensing cannot be attained AV block accompanied by paroxysmal supraventricular tachycardias
VDDR*	Same as for VDD, but when a potential need for ventricular rate-adaptive pacing also exists		Same as for VDD
DDD†	AV block and SND in the CC patient Need for AV synchrony, e.g., to maximize cardiac output, inactive patients	For any rhythm disturbance when atrial sensing and capture are possible, with the exception of AF or atrial flutter, potentially to minimize future AF, reduce morbidity, and improve survival	Chronic AF, atrial flutter, giant inexcitable atrium, or other frequent paroxysmal supraventricular tachyarrhythmias

continues

Table 4–1. (*Continued*)

Mode	Generally agreed-upon indications	Controversial indications	Contraindications
	Previous PM syndrome	For the suppression of tachyarrhythmias by overdrive suppression	When adequate atrial sensing cannot be attained
DDDR	AV block and SND in the CI patient	Same as for DDD	Same as for DDD

AF, atrial fibrillation; AV, atrioventricular; CC, chronotropically competent; CI, chronotropically incompetent; PM, pacemaker; SND, sinus node dysfunction.

*VDDR pacing mode would be more clearly stated as VDD + VVIR. If the patient does not have intrinsic atrial activity, the pacemaker functions as a VVI pacing device or as VVIR if rate-adaptive pacing is triggered.

†DDI and DDIR are not included as separate modes in this table. With widespread availability of DDDR devices, DDI and DDIR are rarely used as the preimplantation modes of choice.

progressive medical illness and marked limitations in activity in whom a decision is made to implant a pacemaker, if VVI pacing results in pacemaker syndrome, the patient may actually feel worse. Although such an outcome may be impossible to predict, it should at least be considered and blood pressures recorded in the native underlying rhythm and with ventricular pacing. If this is done during implantation and a marked decrease in blood pressure occurs with pacing, that is, 15 to 20 mm Hg or more, dual-chamber pacing should be reconsidered.

Atrial Fibrillation With a Slow Ventricular Response

For most patients with bradyarrhythmias requiring pacing who do not have chronic atrial fibrillation, a dual-chamber pacemaker is indicated. If the

Table 4–2.
Trials Assessing the Effect of Pacing Mode on Morbidity and Mortality

Danish study[3]	Cumulative incidence of cardiovascular death, paroxysmal or chronic atrial fibrillation, and thromboembolic events lower with AAI pacing; less severe heart failure with AAI; multivariate analysis: AAI associated with freedom from thromboembolic events and survival from cardiovascular death
PASE[4]	Quality of life improved significantly overall, but no difference between VVIR and DDDR; 26% of patients with VVIR crossed over to DDDR due to pacemaker syndrome; trends of borderline statistical significance in end points favoring DDDR pacing in patients with sinus node dysfunction
CTOPP[5]	No difference in quality of life between VVI and DDD/AAI; no statistically significant difference in mortality or stroke; no difference in number of hospitalizations; 24% decrease in incidence of atrial fibrillation with DDD/AAI
MOST[7]	In progress
UKPACE[8]	In progress
DANPACE[9]	In progress

CTOPP, Canadian Trial of Physiologic Pacing; DANPACE, Danish Pacing Trial; MOST, Mode Selection Trial; PASE, Pacemaker Selection in the Elderly; UKPACE, United Kingdom Pacing and Cardiovascular Events.

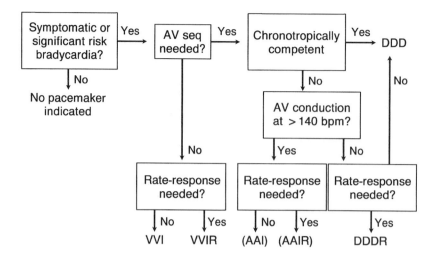

Fig. 4–1. Algorithm for pacing mode selection that includes most available pacing modes. AV, atrioventricular; seq, sequential.

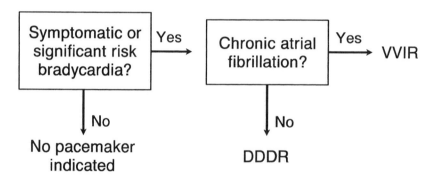

Fig. 4–2. Algorithm for pacing mode selection that includes only DDDR and VVIR pacing modes.

patient has a normal sinus node and normal chronotropic response, a DDD pacemaker is appropriate. If the patient has sinus node disease, which implies associated chronotropic incompetence or the potential for it, a DDDR pacemaker is indicated. Exceptions can be made in either direction. Using DDDR pacemakers in all patients requiring dual-chamber pacing provides the greatest long-term flexibility in programming options. Although DDDR pacemakers are, in general, initially more expensive than DDD pacemakers, long-term cost savings may accrue if a problem develops that can be solved by the pro-

gramming options of a DDDR pacemaker. For example, if chronic atrial fibrillation with a slow ventricular response later develops, the DDDR pacemaker could be reprogrammed to VVIR. A DDD pacemaker, which has no rate-adaptive capability, could be programmed only to VVI, potentially not optimal for the patient.

Pure Sinus Node Dysfunction

For the patient with pure sinus node disease, that is, no documented or provocable abnormalities in atrioventricular

(AV) nodal conduction, AAIR pacing may be appropriate. (Preimplantation criteria for AAI/AAIR pacing are described in Chapter 3.) If preimplantation testing has established normal AV nodal conduction, the annual risk of AV block developing is 1% to 2%.[12] If AV block develops, another procedure is required to implant a ventricular lead and upgrade the pacemaker. This additional procedure is obviated if a DDDR pacemaker is used initially.

Pure Atrioventricular Block

For the patient with pure AV node disease, that is, no documented abnormalities in sinus node behavior, VDD or VDDR pacing may be appropriate.[13] Specifically, the patient with congenital complete heart block may do well with VDD(R) pacing. As before, a problem arises if sinus node dysfunction develops in the future, resulting in a suboptimal pacing mode without reasonable programming options.

Neurocardiogenic Syncope and Carotid Sinus Hypersensitivity

If a patient requires pacing for neurocardiogenic syncope, whether the vasovagal variety or carotid sinus hypersensitivity, dual-chamber pacing is necessary for several reasons.[14–19] In a patient with vasovagal syncope that most likely has some component of vasodepression together with the cardioinhibition that requires pacing, ventricular pacing alone could result in pacemaker syndrome and further aggravate symptoms caused by hypotension. The bradycardia that occurs in patients with carotid sinus hypersensitivity may be due to either AV block or sinus arrest. Therefore, ventricular pacing support is required, and dual-chamber pacing is superior for the reasons already noted.

Cardiomyopathic States

Pacing for hypertrophic and dilated cardiomyopathies is discussed in Chapters 2 and 3. If pacing is used in patients with hypertrophic cardiomyopathy, a dual-chamber pacemaker is required.[20–22] Any hemodynamic advantage of pacing is lost with single-chamber pacing. The only possible exception is the patient with hypertrophic cardiomyopathy and chronic atrial fibrillation. The only pacing mode of choice is VVI(R) if pacing is indicated for associated bradyarrhythmias. If pacing is for hemodynamic improvement alone, few data support VVI(R) pacing in such a situation.

With pacing for hemodynamic improvement in dilated cardiomyopathy, few patients benefit from standard right atrial and right ventricular dual-chamber pacing.[22–24] In this group of patients, either right atrial and biventricular stimulation or right atrial and left ventricular stimulation currently appears to be the most hemodynamically advantageous pacing configuration. More data are needed to determine the superior approach to implanting the system. In the patient with dilated cardiomyopathy and chronic atrial fibrillation, VVIR pacing with biventricular stimulation or possibly a left ventricular pacing site alone may convey hemodynamic improvement.

Cardiac Transplantation

The ideal pacing mode in the patient requiring pacing after cardiac transplantation is controversial.[25] Most patients requiring pacing after cardiac transplantation have sinus node dysfunction. In these patients, arguments can be made for dual-chamber pacing for all the reasons presented earlier in this chapter. Others have argued for an even more elaborate system of placing two atrial leads, one in the recipient atrium and one in the donor atrium.

Conversely, because of the relatively infrequent and short-term (6 months or less) need for pacing in many of the patients, an argument could be made for minimizing the procedure and hardware and implanting a "backup" VVI pacemaker. The patient would still be protected from isolated symptomatic bradycardia.

In a patient with the uncommon occurrence of AV block after cardiac trans-plantation, dual-chamber pacing should be provided.

Choosing Specific Programmable Options

Programming and the wide variety of programmable options available in current devices are covered in Chapter 7. Specific programmable options need to be available for specific conditions. Table 4–3 summarizes these considerations.

Table 4–3.
Programmable Options for Pacemakers

Parameter	Underlying rhythm disturbance or cardiac condition	Justification for use
Hysteresis	Patient in whom pacing will rarely be needed and a clinical decision is made to implant a VVI pacemaker.	Hysteresis allows greater maintenance of sinus rhythm if an initial longer cycle length is required to initiate pacing.
Mode switch	Patients with a history of paroxysmal atrial tachyarrhythmias. (An argument can be made for always providing dual-chamber pacemakers with mode-switch capability should paroxysmal atrial tachyarrhythmia develop in the future or the patient have asymptomatic paroxysmal atrial tachyarrhythmias.)	Allows programming to a tracking mode but prevents tracking if the paroxysmal atrial tachyarrhythmia occurs.
Search hysteresis or Rate Drop Response	Patients with neurocardiogenic syncope.	May help to minimize symptoms associated with neurocardiogenic syncope. The mechanism by which improvement occurs is not clearly understood, but some believe that pacing more rapidly at the onset of symptoms may help to blunt vasodepressor response.
Ventricular rate stabilization algorithms	Patients with atrial fibrillation.	May help to improve tolerance of atrial fibrillation by minimizing variation in ventricular cycle length.
Atrial rate stabilization algorithms	Patients with paroxysmal atrial fibrillation or flutter.	May help to minimize recurrences of these rhythm disturbances.

Choosing the Lead or Leads

A detailed discussion of the merits of various lead types is beyond the scope of this chapter, as is a thorough discussion of the evolution of pacing leads. Rather, the purpose of the chapter is to provide the reader with an understanding of the types of leads that are available and future trends that are likely to be seen.

With the exception of a few specific circumstances, choice of the pacing lead or leads becomes one of personal preference and personal bias. Options that must be considered for all leads are

- Type of insulation: silicone or polyurethane
- Mechanism of fixation: active or passive
- Polarity: unipolar or bipolar
- Compatibity of lead and pulse generator

Choice of an atrial lead must take into account insulation, fixation, polarity, and straight or preformed J type (Fig. 4–3 *A*). The interelectrode distance of a bipolar lead also deserves consideration. This distance affects the duration of the intracardiac electrogram but has little effect on the amplitude and slew rate of the electrogram. A lead with greater distance between electrodes has greater far-field signals. This characteristic may affect mode-switching reliability. In pacing systems with more than one ventricular sensing lead, that is, pacemaker and ICD in the same patient or ICD with biventricular pacing, minimizing far-field signals may also be of increased importance.

The same decisions must be made for choice of the ventricular lead, except that all ventricular leads are straight (Fig. 4–3 *B*).

Although multiple mechanisms have been used to achieve lower thresholds, steroid elution has been the most successful and most widely used method for threshold reduction.[26,27] Steroid elution may be accomplished in several ways, such as from a steroid-saturated silicone plug within the electrode or from a collar around the electrode (Fig. 4–3 *C*). Steroid elution significantly minimizes the threshold evolution that is normal with standard electrodes. The lead contains a very small amount of steroid, for example, 1 mg of dexamethasone sodium phosphate, which does not have any systemic effect. Steroid elution is now available on atrial and ventricular, active and passive leads. In our institution, steroid-eluting leads are used routinely.

Insulation

With few exceptions, the materials that have been used for most pacing leads are silicone rubber and polyurethane. Historically, both have excellent performance records. Table 4–4 compares the basic characteristics of silicone rubber and polyurethane.[28] When first introduced, polyurethane leads were widely used by many implanters because they had a smaller diameter than many of the contemporary silicone rubber leads and were said to handle better when two leads were implanted. Improvements in silicone insulation have made these differences less significant.

Manufacturers often make the same lead available with either silicone or polyurethane outer insulation. Implanters base their choice on past experience, ideally taking into account product surveillance reports that detail the survival of specific leads.

Table 4–4 requires comment. Not all agree on what is advantageous or disadvantageous about the characteristics of the insulating material.

For silicone rubber, "very flexible" may or may not be an advantage. This quality means that something else in the design, such as the conductor coil, must increase the stiffness of the lead to the

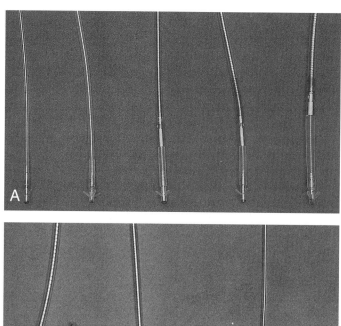

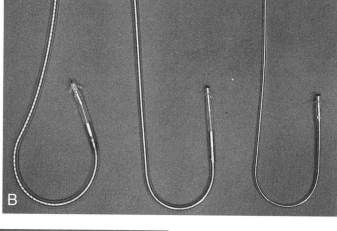

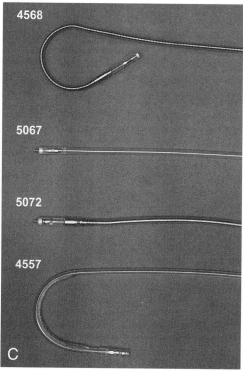

4568

5067

5072

4557

Fig. 4–3. *A,* A variety of passive fixation leads. Passive fixation leads are available in unipolar and bipolar designs. The first three leads, left to right, are bipolar, and the last two leads are unipolar. Electrode spacing in the bipolar leads varies. *B,* A variety of passive fixation preformed J leads. The left and middle leads are bipolar, and the right lead is unipolar. *C,* Active fixation leads may be straight or preformed J, unipolar or bipolar. Preformed J leads are used only in the atrium, and straight active fixation leads may be used in either chamber. The fixation mechanism varies, that is, the screw may be retractable or nonretractable. In some, the nonretractable screw is coated with a material that dissolves once in the bloodstream. This allows the lead to be passed into the heart without an exposed screw catching on the vascular tree. *Continues.*

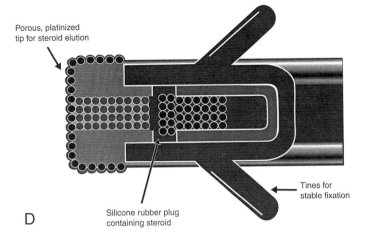

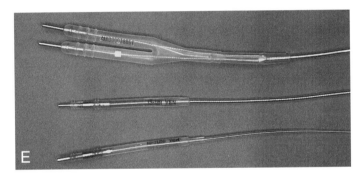

Fig. 4–3 *continued. D,* Diagrammatic representation of a steroid-eluting lead. Steroid (dexa-methasone) is slowly eluted through the porous, platinized tip of a silicone rubber plug. *E,* Three pacemaker lead connectors currently in use. *Top,* Bifurcated bipolar lead. These leads are not commonly used for new systems, but many are still in use. *Middle,* VS-1 in-line bipolar lead. *Bottom,* VS-1 unipolar lead; the ring electrode is inactive.

Table 4–4.
Lead Insulation: Comparison of Silicone Rubber and Polyurethane

Silicone rubber	Polyurethane
Advantages	
• Performance record > 30 years	• High tear strength
• Easy fabrication and molding (?) (see text)	• High cut resistance
• Repairable (?) (see text)	• Low friction in blood
	• High abrasion resistance
	• Inherently less thrombogenic
	• Superior compressive properties
Disadvantages	
• Tears easily	• Relatively stiff (?) (especially 55D) (see text)
• Cuts easily	• Not repairable (?) (see text)
• Higher friction in blood	• Sensitive to manufacturing process
• Subject to cold flow failure	• Potential for environmental stress cracking (true for Pellethane 80A)
• More thrombogenic	• Potential for metal ion oxidation (true for Pellethane 80A and 55D)

optimal value. A lead that is too flexible can damage the heart with excessive movement and can cause dislodgment. A lead that is too stiff can cause perforation or dislodgment. A stiff conductor is more prone to fracture.

"Easy fabrication and molding" is debatable. This might be true for processes that are very low in volume and more expensive. In fact, polyurethane extrusion and molding are much easier, especially for large volumes.

Some sources state that silicone rubber has a manufacturing quality of "low process sensitivity." This is not true, especially for modern platinum-cured materials. They are easily "scorched," and this effect causes embrittlement and propensity to crack.

"Smaller diameter possible" is not included because it is neither an advantage nor a disadvantage. It is the result of the polymer's high tear strength and higher stiffness. That is, even if silicone rubber had the same tear strength as polyurethane, smaller diameter insulation would make a lead like a whipsaw. Higher stiffness allows a thinner tube to maintain high torque strength for implantability, but the thin tube makes the structure flexible in bending. Therefore, an advantage of polyurethane is "higher stiffness" combined with "high tear strength."

Polyurethane has vastly superior compressive properties, specifically low creep or "cold-flow." In addition, many persons agree that polyurethane is inherently less thrombogenic. The ability to use thermoplastic extrusion and molding is a definite manufacturing advantage. Although silicone rubber has been available longer, polyurethane has a record of 24 years in human use as lead insulation.

Silicone rubber is sometimes criticized for "absorbing lipids (calcifications)." Although lipid absorption is reported in the literature for ball and cage heart valves, it has not been proven to be clinically significant in pacing leads and does not appear to result in failures. Lipid absorption and calcification are two different phenomena. Even though mineralization of encapsulating sheaths (extrinsic mineralization) is common, there is no evidence that it causes failure (although it greatly hinders removal of old leads). Mineralization of the silicone rubber per se (intrinsic mineralization) is also seen sometimes, but failures are rare.

For polyurethane, "relatively stiff" is a disadvantage to one who does not know how to make a lead small enough to take advantage of the fact that the bending moment of a tube varies with modulus ("stiffness") and diameter to the fourth power. Today, the higher "stiffness" is an advantage, allowing manufacturers to make small, tough leads that are relatively easy to implant.

"Not repairable" as a disadvantage for polyurethane insulated leads is partially true. Outer insulation repair with medical adhesive and silicone film works well if the repair is done correctly. Terminal pin replacement kits work well on unipolar leads. Repair of inner insulation and replacement of bipolar terminals appear to be hopeless today.

"Sensitive to manufacturing process" is a disadvantage for both materials. Knowledge is required to work with either one. The potential for environmental surface cracking remains true for Pellethane 80A and similar material but is not a significant mechanism of clinical failure in modern leads anymore, especially those using Pellethane 55D. This problem can be designed around. The potential for metal ion oxidation remains an issue, even for Pellethane 55D leads.

In the 1980s, problems arose with specific polyurethane leads that had been implanted in large numbers in the United States.[29,30] These leads had an incidence of failure that was not clinically acceptable. Although several different types of polyurethane were implicated in the failures, the insulation material that accounted for the largest number of failures was Pellethane 80A. The mechanisms of these failures were established and manufacturing processes altered. The reader is referred elsewhere for specific information on these lead failure mechanisms.[31,32] Despite this blemish on polyurethane leads, the overall survival rate for polyurethane leads is excellent.

What is an acceptable rate of lead failure? Ideally, leads would never fail, but it is unlikely that this level of reliability will ever be reached. Most manufacturers strive for a 5-year lead survival rate of 98% or higher.

Lead Polarity

Bipolar leads are used more frequently in the United States. This preference exists largely because of the lower susceptibility to electromagnetic interference when pacemakers are in a bipolar sensing configuration.[33–35] Bipolar leads have had an overall higher incidence of failure than unipolar leads, largely because of the specific bipolar leads that failed in high numbers in the 1980s.[29,30] If these leads were excluded from the analysis, the survival difference between unipolar and bipolar leads would be minimal. The same experts who prefer unipolar leads would argue that improved sensing circuitry in the past decade has minimized interference from electromagnetic sources.

Compatibility of Lead and Pulse Generator

The pacemaker lead or leads and pulse generator selected do not need to be from the same manufacturer. It is fine to "mix and match" leads from company X with a pulse generator from company Y. What is mandatory is that the lead connector be compatible with the header of the pulse generator.

Historically, unipolar leads were 5 or 6 mm in diameter and bipolar leads were of the bifurcated design. Most leads currently used are of "in-line" bipolar design with a 3.2-mm diameter (Fig. 4–3 *D*). In 1986, an international standard for leads and connectors was established. This voluntary standard for leads and connectors incorporating sealing rings on a 3.2-mm lead connector is referred to as VS-1.[36] Subsequently, an industry-wide standard configuration known as IS-1 (international standard 1) was accepted. Figure 4–4 shows the five types of lead connectors available, and Figure 4–5 demonstrates varieties of in-line bipolar

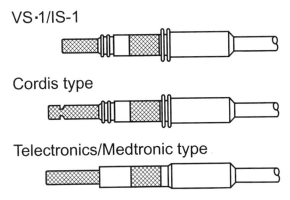

Fig. 4–4. Common varieties of VS-1 leads. *Top diagram,* IS-1, VS-1 lead type. *Middle diagram,* 3.2-mm connector with sealing rings, referred to as the Cordis type. *Bottom diagram,* 3.2-mm connector pin without sealing rings, referred to as the Medtronics or Telectronics type.

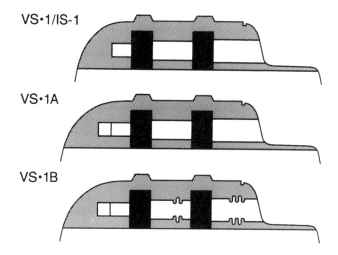

VS·1/IS-1

VS·1A

VS·1B

Fig. 4–5. Available types of in-line pulse generator headers.

pulse generator headers. "Unipolar" leads comply with the same design features, but the ring electrode on a dedicated unipolar lead is electrically inactive.

Epicardial Leads

Epicardial (myocardial) leads are not commonly used. Epicardial pacing may still be necessary in patients with congenital cardiac anomalies that prevent the access needed for transvenous leads, with a prosthetic tricuspid valve, or with other tricuspid valve abnormalities that preclude lead placement across the valve. Figure 4–6 demonstrates available types of epicardial fixation mechanisms. Platinized and steroid-eluting epicardial leads are now available. Epi-

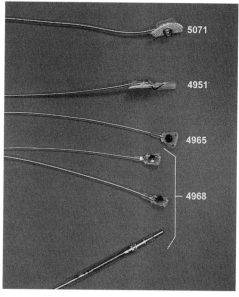

Fig. 4–6. Commonly used epicardial fixation mechanisms. From bottom to top: bipolar "button" lead, Medtronic 4968, which must be sutured to the epicardial surface with contact between the button and the myocardium (the bipolar in-line connector is also shown); epicardial platinized "button" (suture on) unipolar lead, Metronic 4965; epicardial "stab-in" lead, Medtronic 4951; and two-turn screw-in lead, Medtronic 5071.

cardial leads have historically had higher thresholds than transvenous leads. Incorporation of platinized surfaces and steroid elution is an attempt to keep epicardial pacing thresholds lower.[37,38]

Resources for Lead Performance and Survival Data

Lead choice is often determined by the implanter's personal experience or experience during training, that is, the lead choice of the mentor. As new leads become available, it is important to be aware of resources of lead survival and performance. Resources include

- Manufacturers' data
- Published information from individual centers or cooperating centers
- Public databases

Manufacturers are required by law to collect postmarketing surveillance data on hardware performance. Various manufacturers use different approaches for collection and analysis of this information, but performance data should be available from any manufacturer on request. Figure 4–7 is an example of lead performance and survival data from one manufacturer in a report that is regularly updated.

Follow-up data may be obtained from registry information[39] or from centers that publish survival and performance data on individual leads[40,41] (Fig. 4–8). A literature search is likely to yield an implanter with information on many of the most widely used leads.

There is no independent comprehensive database of leads or pulse generators in the United States. Although there have been attempts at developing such a database, it has yet to be accomplished. As of this writing, a database is operational for documenting hardware failures for leads, pacemakers, and ICDs. Because only failures are reported, the database does not provide an incidence with which specific failures might occur, but it may alert one to a potential problem or allow a search to see if others have reported a similar problem. This website, www.pacerandicdregistry.com, is best described by the introduction on the first page:

The purpose of the Registry is to provide physicians, nurses and technicians with information they can use to manage their pacemaker and ICD patients. Our database gathers pacemaker, ICD and lead failure data from clinics and hospitals worldwide. Members are able to search the database and discover which models are failing, when they are failing and why they are failing. We also receive reports about device idiosyncrasies. Idiosyncrasies are behaviors which may cause no harm or necessitate device replacement, but may confuse or mislead a practitioner.

Members have full access to the database. Only members enter information and the Registry reviews data for authenticity and completeness before they are made available to other members. Members may search the Registry's database 24 hours a day. Failure data is categorized according to presentation— expected and unexpected, sign of failure, and reason for failure. Battery depletions for a given model are presented graphically so that follow-up schedules can be adjusted based on actual clinical experience. Members are alerted by e-mail when unexpected pacemaker or ICD failures are reported.

Descriptions of device idiosyncrasies are contained in the database. They encompass a variety of observations, some of which are simply unexplained, or poorly understood. Reports include information as to how the problem was "solved" or at least managed. Members are encouraged to offer their diagnosis and/or solution.

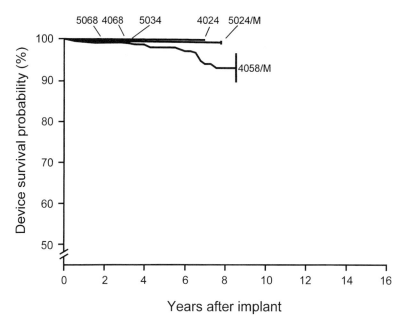

Fig. 4–7. Lead survival data from postmarket surveillance data gathered by Medtronic, Inc. This type of graphic display of performance of leads and pulse generators is made available regularly by the manufacturer. (By permission of Medtronic, Inc.)

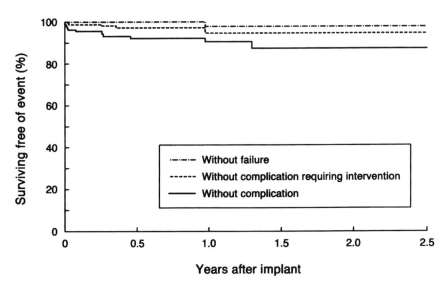

Fig. 4–8. Kaplan-Meier survival curves for a specific transvenous lead from a surveillance study by a single center. The figure designates leads without failure as well as those associated with any other pacing system complication that did or did not require intervention. This information can be obtained by a literature search or from the manufacturer. (From Glikson et al.[41] By permission of Futura Publishing Company.)

Generator and Lead Selection in Defibrillators

Many of the considerations in selecting an appropriate pacing system for a patient—the use of tined or active fixation leads, the need for mode switching or other pacing features—are identical in defibrillator selection and are not repeated here. Other issues, however, either are unique to defibrillators or take on added dimensions, including

- Use of integrated or bipolar sensing
- Pulse generator size in relation to longevity
- Maximum shock output
- Upper pacing rate
- Pacing and defibrillation with a dual- or a single-chamber device and arrhythmia discrimination

Integrated and Bipolar Sensing Compared

The right ventricular lead of a transvenous defibrillator serves three distinct purposes: signal sensing, bradycardia and antitachycardia pacing, and shock delivery. All such leads currently manufactured are tripolar (that is, they have three electrodes), but the distribution of function across the electrodes has varied. In leads with true bipolar sensing, sensing and pacing occur between the tip electrode and a closely spaced dedicated ring (Fig. 4–9). Since the two electrodes of the bipolar pair used for sensing are both small and closely spaced, the physics of the configuration reject far-field signals efficiently. However, because true bipolar leads have only a single defibrillation coil, they must be used with an active can defibrillator or with additional leads containing defibrillation elements. Of note, all defibrillators currently manufactured are available with an active can because of the greater defibrillation efficacy.

Integrated sensing lead systems are constructed with a distal tip electrode for pacing and sensing, a distal coil for both pacing and sensing and for defibrillation, and a proximal coil for defibrillation (Fig. 4–9). This design has the advantage of incorporating two defibrillation coils, which

True bipolar

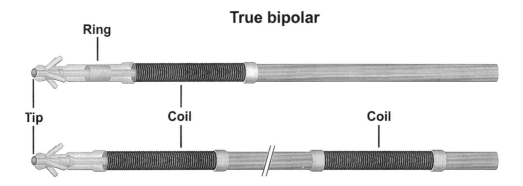

Integrated bipolar

Fig. 4–9. True bipolar (*top*) and integrated bipolar (*bottom*) leads. The true bipolar lead senses between the distal tip and the proximal ring, which are dedicated for pacing and sensing. True bipolar leads have a single coil. In contrast, integrated bipolar leads pace and sense between the tip and the distal coil. The distal coil is used for sensing, pacing, and defibrillation. Integrated bipolar leads also contain a second, proximal coil, increasing the lead surface area for defibrillation.

in conjunction with an active can device most likely lower defibrillation thresholds, although this effect has not been uniformly observed.[42,43] In early lead designs, the distance from the tip to the distal coil was small (6 mm) to minimize detection of far-field signals; however, it was found that with a distally placed coil, the amplitude of the recorded electrogram diminished significantly after a shock, an effect that could on rare occasions lead to failure to redetect continuing ventricular fibrillation if an initial shock was unsuccessful[44,45] (Fig. 4–10). The mechanisms of postshock electrogram diminution include impaired myocyte cellular membrane function due to the proximity of the high-density electrical field to the endocardium, local release of neurotransmitters, electrode polarization (since the shocking electrode is used for sensing), and signal energy effects of the integrated lead design.[45,46] Subsequent to this early experience, integrated leads have been redesigned with a greater distance be-

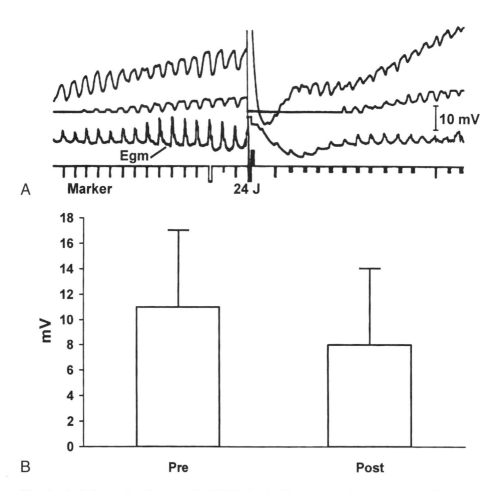

A   Marker   24 J

B   Pre   Post

Fig. 4–10. *A*, Recording from a failed 24-J shock. The endocardial electrogram (Egm) amplitude is diminished by the 24-J shock, although undersensing does not occur in this example from a true bipolar lead. *B*, Mean ventricular fibrillation electrogram amplitude before (Pre) and just after (Post) failed shocks. (Modified from Brady et al.[45] By permission of Excerpta Medica.)

tween the distal coil and the lead tip (12 mm), ameliorating postshock electrogram diminution, so that it is no longer a clinical consideration.[47,48]

Although the greater distance between the tip and the coil has resolved postshock sensing problems, it has introduced problems with oversensing of far-field signals in a small number of patients. The cause is the effectively larger antenna created by the greater intrabipole distance. Moreover, to detect the small-amplitude fibrillation signals that may follow a relatively large R wave, defibrillators utilize dynamic sensing or gain. In most defibrillators, the effective sensitivity after a sensed R wave increases with each passing millisecond until the maximum sensitivity is reached[49] (Fig. 4–11). Thus, patients with slow heart rates—which allow more time after a QRS complex for the effective sensitivity to increase—are at increased risk for this type of oversensing. Since sensitivity (or gain) is rapidly maximized after a paced event, patients with slow rates of pacing are the most likely to experience far-field myopotential oversensing, often because phrenic potentials are oversensed (Fig. 4–12). When it occurs, it can result in suppression of bradycardia pacing or inappropriate detection of ventricular tachyarrhythmias[50] (Fig. 4–12). The stored electrograms resemble those seen with a loose set screw. However, the distinction is important to make, because the oversensing usually responds well to decreasing the programmed sensitivity, although appropriate detection of ventricular fibrillation should be verified.[50]

In summary, for most patients, either integrated or true bipolar sensing leads function well. Patients who are pacemaker-dependent usually have both risks for oversensing—a high frequency of pacing (resulting in maximal effective sensitivity) and a slow pacing rate—so that true bipolar pacing may be preferred, although this has not been formally stud-ied. For patients in whom a high defibrillation threshold is anticipated, an integrated lead may be desirable. Although the literature has been inconsistent on risk factors for an increased threshold, patients with significant hypertrophy (as in hypertrophic cardiomyopathy) or marked dilatation are most likely at risk, particularly if receiving amiodarone.[51–53] However, because increased thresholds are difficult to predict, studies on the benefit of adding a superior vena cava coil are discordant,[42,43] and additional defibrillation elements can be added on separate leads if needed, true bipolar sensing is preferable if a pacemaker-dependent patient appears to be at risk for an increased defibrillation threshold. Moreover, any patient with a concomitant pacemaker should receive a true bipolar sensing lead to minimize the risk that the defibrillator will detect pacing stimuli, which can result in life-threatening device-device interactions.[54]

Size and Longevity

In general, larger devices have greater battery capacity and thus greater longevity. Patient size, particularly in smaller patients or children, may constrain the site of device placement, because of either limited pectoral tissue to support the device or cosmetic concerns. In these situations, the options available are smaller devices with shorter longevity, subpectoral placement, and abdominal placement. When device size becomes a significant factor, the technically simplest solution may be to use the smallest available device and insert it prepectorally, despite potential limits to longevity. In 2000, a 45-cc single-chamber device had a predicted longevity of 7.3 years with 15% pacing and quarterly capacitor charges. A similar device with a 39-cc displacement had a rated longevity of 4.8 years. Technology is rapidly improving, however, and the trade-off is

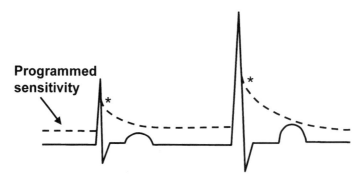

Fig. 4–11. Schematic illustration of dynamic sensing used by many defibrillators. When a QRS event is sensed (*), the sensitivity is decreased to avoid detecting the T wave that follows. The sensitivity progressively increases over time until the next QRS complex is sensed. This progressive sensitivity (or gain adjustment, depending on device) permits defibrillators to detect small fibrillation electrograms and at the same time avoid double counting of QRS complexes and T waves. Because of the progressive increase in gain, the risk of oversensing noncardiac signals is greater with slower heart rates.

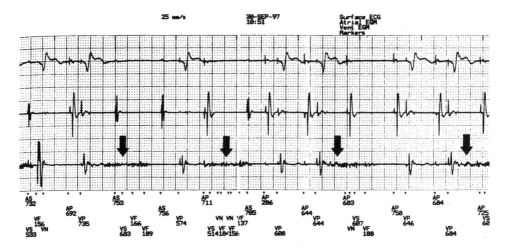

Fig. 4–12. Myopotential oversensing. Real-time recordings are from the surface electrocardiogram, atrial electrogram, and ventricular electrogram (*top* to *bottom*). During labored breathing with the patient at rest, bursts of diaphragmatic myopotential activity (*arrows*) result in inhibition of bradycardia pacing with periods of asystole. Note detection of sensed ventricular fibrillation events in association with oversensing. AP, atrial pace; AS, atrial sense; VF, ventricular fibrillation zone sense; VN, ventricular noise during noise response window; VP, ventricular pace; VS, ventricular sense. (From Deshmukh and Anderson.[50] By permission of Futura Publishing Company.)

becoming smaller. If a dual-chamber system is required, for example, devices as small as 39 cc, available in 2000, have a longevity of 6 years, depending on pacing mode and capacitor charge frequency. Even with selection of the smallest device, alternative insertion sites may be preferable at times. A large study directly comparing subcutaneous and submuscular defibrillator insertion found no significant difference in complication rates.[55] Submuscular placement is discussed in greater detail in Chapter 5. Abdominal placement, on the other hand, should generally be avoided. Not only is it more challenging—requiring two incisions, lead tunneling, abdominal dissection (often necessitating surgical assistance), and general anesthesia—but also it has a greater risk of infection, a threat of peritoneal erosion, and an increased risk of lead fracture, even with totally transvenous systems.[56-58] Further technological advancements will result in progressively smaller devices in the near future. Table 4–5 summarizes device size and longevity for devices commercially available in 2000.

Maximum Shock Output

Maximum shock output may also affect device size, with devices having higher output tending to be larger (Table 4–5). The ability to electrically revert ventricular fibrillation is a function of multiple factors, including lead design, lead position relative to the fibrillating myocardium, waveform, and shock energy. Nonetheless, intuitively it would seem desirable to select a device with a greater output for patients predicted to have an increased defibrillation threshold. This approach faces two significant challenges. First, as noted above, predicting which patients will have an increased defibrillation threshold remains a problem. Studies assessing the influence of left ventricular size, ejection fraction, and left ventricular mass on defibrillation have had discordant results for each factor.[51,59-62] Second, as discussed in detail in Chapter 1, some waveforms are intrinsically more efficient than others. The need for subcutaneous leads may be a marker for borderline defibrillation effectiveness, since they are not typically implanted unless totally transvenous defibrillation thresholds are not acceptable. We found that in biphasic modern devices, the frequency of subcutaneous lead usage was low (less than 4%) and not affected by device out-

put, again suggesting that with current devices, maximum output is an infrequent consideration.[63] Development of smaller, lower output devices could make device output a more important consideration in the future.

Table 4–5 lists the maximum output of devices available in early 2000. As a simple rule, in patients with hypertrophic cardiomyopathy and significantly thickened left ventricular walls or marked dilatation, it is best to choose higher output devices (roughly 35 J or more), although the number of patients in whom this is an active consideration is relatively small. Additionally, if a device with lower output is preferable for other reasons (for example, size, features), defibrillation testing can be performed by connecting the leads to an emulator, determining the threshold, and using the lower output device if the threshold is acceptable. This approach, however, is more cumbersome and rarely needed.

Upper Rate Limit

In patients who do not require bradycardia pacing, the pacing upper rate limit constraints of the defibrillator do not need to be considered. However, in patients who require bradycardia pacing beyond emergency or postshock backup—patients who receive rate-responsive single-chamber systems or dual-chamber systems with or without a sensor—upper rate characteristics can on rare occasions merit consideration. Because defibrillators must be able to sense the small electrograms of fibrillation when it occurs, many devices put constraints on the upper pacing rate to maintain a "quiet" window for detection, free from pacing stimuli. In Medtronic and Guidant devices, for example, the ventriculoatrial interval must be greater than the lowest tachycardia detection interval (in milliseconds) to allow an adequate window of detection

Table 4–5.
Device Size, Longevity, Pacing, and Maximum Output Characteristics (Biphasic, Active Can Systems) for Various Defibrillators*

Manufacturer	Model	Size, cc	Maximum output, J	Single or dual	Rate response	Atrial therapies	Maximum pacing rate	VT rate minus bradycardia URL, bpm	Longevity (15% pacing, quarterly shocks), yr
ELA Medical	9201	75	33	Dual	No	No	172†	Bradycardia URL, not restricted by VT rate; overlap permitted	5.7
Guidant	1783	57	31	Single	No	No	100	5‡	7.6§
	1788	53	36	Single	No	No	100	5‡	7.5§
	1790	39	31	Single	No	No	100	5‡	4.8§
	1774	51	31	Single	Yes	No	175	5‡	4.9–5.2 (depending on pacing mode)§
	1851	39	31	Dual	Yes	No	175	5‡	6.8–7.2 (depending on pacing mode)§
Medtronic	7223	54	30	Single	No	No	120	10∥	7.5¶
	7229	39	30	Single	Yes	No	150	10∥	5.7¶
	7271	62	35	Dual	Yes	No	120	10∥	6.9–9 (depending on EGM storage options)
	7273	39.5	30	Dual	Yes	No	150	10∥	4.6–4.8 (depending on pacing mode)¶
	7250	56	27	Dual	No	Yes; independently programmable atrial defibrillation vectors	120	10∥	5–8

St. Jude	V186	34	32	Single	No	No	90	10#	5.5
	V180	44	31	Single	No	No	90	10#	5.5
	V190								
	C175	57	42	Single	No	No	90	10#	6.1
	C185								

EGM, electrogram; URL, upper rate limit; VT, ventricular tachycardia.

*Not all models from all manufacturers are represented.

†Limited by the total atrial refractory period.

‡A difference greater than 5 bpm may be required. To ensure an adequate detection window, the ventriculoatrial interval (milliseconds) must be greater than the slowest tachycardia detection window (milliseconds). Additionally, the maximum ventricular refractory period (milliseconds) is less than half the maximum sensor rate or the maximum tracking rate, whichever is faster.

§Onset electrogram storage turned on. Recording arrhythmia onset does not adversely affect longevity.

∥A difference greater than 10 bpm may be required. To ensure an adequate detection window, the shortest pacing escape interval must exceed the slowest tachycardia detection interval + 60 msec. For dual-chamber devices, the ventriculoatrial interval matches or exceeds the longest ventricular tachycardia detection interval (milliseconds).

¶Longevity reported with onset electrogram storage turned off. Longevity is adversely affected by turning onset electrograms on.

#The bradycardia refractory period is less than or equal to half the bradycardia pacing interval.

between pacing events (Fig. 4–13). Thus, a small window (approximately 5 to 15 bpm) must be maintained between the pacing upper rate limit and the lowest ventricular tachycardia detection zone, so that bradycardia pacing does not occur in the ventricular tachycardia zone. For example, if the ventricular tachycardia detection is set at 140 bpm, the tracking or sensor-driven upper rate limit cannot exceed approximately 130 bpm (the exact number depends in part on the AV delay).

Depending on the specific algorithm, the upper pacing rate may be further constrained by the use of the safety pacing or mode switch feature. For example, the Medtronic Gem I has an upper rate limit of 120 bpm, and if mode switch and safety pacing are programmed on, this may be further decreased to 111 bpm. In the subsequent version of the device (Gem II), the algorithm was modified to permit an upper rate of 150 bpm. The ELA Medical algorithm, in contrast, permits overlap between the pacing upper rate limit and the slowest tachycardia zone. However, devices approved in the United States (as of early 2000) lack a sensor, so that this feature would be particularly useful only in patients with slow ventricular tachycardias and AV block with preserved sinus function, in whom it may be desirable to permit tracking the sinus node to rates faster than the slowest ventricular tachycardia rate. Specific device algorithms are discussed in greater detail in Chapter 7.

Although upper pacing rate is an infrequent consideration in device selection, it may warrant thought when clinical ventricular tachycardias requiring therapy with rates less than 120 bpm are present in a patient who needs bradycardia pacing support at a similar heart rate. In young patients who need bradycardia support, upper rate may also be a more important consideration. The maximum upper bradycardia pacing rates for various defibrillators are included in Table 4–5.

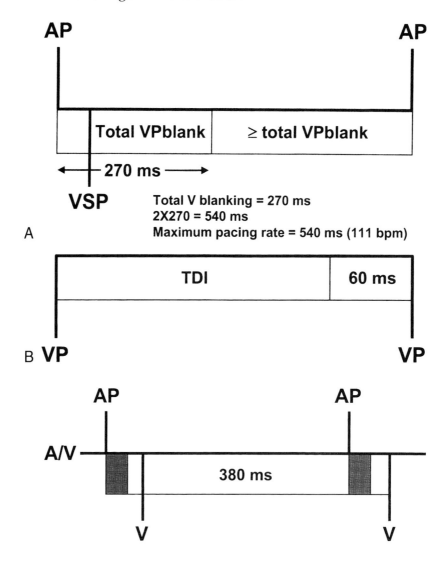

C ▨ = 66 ms ventricular cross-chamber blanking period

Fig. 4–13. Interactions between bradycardia pacing and tachycardia detection. Interactions are algorithm-dependent. *A,* In Medtronic dual-chamber defibrillators, the total ventricular blanking interval (VPblank) can never exceed 50% of the sensing window. If ventricular safety pacing is "on," the entire atrioventricular interval could be blanked. *B,* In Medtronic defibrillators, the maximum pacing rate equals the tachycardia detection interval (TDI) plus 60 msec to ensure an adequate window for detection. For higher pacing rates, dynamic atrioventricular intervals or shorter blanking intervals must be used. *C,* Similarly, in Guidant defibrillators, the lowest tachycardia detection rate interval must be less than the maximum tracking or sensor rate minus the atrioventricular (AV) delay. In the example shown, the maximum tracking or sensor rate = 150 bpm (400 msec), the AV delay = 120 msec, and the difference between 400 msec and 120 msec = 380 msec (or 157 bpm for the ventriculoatrial [VA] interval). Thus, the ventricular tachycardia (VT) detection rate must be greater than 157 bpm (so that the VT detection window "fits" into the VA interval). AP, atrial pacing; V, ventricular event; VP, ventricular pacing; VSP, ventricular sense or pace. (Modified from technical literature from Medtronic, Inc., and Guidant CPI.)

Dual-Chamber or Single-Chamber Device?

The single most important decision in selecting a defibrillator is determining whether to implant a single- or a dual-chamber system. This decision may be influenced by several considerations:

- The need for dual-chamber bradycardia pacing because of a standard indication, such as sinus node dysfunction or AV block
- Specific conditions (for example, long QT syndrome or hypertrophic cardiomyopathy) that may respond to dual-chamber pacing
- Congestive heart failure, which in some situations may favor traditional dual-chamber or, possibly, biventricular pacing
- Paroxysmal atrial arrhythmias—for improved specificity, prevention, and therapy

These are discussed in greater detail below. Table 4–6 summarizes conditions favoring the use of dual-chamber systems. For any given patient, the potential advantages of dual-chamber systems must be weighed against the strengths of single-chamber defibrillators—system simplicity, reduced risk of lead dislodgment, reduced cost, and greater longevity per unit

size. Table 4–7 summarizes the advantages of single-chamber systems.

Bradycardia Pacing

Patients who have a standard bradycardia indication for which dual-chamber pacing is preferred, as detailed earlier in the chapter, should receive implantable defibrillators capable of dual-chamber pacing.[64] Since the rationale for defibrillator use is reduction in mortality, dual-chamber pacing is particularly relevant for patients with sinus node dysfunction, in whom atrial pacing has been shown to reduce mortality.[3] The percentage of defibrillator recipients who need antibradycardia pacing has been estimated to be between 20% and 30%. In our population, 7% of patients have chronic atrial fibrillation at the time of defibrillator implantation, precluding dual-chamber pacing.[65] The availability of atrial defibrillators, however, may reduce the number of patients deemed to have a "chronic" disorder, because greater efforts may be made to restore sinus rhythm.

Specific Conditions

Long QT syndrome and hypertrophic cardiomyopathy are specific disease conditions that can be associated

---

Table 4–6.
Factors Favoring Use of a Dual-Chamber Defibrillator

- Need for dual-chamber bradycardia pacing (strongest indication for a dual-chamber device)
- Specific conditions that may "respond" to dual-chamber pacing (long QT syndrome, hypertrophic cardiomyopathy)
- Congestive heart failure if
    A long PR interval is impairing hemodynamic function
    Medications that impair chronotropic function are needed in a patient with borderline function
    Biventricular pacing is beneficial (not proven as of early 2000)
- Paroxysmal atrial arrhythmias
    Atrial pacing for prevention (not yet established, with possible exception of sinus node dysfunction)
    Improved specificity (i.e., differentiate supraventricular from ventricular arrhythmias)
    Atrial therapy (limited to devices that include specific atrial therapies beyond pacing)

Table 4–7.
Advantages of Single-Chamber Systems

- Simplified implantation
- Greater longevity per unit size
- Less intravascular hardware
- Reduced risk of lead dislodgment
- Reduced cost

with an increased risk of ventricular tachyarrhythmias and that may be independently benefited by dual-chamber pacing. Although patient selection remains challenging, dual-chamber pacing has been advocated for the treatment of symptomatic hypertrophic cardiomyopathy.[66–68] When a defibrillator is warranted in a patient with symptomatic hypertrophic cardiomyopathy, a dual-chamber device is often preferable because it may relieve symptoms or facilitate adjuvant use of β-blocking or calcium channel blocking agents. Exceptions include young children and very small patients, particularly those without an outflow tract gradient, because a smaller pulse generator and limited intravascular hardware then become more important considerations. Pacing or β-adrenergic blockers can prevent or reduce the frequency of ventricular arrhythmias in some patients with long QT syndrome. A dual-chamber defibrillator should be selected when defibrillator therapy is used in this group of patients. This provides the patient with the benefit of pacing therapy (with or without β-adrenergic blockade) and most likely will avoid pacemaker syndrome. Additionally, defibrillators with rate-smoothing algorithms to prevent the short-long-short intervals that can predispose to torsades de pointes in this population may decrease the arrhythmia frequency without the need for continuous overdrive pacing.[69,70]

Congestive Heart Failure

Since the risk of ventricular tachyarrhythmias is increased in patients with ventricular dysfunction,[71] it is not surprising that many patients with implantable defibrillators have congestive heart failure. Indeed, in a recent report, up to 34% of patients with implantable defibrillators had heart failure.[65] Although early studies generated great optimism for the possibility of improved ventricular function with pacing in dilated cardiomyopathy, subsequent more rigorously controlled studies failed to confirm the benefit of routine pacing for this condition.[72,73] Nonetheless, since many patients with heart failure have progressive conduction system disease, have a propensity for atrial fibrillation, and are often treated with digitalis and β-blockers—both of which may impair sinus node or AV nodal function—dual-chamber pacing may be preferable in those who remain in sinus rhythm and who have indications for a defibrillator.[65] In a small subgroup of patients with heart failure and long PR intervals, pacing may also help to relieve heart failure symptoms, although opinion is divided on this issue, so that this is a class IIb indication in the most recent American Heart Association/American College of Cardiology guidelines.[64]

Two important issues should also be considered in patients with heart failure. First, in patients with atrial fibrillation and heart failure, maintenance of sinus rhythm (with amiodarone) has been associated with decreased mortality.[74,75] Whether this benefit will occur with nonpharmacologic therapy has yet to be determined. Nonetheless, available data suggest that maintenance of sinus rhythm may be particularly beneficial in patients with heart failure. Thus, in addition to dual-chamber pacing, atrial defibrillation capabilities (discussed further, below) should be considered in patients with heart failure and atrial fibrillation. The second consideration is biventricular pacing. In nonrandomized pilot studies and in acute hemodynamic studies, biventricular pacing has been shown to improve acute hemodynamic measurements and decrease symptoms of heart failure in patients with impaired intraventricular conduction.[23,76] Several studies under way will determine the role of biventricular pacing for improvement of pump function.[77] Although experimental as of early 2000, device therapy, if it proves to be effective, may be used both to treat arrhythmias and to ameliorate heart failure symptoms in patients with ventricular dysfunction.

Paroxysmal Atrial Arrhythmias

In the Mayo Clinic implantable defibrillator population, 24.5% of patients have a history of paroxysmal atrial fibrillation.[65] Moreover, 33% of recipients of ICDs without a history of atrial arrhythmias have been shown to have such arrhythmias by interrogation of device logs.[78] There are four potential reasons to consider dual-chamber devices for paroxysmal atrial tachyarrhythmias:

- The device may permit continual physiologic pacing with the use of antiarrhythmic drugs
- Greater specificity may avoid inappropriate device therapy when atrial arrhythmias occur
- Atrial pacing can prevent atrial fibrillation episodes in patients with sinus node dysfunction; preventive pacing algorithms might broaden the population in whom atrial pacing inhibits arrhythmias, although this remains unproven
- Some devices include therapies to terminate atrial tachyarrhythmia

In contrast, patients with chronic atrial fibrillation—which has become more a reflection of physician judgment than biologic certainty with the advent of ibutilide-facilitated cardioversion and internal cardioversion—should receive single-chamber defibrillators.

Specificity. Rapidly conducting supraventricular arrhythmias result in inappropriate therapies (often shocks) in 17% to 41% of patients with defibrillators.[79,80] This incidence is important, because most studies have found that patients who receive frequent shocks are more likely to have impaired quality of life and psychosocial stress.[81–83]

Dual-chamber defibrillators can use information regarding atrial activity to look for AV dissociation or to assess atrial rates to better determine whether a tachycardia is atrial or ventricular in origin. Dual-chamber enhancements have been shown to decrease inappropriate therapies by correctly diagnosing 60% to 95% of supraventricular arrhythmia episodes without missing ventricular tachycardia episodes.[84–86] These results are similar to[87,88] or somewhat better than[80,89] those previously published for traditional single-chamber enhancement criteria. Although intuitively superior, data supporting the advantage of dual-chamber algorithms over appropriately programmed single-chamber defibrillators are limited, largely because of the fairly recent introduction of dual-chamber devices. It is clear that any advantage of dual-chamber devices over single-chamber devices for rhythm detection is specific to the device and algorithm.[79,90,91] The specific programming of and clinical results found with various single- and dual-chamber algorithms are reviewed in detail in Chapter 7. In general, dual-chamber defibrillators are preferred for patients with paroxysmal atrial arrhythmias. Importantly, most dual-chamber defibrillators have mode switch capabilities.

Prevention. The role of atrial pacing in the prevention of atrial fibrillation depends on the patient population. In patients with sinus node dysfunction, it is clear that atrial pacing reduces the frequency of atrial fibrillation and most likely of congestive heart failure, thromboembolism, and mortality in comparison with ventricular pacing.[3,92,93] However, in patients with normal sinus node function and more advanced paroxysmal atrial fibrillation awaiting AV node ablation, atrial pacing was found to be of no benefit—possibly because the frequency of pacing in this group was significantly reduced as a result of normal sinus node function.[94] Various algorithms for maintenance of a high percentage of atrial pacing and for prevention of the proarrhythmic pauses after premature atrial complexes (atrial rate stabilization) have been developed, and preliminary results are promising.[95,96] Early data suggest that atrial pacing and prevention therapies decrease the atrial fibrillation burden.[97] However, the advantage of using ICDs with pacing capability in the atrium to prevent atrial arrhythmias in patients other than those with sinus node dysfunction requires further confirmation.

Termination. In addition to providing dual-chamber pacing and specificity, some dual-chamber defibrillators have pacing therapies to terminate atrial arrhythmias. These can include antitachycardia pacing (with burst and ramp protocols similar to those in ventricular therapies), 50-Hz high-frequency burst pacing (which may regionally entrain atrial fibrillation and lead to its termination), and atrial defibrillation.

Results from early studies seem promising. We found that the atrial arrhythmia burden is significantly reduced by atrial therapies—probably because of prompt termination of episodes—and the quick restoration of normal rhythm may result in reversal of abnormal elec-trophysiologic characteristics ("reverse remodeling"), diminishing the frequency of recurrent atrial arrhythmias.[97,98] Importantly, more than 50% of spontaneous atrial tachyarrhythmia episodes were successfully terminated by painless pacing therapies.[97] In contrast to ventricular arrhythmias, atrial fibrillation is not immediately life-threatening. Therefore, atrial defibrillation can be programmed to occur only after sustained episodes (programmable up to 24 hours). Alternatively, atrial defibrillation can be delivered by a patient-controlled activator, or it can be delivered automatically at restricted times of the day.[99–103] The pain associated with atrial defibrillation shocks is highly individualized and variable; many patients have preferred it to continual atrial fibrillation, although a few have had devices explanted or inactivated.[104] Patients with highly symptomatic atrial tachyarrhythmias or frequent episodes that prompt medical attention (at least every 6 months) probably are the best candidates for devices with termination capabilities. Patients with symptomatic episodes occurring more frequently than weekly require adjuvant pharmacologic or catheter ablation therapy to limit the frequency of shocks. Further studies will shed light on the important issues of patient selection and patient toleration of shocks and on the effectiveness of pacing therapies for arrhythmia termination.

Factors Favoring Single-Chamber Defibrillators

Patients with chronic atrial fibrillation or patients who lack the factors favoring dual-chamber devices should receive single-chamber defibrillators. This is particularly true for younger or smaller patients, in whom the greater longevity per unit size and minimal intravascular hardware requirements of single-chamber systems may be more compelling. In addition to simplicity and longevity, single-chamber benefits include fewer complications. Although previous studies suggested no significant difference in overall complication rates between single- and dual-chamber pacemakers, the preponderance of evidence suggests that atrial leads dislodge more frequently than do ventricular leads.[105–108] Unless dislodged atrial leads are electrically abandoned (thus functionally reducing the implanted system to a single-chamber ICD), this increased rate of dislodgment may result in higher reoperation rates for dual-chamber ICDs. Clinical trials of dual-chamber defibrillators have found that rates of atrial lead dislodgment are 4.3% to 7%.[65,109,110] Thus, for patients who have infrequent pacing, who lack episodic atrial arrhythmias, and who do not have specific conditions warranting dual-chamber devices, single-chamber devices are preferred.

Conclusion

The broad array of devices and lead systems now available has broadened the arsenal available to combat bradyarrhythmias and complex life-threatening tachyarrhythmias and has enhanced the opportunity to tailor device therapy to the individual patient.

Pacemaker selection should be made after consideration is given not only to the underlying rhythm disturbance but also to the patient's activity level and need for specific programmable options. For ICD selection, factors such as pacemaker dependency, anticipated defibrillation threshold, need for bradycardia pacing, and paroxysmal or chronic atrial arrhythmias may all affect the choice of system (summarized in Table 4–8). Although most defibrillator systems are suitable for most patients, careful selection of

Table 4–8.
Clinical Factors and Defibrillator Selection

Clinical factor	Lead and device considerations
Pacemaker-dependent patient	• True bipolar sensing preferable • Consider bradycardia upper rate limit, particularly if patient is young
Need for bradycardia pacing	• Confirm that appropriate pacing (sensor, dual-chamber) is made available
Paroxysmal atrial arrhythmias	• Dual-chamber device may enhance specificity • Dual chamber may reduce paroxysmal atrial fibrillation (in sinus node dysfunction; role of algorithms to maintain atrial pacing still being defined) • Consider device that includes atrial defibrillator, depending on frequency of atrial arrhythmia
Chronic atrial fibrillation	• Single-chamber device (VVIR or rarely VVI)
Anticipated elevated defibrillation threshold (previously high defibrillation threshold, hypertrophic cardiomyopathy, marked enlargement)	• Higher output device • Integrated sensing lead (for extra coil)
Small body habitus; younger patient; need for limited intravascular hardware	• Smaller size, single chamber preferable
Very slow ventricular tachycardia	• Consider relationship of upper rate limit to ventricular tachycardia detection zone
Preexisting permanent pacemaker	• True bipolar sensing

system components can provide the best match between patient and device.

References

1. Gregoratos G, Cheitlin MD, Conill A, Epstein AE, Fellows C, Ferguson TB, Jr., Freedman RA, Hlatky MA, Naccarelli GV, Saksena S, Schlant RC, Silka MJ: ACC/AHA Guidelines for Implantation of Cardiac Pacemakers and Antiarrhythmia Devices: Executive Summary—a report of the American College of Cardiology/American Heart Association Task Force on Practice Guidelines (Committee on Pacemaker Implantation). Circulation 97:1325–1335, 1998

2. Andersen HR, Thuesen L, Bagger JP, Vesterlund T, Thomsen PE: Prospective randomised trial of atrial versus ventricular pacing in sick-sinus syndrome. Lancet 344:1523–1528, 1994

3. Andersen HR, Nielsen JC, Thomsen PE, Thuesen L, Mortensen PT, Vesterlund T, Pedersen AK: Long-term follow-up of patients from a randomised trial of atrial versus ventricular pacing for sick-sinus syndrome. Lancet 350:1210–1216, 1997

4. Lamas GA, Orav EJ, Stambler BS, Ellenbogen KA, Sgarbossa EB, Huang SK, Marinchak RA, Estes NA III, Mitchell GF, Lieberman EH, Mangione CM, Goldman L: Quality of life and clinical outcomes in elderly patients treated with ventricular pacing as compared with dual-chamber pacing. Pacemaker Selection in the Elderly Investigators. N Engl J Med 338:1097–1104, 1998

5. Gillis AM, Kerr CD, Connolly SJ, Gent M, Roberts R, for the CTOPP Investigators: Identification of patients most likely to benefit from physiologic pacing (abstract). Pacing Clin Electrophysiol 22:728, 1999

6. Schrepf R, Koller B, Pache J, Hoffman M, Goedel-Meinen L, Schömig A: Results of the randomized prospective DDD vs. VVI trial in patients with paroxysmal atrial fibrillation (abstract). Pacing Clin Electrophysiol 20:1152, 1997

7. Lamas GA: Pacemaker mode selection and survival: a plea to apply the principles of evidence based medicine to cardiac pacing practice. Heart 78:218–220, 1997

8. Toff WD, Skehan JD, De Bono DP, Camm AJ: The United Kingdom Pacing and Cardiovascular Events (UKPACE) trial. United Kingdom Pacing and Cardiovascular Events. Heart 78:221–223, 1997

9. Andersen HR, Nielsen JC: Pacing in sick sinus syndrome—need for a prospective, randomized trial comparing atrial with dual chamber pacing. Pacing Clin Electrophysiol 21:1175–1179, 1998

10. Ausubel K, Furman S: The pacemaker syndrome. Ann Intern Med 103:420–429, 1985

11. Heldman D, Mulvihill D, Nguyen H, Messenger JC, Rylaarsdam A, Evans K, Castellanet MJ: True incidence of pacemaker syndrome. Pacing Clin Electrophysiol 13:1742–1750, 1990

12. Hayes DL, Furman S: Stability of AV conduction in sick sinus node syndrome patients with implanted atrial pacemakers. Am Heart J 107:644–647, 1984

13. Rey JL, Tribouilloy C, Elghelbazouri F, Otmani A: Single-lead VDD pacing: long-term experience with four different systems. Am Heart J 135:1036–1039, 1998

14. Richardson DA, Bexton RS, Shaw FE, Kenny RA: Prevalence of cardioinhibitory carotid sinus hypersensitivity in patients 50 years or over presenting to the accident and emergency department with "unexplained" or "recurrent" falls. Pacing Clin Electrophysiol 20:820–823, 1997

15. Maloney JD, Jaeger FJ, Rizo-Patron C, Zhu DW: The role of pacing for the management of neurally mediated syncope: carotid sinus syndrome and vasovagal syncope. Am Heart J 127:1030–1037, 1994

16. Fitzpatrick A, Theodorakis G, Ahmed R, Williams T, Sutton R: Dual chamber pacing aborts vasovagal syncope induced by head-up 60 degrees tilt. Pacing Clin Electrophysiol 14:13–19, 1991

17. Sra JS, Jazayeri MR, Avitall B, Dhala A, Deshpande S, Blanck Z, Akhtar M: Comparison of cardiac pacing with drug therapy in the treatment of neurocardiogenic (vasovagal) syncope with bradycardia or asystole. N Engl J Med 328:1085–1090, 1993

18. Connolly SJ, Sheldon R, Roberts RS, Gent M: The North American Vasovagal Pacemaker Study (VPS). A randomized trial of permanent cardiac pacing for the prevention of vasovagal syncope. J Am Coll Cardiol 33:16–20, 1999

19. Brignole M, Menozzi C, Lolli G, Bottoni N, Gaggioli G: Long-term outcome of paced and nonpaced patients with severe carotid sinus syndrome. Am J Cardiol 69:1039–1043, 1992

20. Nishimura RA, Hayes DL, Ilstrup DM, Holmes DR, Jr., Tajik AJ: Effect of dual-chamber pacing on systolic and diastolic function in patients with hypertrophic

cardiomyopathy. Acute Doppler echocardiographic and catheterization hemodynamic study. J Am Coll Cardiol 27: 421–430, 1996

21. Kappenberger L, Linde C, Daubert C, McKenna W, Meisel E, Sadoul N, Chojnowska L, Guize L, Gras D, Jeanrenaud X, Ryden L: Pacing in hypertrophic obstructive cardiomyopathy. A randomized crossover study. PIC Study Group. Eur Heart J 18:1249–1256, 1997

22. Hayes DL, Barold SS, Camm AJ, Goldschlager NF: Evolving indications for permanent cardiac pacing: an appraisal of the 1998 American College of Cardiology/American Heart Association Guidelines (editorial). Am J Cardiol 82:1082–1086, 1998

23. Gras D, Mabo P, Tang T, Luttikuis O, Chatoor R, Pedersen AK, Tscheliessnigg HH, Deharo JC, Puglisi A, Silvestre J, Kimber S, Ross H, Ravazzi A, Paul V, Skehan D: Multisite pacing as a supplemental treatment of congestive heart failure: preliminary results of the Medtronic Inc. InSync Study. Pacing Clin Electrophysiol 21:2249–2255, 1998

24. Auricchio A, Stellbrink C, Block M, Sack S, Vogt J, Bakker P, Klein H, Kramer A, Ding J, Salo R, Tockman B, Pochet T, Spinelli J: Effect of pacing chamber and atrioventricular delay on acute systolic function of paced patients with congestive heart failure. The Pacing Therapies for Congestive Heart Failure Study Group. The Guidant Congestive Heart Failure Research Group. Circulation 99:2993–3001, 1999

25. Melton IC, Gilligan DM, Wood MA, Ellenbogen KA: Optimal cardiac pacing after heart transplantation. Pacing Clin Electrophysiol 22:1510–1527, 1999

26. Kruse IM, Terpstra B: Acute and long-term atrial and ventricular stimulation thresholds with a steroid-eluting electrode. Pacing Clin Electrophysiol 8:45–49, 1985

27. Pirzada FA, Moschitto LJ, Diorio D: Clinical experience with steroid-eluting unipolar electrodes. Pacing Clin Electrophysiol 11:1739–1744, 1988

28. Kay GN: Basic concepts of pacing. *In* Cardiac Pacing. Second edition. Edited by KA Ellenbogen. Cambridge, MA, Blackwell Science, 1996, pp 66–84

29. Hayes DL, Holmes DR, Jr., Merideth J, Osborn MJ, Vlietstra RE, Neubauer SA: Bipolar tined polyurethane ventricular lead: a four-year experience. Pacing Clin Electrophysiol 8:192–196, 1985

30. Hayes DL, Graham KJ, Irwin M, Vidaillet H, Disler G, Sweesy M, Osborn MJ, Suman VJ, Neubauer SA, Seebandt M, Kallinen L, Crowson CS: A multicenter experience with a bipolar tined polyurethane ventricular lead. Pacing Clin Electrophysiol 15: 1033–1039, 1992

31. Stokes KB: Polyether polyurethanes: biostable or not? J Biomater Appl 3:228–259, 1988

32. Coury AJ, Slaikeu PC, Cahalan PT, Stokes KB, Hobot CM: Factors and interactions affecting the performance of polyurethane elastomers in medical devices. J Biomater Appl 3:130–179, 1988

33. Jain P, Kaul U, Wasir HS: Myopotential inhibition of unipolar demand pacemakers: utility of provocative manoeuvres in assessment and management. Int J Cardiol 34:33–39, 1992

34. Gabry MD, Behrens M, Andrews C, Wanliss M, Klementowicz PT, Furman S: Comparison of myopotential interference in unipolar-bipolar programmable DDD pacemakers. Pacing Clin Electrophysiol 10:1322–1330, 1987

35. Gross JN, Platt S, Ritacco R, Andrews C, Furman S: The clinical relevance of electromyopotential oversensing in current unipolar devices. Pacing Clin Electrophysiol 15:2023–2027, 1992

36. Calfee RV, Saulson SH: A voluntary standard for 3.2 mm unipolar and bipolar pacemaker leads and connectors. Pacing Clin Electrophysiol 9:1181–1185, 1986

37. Stokes KB: Preliminary studies on a new steroid eluting epicardial electrode. Pacing Clin Electrophysiol 11:1797–1803, 1988

38. Karpawich PP, Stokes KB, Proctor K, Schallhorn R, McVenes R: "In-line" bipolar, steroid-eluting, high impedance, epimyocardial pacing lead. Pacing Clin Electrophysiol 21:503–508, 1998

39. Godin JF, Petitot JC, Pioger G: Stimarec report. Pacing Clin Electrophysiol 21:2157–2158, 1998

40. Hayes DL, Graham KJ, Irwin M, Vidaillet H, Disler G, Sweesy M, Kincaid D, Osborn MJ, Suman VJ, Neubauer SA, Seebandt M, Kallinen L: Multicenter experience with a bipolar tined polyurethane ventricular lead. Pacing Clin Electrophysiol 18: 999–1004, 1995

41. Glikson M, von Feldt LK, Suman VJ, Hayes DL: Clinical surveillance of an active fixation, bipolar, polyurethane insulated pacing lead, Part I: the atrial lead. Pacing Clin Electrophysiol 17:1399–1404, 1994

42. Gold MR, Foster AH, Shorofsky SR: Lead system optimization for transvenous

defibrillation. Am J Cardiol 80:1163–1167, 1997

43. Bardy GH, Dolack GL, Kudenchuk PJ, Poole JE, Mehra R, Johnson G: Prospective, randomized comparison in humans of a unipolar defibrillation system with that using an additional superior vena cava electrode. Circulation 89:1090–1093, 1994

44. Jung W, Manz M, Moosdorf R, Luderitz B: Failure of an implantable cardioverter-defibrillator to redetect ventricular fibrillation in patients with a nonthoracotomy lead system. Circulation 86:1217–1222, 1992

45. Brady PA, Friedman PA, Stanton MS: Effect of failed defibrillation shocks on electrogram amplitude in a nonintegrated transvenous defibrillation lead system. Am J Cardiol 76:580–584, 1995

46. Goldberger JJ, Horvath G, Donovan D, Johnson D, Challapalli R, Kadish AH: Detection of ventricular fibrillation by transvenous defibrillating leads: integrated versus dedicated bipolar sensing. J Cardiovasc Electrophysiol 9:677–688, 1998

47. Isbruch FM, Block M, Bocker D, Dees H, Hammel D, Borggrefe M, Scheld HH, Breithardt G: Improved sensing signals after endocardial defibrillation with a redesigned integrated sense pace defibrillation lead. Pacing Clin Electrophysiol 19:1211–1218, 1996

48. Cooklin M, Tummala RV, Peters RW, Shorofsky SR, Gold MR: Comparison of bipolar and integrated sensing for redetection of ventricular fibrillation. Am Heart J 138:133–136, 1999

49. Friedman PA, Stanton MS: The pacer-cardioverter-defibrillator: function and clinical experience. J Cardiovasc Electrophysiol 6:48–68, 1995

50. Deshmukh P, Anderson K: Myopotential sensing by a dual chamber implantable cardioverter defibrillator: two case reports. J Cardiovasc Electrophysiol 9:767–772, 1998

51. Friedman PA, Stanton MS: Predictors of defibrillation efficacy in a dilated cardiomyopathy model (abstract). Pacing Clin Electrophysiol 18:1796, 1995

52. Gold MR, Khalighi K, Kavesh NG, Daly B, Peters RW, Shorofsky SR: Clinical predictors of transvenous biphasic defibrillation thresholds. Am J Cardiol 79:1623–1627, 1997

53. Khalighi K, Daly B, Leino EV, Shorofsky SR, Kavesh NG, Peters RW, Gold MR: Clinical predictors of transvenous defib-

rillation energy requirements. Am J Cardiol 79:150–153, 1997

54. Glikson M, Trusty JM, Grice SK, Hayes DL, Hammill SC, Stanton MS: A stepwise testing protocol for modern implantable cardioverter-defibrillator systems to prevent pacemaker-implantable cardioverter-defibrillator interactions. Am J Cardiol 83: 360–366, 1999

55. Gold MR, Peters RW, Johnson JW, Shorofsky SR: Complications associated with pectoral cardioverter-defibrillator implantation: comparison of subcutaneous and submuscular approaches. Worldwide Jewel Investigators. J Am Coll Cardiol 28:1278–1282, 1996

56. Reddy RK, Bardy GH: Unipolar pectoral defibrillation systems. Pacing Clin Electrophysiol 20:600–606, 1997

57. Brady PA, Friedman PA, Trusty JM, Grice S, Hammill SC, Stanton MS: High failure rate for an epicardial implantable cardioverter-defibrillator lead: implications for long-term follow-up of patients with an implantable cardioverter-defibrillator. J Am Coll Cardiol 31:616–622, 1998

58. Luria D, Rasmussen MJ, Hammill SC, Friedman PA: Frequency and mode of detection of nonthoracotomy implantable defibrillator lead failure (abstract). Pacing Clin Electrophysiol 22:705, 1999

59. Bardy GH, Hofer B, Johnson G, Kudenchuk PJ, Poole JE, Dolack GL, Gleva M, Mitchell R, Kelso D: Implantable transvenous cardioverter-defibrillators. Circulation 87:1152–1168, 1993

60. Haberman RJ, Mower MM, Veltri EP: LV mass and defibrillation threshold (letter). Am Heart J 115:1340–1341, 1988

61. Hillsley RE, Wharton JM, Cates AW, Wolf PD, Ideker RE: Why do some patients have high defibrillation thresholds at defibrillator implantation? Answers from basic research. Pacing Clin Electrophysiol 17:222–239, 1994

62. Klein GJ, Jones DL, Sharma AD, Kallok MJ, Guiraudon GM: Influence of cardiopulmonary bypass on internal cardiac defibrillation. Am J Cardiol 57:1194–1195, 1986

63. Trusty JM, Hayes DL, Stanton MS, Friedman PA: Factors affecting the frequency of subcutaneous lead usage in implantable defibrillators. Pacing Clin Electrophysiol 23:842–846, 2000

64. Gregoratos G, Cheitlin MD, Conill A, Epstein AE, Fellows C, Ferguson TB Jr, Freedman RA, Hlatky MA, Naccarelli GV, Saksena S, Schlant RC, Silka MJ, Ritchie JL,

Gibbons RJ, Eagle KA, Gardner TJ, Lewis RP, O'Rourke RA, Ryan TJ, Garson A Jr: ACC/AHA guidelines for implantation of cardiac pacemakers and antiarrhythmia devices: a report of the American College of Cardiology/American Heart Association Task Force on Practice Guidelines (Committee on Pacemaker Implantation). J Am Coll Cardiol 31:1175–1209, 1998

65. Best PJ, Hayes DL, Stanton MS: The potential usage of dual chamber pacing in patients with implantable cardioverter defibrillators. Pacing Clin Electrophysiol 22:79–85, 1999

66. Gadler F, Linde C, Daubert C, McKenna W, Meisel E, Aliot E, Chojnowska L, Guize L, Gras D, Jeanrenaud X, Kappenberger L: Significant improvement of quality of life following atrioventricular synchronous pacing in patients with hypertrophic obstructive cardiomyopathy. Data from 1 year of follow-up. PIC study group. Pacing In Cardiomyopathy. Eur Heart J 20:1044–1050, 1999

67. Maron BJ, Nishimura RA, McKenna WJ, Rakowski H, Josephson ME, Kieval RS: Assessment of permanent dual-chamber pacing as a treatment for drug-refractory symptomatic patients with obstructive hypertrophic cardiomyopathy. A randomized, double-blind, crossover study (M-PATHY). Circulation 99:2927–2933, 1999

68. Nishimura RA, Trusty JM, Hayes DL, Ilstrup DM, Larson DR, Hayes SN, Allison TG, Tajik AJ: Dual-chamber pacing for hypertrophic cardiomyopathy: a randomized, double-blind, crossover trial. J Am Coll Cardiol 29:435–441, 1997

69. Viskin S: Long QT syndromes and torsade de pointes. Lancet 354:1625–1633, 1999

70. Viskin S, Fish R, Roth A, Copperman Y: Prevention of torsade de pointes in the congenital long QT syndrome: use of a pause prevention pacing algorithm. Heart 79:417–419, 1998

71. Bigger JT Jr, Fleiss JL, Kleiger R, Miller JP, Rolnitzky LM: The relationships among ventricular arrhythmias, left ventricular dysfunction, and mortality in the 2 years after myocardial infarction. Circulation 69:250–258, 1984

72. Hochleitner M, Hortnagl H, Fridrich L, Gschnitzer F: Long-term efficacy of physiologic dual-chamber pacing in the treatment of end-stage idiopathic dilated cardiomyopathy. Am J Cardiol 70:1320–1325, 1992

73. Gold MR, Feliciano Z, Gottlieb SS, Fisher ML: Dual-chamber pacing with a short atrioventricular delay in congestive heart failure: a randomized study. J Am Coll Cardiol 26:967–973, 1995

74. Dries DL, Exner DV, Gersh BJ, Domanski MJ, Waclawiw MA, Stevenson LW: Atrial fibrillation is associated with an increased risk for mortality and heart failure progression in patients with asymptomatic and symptomatic left ventricular systolic dysfunction: a retrospective analysis of the SOLVD trials. Studies of Left Ventricular Dysfunction. J Am Coll Cardiol 32: 695–703, 1998

75. Deedwania PC, Singh BN, Ellenbogen K, Fisher S, Fletcher R, Singh SN: Spontaneous conversion and maintenance of sinus rhythm by amiodarone in patients with heart failure and atrial fibrillation: observations from the Veterans Affairs Congestive Heart Failure Survival Trial of Antiarrhythmic Therapy (CHF-STAT). The Department of Veterans Affairs CHF-STAT Investigators. Circulation 98:2574–2579, 1998

76. Blanc JJ, Etienne Y, Gilard M, Mansourati J, Munier S, Boschat J, Benditt DG, Lurie KG: Evaluation of different ventricular pacing sites in patients with severe heart failure: results of an acute hemodynamic study. Circulation 96:3273–3277, 1997

77. Saxon LA, Boehmer JP, Hummel J, Kacet S, De Marco T, Naccarelli G, Daoud E: Biventricular pacing in patients with congestive heart failure: two prospective randomized trials. The VIGOR CHF and VENTAK CHF Investigators. Am J Cardiol 83:120D-123D, 1999

78. Stein K, Hess M, Hannon C, Mehra R, Mittal S, Markowitz S, Lerman B: Atrial arrhythmias in ICD recipients: incidence and efficacy of atrial antitachycardia pacing (abstract). Pacing Clin Electrophysiol 22: 824, 1999

79. Kuhlkamp V, Dornberger V, Mewis C, Suchalla R, Bosch RF, Seipel L: Clinical experience with the new detection algorithms for atrial fibrillation of a defibrillator with dual chamber sensing and pacing. J Cardiovasc Electrophysiol 10: 905–915, 1999

80. Brugada J, Mont L, Figueiredo M, Valentino M, Matas M, Navarro-Lopez F: Enhanced detection criteria in implantable defibrillators. J Cardiovasc Electrophysiol 9:261–268, 1998

81. Namerow PB, Firth BR, Heywood GM, Windle JR, Parides MK: Quality-of-life six months after CABG surgery in patients randomized to ICD versus no ICD therapy:

findings from the CABG Patch Trial. Pacing Clin Electrophysiol 22:1305–1313, 1999

82. Heller SS, Ormont MA, Lidagoster L, Sciacca RR, Steinberg S: Psychosocial outcome after ICD implantation: a current perspective. Pacing Clin Electrophysiol 21:1207–1215, 1998

83. Chevalier P, Verrier P, Kirkorian G, Touboul P, Cottraux J: Improved appraisal of the quality of life in patients with automatic implantable cardioverter defibrillator: a psychometric study. Psychother Psychosom 65:49–56, 1996

84. Wilkoff BL, Kühlkamp V, Gillberg JM, Brown AB, Cuijpers A, DeSouza CM, and the 7271 Gem DR Worldwide Investigators: Performance of a dual chamber detection algorithm (PR logic™) based on the worldwide Gem DR clinical results (abstract). Pacing Clin Electrophysiol 22:720, 1999

85. Swerdlow CD, Gunderson BD, Gillberg JM, Pietersen AH, Volosin KJ, Stadler RW, Olson WH: Discrimination of concurrent atrial and ventricular tachyarrhythmias from rapidly-conducted atrial arrhythmias by dual-chamber ICD (abstract). Pacing Clin Electrophysiol 22:775, 1999

86. Lavergne T, Daubert JC, Chauvin M, Dolla E, Kacet S, Leenhardt A, Mabo P, Ritter P, Sadoul N, Saoudi N, Henry C, Nitzsche R, Ripart A, Murgatroyd F: Preliminary clinical experience with the first dual chamber pacemaker defibrillator. Pacing Clin Electrophysiol 20:182–188, 1997

87. Swerdlow CD, Ahern T, Chen PS, Hwang C, Gang E, Mandel W, Kass RM, Peter CT: Underdetection of ventricular tachycardia by algorithms to enhance specificity in a tiered-therapy cardioverter-defibrillator. J Am Coll Cardiol 24:416–424, 1994

88. Swerdlow CD, Chen PS, Kass RM, Allard JR, Peter CT: Discrimination of ventricular tachycardia from sinus tachycardia and atrial fibrillation in a tiered-therapy cardioverter-defibrillator. J Am Coll Cardiol 23:1342–1355, 1994

89. Barold HS, Newby KH, Tomassoni G, Kearney M, Brandon J, Natale A: Prospective evaluation of new and old criteria to discriminate between supraventricular and ventricular tachycardia in implantable defibrillators. Pacing Clin Electrophysiol 21:1347–1355, 1998

90. Nair M, Saoudi N, Kroiss D, Letac B: Automatic arrhythmia identification using analysis of the atrioventricular association. Application to a new generation of implantable defibrillators. Participating Centers of the Automatic Recognition of Arrhythmia Study Group. Circulation 95:967–973, 1997

91. Swerdlow CD, Sheth NV, Olson WH, for the Worldwide Jewel AF Investigators: Clinical performance of a pattern-based, dual-chamber algorithm for discrimination of ventricular from supraventricular arrhythmias (abstract). Pacing Clin Electrophysiol 21:800, 1998

92. Stabile G, Senatore G, De Simone A, Turco P, Coltorti F, Nocerino P, Vitale DF, Chiariello M: Determinants of efficacy of atrial pacing in preventing atrial fibrillation recurrences. J Cardiovasc Electrophysiol 10:2–9, 1999

93. Delfaut P, Saksena S, Prakash A, Krol RB: Long-term outcome of patients with drug-refractory atrial flutter and fibrillation after single- and dual-site right atrial pacing for arrhythmia prevention. J Am Coll Cardiol 32:1900–1908, 1998

94. Gillis AM, Wyse DG, Connolly SJ, Dubuc M, Philippon F, Yee R, Lacombe P, Rose MS, Kerr CD: Atrial pacing periablation for prevention of paroxysmal atrial fibrillation. Circulation 99:2553–2558, 1999

95. Garrigue S, Barold SS, Cazeau S, Gencel L, Jais P, Haissaguerre M, Clementy J: Prevention of atrial arrhythmias during DDD pacing by atrial overdrive. Pacing Clin Electrophysiol 21:1751–1759, 1998

96. Murgatroyd FD, Nitzsche R, Slade AK, Limousin M, Rosset N, Camm AJ, Ritter P: A new pacing algorithm for overdrive suppression of atrial fibrillation. Chorus Multicentre Study Group. Pacing Clin Electrophysiol 17:1966–1973, 1994

97. Friedman PA, Stein KM, Wharton JM, Hammill SC: Reduced atrial fibrillation burden with prompt treatment by an implantable arrhythmia management device: evidence of reverse remodeling? (Abstract.) Circulation 100:I-69, 1999

98. Timmermans C, Wellens HJJ, for the Metrix Investigators: Effect of device-mediated therapy on symptomatic episodes of atrial fibrillation (abstract). J Am Coll Cardiol 31 Suppl A:331A, 1998

99. Ayers GM, Griffin JC: The future role of defibrillators in the management of atrial fibrillation. Curr Opin Cardiol 12: 12–17, 1997

100. Ammer R, Alt E, Ayers G, Lehmann G, Schmitt C, Pasquantonio J, Putter K, Schmidt M, Schomig A: Pain threshold for low energy intracardiac cardiover-

sion of atrial fibrillation with low or no sedation. Pacing Clin Electrophysiol 20:230–236, 1997

101. Cooper RA, Plumb VJ, Epstein AE, Kay GN, Ideker RE: Marked reduction in internal atrial defibrillation thresholds with dual-current pathways and sequential shocks in humans. Circulation 97:2527–2535, 1998

102. Heisel A, Jung J, Fries R, Schieffer H, Ozbek C: Atrial defibrillation: can modifications in current implantable cardioverter-defibrillators achieve this? Am J Cardiol 78:119–127, 1996

103. Heisel A, Jung J: The atrial defibrillator: a stand-alone device or part of a combined dual-chamber system? Am J Cardiol 83:218D–226D, 1999

104. Wellens HJ, Lau CP, Luderitz B, Akhtar M, Waldo AL, Camm AJ, Timmermans C, Tse HF, Jung W, Jordaens L, Ayers G: Atrioverter: an implantable device for the treatment of atrial fibrillation. Circulation 98:1651–1656, 1998

105. Markewitz A, Hemmer W, Weinhold C: Complications in dual chamber pacing: a six-year experience. Pacing Clin Electrophysiol 9:1014–1018, 1986

106. Aggarwal RK, Connelly DT, Ray SG, Ball J, Charles RG: Early complications of permanent pacemaker implantation: no difference between dual and single chamber systems. Br Heart J 73:571–575, 1995

107. Chauhan A, Grace AA, Newell SA, Stone DL, Shapiro LM, Schofield PM, Petch MC: Early complications after dual chamber versus single chamber pacemaker implantation. Pacing Clin Electrophysiol 17:2012–2015, 1994

108. Mueller X, Sadeghi H, Kappenberger L: Complications after single versus dual chamber pacemaker implantation. Pacing Clin Electrophysiol 13:711–714, 1990

109. Model 7250 Jewel AF Arrhythmia Management Device, Clinical Summary, Medtronic, Inc., 1999

110. Kopp DE, Lin AC, Burke MC, Kall JG, Verdino RJ, Johnson CT, Wilber DJ: Adverse events with dual chamber implantable cardioverter-defibrillators (abstract). Pacing Clin Electrophysiol 22: 896, 1999

5

Implantation Techniques

David L. Hayes, M.D.

Once performed only by surgeons, pacemaker and defibrillator implantations in the United States are now usually done by cardiologists. Regardless of who implants the device, this person should have a thorough working knowledge of cardiac pacing and defibrillation as well as a complete understanding of sterile technique and the specific surgical skills necessary for pacemaker implantation.[1-3] Guidelines for training have been established by the North American Society of Pacing and Electrophysiology.[4]

Because virtually all implantations of the implantable cardioverter-defibrillator (ICD) are now nonthoracotomy procedures with the ICD placed in the prepectoral position, the same as pacemakers, this chapter addresses the implantation of both types of devices. Throughout the chapter, the device is simply referred to as "pulse generator," implying either pacemaker or ICD unless a specific difference applies.

Implant-related complications are discussed in Chapter 10.

Implantation Facility

Pulse generators should be implanted in a surgical environment, whether a specially equipped operating room or a catheterization suite (Fig. 5–1). Requirements include excellent fluoroscopy, electrocardiographic monitoring, oxygen saturation monitoring (by finger plethysmography), and standby defibrillator and life-support equipment. Additional desirable features are facilities for lateral and anteroposterior fluoroscopy projection, a fluoroscopy table capable of tilting, and intra-arterial pressure equipment.

Anesthesia

Local anesthesia is used for all patients unless contraindicated. Pediatric patients, uncooperative or confused patients undergoing permanent pacing, and special circumstances may require general anesthesia. Supplemental parenteral sedatives are used as needed for patient comfort.[5] We commonly use intravenously administered midazolam and fentanyl, the dose depending on individual patient requirements, associated cardiopulmonary disease, and age.

Lead extraction, discussed in Chapter 10, is usually performed under general anesthesia.

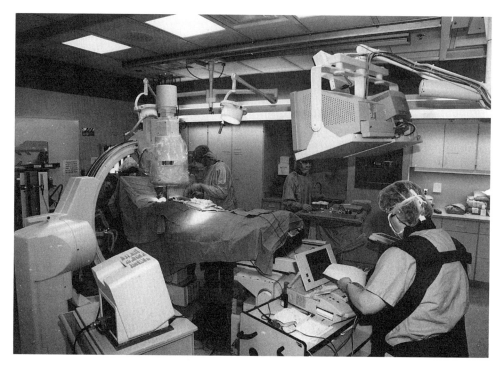

Fig. 5–1. Pacemaker and implantable cardioverter-defibrillator implantation suite.

The Pulse Generator Pocket

Forming the pulse generator pocket is an integral part of pulse generator implantation. The pocket is commonly developed in the prepectoralis fascia (Fig. 5–2). It should be large enough to allow for easy placement of the pulse generator and leads. It is important to avoid a tight pocket, which can cause erosion, or a loose pocket, which can permit excessive movement and migration.

The site of placement of the pulse generator is extremely important in providing long-term comfort and complete mobility for the adjacent shoulder. The pulse generator should be implanted in the subcutaneous tissue, deep to the fatty layer of the pectoral region. An inexperienced operator may not find the plane between the subcutaneous tissue and the pectoral fascia. Occasionally, the space developed may be subcuticular, with the subcutaneous fatty layer deep to the pulse generator. In that situation, the pulse generator presses on the undersurface of the skin and the wound may be continually painful. Characteristically, light touch of the overlying skin produces exquisite pain. An equally inexperienced evaluator of this circumstance may not understand the problem, which can be solved by repositioning the pulse generator into a deeper and subcutaneous site.

The pulse generator should be sufficiently inferior to the clavicle so that a full range of shoulder motion is not restricted by its impingement against the clavicle. The device should be sufficiently medial to keep it from approaching the anterior axillary fold. Otherwise, every anterior movement of the arm past the pulse generator will be uncomfortable.

After dissection and development of

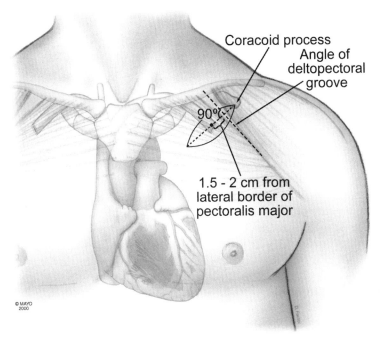

Coracoid process
Angle of
deltopectoral
groove

90°

1.5 - 2 cm from
lateral border of
pectoralis major

© MAYO
2000

Fig. 5–2. Location of pacemaker pocket in upper left aspect of chest. Note that the incision is made parallel to and several centimeters below the lower clavicular margin. (By permission of Mayo Foundation.)

the pocket, a sponge soaked with antibiotic solution may be kept within the pocket during placement of the leads, but its removal is mandatory before wound closure.

In general, the smallest pulse generator appropriate for the patient should be selected. This choice is of particular importance in pediatric patients, young adults, and thin patients. If the prepectoral position is not suitable because the optimal pulse generator is too large or because cosmetic or other considerations predominate, other choices are possible. Although rarely necessary, the pulse generator can be placed deep to the pectoral muscle. This location may result in a higher incidence of pectoral muscle stimulation or muscle inhibition with a unipolar system; therefore, in this situation, a bipolar system is preferred.

Retromammary pacemaker placement, another option, could be used for cosmetic purposes or, in a thin person, for protection of the implant site by the fatty layer of the breast. However, current pacemakers are small enough to be implanted without causing any significant cosmetic concern. In addition, the retromammary pulse generator has been reported to cause lactation abnormalities in selected cases.

Although ICDs are still larger than pacemakers and may cause more cosmetic concerns, placing the ICD in a retromammary position could significantly impair optimal mammography and therefore be of clinical concern. In fact, ICDs should be implanted in such a way that the device obscures the minimum of breast tissue. It is also reasonable to be certain that a female patient has had recent mammography before ICD implantation.

Venous Approaches

Before 1979, transvenous pacing leads were almost always placed through a cephalic vein cutdown in the deltopectoral groove. If the cephalic vein was too small or friable or had previously been used for implantation or if a second lead was required, the ipsilateral external or internal jugular vein was used. Rarely, subclavian or axillary vein cutdowns were performed. Deep dissection demanded precise surgical techniques— techniques in which cardiologists are not often skilled.

Each venous approach has its own particular advantages and disadvantages. The subclavian puncture and cephalic cutdown approaches are most commonly used today. Placement through the external or internal jugular veins, in addition to more local dissection, requires the operator to tunnel the lead over or under the clavicle to the pulse generator. Techniques for permanent lead placement via the iliac vein have also been described, and although not used at our institution, they should be considered when there is limited venous access.

Subclavian Approach

The introducer approach for subclavian venipuncture is frequently used because this technique is fast, usually causes minimal trauma, and facilitates placement of multiple leads.[6] The basic procedure, a modification of the Seldinger technique, requires detailed knowledge about the route of the subclavian vein and the relationship of the vein to the clavicle, first rib, subclavian artery, and apex of the lung (Fig. 5–3). The ease, efficacy, and safety of the technique are directly related to adherence to specific guidelines (Table 5–1) and to the expertise of the physician performing the venipuncture.

Prepackaged kits containing a nee-

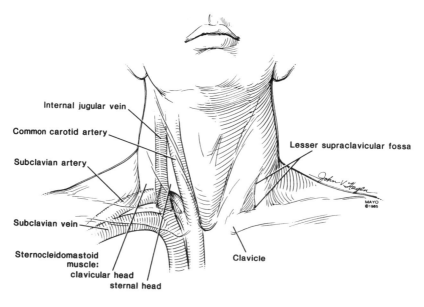

Fig. 5–3. Relationships of clavicle, subclavian artery and vein, carotid artery, and internal jugular vein. (From Holmes DR Jr: Permanent pacemaker implantation. *In* A Practice of Cardiac Pacing. Edited by S Furman, DL Hayes, DR Holmes Jr. Mount Kisco, NY, Futura Publishing Company, 1986, pp 97–127. By permission of Mayo Foundation.)

Table 5–1.
Principles of Subclavian Puncture

- Know the anatomy
- Distend the subclavian vein
- Ensure that hydration is adequate
- Place the patient in the Trendelenburg position
- Use as small a needle as possible (18 gauge)
- Approach the vein as laterally as possible
- Avoid repeated punctures
- Consider peripherally administered contrast venography to facilitate puncture

dle, guide wire, dilator, and peel-away sheath are available for subclavian puncture. The subclavian vein is entered through the incision with an 18-gauge needle (Fig. 5–4). Placing the patient in the Trendelenburg position may facilitate entry because the subclavian vein may be less distended in the recumbent patient with normal venous pressure. Entry is even more of a problem if the patient has been fasting for several hours before the procedure and is volume-depleted. Historically, it was taught that the vein was entered at the junction of the middle and inner thirds of the clavicle or even with a very medial approach, which was referred to as the "safe introducer technique." A very medial approach predisposes the lead or leads to crush injury between the clavicle and the first rib.[7] Conversely, if the venous approach is very lateral, it is possible to enter the axillary vein, which is extrathoracic[8] (Fig. 5–5). This eliminates the possibility of a pneumothorax. A technique has been described whereby the needle is "walked along" the first rib in an attempt to locate the axillary vein.

Subclavian venipuncture should be performed with a syringe with saline or

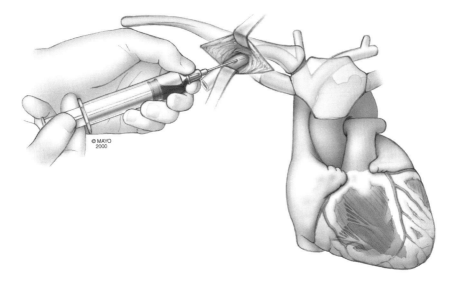

© MAYO 2000

Fig. 5–4. The subclavian vein can be used for single- or dual-lead placement. The first step is to puncture the vein with an 18-gauge needle. Blood is aspirated to ensure proper positioning in the venous structure. (By permission of Mayo Foundation.)

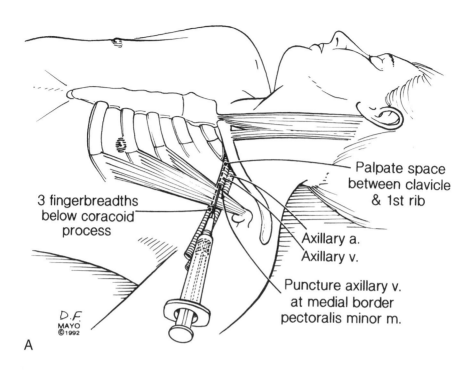

3 fingerbreadths
below coracoid
process

Palpate space
between clavicle
& 1st rib

Axillary a.
Axillary v.

Puncture axillary v.
at medial border
pectoralis minor m.

D.F.
MAYO
©1992

A

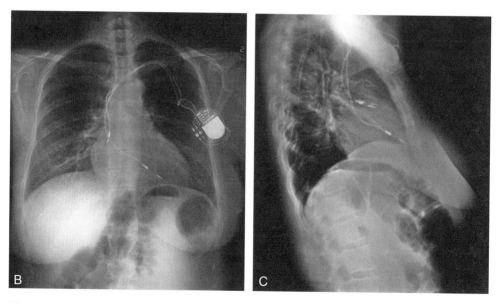

B

C

Fig. 5–5. Anatomical landmarks (A) used for true axillary venipuncture. Posteroanterior (B) and lateral (C) chest radiographs from a patient with a pacemaker implanted in an axillary position. (A, From Hayes et al.[3] By permission of Mayo Foundation.)

1% lidocaine attached to the needle. As the puncture is performed, a slight vacuum should be maintained on the syringe. The syringe should be constantly observed for the aspiration of air, blood, or other fluids.

Once the vein is successfully punctured, the guide wire is advanced through the needle and into the right side of the heart under fluoroscopic control (Fig. 5–6). On occasion, this guide wire enters the jugular system and ascends. This error can be corrected by manipulation under fluoroscopy. After removal of the needle, the introducer, dilator, and peel-away sheath are advanced over the guide wire into the central circulation (Fig. 5–7). Selection of the appropriate-sized introducer (from 7F to 12F) is based on the size of the lead or leads to be used. After removal of the dilator and guide, the pacing lead or leads are advanced through the sheath into the right side of the heart. One should take care to avoid

air embolism during this procedure by having the patient hold respiration until passage of the lead into the right side of the heart. The sheath is then peeled away (Fig. 5–8).

Potential complications of subclavian vein puncture that have been described include pneumothorax, hemopneumothorax, lung laceration, inadvertent arterial puncture, air embolism, arteriovenous fistula, thoracic duct injury, and brachial plexus injury. Pneumothorax is the most common complication, and use of contrast venography minimizes this risk. Contrast venography also lessens the risk of inadvertent subclavian artery puncture. Meticulous attention is required to minimize any of these risks.

Contrast venography requires no additional preparation with the exception of determining that the patient does not have a contrast allergy and placing an intravenous line (20 gauge or larger) in the arm on the side of the pulse generator

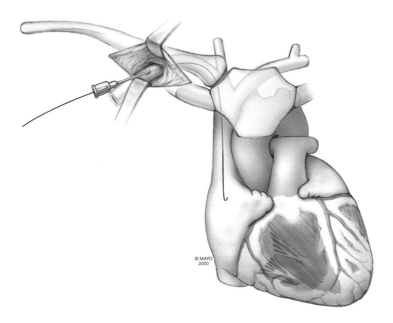

Fig. 5–6. The syringe is removed, the flexible guide wire is passed through needle, and the proximal end of the wire is directed into the region of the right atrium. (By permission of Mayo Foundation.)

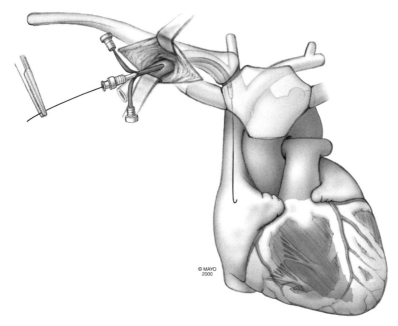

Fig. 5–7. With the guide wire in place, the needle is pulled back and off the guide wire. The dilator and peel-away sheath are then placed over the guide wire and passed into the subclavian vein. As the dilator and sheath are being passed into the vein, a hemostat is placed on the guide wire to prevent loss of the wire into the venous circulation. (By permission of Mayo Foundation.)

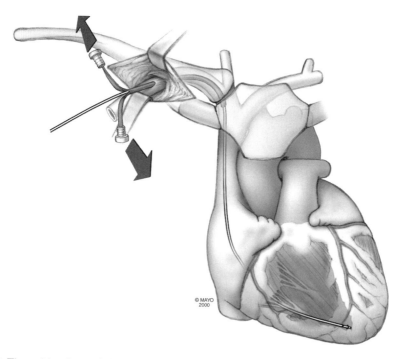

Fig. 5–8. The guide wire and dilator are removed from the sheath, and the pacing lead is quickly passed through the sheath into the right atrium. *Arrows* indicate pulling of the peel-away introducer from the lead. (By permission of Mayo Foundation.)

implantation.[9] The intravenous line should be checked for patency before injection of contrast medium. Some implanters prefer to use contrast venography routinely. Alternatively, in patients with normal costoclavicular relationships, no prior permanent pacing leads, and no venous thrombosis, a "blind" venipuncture can be first attempted as previously described. If the subclavian vein is not punctured on the initial attempts, a contrast agent is used to assist in localizing the vein. In patients who may have unusual venous anatomy, it may be desirable to use contrast venography before the initial attempt to ensure venous patency and location. Such patients might include those with kyphoscoliosis, prior clavicular fracture, or previous lead implantation.

The contrast injection can be done by anyone in the room with access to the peripheral, ipsilateral intravenous line. Approximately 14 to 20 mL of ionic or nonionic iodinated contrast medium is rapidly injected through the intravenous line in the forearm. A saline bolus may be used to flush the contrast agent into the venous system if necessary. It may also be helpful to massage the arm to assist in venous return and venous visualization. This can be done either under the sterile drapes by an assistant or over the sterile drapes by the implanter. The subclavicular area is monitored with fluoroscopy for the appearance of contrast, which usually takes from 5 to 20 seconds (Fig. 5–9).

With contrast medium in the vein, the venipuncture needle can be positioned directly into the subclavian vein with fluoroscopic guidance (Fig. 5–10). The anteroposterior location of the subclavian vein

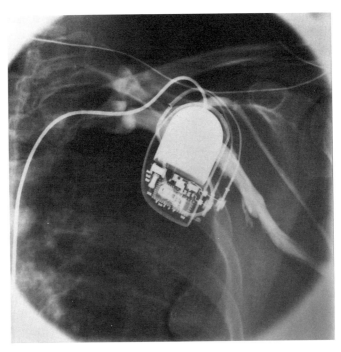

Fig. 5–9. Contrast venogram shows an occluded right subclavian vein in a patient with a long-term pacing lead in the subclavian vein. The venogram was obtained before attempted placement of an atrial lead and a dual-chamber pacemaker. The image was obtained approximately 15 to 20 seconds after contrast injection. (From Holmes DR Jr: Permanent pacemaker implantation. *In* A Practice of Cardiac Pacing. Edited by S Furman, DL Hayes, DR Holmes Jr. Mount Kisco, NY, Futura Publishing Company, 1986, pp 97–127. By permission of the publisher.)

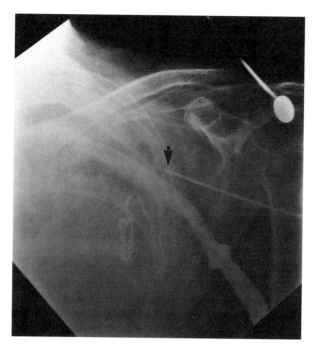

Fig. 5–10. Contrast venogram obtained during subclavian venipuncture. With contrast in the vein, the venipuncture needle (*arrow*) can be positioned directly into the subclavian vein under fluoroscopic guidance.

is not appreciated with anteroposterior fluoroscopy. Needle passes may occasionally be too anterior or posterior despite appearing to be within the column of contrast. Repeat injections are given as needed. Alternatively, if the contrast venogram demonstrates a nonpatent or small subclavian vein, the implanting physician may choose a different venous route.

Cephalic Approach

Some institutions prefer the cephalic or jugular approach, which avoids the risks of subclavian venipuncture.[10] The cephalic vein always lies within the deltopectoral groove. The deltopectoral groove is a constant anatomical site between the deltoid and pectoralis major muscles. The cephalic vein usually always accommodates a single lead and often accommodates two leads. The operative skills required for the cephalic approach are modest and can be readily taught to anyone sufficiently skilled to perform subclavian puncture or other invasive cardiovascular procedures. Cannulation of the cephalic vein is free of significant complications. If damaged, the vein can be ligated, with prompt cessation of bleeding. In addition, the normal venous pressure and the venous valves prevent aspiration of air into the central circulation.

If the cephalic vein is too small to accommodate even a single lead, a guide wire technique may be useful. For this technique, the cephalic vein is opened in the usual manner, but instead of attempting to pass the lead, the implanter places a guide wire through the opening into the superior vena cava or right atrium. The introducer is then placed over the guide wire, as in a conventional subclavian approach, and a lead or leads are introduced (Fig. 5–11).

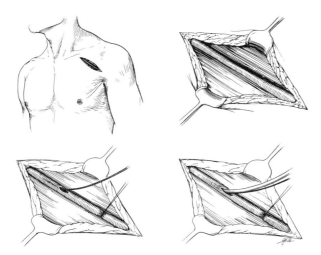

Fig. 5–11. A partial cephalic cutdown and introducer technique involves exposure of the cephalic vein in the deltopectoral groove (*upper left* and *upper right*). If the vein is too small to accept a lead, a guide wire is placed (*lower left*) and an introducer over it (*lower right*). (From Holmes DR, Hayes DL, Furman S: Permanent pacemaker implantation. *In* A Practice of Cardiac Pacing. Second revised and enlarged edition. Edited by S Furman, DL Hayes, DR Holmes Jr. Mount Kisco, NY, Futura Publishing Company, 1989, pp 239–287. By permission of Mayo Foundation.)

Jugular Approach

If the external or internal jugular vein is selected, two incisions are required. An incision is made immediately above the clavicle, over the area between the posterior border of the sternocleidomastoid muscle and the anterior border of the trapezius muscle.[2,3] External jugular access to the heart usually is easier by the right external jugular vein than by the left, because the vessel is often less tortuous. If no satisfactory external jugular vessel is found, the incision is extended to a point anterior to the sternal head of the sternocleidomastoid muscle. The carotid sheath is exposed after the superficial fascia is opened behind the posterior border of the sternocleidomastoid muscle. The muscle is then elevated to visualize the carotid sheath optimally. On occasion, the clavicular head of the sternocleidomastoid muscle must be divided to expose the carotid sheath (Fig. 5–12). The carotid sheath is then opened; the internal jugular vein is identified and isolated with nonabsorbable ligatures. After venotomy, the lead or leads can be introduced. Use of either the external or the internal jugular vein requires that the lead be tunneled down to the pulse generator site, either superficial or deep to the clavicle. In addition, the internal jugular procedure requires more extensive dissection with the possibility of damage to the subclavian artery and vein and the recurrent laryngeal nerve. Should the cutdown route be attempted before subclavian puncture, use of the cephalic and external jugular veins for introduction of lead systems remains consistent and reliable.

Iliac Vein Approach

Although not used at this institution to date, the iliac vein approach is worth knowing in the event that the more commonly used venous routes are not accessible (Fig. 5–13).

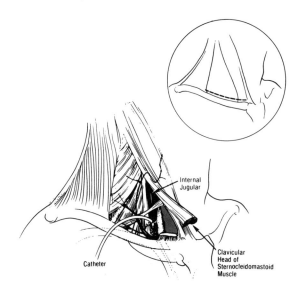

Fig. 5–12. Approach to the internal jugular vein. An incision (*inset*) is made immediately above the clavicle. The carotid sheath is exposed and then opened (see text for details). (From Brodman R, Furman S: Pacemaker implantation through the internal jugular vein. Ann Thorac Surg 29:63–65, 1980. By permission of The Society of Thoracic Surgeons.)

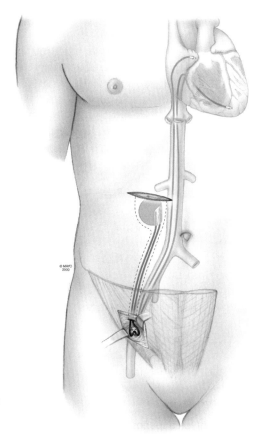

Fig. 5–13. Schematic approach to the iliac vein and pulse generator positioning. (By permission of Mayo Foundation.)

The recommended procedure is to puncture the iliac vein with standard puncture technique after making a small incision just above the inguinal ligament and to carry the dissection down to the fascia above the vein. After the puncture is made and lead or leads placed, a purse-string suture is placed to provide hemostasis. A pocket, superficial to the rectus sheath, is created lateral to the umbilicus.[2,11]

Ventricular Lead Placement

Successful placement of a reliable right ventricular pacing system requires knowledge of, and experience with, the specific lead used as well as knowledge of right heart anatomy and catheterization techniques. Great care must be taken during implantation to avoid damage to the lead. The lead stylet, in particular, should not be forced, because forcing may result in perforation of the stylet through the conductor coil and into the insulation. Keeping the stylet clean, free of blood, and moistened with saline helps avoid trauma to the lead during multiple stylet changes. Several placement techniques are used; all must result in a stable right ventricular catheter position with adequate pacing and sensing thresholds. Traditionally, the lead is positioned in the right ventricular apex. Currently, however, a great deal of controversy exists over whether other positions, such as high septal or outflow tract, may be hemodynamically superior. Other sites, for example, the right ventricular outflow tract, may also need to be considered preferentially over the apex because of local myocardial problems, such as previous inferoapical infarction.

When any lead is initially advanced into the central circulation, it should first be seen to pass to the right of the vertebral column through the superior vena cava. If the lead is introduced from the left side and passes to the left of the vertebral column, it is probably within a persistent left superior vena cava (Fig. 5–14). If this occurs, there are two options. One is to continue to advance the lead or leads through the coronary sinus and back into the heart. Although this approach has been reported many times, it can be difficult. The alternative is to abandon the procedure and then perform contrast

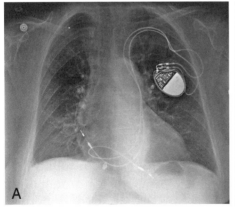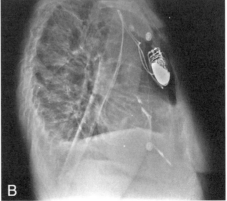

Fig. 5–14. Posteroanterior (*A*) and lateral (*B*) chest radiographs show leads placed through a persistent left superior vena cava.

venography from a peripheral intravenous line in the right arm to determine whether a right-sided superior vena cava also exists. If it does, the implant site can be moved to the right and leads placed in a traditional manner. One should be more alert to the possibility of a persistent left superior vena cava in a patient with associated congenital anomalies.

The lead can be initially passed through the introducer with a straight or a curved stylet in place. A curved stylet is helpful in introducing the lead across the tricuspid valve and into the pulmonary outflow tract. (A curved stylet is accomplished by wetting the stylet and the gloved index finger and thumb and pulling the stylet through the apposed fingers while rotating the fingers to impart a curve to the wire.) Initially placing the lead in the outflow tract assures that the lead is indeed in the right ventricle and not in the coronary sinus or in an extracardiac vessel, such as the hepatic vein. The lead may cause several premature ventricular contractions as it passes through the outflow tract, but these usually cease as the catheter passes into the main pulmonary artery. Once the lead tip is in the outflow tract, the curved guide wire should be replaced by a straight stylet. The straight stylet is not passed completely into the lead initially. The lead should be slowly withdrawn from the outflow tract, allowing the lead tip to fall toward the right ventricular apex. The stylet should be simultaneously advanced as the lead is slowly withdrawn, allowing the straightened lead to fall toward the apex. Once the lead falls from the outflow tract and is directed toward the apex, the lead, with stylet in place, should be advanced toward the apex. This maneuver may be assisted by asking the patient to breathe deeply, causing the right ventricular apex to descend with the diaphragm, at which point the lead can be advanced.

It is sometimes also possible to position the lead without a curved stylet. Once the lead is in the right atrium, the straight stylet should be withdrawn about 5 cm and the lead moved inferiorly. It will often catch in the right atrium and be deflected toward the tricuspid valve (Fig. 5–15). If the lead passes the tri-

Fig. 5–15. Intracardiac manipulation is basic to successful pacemaker implantation. Implantation of a dual-chamber pacemaker involves placement of an atrial and a ventricular lead. *A,* Both leads may be introduced via the subclavian, cephalic, or external jugular vein. Initially, both are in the superior vena cava or the right atrial appendage. *B,* Because ventricular stimulation is usually more important than atrial stimulation, the ventricular lead is positioned first. The atrial lead can be introduced immediately after or simultaneously with the ventricular lead or introduced after the ventricular lead is positioned. If the atrial lead is introduced before ventricular lead positioning, the atrial lead can be left in the upper inferior vena cava or low right atrium until time to position the lead. *C,* Once the ventricular lead is past the tricuspid valve and in the midright ventricle, it should be advanced into the pulmonary artery so that it is clear that it has not entered the coronary sinus (panel 6). *D,* If the lead tip will not pass the tricuspid valve, entry by deflection from the lateral atrial wall may be successful. *E,* Advancing the bowed lead in the right ventricle and then the guide wire within the bow can flip the lead tip into the right ventricular outflow tract. Note that during this entire maneuver, the atrial lead is "parked" in the inferior vena cava. *F,* As above, the lead is passed into the pulmonary artery. *G,* Once there, the lead is slowly withdrawn so that it falls toward the right ventricular apex. *H,* Once at the diaphragmatic surface of the ventricle, the lead is advanced into the apex. A deep breath angulates the apex downward and allows easier access. *I,* When the ventricular lead has been positioned properly, the guide wire is allowed to remain withdrawn about 1 inch from the tip to hold it in position while the atrial lead is being manipulated. *J,* Because the two leads often adhere lightly to each other, when one lead is manipulated, the other should be held so that it is not inadvertently displaced. The atrial lead should be pulled into the low right atrium and the guide wire withdrawn about 7 cm; the J will form. *K,* The atrial lead should then be pulled upward slowly. Entry into the base of the atrial appendage is recognized by straightening of the J with gentle traction on the lead. *L,* Additional traction is stopped, and the lead is advanced into the tip of the atrial appendage. (By permission of Mayo Foundation.)

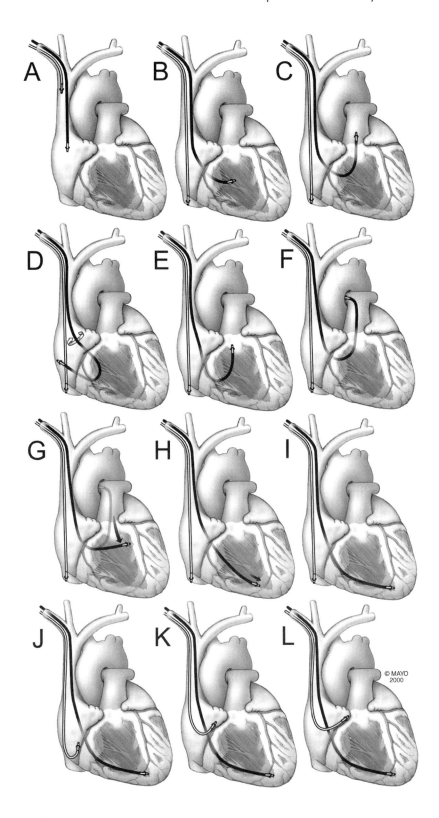

cuspid valve, it will be in the inflow tract of the right ventricle. These maneuvers are readily visible fluoroscopically and, if seen, assure that the lead has traversed the right ventricle. The lead occasionally enters the coronary sinus from the right atrium. A lead within the coronary sinus may appear to be within the right ventricle, but the passage is not superiorly but rather more laterally toward the left cardiac border. Should the lead begin to curl about the left cardiac border, it is certainly in the coronary sinus. In addition, no ventricular ectopy exists if the lead is in the coronary sinus. Attempts at entering the pulmonary artery will be unsuccessful, but the most important clue is in the lateral fluoroscopic view. The outflow tract of the right ventricle is an anterior structure, and a lead in it is seen in the retrosternal position. The coronary sinus is on the posterior wall of the heart, and a lead within it is visualized on the posterior cardiac border.

Alternatively, with the straight stylet withdrawn approximately 5 cm, the lead tip can be projected against the lateral atrial wall and the curved portion of the lead backed into the tricuspid valve.

The ventricular lead is usually positioned in the right ventricular apex. Radiographically, the end of the ventricular lead appears on the posteroanterior projection to be between the left border of the vertebral column and the cardiac apex. The position of the heart, vertical or relatively more horizontal, largely determines the position of the lead in relation to the cardiac apex and varies among patients. The lateral view is necessary to distinguish among apical positions in which the lead tip is anterior and caudally directed, is directed posteriorly in the right ventricle, and is on the posterior surface of the heart, that is, within the coronary sinus. On the posteroanterior radiographic view, the ventricular lead should have a gentle curve along the lateral wall of the right atrium and cross the tricuspid valve to the ventricular apex (Fig. 5–16).

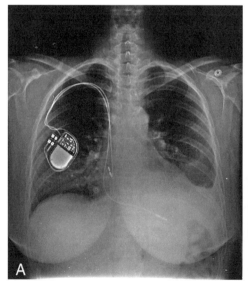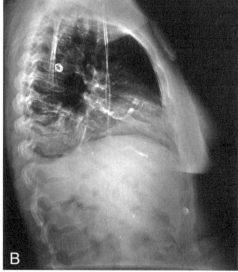

Fig. 5–16. Posteroanterior (*A*) and lateral (*B*) chest radiographs demonstrating gentle curve of the ventricular lead as it passes across the tricuspid lead.

If an atrial lead is not to be implanted, the guide wire can be removed from the ventricular lead and the lead can be checked for stability by deep breathing or coughing and by assessment of pacing and sensing thresholds. In addition, diaphragmatic stimulation should be assessed. Our technique is to pace at 10 V, the maximum voltage available on the pacing system analyzer used. During 10-V pacing, the left hemidiaphragm is assessed fluoroscopically for detection of pacing-induced excursions of the diaphragm. If an atrial lead is being assessed, the right hemidiaphragm is assessed fluoroscopically. Alternatively, a hand can be placed over the appropriate hemidiaphragm to feel for diaphragmatic stimulation. If diaphragmatic stimulation occurs, the lead should be repositioned.

If a single lead is being implanted as part of a "single-pass VDD" pacing system, special attention is necessary during lead placement. The tip of the lead is positioned in a standard manner to achieve a stable position with adequate ventricular pacing and sensing thresholds. How-ever, one must note the positioning of the atrial sensing electrodes that are incorporated within the lead. These electrodes need to be positioned within the atrium. To achieve this, it may be necessary to alter the usual curvature or redundancy of the lead (Fig. 5–17).

As previously noted, it may be desirable to position the lead somewhere other than in the right ventricular apex. The hemodynamic superiority of one position over the other has not yet been firmly established. However, so long as pacing and sensing thresholds are acceptable and the lead is secure, it can be positioned anywhere within the right ventricle.

Because of the difficulty in comparing different ventricular pacing sites, nomenclature has been proposed to describe alternative right ventricular pacing sites (other than for apical pacing).[12] The proposed sites are as follows:

- *Right ventricular inlet septal pacing.* Pacing above, on, or beneath the annulus of the septal-anterior tricus-

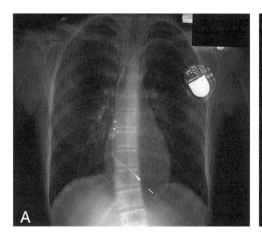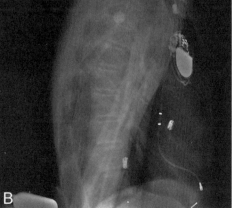

Fig. 5–17. Posteroanterior (*A*) and lateral (*B*) chest radiographs show a single-pass VDD lead system. The atrial sensing electrodes can be visualized in the vicinity of the right atrium.

pid valve leaflets, yielding relatively normal QRS morphology and axis ("A" in Fig. 5–18).

- *Right ventricular infundibular septal pacing.* Pacing proximal to the pulmonic valve and distal to, or near, the crista supraventricularis, yielding left bundle branch block and a vertical axis ("B" in Fig. 5–18).
- *Right ventricular outflow septal pacing.* Pacing site, most commonly referred to as "RVOT," near the septal-moderator band insertion at a midposition on the right ventricular septum, yielding left bundle branch block and a vertical axis ("C" in Fig. 5–18).
- *Right ventricular apical septal pacing.* Pacing proximal to the septal-moderator band continuity that does not typically produce a vertical QRS axis ("D" in Fig. 5–18).

If pacing is for hemodynamic relief of medically refractory hypertrophic car-

diomyopathy, it is crucial that the ventricular lead be positioned as apically as possible for maximum hemodynamic benefit.

Coronary sinus lead placement for left ventricular stimulation is also being used increasingly for patients with congestive heart failure. The hemodynamic implications of biventricular stimulation or cardiac resynchronization are discussed in detail in Chapter 2.

When a coronary sinus lead is implanted, it is introduced into the central venous circulation by the techniques already described. Several techniques are successful in cannulating the coronary sinus and passing the lead into a distal vessel to accomplish left ventricular stimulation. These options include

- Passing of the lead only, attempting to negotiate the coronary sinus os.
- A long sheath or delivery system through which the lead is passed and through which a balloon

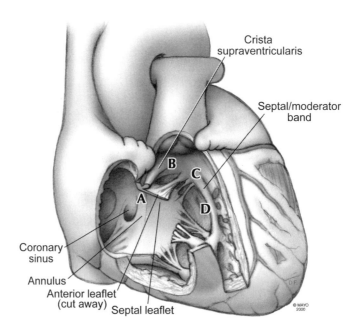

Fig. 5–18. Schematic representation of alternative right ventricular pacing sites proposed by Giudici and Karpawich[12] (see text for explanation of A through D). (By permission of Mayo Foundation.)

catheter can be passed to allow occlusion of the coronary sinus while a venogram is obtained.

- A specially designed over-the-wire pacing lead that allows the coronary sinus and tributaries to be negotiated in the same manner as that used for percutaneous coronary angiography (Fig. 5–19).

It is crucial that the physician placing the coronary sinus lead have a thorough understanding of coronary venous anatomy and appreciation of the marked interindividual variability of this anatomy (Fig. 5–20). Although much is yet to be learned about ideal coronary sinus lead placement when the goal is cardiac resynchronization, current thinking suggests a preference for

- Positioning in the lateral cardiac vein as the first choice (Fig. 5–21).
- A wide bipole between the right ventricular and the left ventricular lead tips.
- A measurable narrowing of the QRS width during pacing from the left ventricle or during simultaneous right ventricular and left ventricular pacing.

The ventricular lead of an ICD system, whether single- or dual-chamber, is placed in exactly the same manner as described above. However, alterations in technique may be required if defibrillation thresholds are unacceptable. Our approach is to first place the lead as apically as possible, so long as pacing and sensing thresholds are acceptable. If the defibrillation thresholds

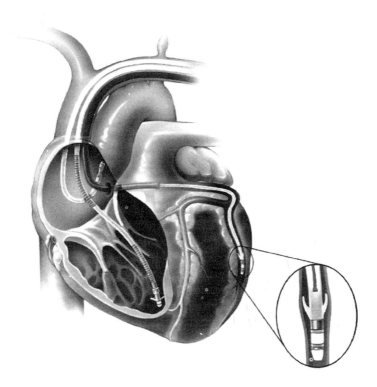

Fig. 5–19. Schematic drawing of pacing leads in the right atrium, right ventricle, and coronary sinus. The close-up view of the coronary sinus lead shows small tines that wedge the lead in the coronary vein. The coronary sinus lead in this illustration is implanted by an over-the-wire technique. (Courtesy of Guidant/CPI.)

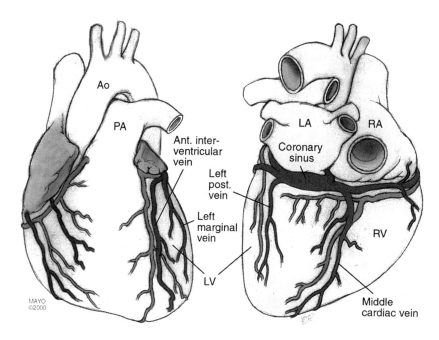

Fig. 5–20. Schematic drawing of the coronary venous anatomy. (By permission of Mayo Foundation.)

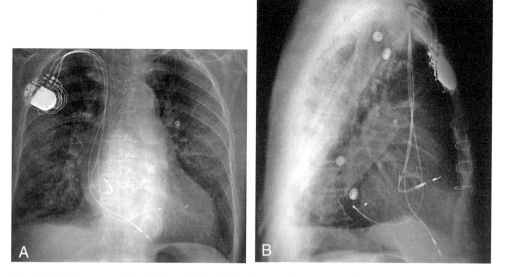

Fig. 5–21. Posteroanterior (*A*) and lateral (*B*) chest radiographs with pacing leads positioned in the right atrial appendage, right ventricular apex, and lateral coronary vein.

are unacceptable, the lead is usually repositioned to an alternative right ventricular site where thresholds are again acceptable. Acceptable thresholds can be obtained with a single-coil right ventricular lead in more than 90% of patients.

If adequate defibrillation thresholds cannot be achieved despite repeated repositioning of the right ventricular lead, and if this lead is a single-coil lead, a superior vena cava lead can be placed and threshold testing repeated with both leads (Fig. 5–22). This should result in acceptable defibrillation thresholds for most patients in whom a single coil failed to achieve acceptable ones. However, if thresholds are still unacceptable, a subcutaneous array can be considered.

A subcutaneous array (Fig. 5–23) consists of three electrically common multifilar coils that form one electrode. The coils come together in an insulated cable that is connected to a terminal pin that can be connected to the connector block. The "array" provides a greater surface area over the lateral chest to facilitate defibrillation (Fig. 5–24). Our approach is to make an incision near the midaxillary line at the level of the nipple. Dissection is carried to the level of the muscle. With a trochar that is supplied with the array, three tunnels are formed, one at a time, with a peelaway introducer over the trochar. The trochar is removed, and one of the three coils is placed within the sheath, which is carefully peeled away. Once all three are placed, each coil is secured to the underlying tissue with the sleeve provided, and the "yoke," or point where the three coils join, is secured to the underlying tissue as well. The insulated cable is then passed into the inferior portion of the previously formed prepectoral pocket and connected to the ICD.

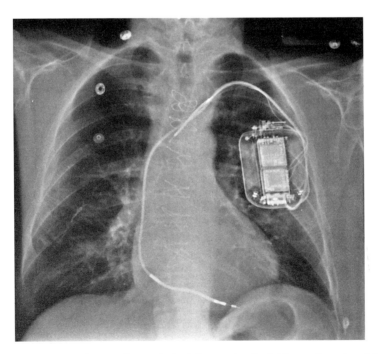

Fig. 5–22. Posteroanterior chest radiograph depicting an implantable cardioverter-defibrillator system that has a superior vena cava lead in addition to the right ventricular lead.

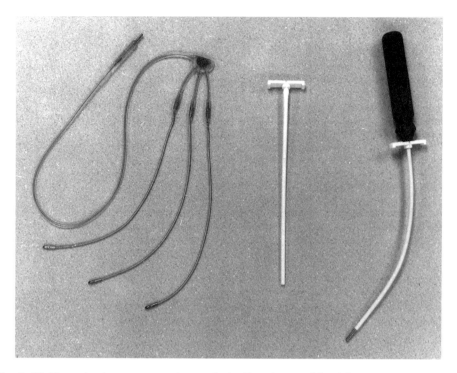

Fig. 5–23. The subcutaneous array is supplied with a three-coil lead that connects to a single body for connection to the cardioverter-defibrillator (*left*), peel-away sheaths for each of the three coils (*center*), and a trochar for lead placement (*right*).

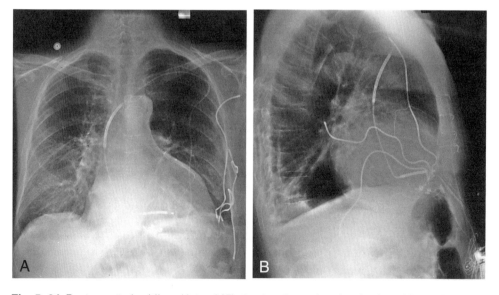

Fig. 5–24. Posteroanterior (*A*) and lateral (*B*) chest radiographs of an implantable cardioverter-defibrillator system that incorporates a subcutaneous array. Adequate defibrillation thresholds could not be achieved without the array.

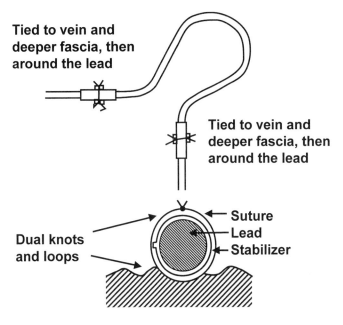

Fig. 5–25. Implantable cardioverter-defibrillator lead secured with two sleeves in a configuration to provide a strain-relief loop.

Securing the Lead

If pacing and sensing thresholds are satisfactory and there is no diaphragmatic stimulation measured with pacing at 10 V, the silicone rubber sleeve provided on the lead is positioned over the lead at the point of entry into the vein. Synthetic nonabsorbable ligature is used to fix the sleeve to the lead and to the muscle or the vein itself. It is essential to use the sleeve and not affix the lead directly to the adjacent tissue. Ligatures applied directly to the lead may damage the insulation and act as a fulcrum, with eventual lead fracture at the fixation.

Some ICD leads are manufactured with two sleeves. The use of the second sleeve is optional. The original rationale behind two sleeves on ICD leads was to allow additional anchoring support for the heavier pulse generator. If both sleeves are used, they should be secured to the lead in the manner described and then secured to the underlying tissue in such a way as to form a "strain-relief" loop (Fig. 5–25). Again, with the rapid decrease in weight and volume of ICDs, clinically important use of the second sleeve is relatively uncommon.

Dual-Chamber Pulse Generator Implantation

The subclavian introducer technique can be used to place two leads. Three variations of the technique can be selected. Two subclavian venipunctures can be made, one for each catheter to be inserted, the ventricular lead being placed first (Fig. 5–26). This technique reduces the potential for displacement of one lead while the other is being positioned but requires two separate venipunctures. In the second variation, one venipuncture is made and one lead is introduced, and the guide wire is reintroduced or retained before the sheath is peeled away (Fig. 5–27 *A*); a new intro-

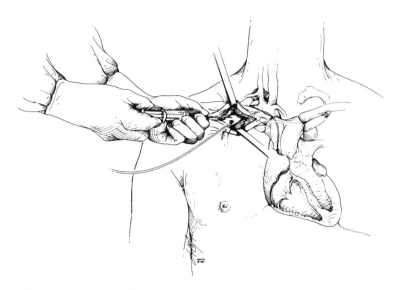

Fig. 5–26. If a second lead is to be used, a second subclavian puncture can be made parallel to the already placed pacing lead or the second puncture can be accomplished after the first guide wire is in place but before the first pacing lead is inserted. If the second puncture is made after the initial lead is in place, care should be taken to avoid puncturing the indwelling lead. The potential for damage can be minimized by placing the puncture medial to the existing lead. (From Holmes DR, Hayes DL, Furman S: Permanent pacemaker implantation. *In* A Practice of Cardiac Pacing. Second revised and enlarged edition. Edited by S Furman, DL Hayes, DR Holmes Jr. Mount Kisco, NY, Futura Publishing Company, 1989, pp 239–287. By permission of Mayo Foundation.)

ducer is placed over the retained guide wire to accommodate the second lead (Fig. 5–27 *B*). In the third variation, two leads (one for atrial and one for ventricular placement) can be advanced through the same introducer sheath into the right side of the heart (Fig. 5–28). (The size of the introducer required to introduce two leads depends on the additive size of the two leads. With current leads, it should be possible to accommodate two bipolar leads in a 12F introducer.)

Our preference is to position the ventricular lead and then pass the atrial lead. Alternatively, both leads can be passed into the right heart and the atrial lead held in a stable position in the right atrium while the ventricular lead is positioned in the right ventricular apex. After stable ventricular placement is achieved, the atrial lead is positioned.

Placement of the atrial lead is identi-cal for either single-chamber or dual-chamber pulse generators. Although the atrial lead is most commonly positioned in the right atrial appendage, satisfactory pacing can be achieved from multiple positions within the right atrium. In patients with previous cardiac surgery in whom the appendage has been cannulated or amputated, finding a stable position in the atrial appendage may be more difficult but is usually possible.

Technique varies, depending on whether a preformed atrial J lead or a nonpreformed lead, that is, a standard straight lead that can be used in either the atrium or the ventricle, is used. If a preformed J lead is chosen, a straight stylet is placed in the lead to straighten it, and the lead is passed into the middle to low right atrium (Fig. 5–29 *A*). The straight stylet is withdrawn approximately 10 cm, and the lead assumes the J shape (Fig. 5–29 *B*). The

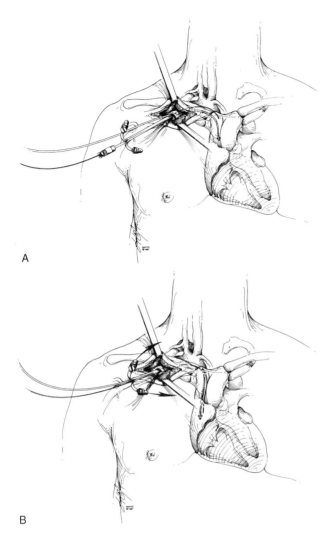

A

B

Fig. 5–27. Two leads can be placed without a second subclavian puncture and without simultaneously passing the leads. *A,* As the dilator and guide wire are removed and the initial pacing lead is passed into the right heart, the guide wire is reinserted through the peel-away introducer alongside the pacing lead. The introducer is then peeled away, and the pacing lead and guide wire are left in place. *B,* A second introducer is then passed over the reintroduced guide wire, and the second lead is placed. (From Holmes DR, Hayes DL, Furman S: Permanent pacemaker implantation. *In* A Practice of Cardiac Pacing. Second revised and enlarged edition. Edited by S Furman, DL Hayes, DR Holmes Jr. Mount Kisco, NY, Futura Publishing Company, 1989, pp 239–287. By permission of Mayo Foundation.)

lead is gradually withdrawn in an effort to secure the lead tip against the endocardial surface (Fig. 5–29 C). If the lead tip is securely against the atrial wall when the J begins to straighten, the lead should again be advanced slowly to allow the appropriate J to occur. If the lead has active fixation, the fixation mechanism should then be secured. Sensing and pacing thresholds should be checked. If they are adequate, the lead should be secured with the sleeve provided, as previously described.

Entry into the atrial appendage is indicated by a rhythmic to and fro medial and lateral motion of the J portion of the lead. The posteroanterior fluoroscopic projection may show that the lead is medial or lateral, and a lateral projection shows the lead to be anterior at approximately the same level as a lead in the right ventricular apex. If the atrial lead is being placed as part of a dual-chamber implant, the ventricular lead should be carefully observed so that it is not inadvertently displaced.

If a straight active fixation lead is used, a J curved stylet is needed to enter the atrial appendage. The stylet is introduced into the atrial lead in the low right atrium, and the lead is pulled into the

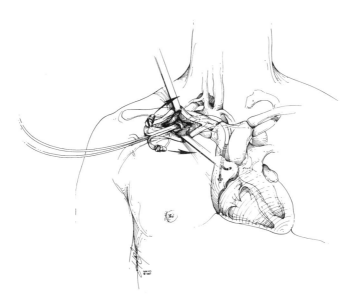

Fig. 5–28. If two pacing leads are necessary, they can be inserted simultaneously through a peel-away introducer large enough to accommodate both of them. With straight stylets in place, one lead is staggered 1 to 2 cm behind the other lead, and they are passed simultaneously into the right heart, whereupon the introducer is peeled away. (From Holmes DR, Hayes DL, Furman S: Permanent pacemaker implantation. *In* A Practice of Cardiac Pacing. Second revised and enlarged edition. Edited by S Furman, DL Hayes, DR Holmes Jr. Mount Kisco, NY, Futura Publishing Company, 1989, pp 239–287. By permission of Mayo Foundation.)

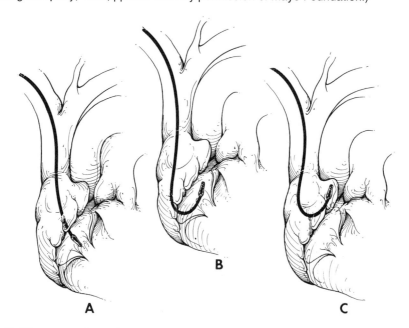

Fig. 5–29. Placement of a preformed atrial J lead. *A,* The lead is at the middle of the right atrium with a straight stylet in place. *B,* The straight stylet is removed; removal allows the catheter to assume the preformed J configuration. *C,* The entire lead is pulled back, and the tip of the electrode is allowed to enter the right atrial appendage. The lead has a characteristic to-and-fro motion when positioned in the right atrial appendage. (From Holmes DR, Hayes DL, Furman S: Permanent pacemaker implantation. *In* A Practice of Cardiac Pacing. Second revised and enlarged edition. Edited by S Furman, DL Hayes, DR Holmes Jr. Mount Kisco, NY, Futura Publishing Company, 1989, pp 239–287. By permission of Mayo Foundation.)

right atrial appendage. The active fixation lead is fixed in place, and the J guide wire is gently withdrawn to avoid displacing the lead from the point of attachment. Again, sensing and pacing thresholds should be checked. If they are adequate, the lead should be secured with the sleeve provided, as previously described.

Regardless of whether a preformed J or a straight lead is implanted in the atrium, with implantation in the right atrial appendage the J portion of the lead is slightly medial on the posteroanterior projection and anterior on the lateral projection. Optimally, the limits of the J should be no greater than approximately 80° apart. Redundancy proximal to the J within the atrium or superior vena cava should not be seen.

As noted above, locations other than the right atrial appendage may be used for atrial lead positioning, and their use is increasing. The right atrium can be explored, particularly when lateral fluoroscopy is available, to find optimal positioning for lead placement. With active fixation leads, the lead can be placed in the atrial septum or in the free atrial wall (Fig. 5–30).

Atrial leads are being positioned in the coronary sinus, adjacent to the coronary sinus os, and in septal positions to prevent recurrent atrial fibrillation and flutter.[13–15] The hemodynamic implications of dual-site atrial pacing are discussed in detail in Chapter 2.

The technical details of introduction of a coronary sinus lead have previously been described. Obviously, for atrial pacing, the coronary sinus lead needs to be positioned in a tributary of the coronary sinus that will afford adequate and stable atrial pacing and sensing. The ideal position is probably in the vein of Marshall (Fig. 5–31). Once again, because of the individual variability in coronary venous anatomy, not all patients have a true vein of Marshall.

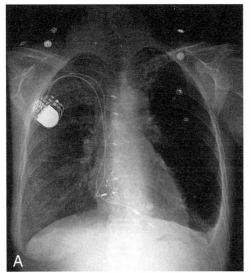 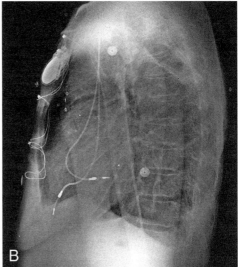

Fig. 5–30. Posteroanterior (*A*) and lateral (*B*) views of placement of an active fixation atrial lead in the lateral wall of the atrium.

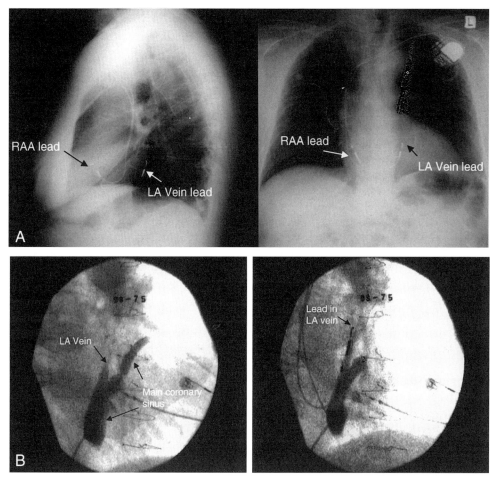

Fig. 5–31. Chest radiographs (*A*) and coronary venograms (*B*) depicting the vein of Marshall, a coronary venous position for left atrial pacing. LA, left atrial; RAA, right atrial appendage. (Courtesy of Dr. Anthony Tang, Ottawa Heart Institute, Ottawa, Ontario, Canada.)

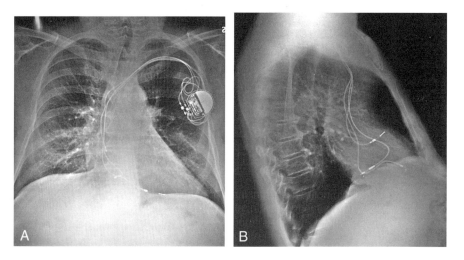

Fig. 5–32. Posteroanterior (*A*) and lateral (*B*) chest radiographs from a patient with paroxysmal atrial fibrillation in whom a dual-chamber pacemaker with dual-site atrial pacing has been implanted.

To position an active fixation atrial lead near the coronary sinus os, the lead is passed into the coronary sinus and then gently withdrawn and secured after exiting the coronary sinus. (A straight lead is required; a preformed J should not be used.) Fluoroscopic imaging in a right anterior oblique position may allow one to better visualize the posterior and septal position desirable (Fig. 5–32). The left anterior oblique fluoroscopic view is helpful subsequently to verify the location of the lead.

Special circumstances may call for innovative placement of the atrial lead. An atrial endocardial lead was placed through the atrial wall at the time of open heart surgery, and stable atrial pacing was maintained without complication (Fig. 5–33).

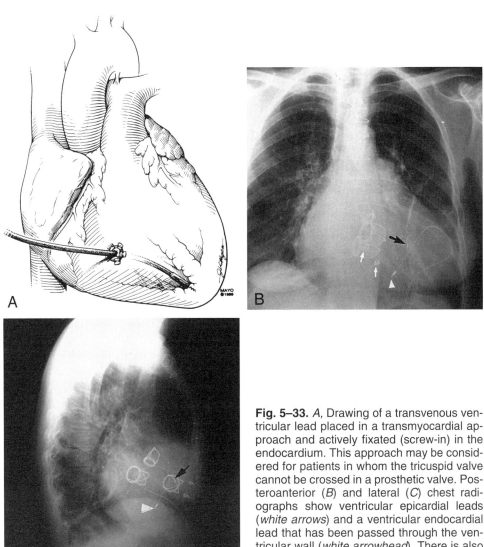

Fig. 5–33. *A*, Drawing of a transvenous ventricular lead placed in a transmyocardial approach and actively fixated (screw-in) in the endocardium. This approach may be considered for patients in whom the tricuspid valve cannot be crossed in a prosthetic valve. Posteroanterior (*B*) and lateral (*C*) chest radiographs show ventricular epicardial leads (*white arrows*) and a ventricular endocardial lead that has been passed through the ventricular wall (*white arrowhead*). There is also a portion of a fractured epicardial lead (*black arrow*). (From Hayes et al.[3] By permission of Mayo Foundation.)

Measurement of Pacing and Sensing Thresholds

Knowledge and measurement of pacing and sensing thresholds are integral parts in the placement of a permanent pacemaker or ICD. The equipment used and measurements made vary from laboratory to laboratory. In most institutions, pacing system analyzers are used. These are available from the pulse generator manufacturers. Most centers use an analyzer from a single manufacturer. (Although of historical concern, use of a mismatched pacing system analyzer and pulse generator rarely, if ever, results in any clinical problem.) In some laboratories, physiologic recorders with bandwidths of 0.1 to 2,000 Hz are used to assess intracardiac electrograms. Measurements necessary during device implantation are listed in Table 5–2.

Determination of Pacing Threshold

The pacing threshold is the minimal electrical stimulus required to produce consistent cardiac depolarization. It should be measured with the same electrode configuration (unipolar or bipolar) as the lead and pulse generator that are to be used. During pacing, the output of the pacing system analyzer is gradually decreased from 5 V to the point at which loss of capture is documented. The pacing rate selected during this measurement is important. The rate should be just fast enough (approximately 10 bpm faster) to override the intrinsic rhythm. In some patients, pacing during measurement of thresholds suppresses intrinsic rhythm and results in the lack of a stable ventricular escape focus, or even asystole, when pacing is discontinued. The implanting physician may decide to position a temporary pacemaker in these patients. The lower the stimulation threshold, the better. Acceptable acute thresholds are less than 1 V for both ventricular and atrial leads at 0.5 msec pulse duration. Typical acute thresholds for ventricular leads at 0.5 msec pulse duration are approximately 0.5 V and 1.4 mA, and typical thresholds for atrial leads are 0.9 V and 1.8 mA.

If active fixation leads are used, thresholds checked immediately after deployment of the fixation mechanism may

---

Table 5–2.
Measurements During Pacemaker or Cardioverter-Defibrillator Implantation

---

Threshold of stimulation
  Atrium*
  Ventricle
Sensing threshold
  Atrium†
  Ventricle
Measurement of electrogram‡
  Atrium*
  Ventricle
Measurement of antegrade conduction§
  Wenckebach-block point
Defibrillation threshold‖

---

*Necessary only when an atrial lead is being placed.

†Necessary only when an atrial lead or a single-pass VDD lead is used.

‡Considered optional by many, and these measurements can be accomplished noninvasively with many devices.

§Necessary only when an AAI implant is considered.

‖For cardioverter-defibrillator implantation only.

not reflect true thresholds. If the lead position looks good and the initial thresholds are high, it is worthwhile waiting for a short time, for example, 1 minute, and repeating the measurements to see whether the thresholds are now acceptable.

The impedance of the pacing electrode is also measured, usually by Ohm's law, in which volts equal current times resistance. Measurement of volts and current allows calculation of the lead resistance, which varies greatly depending on the lead used. A range from 300 to 1,500 Ω may be seen, depending on lead type. Impedances should always be measured under standardized conditions of output and pulse duration. The finding of unsuspected low impedance raises the possibility of an insulation failure in the lead and that of high impedance the possibility of a poor connection or lead fracture.

Determination of Sensing Threshold

Measurement of sensing thresholds is equally important. Adequate sensing thresholds are essential to avoid the problem of undersensing or oversensing after implantation. The pulse generator senses intracardiac events, not the events seen on the surface electrocardiogram (Fig. 5–34). The intrinsic deflection is that component of the intracardiac electrogram that is sensed.[16] It is the amplitude of this intracardiac signal in the chamber to be paced that is measured. The result is expressed as a voltage. The ventricular electrogram sensed for adequate long-term sensing should be more than 4 mV. More commonly, the ventricular signal is 6 to 20 mV, a range that provides excellent sensing. For atrial sensing, a signal of at least 2 mV is desirable. However, with current pacemakers that offer programmable options for atrial sensing as low as 0.18 mV and with ICDs that incorporate autosensing to vary sensitivity values, lower atrial sensing thresholds can at times be accepted. Still, the goal should be a measured P wave of at least 2 mV.

In addition to peak amplitude, other aspects of sensing should be considered. The change in voltage with time (dV/dt), the slew rate, of the intrinsic deflection may be clinically important. Usually, this

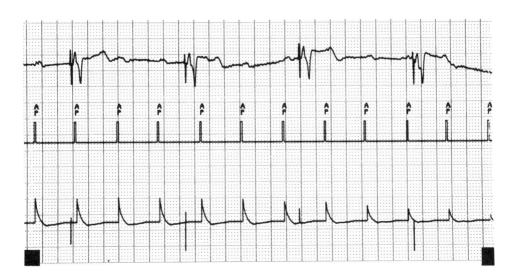

Fig. 5–34. Intracardiac electrograms obtained at the time of pacemaker implantation in a patient with complete heart block. Pacemakers sense intracardiac electrograms, specifically intrinsic deflection of either ventricle or atrium. The slew rate is a measure of dV/dt (see text for details).

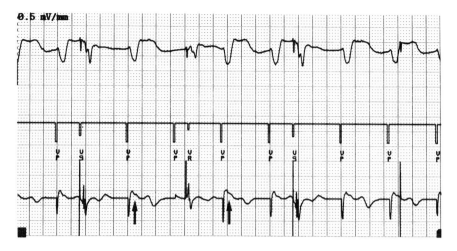

Fig. 5–35. Intracardiac electrograms at the time of pacemaker implantation. In addition to assessment of magnitude and relationship of intrinsic deflection of atrium and ventricle, a current of injury is identified (*arrows*). This current of injury, manifested as an increase in electrical potential after intrinsic deflection, indicates adequate endocardial contact.

is most important in patients with borderline sensing voltages. In patients with low voltages (< 5 mV), the slew rate measurement may be helpful and with current pacing system analyzers is easy to obtain. Some patients with a QRS of 3 mV but a slow slew rate may have undersensing, whereas other patients with a QRS of 3 mV but a normal slew rate have normal sensing.

Few institutions currently assess electrograms. If electrograms are assessed, an added feature is evaluation of current of injury at the time of lead placement. The current, appearing as an increase in the electrical potential that immediately follows the intrinsic deflection, represents a small area of damaged endocardium (Fig. 5–35). This finding indicates adequate contact with the endocardium.

Additional Measurements

Assessment of atrioventricular (AV) nodal conduction is necessary if an AAI pacemaker is to be implanted. In this situation, the atrial lead is positioned and the atrium is paced at rates nearly equal to the sinus rate and then at incremental rates up to approximately 150 bpm. A typical sequence might be 80, 100, 120, 140, and 160 bpm. The pacing rate at which Wenckebach, or higher grade, AV block occurs is recorded, as is the AR interval (paced atrial event to intrinsic QRS). To proceed with AAI pacing, the patient should have 1:1 conduction to rates of 130 to 140 bpm without any significant prolongation of the AR interval.

Epimyocardial Systems

Epimyocardial systems account for no more than 5% of pacemaker implantation procedures. Three groups of patients still undergo placement of epicardial systems.

1. Patients undergoing cardiac surgery for another indication. In these patients, permanent epicardial leads may be placed at the time of surgery. Alternatively, some of these patients have temporary pacing until recovery from open-heart surgery. Before dismissal from the hospital, they may undergo placement of a trans-

venous pacing system. This latter approach is preferable, since transvenous leads have proven to be more reliable than epimyocardial leads.

2. Patients with a prosthetic tricuspid valve, a congenital anomaly, or atresia of the tricuspid valve. In these patients, epimyocardial ventricular leads are usually required. Bioprosthetic valves are, however, compatible with transvenous implantation. In our experience, we have not seen any adverse outcomes from placing a transvenous lead across a bioprosthetic valve.

3. Patients with ventricular septal defects or patients with right-to-left shunts in whom the possibility for systemic embolization exists.

Two surgical procedures have been described for the placement of epimyocardial leads: (1) subxiphoid, or left costal, approach and (2) left lateral thoracotomy. Such procedures obviously require a trained surgeon, and the reader is referred to cardiovascular surgical texts for details of these approaches.

Hardware Adaptations

The "pin" of the implanted lead connects to the "header" of the pulse generator to provide the permanent but reversible connection between the two. The portion of the connector on the header holds the portion that is the extravascular end of the lead.

Although some bifurcated bipolar leads are still in service, most contemporary leads, whether unipolar or bipolar and whether coaxial or some other conductor design, are of the "in-line" variety. They conform to a formal, international pacing connector standard, the "international standard," or IS-1, design.

VS (voluntary standard)-1/IS-1 pacing leads are 3.2 mm in diameter, have sealing rings on the lead, and have a short (0.508 cm) terminal pin (Fig. 5–36).

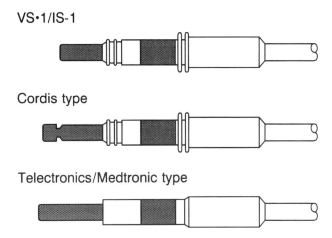

VS·1/IS-1

Cordis type

Telectronics/Medtronic type

Fig. 5–36. VS-1/IS-1 connectors are intended to restore universal interconnection of all leads and pulse generators via the standardized 3.2-mm connectors. The pin is connected to the negative output and the ring to the positive terminal in the pulse generator header. Unipolar leads of similar configuration exist, but without a positive terminal, and are of the same size as and interchangeable with a bipolar receptacle. The ridges represent the sealing rings, which prevent the ingress of fluid into the header. The leads with longer pins have been commonly referred to by the manufacturer's name (see text).

Table 5–3.
Pacemaker Connector Block Variations

VS-1/IS-1	Accepts only VS-1/IS-1 leads
VS-1A/IS-1A	Accepts VS-1/IS-1 leads and 3.2-mm in-line leads with a longer pin
VS-1B/IS-1B	Accepts VS-1/IS-1 leads and 3.2-mm in-line leads that have a longer pin and sealing rings

VS-1/IS-1 pacing leads fit all 3.2-mm pacemakers. VS-1/IS-1 pacemaker headers are 3.2 mm in diameter, have *no* sealing rings, have a short (5.08 cm) receptacle for the lead terminal, and accept only VS-1/IS-1 pacing leads. Table 5–3 provides an abbreviated compatibility guide for various pacing leads and pacemaker headers.

Pacemaker headers with the designations VS-1A and VS-1B still exist as a point of confusion (Fig. 5–37). Pacemakers designated VS-1A are 3.2 mm in diameter, have no sealing rings, and have a long (0.851 cm) receptacle for the lead terminal. Pacemakers with the VS-1B designation have sealing rings in the header but are otherwise like the VS-1A designation (Fig. 5–37). This terminology need not be confusing. Dimensions are the same for both unipolar and bipolar VS-1/IS-1 leads and pacers. There is only one configuration for VS-1 and IS-1 lead connectors. The VS-1 and IS-1 designs have provisions within the pacer connector for three functional options.

Many older connector leads remain in use; therefore, as pulse generator replacement is required, adapters will be necessary. Some pulse generators are now made specifically to accommodate pulse generator replacement. Some pacemakers are available in a variety of connector formats: (1) in-line bipolar, that is, 3.2 mm; (2) 3.2 mm IS-1 unipolar; (3) unipolar to accept an older 5-mm lead only; and (4) unipolar to accept a 5- or 6-mm lead.

An attempt should be made to match polarity and design of the pacing lead and pulse generator, for example, a bipolar in-

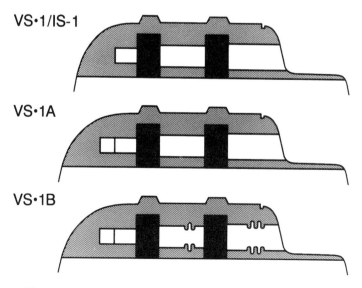

Fig. 5–37. Variations in pacemaker headers. See text.

Table 5–4.
Specific Adaptor for Specific Combination

	Lead		
Pulse generator	Unipolar	In-line bipolar	Bifurcated bipolar
Unipolar	ō	Low-profile adaptor sleeve (1)	End cap (2)
In-line bipolar	Low-profile lead to bifurcated pulse generator (5) and an indifferent electrode (4)	ō	Bifurcated lead to in-line generator adaptor (3)
Bipolar with bifurcated connector	Indifferent electrode (4)	Low-profile lead to bifurcated pulse generator adaptor (5)	ō

From Holmes DR, Hayes DL, Furman S: Permanent pacemaker implantation. *In* A Practice of Cardiac Pacing. Second revised and enlarged edition. Edited by S Furman, DL Hayes, DR Holmes Jr. Mount Kisco, NY, Futura Publishing Company, 1989, p 276. By permission of the publisher.

line lead to a bipolar in-line pulse generator and a bifurcated bipolar lead to a bipolar pulse generator. Special adaptors are necessary to allow use of polarity-mismatched lead and pulse generator. Table 5–4 outlines possible combinations and adaptors necessary. Each adaptor is numbered, and the numbers correspond to the numbers in Figure 5–38, which shows the adaptors. Again, every attempt should be

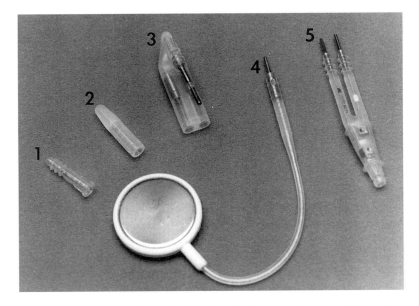

Fig. 5–38. Various adaptors used for pacing lead and pulse generator mismatches. The numbers (1 to 5) correspond to those in Table 5–4, which outlines specific adaptors needed for specific combinations. 1 = bipolar in-line sleeve adaptor; 2 = end cap; 3 = bifurcated lead to in-line connector; 4 = indifferent electrode; and 5 = in-line lead to bifurcated connector. (From Holmes DR, Hayes DL, Furman S: Permanent pacemaker implantation. *In* A Practice of Cardiac Pacing. Second revised and enlarged edition. Edited by S Furman, DL Hayes, DR Holmes Jr. Mount Kisco, NY, Futura Publishing Company, 1989, pp 239–287. By permission of Mayo Foundation.)

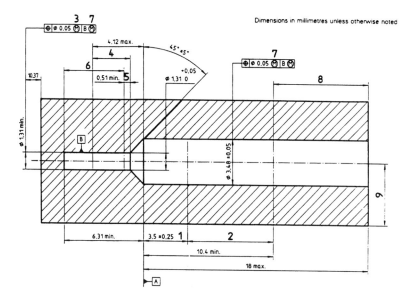

Fig. 5–39. Schematic representation of the DF-1 connector for implantable cardioverter-defibrillator leads.

made to match lead and pulse generator hardware configuration.

ICD leads currently follow a different standard, known as DF-1, than that for pacing leads[17] (Fig. 5–39). At present, ICD leads from major United States manufacturers are compatible with the DF-1 standard. Pacing and ICD lead selection is discussed in Chapter 4.

Special Considerations in Pediatric Patients

Permanent pacing in the pediatric population raises specific issues, including the size and expected growth of the patients, whether congenital heart disease is associated, the need for long-term pacing, and often a need for dual-chamber pacing systems.

Transvenous systems are used most frequently and have been shown to be superior to epicardial systems. Previous studies showed that survival of endocardial leads was superior to that of myoepicardial leads in pediatric patients.

In the pediatric patient with congeni-tal cardiovascular anomalies who is undergoing permanent pacing, it is helpful to know before implantation whether the child has an associated persistent left superior vena cava. This can usually be determined echocardiographically. If concern exists, angiography is diagnostic. Advancing the pacing lead into a persistent left superior vena cava results in traversing the coronary sinus to the right ventricle. To avoid the problems associated with a persistent left superior vena cava, the right subclavian vein should be used if there is any doubt about whether the patient has a persistent left superior vena cava. Even with a left superior vena cava, the patient usually has a right superior vena cava.

For lead placement, there are two potential approaches. The first is to allow more lead redundancy than would usually be left in an adult patient but to otherwise use standard techniques to place the lead, including securing the lead with the sleeve provided. However, instead of securing the sleeve with nonabsorbable suture, as is our usual practice, some believe that the use of absorbable suture may allow the lead to advance as the child grows.

The additional redundancy of the lead allows for growth of the pediatric patient (Fig. 5–40). If this approach is taken, the leads must be evaluated periodically during follow-up. If the child "outgrows" the lead, that is, there is radiographic evidence of straightening of the lead, it is necessary to place a new lead. Because of entrapment of the lead in the venous system and cardiac chambers, the lead may not "advance" on its own, and lead advancement may not even be possible with a stylet in place after the lead has been in place for a long period. Although a variety of clinical situations may occur when the patient truly "outgrows" the pacing system, most commonly, intermittent sensing abnormalities occur as tension develops on the lead at the electrode-tissue interface.

It is of particular importance to select the smallest pulse generator that allows the desired pacing mode for the pediatric patient. The small weight and dimensions of

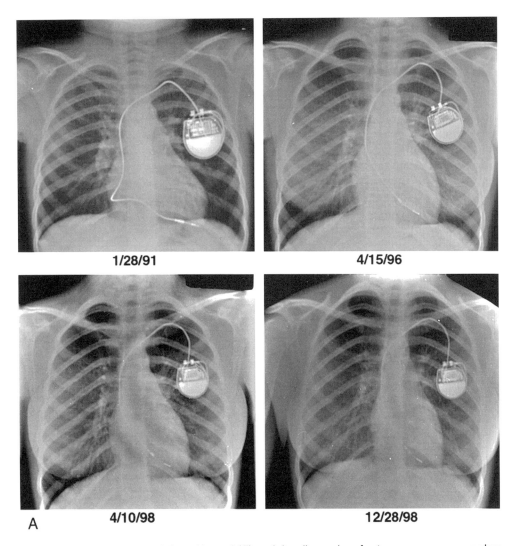

1/28/91

4/15/96

A   4/10/98

12/28/98

Fig. 5–40. Posteroanterior (*A*) and lateral (*B*) serial radiographs of a transvenous pacemaker in a child show that initial lead redundancy decreases with growth. *Continues.*

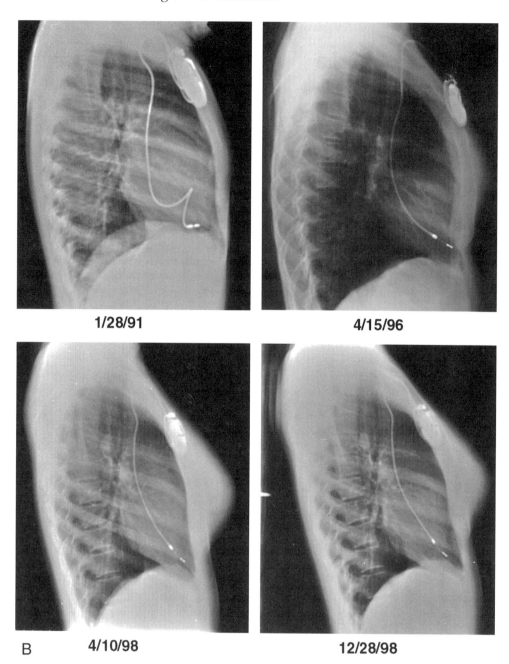

1/28/91

4/15/96

B   **4/10/98**

12/28/98

Fig. 5–40 *continued.*

current pulse generators allow implantation in a prepectoral position in a patient of almost any size. In very small infants, if there is a concern that there is not enough subcutaneous tissue to protect the pacemaker, consideration may be given to placing the pacemaker in a subpectoral position. In our experience, this placement is not often necessary with pacemakers but has been necessary occasionally for ICDs. Before the advent of very small pulse generators, the transvenous lead was occasionally tunneled subcutaneously from the pectoral entry site to an area in the abdomen or flank where the pulse generator could be placed more easily. This approach, too, is rarely necessary with the small size of currently available pulse generators.

Traditional venous routes can be used in the pediatric patient. That is, the subclavian puncture technique with placement of one or two leads via the subclavian vein is usually possible. Two leads can often be placed via the cephalic vein as well. Use of a single-pass VDD pacing system should be considered in the pediatric patient with AV block. Such a system minimizes hardware but still accomplishes AV synchrony and maintains P-synchronous rate adaptation if the sinus node is intact.

Although any standard pacing lead can be used in pediatric patients, active fixation leads are generally preferred for specific reasons. Active fixation may allow additional stability of the lead in the immediate postimplantation period, when it is difficult to control the activities of a pediatric patient. The pediatric patient may require several pacing systems during the growth years. Although a noninfected lead may be abandoned and left in place, it is reasonable to attempt removal of abandoned leads in the pediatric patient so that an excessive amount of hardware does not accumulate in the patient throughout a lifetime. Some preference has therefore been given to active fixation leads, because they are generally easier to remove than a long-term passive fixation (tined) lead.

Finally, active fixation leads can be placed in a greater variety of positions than passive fixation leads. This advantage is important in the patient with associated congenital heart disease, because the anatomy may be quite distorted. An active fixation lead allows placement in all portions of the atrium, not the atrial appendage alone. Active fixation leads have been used in patients after the Mustard procedure, with the leads placed across the intra-atrial baffle and pacing in the left atrium (see Chapter 11).

A specific problem in pediatric pacing involves cardiac pacing after the Fontan procedure. Because the postoperative

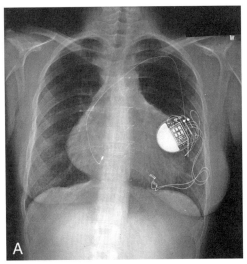 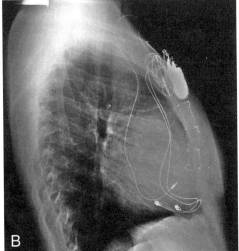

Fig. 5–41. Posteroanterior (*A*) and lateral (*B*) radiographs from a patient with a dual-chamber pacemaker. The ventricle is paced from the epimyocardial position, and the atrium is paced from the endocardial position. The atrial lead is then tunneled subcutaneously to the site of the pulse generator.

anatomy precludes transvenous endocardial ventricular pacing, dual-chamber pacing in these patients has been accomplished by placing a ventricular epicardial lead at the time of surgery and subsequently placing an atrial endocardial lead and tunneling the two leads to a common prepectoral position for attachment to a dual-chamber pacemaker (Fig. 5–41).

Permanent Pacing After Cardiac Transplantation

As more cardiac transplantations are performed, information is emerging on the special considerations for pacing in these patients. After cardiac transplantation, the donor atrium can no longer receive stimuli from the intrinsic or native (recipient) sinoatrial node. The sinoatrial node remains in continuity with the recipient atrium and may drive the recipient atrium at a normal rate or at a rate more rapid than normal. The suture line between the free wall of the donor atrium and the recipient atrium is a barrier to the passage of stimuli, which normally traverse the atrium to reach the AV node and bundle of His. After transplantation, the patient has two atrial rhythms, that of the donor atrium and that of the recipient atrium, both of which may be visible on the electrocardiogram.

Several approaches have been used for pacing in cardiac transplant recipients, some of which are quite complex. We have taken a conservative and simple approach. Because normal AV conduction usually exists between the donor atrium and ventricle, atrial pacing could be used both to preserve the AV sequence and to modulate the rate appropriately. Also, in many transplant recipients, sinus node dysfunction, a potential clinical problem from 1 month to 6 months after transplantation, often resolves. Nevertheless, our approach has been to implant a standard dual-chamber pacemaker and to position the atrial lead in the donor atrium. Even if there is no clinical manifestation of AV conduction disease, we are more comfortable placing a dual-chamber pacemaker for the unlikely event of late AV block.

Hospital Stay After Implantation

The length of time the patient should be kept in the hospital after pulse generator implantation varies among institutions. We currently admit patients the morning of the procedure and dismiss them the next morning. The patient is monitored during the overnight stay. If the patient is pacemaker-dependent, we tend to continue bed rest for most of the day after implantation. The next morning, the patient is sent to the radiology department for posteroanterior and lateral chest radiographs. Patients who are not pacemaker-dependent are allowed to walk 4 hours after the procedure and are dismissed the following morning. For nondependent patients, the chest radiograph is obtained after they are ambulatory. Before dismissal, thresholds are documented and the pulse generator is programmed to its final settings. If a rate-adaptive pacemaker has been implanted, informal exercise is performed the morning after implantation and the rate-responsive settings are adjusted to fit the needs of the patient. When the patient's pulse generator reaches battery depletion, the pulse generator is replaced during an outpatient procedure.

Some institutions now perform initial pacemaker or ICD implantation as an outpatient procedure. Large series of ambulatory pacemaker implantations have been reported. Some physicians restrict outpatient implantation to non-pacemaker-dependent patients, whereas others perform outpatient procedures regardless of dependency status. Some third-party payers now insist that device implantation be accomplished as an outpatient procedure or that the hospital stay be less than 24 hours.

Homegoing Instructions

After implantation, the incision is covered with sterile gauze and tape or a "coverlet." This is generally removed the next morning, and if the incision is dry, it is left uncovered. Patients are allowed to bathe 48 hours after implantation.

Postoperatively, a patient may want to restrict the movement of the ipsilateral shoulder. Movement should be encouraged, because immobility may cause pain later when full mobilization is attempted, with consequent further restriction of movement. Movement of the shoulder should be encouraged on the first postoperative day. Early movement will not displace a well-placed and secure lead system. We do recommend that the patient avoid lifting the arm on the side of the pulse generator higher than shoulder level for the first few weeks after implantation. This restriction may be overcautious, but it serves to remind the patient to avoid aggressive activities while at the same time does not significantly limit arm or shoulder motion or activities of daily living.

For medicolegal reasons, we recommend that the patient not drive for 2 weeks after receiving a pacemaker implant. Return to driving after ICD implantation is a more complex issue and depends on the clinical history, rhythm disturbance requiring the ICD, and applicable state or country regulations. This is discussed in greater detail in Chapter 13.

References

1. Smyth NP: Pacemaker implantation: surgical techniques. Cardiovasc Clin 14: 31–44, 1983
2. Belott PH, Reynolds DW: Permanent pacemaker implantation. *In* Clinical Cardiac Pacing. Edited by KA Ellenbogen, GN Kay, BL Wilkoff. Philadelphia, WB Saunders Company, 1995, pp 447–490
3. Hayes DL, Holmes DR Jr, Furman S: Permanent pacemaker implantation. *In* A Practice of Cardiac Pacing. Third edition. Edited by S Furman, DL Hayes, DR Holmes Jr. Mount Kisco, NY, Futura Publishing Company, 1993, pp 261–307
4. Hayes DL, Naccarelli GV, Furman S, Parsonnet V: Report of the NASPE Policy Conference training requirements for permanent pacemaker selection, implantation, and follow-up. North American Society of Pacing and Electrophysiology. Pacing Clin Electrophysiol 17:6–12, 1994
5. Bubien RS, Fisher JD, Gentzel JA, Murphy EK, Irwin ME, Shea JB, Dick M II, Ching E, Wilkoff BL, Benditt DG: NASPE expert consensus document: use of i.v. (conscious) sedation/analgesia by nonanesthesia personnel in patients undergoing arrhythmia specific diagnostic, therapeutic, and surgical procedures. Pacing Clin Electrophysiol 21:375–385, 1998
6. Miller FA Jr, Holmes DR Jr, Gersh BJ, Maloney JD: Permanent transvenous pacemaker implantation via the subclavian vein. Mayo Clin Proc 55:309–314, 1980
7. Magney JE, Staplin DH, Flynn DM, Hunter DW: A new approach to percutaneous subclavian venipuncture to avoid lead fracture or central venous catheter occlusion. Pacing Clin Electrophysiol 16:2133–2142, 1993
8. Byrd CL: Clinical experience with the extrathoracic introducer insertion technique. Pacing Clin Electrophysiol 16:1781–1784, 1993
9. Higano ST, Hayes DL, Spittell PC: Facilitation of the subclavian-introducer technique with contrast venography. Pacing Clin Electrophysiol 13:681–684, 1990
10. Furman S: Venous cutdown for pacemaker implantation. Ann Thorac Surg 41:438–439, 1986
11. Ellestad MH, French J: Iliac vein approach to permanent pacemaker implantation. Pacing Clin Electrophysiol 12:1030–1033, 1989
12. Giudici MC, Karpawich PP: Alternative site pacing: it's time to define terms (editorial). Pacing Clin Electrophysiol 22: 551–553, 1999
13. Delfaut P, Saksena S, Prakash A, Krol RB: Long-term outcome of patients with drug-refractory atrial flutter and fibrillation after single- and dual-site right atrial

pacing for arrhythmia prevention. J Am Coll Cardiol 32:1900–1908, 1998

14. Giudici MC, Paul DL, Devlin TA, Meier-bachtol CJ, Walton MC, Orias DW: Bach-mann's bundle permanent pacing short-ens intra-atrial conduction time. Will it decrease paroxysmal atrial fibrillation? (Abstract.) J Am Coll Cardiol 29 (Suppl A):253A, 1997

15. Spencer WH III, Zhu DW, Markowitz T, Badruddin SM, Zoghbi WA: Atrial septal pacing: a method for pacing both atria si-multaneously. Pacing Clin Electrophysiol 20:2739–2745, 1997

16. Furman S: Sensing and timing the cardiac electrogram. *In* A Practice of Cardiac Pac-ing. Third edition. Edited by S Furman, DL Hayes, DR Holmes Jr. Mount Kisco, NY, Futura Publishing Company, 1993, pp 89–133

17. Cardiac defibrillators—Connector as-sembly for implantable defibrillators—Dimensional and test requirements. ISO 11318:1993/Amd. 1:1996(E)

6

Pacemaker Timing Cycles and Pacemaker Electrocardiography

David L. Hayes, M.D.

An understanding of the basic concepts of cardiac pacing (Chapter 1) and comprehension of the pacemaker timing cycles of cardiac pacing are fundamental before one approaches the paced electrocardiogram (ECG). This chapter begins with a detailed description of "timing cycles" and then outlines assessment of the paced ECG.

Paced electrocardiography must be approached systematically, much as nonpaced electrocardiography, chest radiography, or any other diagnostic procedure. Knowing the type of pacemaker, the programmed parameters, and the underlying rhythm necessitating pacing is important in interpreting the paced ECG. Obviously, this information makes the interpretation much easier, but it is frequently not available.

Pacemaker timing cycles include all potential variations of a single complete pacing cycle[1] (Table 6–1). This could mean the time from paced ventricular beat to paced ventricular beat; from paced ventricular beat to an intrinsic ventricular beat, whether it be a conducted R wave or a premature ventricular contraction; from paced atrial beat to paced atrial beat; from intrinsic atrial beat to paced atrial beat; from intrinsic ventricular beat to paced ventricular beat; and so forth. Various aspects of each of these cycles include events sensed, events paced, and periods when the sensing circuit or circuits are refractory. Each portion of the pacemaker timing cycle should be considered in milliseconds (msec) and not in paced beats per minute (ppm). Although it may be easier to think of the patient's pacing rate in paced beats per minute, portions of the timing cycle are too brief to be considered in any unit but milliseconds.

If one knows the relation between the various elements of the paced ECG, understanding pacemaker rhythms becomes less complicated.[2] Although a native rhythm may be affected by multiple unknown factors, each timing circuit of a pacemaker can function in only one of two states. A given timer can proceed until it completes its cycle; completion results in either the release of a pacing stimulus or the initiation of another timing cycle. Alternatively, a given timer can be reset, at which point it starts the timing period all over again.

Table 6–1.
Abbreviations for Native and Paced Events and Portions of the Timing Cycle

P	Native atrial depolarization
A	Atrial paced event
R	Native ventricular depolarization
V	Ventricular paced event
I	Interval
AV	Sequential pacing in the atrium and ventricle
AVI	Programmed atrioventricular pacing interval
AR	Atrial paced event followed by intrinsic ventricular depolarization
ARP	Atrial refractory period
PV	Native atrial depolarization followed by a paced ventricular event, P-synchronous pacing
LRL	Lower rate limit
URL	Upper rate limit
MTR	Maximum tracking rate
MSR	Maximum sensor rate
PVARP	Postventricular atrial refractory period
RRAVD	Rate-responsive atrioventricular delay
VA interval	Interval from a ventricular sensed or paced event to an atrial paced event
VRP	Ventricular refractory period

Pacing Modes

Ventricular Asynchronous Pacing, Atrial Asynchronous Pacing, and Atrioventricular Sequential Asynchronous Pacing

Ventricular asynchronous (VOO) pacing is the simplest of all pacing modes because there is no sensing and no mode of response. The timing cycle is shown in Figure 6–1. Irrespective of any other events, the ventricular pacing artifacts occur at the programmed rate. The timing cycle cannot be reset by any intrinsic event. Without sensing, there is no defined refractory period.

Atrial asynchronous (AOO) pacing behaves exactly like VOO except that the pacing artifacts occur in the atrial chamber.

Dual-chamber, or atrioventricular

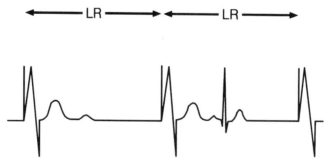

Fig. 6–1. The VOO timing cycle consists of only a defined rate. The pacemaker delivers a ventricular pacing artifact at the defined rate regardless of intrinsic events. In this example, an intrinsic QRS complex occurs after the second paced complex, but because there is no sensing in the VOO mode, the interval between the second and the third paced complex remains stable. LR, lower rate [limit]. (From Hayes and Levine.[1] By permission of Blackwell Scientific Publications.)

(AV) sequential asynchronous (DOO), pacing has an equally simple timing cycle. The interval from atrial artifact to ventricular artifact (atrioventricular interval, AVI) and the interval from the ventricular artifact to the subsequent atrial pacing artifact (ventriculoatrial, or atrial escape, interval, VA interval) are fixed. The intervals never change, because the pacing mode is insensitive to any atrial or ventricular activity, and the timers are never reset (Fig. 6–2).

Ventricular Inhibited Pacing

By definition, ventricular inhibited (VVI) pacing incorporates sensing on the ventricular channel, and pacemaker output is inhibited by a sensed ventricular event (Fig. 6–3). VVI pacemakers are refractory for a period after a paced or sensed ventricular event, the ventricular refractory period (VRP). Any ventricular event occurring within the VRP is not sensed and does not reset the ventricular timer (Fig. 6–4). (Every pacemaker capable of sensing must include a refractory period in its basic timing cycle. Refractory periods prevent the sensing of early

inappropriate signals, such as the evoked potential and repolarization [T wave].)

Atrial Inhibited Pacing

Atrial inhibited (AAI) pacing, the atrial counterpart of VVI pacing, incorporates the same timing cycles, with the obvious difference that pacing and sensing occur from the atrium and pacemaker output is inhibited by a sensed atrial event (Fig. 6–5). An atrial paced or sensed event initiates a refractory period during which nothing is sensed by the pacemaker. Confusion can arise when multiple ventricular events occur while there is atrial pacing. For example, in addition to the intrinsic QRS that occurs in response to the paced atrial beat, if a premature ventricular beat follows, it does not inhibit an atrial pacing artifact from being delivered (Fig. 6–6). When the AA timing cycle ends, the atrial pacing artifact is delivered regardless of ventricular events, because an AAI pacemaker should not sense anything in the ventricle. An exception to this rule is far-field sensing; that is, the ventricular signal is large enough to be inappropriately sensed by

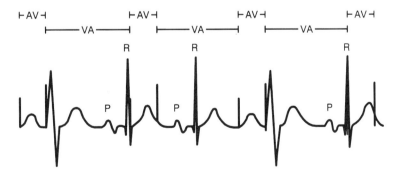

Fig. 6–2. The DOO timing cycle consists of only defined atrioventricular (AV) and VV intervals. The ventriculoatrial (VA) interval is a function of the AV and VV intervals. An atrial pacing artifact is delivered, and the ventricular artifact follows at the programmed AV interval. The next atrial pacing artifact is delivered at the completion of the VA interval. There is no variation in the intervals because no activity is sensed; that is, nothing interrupts or resets the programmed cycles. (From Hayes and Levine.[1] By permission of Blackwell Scientific Publications.)

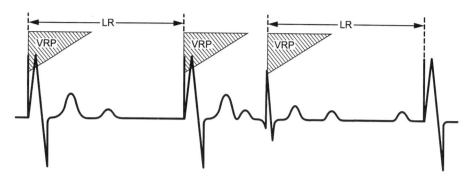

Fig. 6–3. The VVI timing cycle consists of a defined lower rate (LR) limit and a ventricular refractory period (VRP, represented by triangle). When the LR limit timer is complete, a pacing artifact is delivered in the absence of a sensed intrinsic ventricular event. If an intrinsic QRS occurs, the LR limit timer is started from that point. A VRP begins with any sensed or paced ventricular activity. (From Hayes DL, Zipes DP: Cardiac pacemakers and cardioverter-defibrillators. *In* Heart Disease: A Textbook of Cardiovascular Medicine. Sixth edition. Edited by E Braunwald, DP Zipes, P Libby. Philadelphia, WB Saunders Company [in press]. By permission of the publisher.)

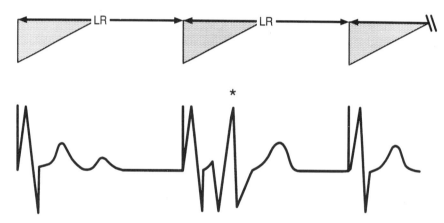

Fig. 6–4. If, in the VVI mode, an intrinsic ventricular event (*) occurs during the ventricular refractory period (VRP, represented by triangle), it is not sensed and therefore does not reset the lower rate (LR) limit timer. (From Hayes and Levine.[1] By permission of Blackwell Scientific Publications.)

the atrial lead (Fig. 6–7). In this situation, the atrial timing cycle is reset. Sometimes this anomaly can be corrected by making the atrial channel less sensitive or by lengthening the refractory period.

Single-Chamber Triggered-Mode Pacing

Initially developed as a way to defeat the problem associated with oversensing in the inhibited demand mode, the triggered mode has its own unique advantages as well as disadvantages. In single-chamber triggered-mode pacing, the pacemaker releases an output pulse every time a native event is sensed. This feature increases the current drain on the battery, accelerating its rate of depletion. This mode of pacing also deforms the native signal, compromising interpretation of the ECG. However, it can serve as an excellent marker for the site of sensing within a complex. It can also prevent inappropriate inhibition from oversensing when the patient does not have a stable native escape rhythm. Additionally,

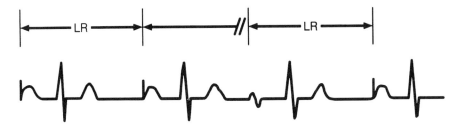

Fig. 6–5. The AAI timing cycle consists of a defined lower rate (LR) limit and an atrial refractory period. When the LR limit timer is complete, a pacing artifact is delivered in the atrium in the absence of a sensed atrial event. If an intrinsic P wave occurs, the LR limit timer is started from that point. An atrial refractory period begins with any sensed or paced atrial activity. (From Hayes and Levine.[1] By permission of Blackwell Scientific Publications.)

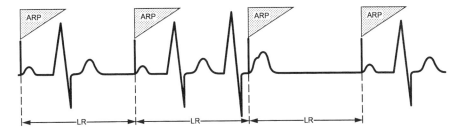

Fig. 6–6. In the AAI mode, only atrial activity is sensed. In this example, it may appear unusual for paced atrial activity to occur so soon after intrinsic ventricular activity. Because sensing occurs only in the atrium, ventricular activity would not be expected to reset the pacemaker's timing cycle. ARP, atrial refractory period; LR, lower rate [limit]. (From Hayes DL, Zipes DP: Cardiac pacemakers and cardioverter-defibrillators. *In* Heart Disease: A Textbook of Cardiovascular Medicine. Sixth edition. Edited by E Braunwald, DP Zipes, P Libby. Philadelphia, WB Saunders Company [in press]. By permission of the publisher.)

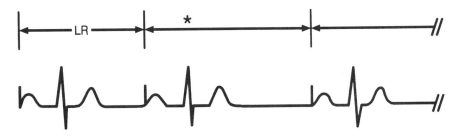

Fig. 6–7. In this example of AAI pacing, the AA interval is 1,000 msec (60 ppm). The interval between the second and the third paced atrial events exceeds 1,000 msec. The interval from the second QRS complex to the subsequent atrial pacing artifact is 1,000 msec. This occurs because the second QRS complex (*) has been sensed on the atrial lead (far-field sensing) and has inappropriately reset the timing cycle. LR, lower rate [limit]. (From Hayes and Levine.[1] By permission of Blackwell Scientific Publications.)

it can be used for noninvasive electrophysiologic studies, with the already implanted pacemaker tracking chest wall stimuli created by a programmable stimulator. A special requirement if one is to use the triggered mode for noninvasive electrophysiologic studies is to shorten the refractory period intentionally, allowing the implanted pacemaker to track the external chest wall stimuli to rapid rates and close coupling intervals. Normally, the refractory mode is at or near 400 msec to minimize the chance of sensing its own T wave and triggering another output pulse into the vulnerable zone of myocardial repolarization.

Rate-Modulated Pacing

Single-Chamber Rate-Modulated Pacing

Single-chamber pacemakers capable of rate-modulated (SSIR) pacing can be implanted in the ventricle (VVIR) or atrium (AAIR). The timing cycles for SSIR pacemakers are not significantly different from those of their non-rate-modulated counterparts. The timing cycle includes the basic VV or AA interval and a refractory period from the paced or sensed event. The difference lies in the variability of the VV or AA interval (Fig. 6–8). Depending on the sensor incorporated and the level of exertion of the patient, the basic interval shortens from the programmed lower rate limit (LRL).

Shortening requires that an upper rate limit (URL) be programmed to define the absolute shortest cycle length allowable. Most approved SSIR pacemakers incorporate a fixed refractory period; that is, regardless of whether the pacemaker is operating at the LRL or URL, the refractory period remains the same. Thus, at the higher rates under sensor drive, the pacemaker may effectively become SOOR, since the alert period during which sensing can occur is so abbreviated. Native beats falling during the refractory period are not sensed. Hence, in SSIR pacing systems, if the refractory period is programmable, it should be programmed to a short interval to maximize the sensing period at both the low and the high sensor-controlled rates. Rate-variable or rate-adaptive refractory period as a programmable option—that is, as the cycle length shortens, the refractory period shortens appropriately, analogous to the QT interval of the native ventricular depolarization—probably will become more commonly available in subsequent generations of SSIR pacemakers.

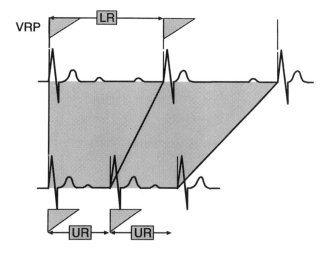

Fig. 6–8. The VVIR timing cycle consists of a lower rate (LR) limit, an upper rate (UR) limit, and a ventricular refractory period (VRP, represented by triangle). As indicated by sensor activity, the VV cycle length shortens accordingly. (The shaded area represents the range of sensor-driven VV cycle lengths.) In most VVIR pacemakers, the VRP remains fixed despite the changing VV cycle length. In selected VVIR pacemakers, the VRP shortens as the cycle length shortens. (Modified from Hayes and Levine.[1] By permission of Blackwell Scientific Publications.)

Single-Chamber Rate-Modulated Asynchronous and Dual-Chamber Rate-Modulated Asynchronous Pacing

If rate modulation is incorporated in an asynchronous pacing mode, the basic cycle length is altered by sensor activity. In the single-chamber rate-modulated asynchronous (AOOR and VOOR) pacing modes, any alteration in cycle length is due to sensor activity and not to the sensing of intrinsic cardiac depolarizations. In the dual-chamber rate-modulated asynchronous (DOOR) pacing mode, the pacing rate changes in response to the sensor input signal but not to the native P or R wave.

Atrioventricular Sequential, Ventricular Inhibited Pacing

AV sequential, ventricular inhibited (DVI) pacing is rarely used as the preimplantation pacing mode of choice, but it remains a programmable option in most dual-chamber pacemakers. In addition, a small number of patients still have dedicated DVI pacemakers. For these reasons, it is important to understand the timing cycles for DVI pacing.

By definition, DVI provides pacing in both the atrium and the ventricle (D) but sensing only in the ventricle (V). The pacemaker is inhibited and reset by sensed ventricular activity but ignores all intrinsic atrial complexes.

The timing cycle (VV) consists of the AVI and the VA interval. The basic cycle length (VV), or LRL, is programmable, as is the AVI. The difference, VV - AV, is the VA interval. During the initial portion of the VA interval, the sensing channel is refractory. (The refractory period is almost always a programmable interval.) After the refractory period, the ventricular sensing channel is again operational, or "alert." If ventricular activity is not sensed by the expiration of the VA interval, atrial pacing oc-

curs, followed by the AVI. If intrinsic ventricular activity occurs before the VA interval is completed, the timing cycle is reset.

Atrioventricular Sequential, Non-P-Synchronous Pacing With Dual-Chamber Sensing

AV sequential pacing with dual-chamber sensing, non-P-synchronous (DDI) pacing can be thought of as DDD pacing without atrial tracking.[3] The difference between DVI and DDI is that DDI incorporates atrial sensing as well as ventricular sensing. This prevents competitive atrial pacing that can occur with DVI pacing. The DDI mode of response is inhibition only; that is, no tracking of P waves can occur. Therefore, the paced ventricular rate cannot be greater than the programmed LRL. The timing cycle consists of the LRL, AVI, postventricular atrial refractory period (PVARP), and VRP. The PVARP is the period after a sensed or paced ventricular event during which the atrial sensing circuit is refractory. Any atrial event occurring during the PVARP will not be sensed by the atrial sensing circuit. If a P wave occurs after the PVARP and is sensed, no atrial pacing artifact is delivered at the end of the VA interval. The subsequent ventricular pacing artifact cannot occur until the VV interval has been completed; that is, the LRL cannot be violated (Fig. 6–9).

It bears repeating that because P-wave tracking does not occur with the DDI mode, the paced rate is never greater than the programmed LRL. A slight exception to this statement occurs when an intrinsic ventricular complex takes place after the paced atrial beat (AR) and inhibits paced ventricular output before completion of the programmed AVI; that is, AR < AV. In this situation, the cycle length from A to A is shorter than the programmed LRL by the difference between the AR and the programmed AVI.

Fig. 6–9. The timing cycle in DDI consists of a lower rate (LR) limit, an atrioventricular (AV) interval, a ventricular refractory period (VRP), and an atrial refractory period (ARP). The VRP is initiated by any sensed or paced ventricular activity, and the ARP is initiated by any sensed or paced atrial activity. DDI can be thought of as DDD pacing without the capability of P-wave tracking or DVI without the potential for atrial competition by virtue of atrial sensing. The LR limit

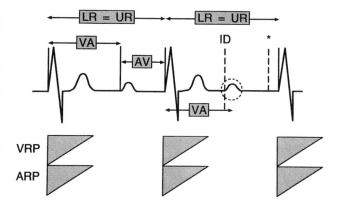

cannot be violated even if the sinus rate is occurring at a faster rate. For example, the LR limit is 1,000 msec, or 60 ppm, and the AV interval is 200 msec. If a P wave occurs 500 msec after a paced ventricular complex, the AV interval is initiated; but at the end of the AV interval, 700 msec from the previous paced ventricular activity, a ventricular pacing artifact cannot be delivered, because it would violate the LR limit (*). ID, intrinsic deflection; UR, upper rate [limit]; VA, ventriculoatrial [interval]. (Modified from Hayes and Levine.[1] By permission of Blackwell Scientific Publications.)

Atrioventricular Sequential, Non-P-Synchronous, Rate-Modulated Pacing With Dual-Chamber Sensing

The timing cycles for non-P-synchronous, rate-modulated AV sequential (DDIR) pacing are the same as those described above for DDI pacing except that paced rates can exceed the programmed LRL through sensor-driven activity.

Atrial Synchronous (P-Tracking) Pacing

Atrial synchronous (P-tracking) (VDD) pacemakers pace only in the ventricle (V), sense in both atrium and ventricle (D), and respond both by inhibition of ventricular output by intrinsic ventricular activity (I) and by ventricular tracking of P waves (T). The VDD mode has also become increasingly available as a single-lead pacing system. In this system, a single lead is capable of pacing in the ventricle in response to sensing atrial activity by way of a remote electrode situated on the intra-atrial portion of the ventricular pacing lead.

The timing cycle is composed of LRL, AVI, PVARP, VRP, and URL. A sensed atrial event initiates the AVI. If an intrinsic ventricular event occurs before the termination of the AVI, ventricular output is inhibited and the LRL timing cycle is reset. If a paced ventricular beat occurs at the end of the AVI, this beat resets the LRL. If no atrial event occurs, the pacemaker escapes with a paced ventricular event at the LRL; that is, the pacemaker displays VVI activity in the absence of a sensed atrial event (Fig. 6–10).

Dual-Chamber Pacing and Sensing With Inhibition and Tracking

Although it involves more timers, standard dual-chamber pacing and sensing with inhibition and tracking (DDD) is reasonably easy to comprehend if one understands the timing cycles already discussed.[4] The basic timing circuit associated with LRL pacing is divided into two sections. The first is the interval from a ventricular sensed or paced event to an atrial event. This is the VA interval. The second interval begins with an atrial sensed or paced event and extends to a ventricular event. This interval may be

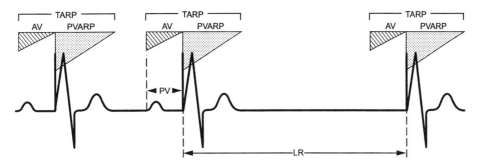

Fig. 6–10. The timing cycle of VDD consists of a lower rate (LR) limit, an atrioventricular interval (AVI), a ventricular refractory period, a postventricular atrial refractory period (PVARP), and an upper rate limit. A sensed P wave initiates the AVI (during the AVI, the atrial sensing channel is refractory). At the end of the AVI, a ventricular pacing artifact is delivered if no intrinsic ventricular activity has been sensed, that is, P-wave tracking. Ventricular activity, paced or sensed, initiates the PVARP and the ventriculoatrial interval (the LR limit interval minus the AVI). If no P-wave activity occurs, the pacemaker escapes with a ventricular pacing artifact at the LR limit. PV, native atrial depolarization followed by paced ventricular event; TARP, total atrial refractory period. (From Hayes DL, Zipes DP: Cardiac pacemakers and cardioverter-defibrillators. *In* Heart Disease: A Textbook of Cardiovascular Medicine. Sixth edition. Edited by E Braunwald, DP Zipes, P Libby. Philadelphia, WB Saunders Company [in press]. By permission of the publisher.)

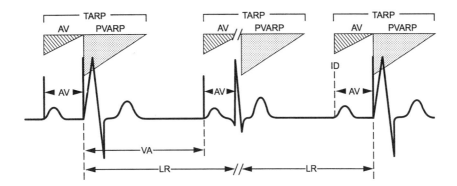

Fig. 6–11. The timing cycle in DDD consists of a lower rate (LR) limit, an atrioventricular (AV) interval, a ventricular refractory period, a postventricular atrial refractory period (PVARP), and an upper rate limit. If intrinsic atrial and ventricular activity occur before the LR limit times out, both channels are inhibited and no pacing occurs. In the absence of intrinsic atrial and ventricular activity, AV sequential pacing occurs (first cycle). If no atrial activity is sensed before the ventriculoatrial (VA) interval is completed, an atrial pacing artifact is delivered, which initiates the AV interval. If intrinsic ventricular activity occurs before the termination of the AV interval, the ventricular output from the pacemaker is inhibited, that is, atrial pacing (second cycle). If a P wave is sensed before the VA interval is completed, output from the atrial channel is inhibited. The AV interval is initiated, and if no ventricular activity is sensed before the AV interval terminates, a ventricular pacing artifact is delivered, that is, P-synchronous pacing (third cycle). ID, intrinsic deflection; TARP, total atrial refractory period. (From Hayes DL, Zipes DP: Cardiac pacemakers and cardioverter-defibrillators. *In* Heart Disease: A Textbook of Cardiovascular Medicine. Sixth edition. Edited by E Braunwald, DP Zipes, P Libby. Philadelphia, WB Saunders Company [in press]. By permission of the publisher.)

defined by a paced AVI, PR interval, AR interval, AR interval, or PV interval. An atrial sensed event that occurs before completion of the VA interval terminates this interval and initiates an AVI, and the result is P-wave synchronous ventricular pacing. If the intrinsic sinus rate is less than the programmed LRL, AV sequential pacing at the programmed rate or functional single-chamber atrial (AR) pacing occurs (Fig. 6–11).

In a DDD system, a sensed or paced atrial event initiates an atrial refractory period (ARP) and also initiates the AVI (Fig. 6–11). During this portion of the timing cycle, the atrial channel is refractory to any sensed events; nor will atrial pacing occur during this period. A sensed or paced ventricular event initiates a VRP. (A VRP is always part of the timing cycle of any pacing system with ventricular pacing and sensing.) The VRP prevents sensing of the evoked potential and the

resultant T wave on the ventricular channel of the pacemaker. A sensed or paced ventricular event also initiates a PVARP. The PVARP prevents atrial sensing of a retrograde P wave (see "Endless-Loop Tachycardia," below) and also prevents sensing of far-field ventricular events.

A dual-chamber pacemaker can track the atrial rhythm to a defined maximum tracking rate (MTR). The combination of the PVARP and the AVI forms the total atrial refractory period (TARP). The TARP, in turn, is the limiting factor for the maximum sensed atrial rate that the pacemaker can reach. For example, if the AVI is 150 msec and the PVARP is 250 msec, the TARP is 400 msec, or 150 ppm. In this case, a paced ventricular event initiates the 250-msec PVARP, and only after this interval has ended can an atrial event be sensed. If an atrial event is sensed immediately after the termination of the PVARP, the sensed atrial event initiates

Fig. 6–12. When the sinus rate exceeds the programmed maximum tracking rate, several upper rate (UR) behaviors can occur. In the *top panel,* pseudo-Wenckebach behavior is seen. If a P wave occurs outside the postventricular atrial refractory period (PVARP) and is sensed, the atrioventricular interval (AVI) is initiated. However, a ventricular pacing artifact cannot be delivered at the end of the programmed AVI if this would violate the programmed maximum tracking rate. Instead, the AVI would be lengthened and the ventricular pacing artifact would occur when the maximum tracking rate had "timed out." For example, if the maximum tracking rate is 120 bpm, or an interval of 500 msec, the AVI is 150 msec, the PVARP is 250 msec, and the P wave is sensed 10 msec after completion of the PVARP, or 260 msec after the preceding ventricular event, the next ventricular pacing artifact could not be delivered

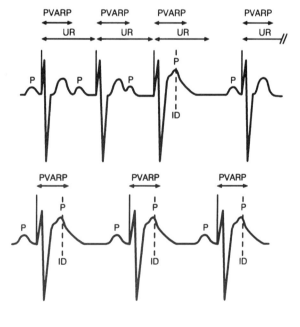

for 240 msec (500 - 260). In the *bottom panel,* 2:1 UR behavior occurs when every other sinus beat falls in the PVARP. ID, intrinsic deflection. (From Hayes DL: DDDR timing cycles: upper rate behavior. *In* New Perspectives in Cardiac Pacing, 3. Edited by SS Barold, J Mugica. Mount Kisco, NY, Futura Publishing Company, 1993, pp 233–257. By permission of the publisher.)

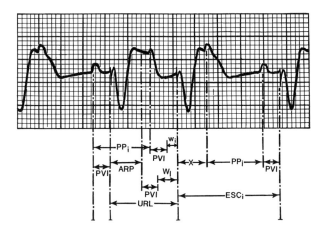

Fig. 6–13. Electrocardiographic tracing from a patient with pseudo-Wenckebach upper rate behavior (see Fig. 6–12). ARP, atrial refractory period; ESC_i, escape interval; PP_i, atrial rate; PVI, interval from P wave to ventricular stimulus; URL, upper rate limit; W_i, interval from beat-to-beat prolongation of the P wave to ventricular stimulus; W_l, URL-TARP (total atrial refractory period), representing the theoretical maximum increment in PV interval allowed; X, time from the ventricular stimulus to the first P wave that has fallen in the postventricular atrial refractory period. (From Higano and Hayes[24] By permission of Futura Publishing Company.)

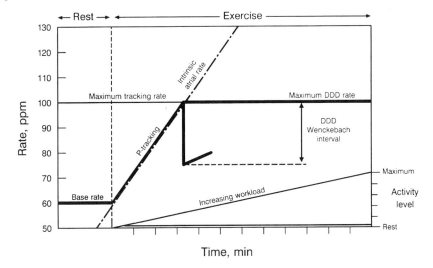

Fig. 6–14. Schema of the rate response of a DDD pacemaker with pseudo-Wenckebach type block at the upper rate limit (100 ppm). The dashed-dotted line represents the intrinsic atrial rate, and the heavy black line represents the ventricular paced rate, assuming pseudo-Wenckebach block as the atrial rate exceeds the maximum tracking rate. (From Higano et al.[25] By permission of Futura Publishing Company.)

the AVI of 150 msec. On termination of the AVI, in the absence of an intrinsic R wave, a paced ventricular event occurs, resulting in a VV cycle length of 400 msec, or 150 ppm. Programming a long PVARP limits the upper rate by limiting the maximum sensed atrial rate (Fig. 6–12, *top*). If the native atrial rate were 151 beats per minute

(bpm), every other P wave would coincide with the PVARP, not be sensed, and hence not be tracked, so that the effective paced rate would be approximately 75 ppm, or half the atrial rate (Fig. 6–12, *bottom*). Pseudo-Wenckebach behavior is explained in Figure 6–13. The pseudo-Wenckebach interval can be quantitated by mathematical equations.[5] Figure 6–14 schematically displays the relationship of the effective paced ventricular rate and the atrial rate.

Portions of Pacemaker Timing Cycles

Atrioventricular Interval

The AVI is often poorly understood. The AVI should be considered as a single interval with two subportions (Fig. 6–15 A). The blanking period accounts for the earliest portion of the AVI. The blanking period can be defined as the time during and after a pacemaker stimulus when the opposite channel of a dual-chamber pacemaker is insensitive. The purpose of this period is to avoid sensing the electronic event of one channel in the opposite channel.

If the atrial pacing artifact were sensed by the ventricular sensing circuit, ventricular output inhibition would result. This is termed "crosstalk." To prevent this, the leading edge of the atrial pacing artifact is masked, or blanked, by rendering the ventricular sensing circuit

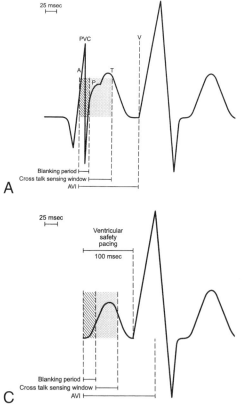

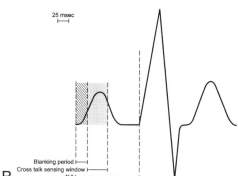

Fig. 6–15. *A,* The atrioventricular interval (AVI) should be considered as a single interval with two subportions. The entire AVI corresponds to the programmed value, that is, the interval following a paced or sensed atrial beat allowed before a ventricular pacing artifact is delivered. The initial portion of the AVI is the blanking period. This interval is followed by the crosstalk sensing window. *B,* If the ventricular sensing circuit senses activity during the crosstalk sensing window, a ventricular pacing artifact is delivered early, usually at 100 to 110 msec after the atrial event. This has been referred to as "ventricular safety pacing," "110-msec phenomenon," and "nonphysiologic AV delay." *C,* The initial portion of the AVI in most dual-chamber pacemakers is designated as the blanking period. During this portion of the AVI, sensing is suspended. The primary purpose of this interval is to prevent ventricular sensing of the leading edge of the atrial pacing artifact. Any event that occurs during the blanking period, even if it is an intrinsic ventricular event, as shown in this figure, is not sensed. In this example, the ventricular premature beat that is not sensed is followed by a ventricular pacing artifact delivered at the programmed AVI and occurring in the terminal portion of the T wave. PVC, premature ventricular contraction. (From Hayes and Levine.[1] By permission of Blackwell Scientific Publications.)

refractory during the very early portion of the AVI (Fig. 6–15 *B*). In current DDD pacemakers, the blanking period may be programmable, ranging from 12 to 125 msec. The blanking period is traditionally of short duration because it is important for the ventricular sensing circuit to be returned to the "alert" state relatively early during the AVI so that intrinsic ventricular activity can inhibit pacemaker output if it occurs before the AVI ends. The potential exists for signals other than those of intrinsic ventricular activity to be sensed and to inhibit ventricular output. The greatest concern is crosstalk. Even though the leading edge of the atrial pacing artifact is effectively ignored because of the blanking period, the trailing edge of the atrial pacing artifact occurring after the blanking period can at times be sensed on the ventricular channel. In a pacemaker-dependent patient, inhibition of ventricular output by crosstalk would result in asystole. A safety mechanism is present to prevent such an outcome.

If activity is sensed on the ventricular sensing circuit in a given portion of the AVI immediately after the blanking pe-riod (the second portion of the AVI has been called the "ventricular triggering period" or the "crosstalk sensing window"), it is assumed that crosstalk cannot be differentiated from intrinsic ventricular activity. To prevent catastrophic ventricular asystole, a ventricular pacing artifact is delivered early, that is, at an AVI of 100 to 120 msec, although in some pacemakers this interval is programmable for 50 to 150 msec (Fig. 6–15 *C*). If the signal sensed is indeed crosstalk, a paced ventricular complex at the abbreviated interval prevents ventricular asystole. If, on the other hand, intrinsic ventricular activity occurs during the early portion of the AVI, the safety mechanism results in delivery of a ventricular pacing artifact within or immediately after the intrinsic beat. This delivery is safe because the ventricle is refractory, no depolarization results from the pacing artifact, and the pacing artifact is delivered too early to coincide with ventricular repolarization or a vulnerable period. This event has been referred to as "ventricular safety pacing," "nonphysiologic AV delay," or the "110-msec phenomenon."

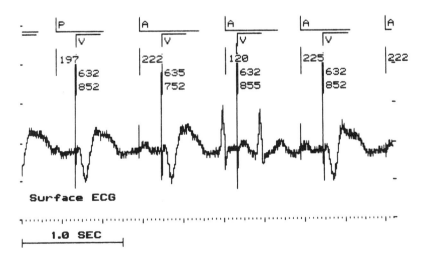

Fig. 6–16. Differential atrioventricular interval (AVI) timing is present with a PV interval of 197 and an AVI of 222 to 225 msec. Also noted on this telemetered tracing, the third ventricular event occurs in the crosstalk sensing window and results in ventricular safety pacing, with an AVI of 120 msec.

Differential Atrioventricular Interval

If there is a consistent difference between AVIs initiated by a sensed event and those triggered by a paced event, the most likely explanation is a differential AVI. This is an attempt to provide an interatrial conduction time of equal duration whether the atrial contraction is paced or sensed.[6,7] The PV interval initiated with atrial sensing begins at the time of atrial depolarization. Conversely, the AVI initiated with atrial pacing commences with the pacing artifact, not with atrial depolarization. The AVI following a sensed atrial event should therefore be shorter than that following a paced atrial event (Fig. 6–16). In some pacemakers, the AVI differential is programmable; in others, a preset differential is used.

Rate-Variable or Rate-Adaptive Atrioventricular Interval

Many DDDR pacemakers may have the capability of shortening the AVI during AV sequential sensor-driven pacing.[8–10] Rate-adaptive or rate-variable AVI is intended to optimize cardiac output by mimicking the normal physiologic decrease in the PR interval that occurs in the normal heart as the atrial rate increases (Fig. 6–17). The rate-related shortening of the AVI may also improve atrial sensing by shortening the TARP and thereby giving more time for the atrial sensing window.

There are many variations of rate-adaptive AVI, but linear shortening of the AVI from a programmed baseline AVI to a programmed minimum AVI is the most common.

Atrioventricular Interval Hysteresis

This term is most commonly used to note an alteration of the AVI depending on the patient's native AV conduction. There is not complete agreement on the terminology.

Positive AVI hysteresis is usually used to describe a lengthening of the AVI in an effort to maintain intrinsic AV nodal conduction.[11,12] A variety of algorithms are used for this function. It basically involves a gradual lengthening of the programmed AVI to determine if an intrinsic ventricular depolarization will occur within a certain interval. If criteria are met, the extended AVI persists unless there is lengthening of the AR or PR interval beyond preset limits, which would once again invoke the programmed AVI (Fig. 6–18).

Negative AVI hysteresis is usually used to describe a shortening of the AVI

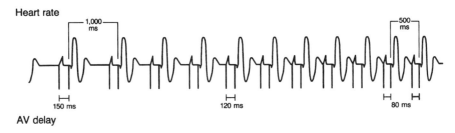

Fig. 6–17. Schematic representation of rate-adaptive atrioventricular (AV) interval. As the ventricular rate increases, the AV interval progressively shortens. (Reproduced with permission from Siemens-Pacesetter.)

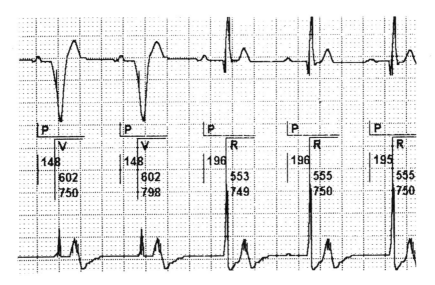

Fig. 6–18. Simulated electrocardiographic tracing demonstrating "positive" atrioventricular interval (AVI) hysteresis. The AVI is prolonged to allow intrinsic atrioventricular nodal conduction.

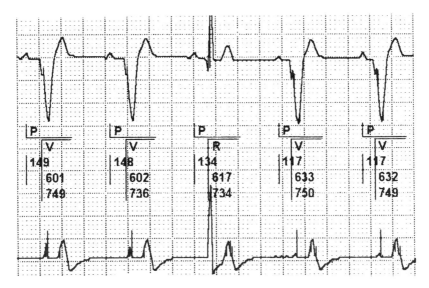

Fig. 6–19. Simulated electrocardiographic tracing demonstrating "negative" atrioventricular interval (AVI) hysteresis. After two cycles of P-synchronous pacing, the next P wave is followed by an intrinsic QRS at a PR interval of 134. The AVI is subsequently shortened to promote paced ventricular depolarization.

in an effort to maintain paced ventricular depolarization (Fig. 6–19). This may be hemodynamically desirable for some patients, such as those with hypertrophic cardiomyopathy.

Atrial- and Ventricular-Based Timing Compared

The way a pacemaker behaves in response to a sensed ventricular signal varies among manufacturers and among devices from the same manufacturer. Dual-chamber pacemakers may have a ventricular-based timing system, an atrial-based timing system, or a hybrid of these two systems.[13–15] The difference between contemporary atrial- and ventricular-based dual-chamber pacemakers is of little clinical importance, although the difference could create confusion in interpretation of paced ECGs. Regardless of the timing system used, most manufacturers have modified the timing systems in such a way that the function and ECG manifestations are very similar.

Ventricular-Based Timing

In a pure ventricular-based timing system, the VA interval is "fixed." A ventricular sensed event occurring during the VA interval resets this timer, causing it to start all over again (Fig. 6–16). A ventricular sensed event occurring during the AVI both terminates the AVI and initiates a VA interval (Fig. 6–20, *top*). If there is intact conduction through the AV node after an atrial pacing stimulus such that the AR interval (atrial stimulus to sensed R wave) is shorter than the programmed AVI, the resulting paced rate accelerates. When this occurs at the LRL, as demonstrated in Figure 6–20 (*top*), the rate acceleration is minimal. In this example, it is assumed that the pacemaker is programmed to an LRL of 60 bpm (a pacing interval of 1,000 msec). With a programmed AVI of 200 msec, the VA interval is 800 msec (VA interval = LRL - AVI). If AV nodal function permits conduction in 150 msec (AR interval = 150 msec), the conducted or sensed R wave inhibits the ventricular output. This, in turn, resets the VA interval, which remains stable at 800 msec. The resulting interval between consecutive atrial pacing stimuli is 950 msec (VA interval + AR interval). This

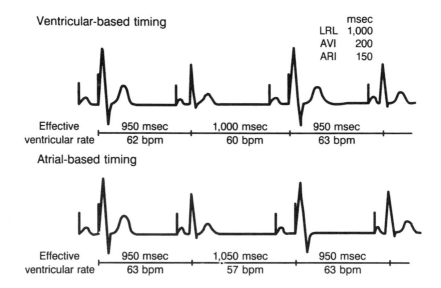

Fig. 6–20. *Top,* With ventricular-based timing in patients with intact atrioventricular (AV) nodal conduction after atrial (AR) pacing, the sensed R wave resets the ventriculoatrial (VA) interval. The base pacing interval consists of the sum of the AR and the VA intervals; thus, it is shorter than the programmed minimum rate interval. *Bottom,* With atrial-based timing in patients with intact AV nodal conduction after AR pacing, the sensed R wave inhibits the ventricular output but does not reset the basic timing of the pacemaker. There is AR pacing at the programmed base rate. ARI, interval from paced atrial event to intrinsic QRS; AVI, atrioventricular interval; LRL, lower rate limit. (Reproduced with permission from Siemens-Pacesetter.)

is equivalent to a rate of 63 bpm, which is slightly faster than the programmed LRL. When a native R wave occurs—for example, a ventricular premature beat during the VA interval—the VA interval is also reset. The pacemaker then recycles, and the result is a rate defined by the sum of the VA interval and the AVI. This escape interval is therefore equal to the LRL (Fig. 6–20, *top*). In both cases, the sensed ventricular event, an R wave, regardless of where it occurs, resets the VA interval.

Atrial-Based Timing

In an atrial-based timing system, the AA interval is fixed. This is in contrast to a ventricular-based system, in which the VA interval is fixed. As long as there is stable LRL pacing, there will be no discernible difference between the two timing systems.

In a system with pure atrial-based timing, a sensed R wave occurring during the AVI inhibits the ventricular output but does not alter the basic AA timing. Hence, the rate stays at the programmed LRL (Fig. 6–20, *bottom*) during effective single-chamber atrial pacing. When a ventricular premature beat is sensed during the VA interval, the timers are also reset, but now it is the AA interval rather than the VA interval that is reset. The pacemaker counts out an AA interval and then adds the programmed AVI, attempting to mimic the compensatory pause commonly seen in normal sinus rhythm with ventricular ectopy. Atrial-based timing at the lower rate is demonstrated by example in Figure 6–17. This schema begins with AV sequential pacing and is followed by an atrial paced event at 1,000 msec from the previous paced atrial event. However, intrinsic ventricular conduction occurs at 150 msec, resulting in an effective ventricular rate of 950 msec, or 63 bpm, that is, an 800-msec VA interval plus a 150-msec AR interval. The next paced atrial event is still delivered at 1,000 msec after the preceding paced atrial event, as defined by atrial-based timing. This time, the programmed AVI expires and a paced ventricular complex occurs. This results in an effective ventricular rate of 850 msec; the VA interval, which was lengthened by 50 msec because of the preceding intrinsic ventricular activity; and the 200-msec AVI, for a cycle length of 1,050 msec, or 57 bpm.

Most contemporary pacemakers are ventricular-based with modifications, that is, there are some alterations in strict ventricular-based timing to prevent any significant ventricular rate acceleration above the programmed rate limit.[16] Although some published information is available on variations in timing systems, the best source is the technical manual for the specific dual-chamber pacemaker in question.

Mode Switching

Mode switching refers to the ability of the pacemaker to automatically change from one mode to another in response to an inappropriately rapid atrial rhythm. This may alter the ECG "timing" in a significant way. When the pacemaker is programmed to a pacing mode with ventricular tracking of atrial events, mode-switching algorithms automatically reprogram the device to a nontracking mode if the pacemaker meets specific criteria for what it considers a pathologic atrial rhythm.[17–20] Mode switching is particularly useful for patients with paroxysmal supraventricular rhythm disturbances. In the DDD or DDDR pacing modes, if a supraventricular rhythm disturbance occurs and the pacemaker senses the pathologic atrial rhythm, rapid ventricular pacing may occur (Fig. 6–21). Any pacing mode that eliminates tracking of the pathologic rhythm, that is, DDI, DDIR, DVI, or DVIR, also eliminates the ability to track normal sinus rhythm, which is usually the predominant rhythm (Fig. 6–22).

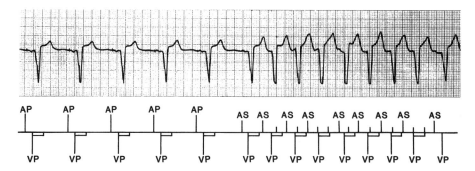

Fig. 6–21. Electrocardiographic tracing with Marker Channel-like diagram from a patient with a DDDR pacemaker. Atrial tachyarrhythmia develops, and in the absence of mode switching, rapid ventricular tracking of the tachyarrhythmia occurs. AP, atrial pacing; AS, atrial sensing; VP, ventricular pacing.

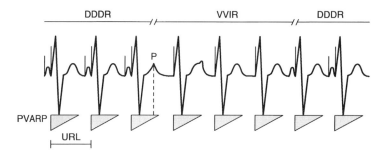

Fig. 6–22. Electrocardiographic appearance of mode switching. The first three cardiac cycles are due to sensor-driven atrioventricular (AV) sequential pacing, that is, DDDR pacing. After the third paced ventricular complex, a P wave occurs during the postventricular atrial refractory period (PVARP) (triangles) and initiates mode switching to the VVIR mode because the atrial rate has exceeded the upper rate limit (URL). The pacing mode reverts to DDDR when the atrial rate falls below the programmed URL; that is, P waves fall outside the PVARP. (From Barold and Mond.[17] By permission of Futura Publishing Company.)

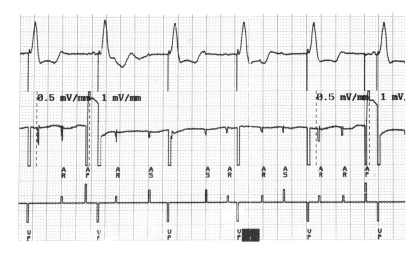

Fig. 6–23. Electrocardiographic tracing with Marker Channel from a patient with mode switching. The Marker Channel reveals atrial tachycardia, and the electrocardiogram is compatible with mode switching to the DDI pacing mode. AP, atrial pacing; AR, atrial event in refractory period; AS, atrial sensing; VP, ventricular pacing.

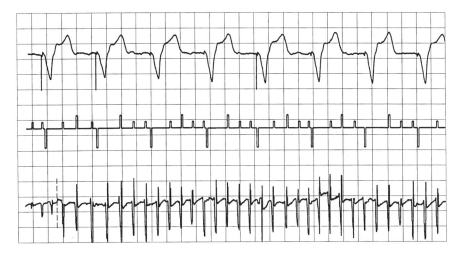

Fig. 6–24. Pacemaker programmer recording obtained during mode switching. The *top tracing* is the surface electrocardiogram, which shows VVI pacing. The *middle tracing* is the "event channel," and the *bottom tracing* is the atrial electrogram, which is consistent with atrial fibrillation.

Mode switching avoids this limitation. Examples of mode switching are shown in Figures 6–23 and 6–24.

Dual-Chamber Rate-Modulated Pacemakers: Effect on Timing Cycles

DDDR pacing systems further increase the complexity of the upper rate behavior because the pacemaker can be driven by intrinsic atrial activity to cause PV (native atrial depolarization followed by a paced ventricular event) pacing or by a sensor whose input signal is not identifiable on the ECG, or by both, to result in AV or AR pacing.[21,22] The eventual upper rate also depends on the type of sensor incorporated in the pacemaker and how the sensor is programmed. Between the programmed LRL and the programmed URL, there may be stable P-wave synchronous pacing, P-wave synchronous pacing alternating with AV sequential pacing, or stable AV sequential pacing at rates exceeding the base rate (Fig. 6–25). AV sequential pacing rates may increase as high as the programmed maximum sensor rate (MSR).

Although the MSR and MTR are closely related, they are not identical. The tracking rate refers to the rate when the pacemaker is sensing and tracking intrinsic atrial activity. The MTR is the maximum ventricular paced rate that is allowed in response to sensed atrial rhythms. This may result in fixed-block, Wenckebach, fallback, or rate-smoothing responses, depending on the design of the system.[23,24] The sensor-controlled rate is the rate of the pacemaker that is determined by the sensor input signal. The MSR is the maximum rate that the pacemaker is allowed to achieve under sensor control. In some units in which MTR and MSR can be independently programmed, the ventricular paced rate under sensor drive might exceed that attained when intrinsic atrial activity is being tracked.

Whether at the MTR or during rate acceleration below the MTR, the rhythm that results may be in part sensor-driven and in part sinus-driven (P-wave tracking) and not purely one or the other (Fig. 6–26). Which of these mechanisms predominates depends on the integrity of the sinus node and the sensor and how the pacemaker is programmed. DDDR pac-

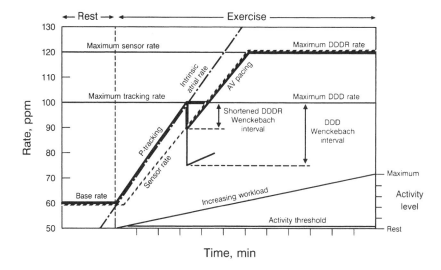

Fig. 6–25. Diagram illustrating the rate response of a DDDR pacemaker and its behavior at both the maximum tracking and the maximum sensor rates. The dashed-dotted line represents the intrinsic atrial rate, and the diagonal dashed line represents the sensor rate during progressively increasing workloads. The heavy black line shows the ventricular paced rate, assuming complete heart block as it progresses from the P-tracking mode to atrioventricular (AV) sequential pacing through a period of pseudo-Wenckebach block. Note that the DDD pseudo-Wenckebach interval is shortened by sensor-driven pacing. Maximal shortening of the pseudo-Wenckebach period is accomplished by optimal programming of the sensor rate-adaptive variables. (From Higano et al.[25] By permission of Futura Publishing Company.)

ing can result in a type of rate smoothing. If the sensor is optimally programmed, as the atrial rate exceeds the MTR, the RR interval will display minimal variation between sinus-driven and sensor-driven pacing[25] (Fig. 6–27). If the rate-responsive circuitry is programmed to mimic the native atrial rate, the paced ventricular rate will not demonstrate the 2:1, or Wenckebach-type, behavior. Conversely, if the rate-responsive circuitry is programmed to very low levels of sensor-driven pacing, little or no rate smoothing will take place.

Maximum sensor-driven rate smoothing requires optimal programming of the rate-adaptive sensor. Thus, sensor-modulated rate smoothing occurs only when the rate-adaptive sensor is driving the pacemaker, when the intrinsic atrial rate exceeds the programmed MTR. As shown in Figure 6–27, the variation in RR interval is markedly lessened with the sensor "on" (DDDR) rather than "passive" (DDD). In the DDDR mode, the RR interval is allowed to lengthen only as much as the difference between the MTR and the activity sensor rate interval. For example, if a device is programmed to a P-wave tracking limit of 120 ppm and the patient's atrial rate exceeds this, the pacemaker will operate in a Wenckebach-type block. If the sensor-indicated rate at this time is 100 ppm, the paced rate will drop from 120 ppm (500 msec) to an AV sequential paced rate of 100 ppm (600 msec) for the Wenckebach cycle and then return to P-wave tracking at a rate of 120 ppm. This situation usually shortens the DDD Wenckebach interval, but this interval depends on the atrial rate and the programmed values for the MTR and the TARP.

Another aspect of DDDR timing cycles is the atrial-sensing window (ASW).[26] The portion of the RR cycle that is not part of the PVARP or the AVI is the period during which the atrial-sensing channel is alert, the ASW. If the PVARP or AVI (or both) is extended, there may

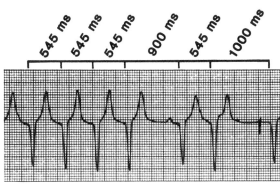

Base rate = 60 ppm
Maximum tracking rate = 110 ppm

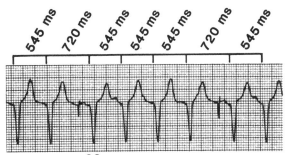

Base rate = 60 ppm
Maximum tracking rate = 110 ppm
Maximum sensor rate = 140 ppm

Fig. 6–26. *Top panel,* Electrocardiographic tracing from a patient with a DDDR pacemaker programmed to the DDD mode. During exercise, when the maximum tracing rate is exceeded, there are marked variations in VV cycle length as the pacemaker either waits until the ventriculoatrial interval "times out" to deliver an atrial pacing artifact or tracks an intrinsic atrial event that occurs. *Bottom panel,* Electrocardiographic tracing from the same patient, whose pacemaker is now programmed to the DDDR mode. Sensor-driven pacing during exercise minimizes the variation in VV cycle length. This effect has been called "sensor-driven rate smoothing." (From Hayes et al.[22] By permission of Futura Publishing Company.)

RR = 461 ms

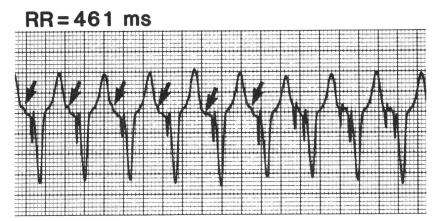

Maximum tracking rate = 130 ppm
Maximum sensor rate = 130 ppm

Fig. 6–27. Electrocardiographic tracing from a patient with a DDDR pacemaker programmed to maximum sensor and tracking rates of 130 ppm. The tracing initially demonstrates P-synchronous pacing (*arrows* indicate P waves), which is followed by atrioventricular sequential or sensor-driven pacing at an almost identical rate. Minimizing the variation in cycle length between sinus-driven and sensor-driven pacing is the goal of optimal programming, that is, "sensor-driven rate smoothing." (From Hayes et al.[22] By permission of Futura Publishing Company.)

Fig. 6–28. In this electrocardiographic example from a DDDR pacemaker, the maximum sensor rate is 150 ppm (400 msec), the atrial refractory period (ARP) is 350 msec, and the atrioventricular (AV) interval is 100 msec. As illustrated in the block diagrams above the electrocardiogram, the two sensor-driven atrial pacing artifacts both occur during the terminal portion of the postventricular atrial refractory period (PVARP). Even though no atrial sensing can occur during the PVARP, as can be seen in this example by the intrinsic P wave that occurs immediately after the first paced ventricular depolarization, a sensor-driven atrial pacing artifact is not prevented by the PVARP. Whether a sensor-driven atrial pacing artifact is delivered depends on the sensor-indicated rate at that time and not on the PVARP. VA, ventriculoatrial. (From Hayes and Higano.[27] By permission of Futura Publishing Company.)

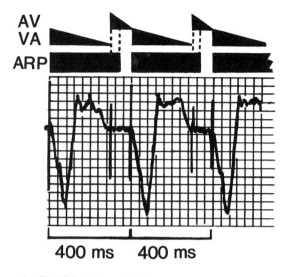

Fig. 6–29. Diagram showing how an appropriately timed P wave can inhibit the sensor-driven A spike and result in apparent P-wave tracking above the maximum tracking rate (MTR). In this example, the MTR is 100 ppm, or 600 msec. The second and third complexes are preceded by intrinsic P waves that occurred during the atrial sensing window (ASW). This resulted in A-spike inhibition, or P-wave tracking above the MTR. The fourth complex was initiated by atrial pacing, because the preceding native P wave occurred outside the ASW in the atrial refractory period (ARP, 275 msec). Note the short P-stimulus interval produced by the subsequent atrial spike. Also shown are the ASW (65 msec), atrioventricular interval (AVI, 100 msec), and variable PV interval. The intrinsic atrial rate is 143 bpm (420 msec). The sensor rate is 136 ppm (440 msec). A diagram in Marker Channel (Medtronic, Inc., Minneapolis, MN) fashion demonstrates the electrocardiographic findings. AP, atrial paced event; AS, atrial sensed event; VP, ventricular paced event. (From Higano and Hayes.[26] By permission of Futura Publishing Company.)

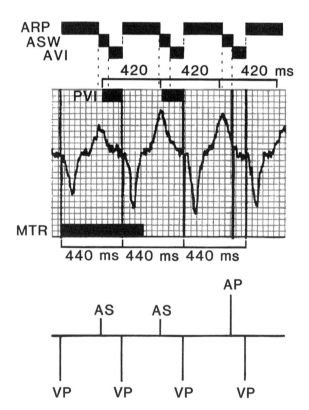

effectively be no ASW and even a DDD pacemaker functions effectively as a DVI system. Conversely, if a DDDR pacemaker has exceeded the programmed MTR and is pacing at faster rates based on sensor activation, an appropriately timed intrinsic P wave can still inhibit the sensor-driven atrial pacing artifact and give the appearance of P-wave tracking at rates greater than the MTR[27] (Fig. 6–28). Although the MTR is programmed to a single value in DDDR pacing, it behaves as if it were variable and equal to the sensor-driven rate when the sensor-driven rate exceeds the programmed MTR (if a P wave occurs during the ASW to inhibit output of an atrial pacing artifact) (Fig. 6–29).

Endless-Loop Tachycardia

Endless-loop tachycardia is not a portion of the timing cycle, but under-standing the timing cycle of dual-chamber pacing is crucial to understanding endless-loop tachycardia and vice versa. Endless-loop tachycardia has also been referred to as "pacemaker-mediated tachycardia," "pacemaker-mediated re-entry tachycardia," and "pacemaker circus movement tachycardia." Endless-loop tachycardia has been de-fined as a reentry arrhythmia in which the dual-chamber pacemaker acts as the antegrade limit of the tachycardia and the natural conduction pathway acts as the retrograde limit[28] (Fig. 6–30).

If AV synchrony is uncoupled, that is, if the P wave is displaced from its normal relation to the QRS complex, the subsequent ventricular event may result in retrograde atrial excitation if retrograde or VA conduction is intact. If the retrograde P wave is sensed, the AVI of the pacemaker is initiated. On termination of

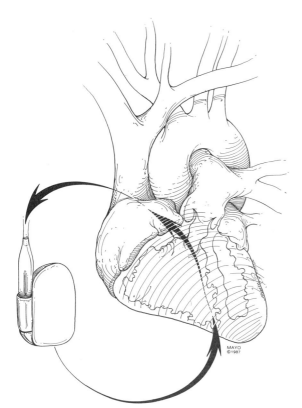

Fig. 6–30. Schematic representation of pacemaker-mediated tachycardia. The intrinsic conduction system acts as the retrograde pathway and the pacemaker as the antegrade pathway. (From Hayes.[28] By permission of Mayo Foundation.)

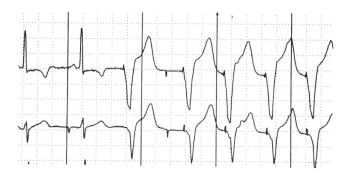

Fig. 6–31. Electrocardiographic tracing from an ambulatory monitor worn by a patient complaining of intermittent tachycardia. The tracing begins with two native QRS events followed by ventricular pacing. The first paced ventricular event presumably follows some event sensed on the atrial channel, but this cannot be identified. A subsequent atrial pacing artifact fails to capture. After the programmed AVI, the ventricle is paced and retrograde conduction occurs to a vulnerable atrium; the retrograde P wave is sensed and initiates pacemaker-mediated tachycardia.

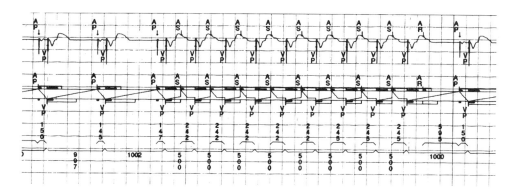

Fig. 6–32. Telemetered tracing of an episode of pacemaker-mediated tachycardia (PMT) and termination by the PMT algorithm. The PMT is initiated by atrial failure to capture and subsequent retrograde conduction after the paced ventricular event. In the ninth cycle, the atrial refractory period is extended and the PMT is terminated. AP, atrial pacing; AR, atrial event in refractory period; AS, atrial sensing; VP, ventricular pacing.

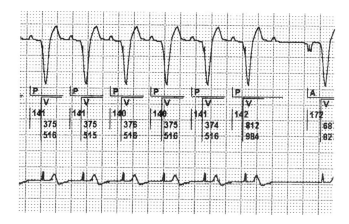

Fig. 6–33. Electrocardiographic tracing demonstrating the termination of pacemaker-mediated tachycardia (PMT). In this pacemaker, if the PMT algorithm is activated (i.e., criteria are met for a PMT), after 10 beats at the maximum tracking rate, the postventricular atrial refractory period (PVARP) is extended. The result is that the next retrograde P wave falls in the PVARP and the PMT cycle is interrupted.

the AVI and MTR interval, a ventricular pacing artifact is delivered, which could once again be conducted in a retrograde fashion. Once established, this reentrant mechanism continues until interrupted or until the retrograde limb of the circuit is exhausted (Fig. 6–31). The paced VV interval cannot violate the programmed maximum limit, or URL, of the pacemaker, and the endless-loop tachycardia often occurs at the URL. Many mechanisms have been adopted to prevent or minimize endless-loop tachycardia (Fig. 6–32 and 6–33).

Initial Electrocardiographic Interpretation

In reviewing an ECG from a patient with an implanted pacemaker, one should carefully assess the underlying rhythm and its relationship to the pacemaker artifacts.[2] The first step is to find any portion of the ECG during which the heart is not paced, that is, identify the intrinsic cardiac rhythm. That portion of the ECG should be interpreted as any ECG would be: PR, QRS, and QT intervals; rate; axis; voltage;

and so forth. If no intrinsic rhythm is apparent, the patient may be pacemaker-dependent or the pacemaker may be programmed to stimulate faster (that is, at a shorter cycle length) than the intrinsic rhythm. After determining the spontaneous atrial and ventricular rhythms, one should look for any relationship between the two; for example, does a P wave result in a QRS complex, indicating intact AV conduction? After the intrinsic rhythm has been carefully scrutinized, pacemaker activity should be assessed. If pacemaker activity is present, is there one stimulus or are there two stimuli? If only one stimulus is present, does it result in atrial (Fig. 6–34) or ventricular (Fig. 6–35) depolarization? Is there an apparent relationship between pacemaker activity and atrial activity or ventricular activity, or both? If pacing artifacts are occurring only in the ventricle, there is no relationship between the pacemaker stimulus and a preceding P wave, and the pacemaker stimulus follows the intrinsic QRS complex at a consistent cycle length, ventricular sensing as part of ventricular inhibited (VVI) pacing is present (Fig. 6–36). If a pacemaker artifact is

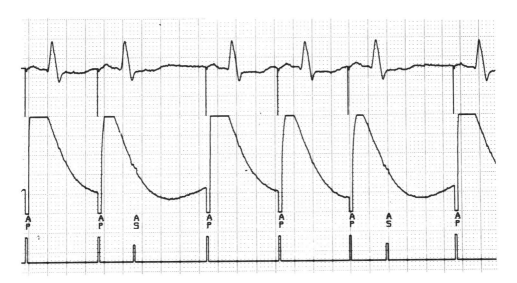

Fig. 6–34. Electrocardiographic tracing demonstrating atrial pacing (AP) with far-field sensing. On the Marker Channel, two of the native QRS complexes are identified as sensed atrial events (AS). This resets the timing cycle.

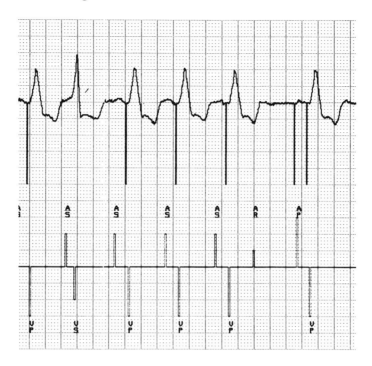

Fig. 6–35. Electrocardiographic tracing and diagnostic interpretation markers compatible with DDD pacing. The markers confirm atrial sensing (AS) and pacing (AP), ventricular sensing (VS) and pacing (VP), and an atrial event occurring in the refractory period (AR).

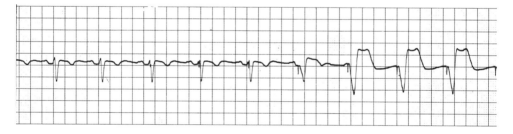

Fig. 6–36. Electrocardiographic tracing from a patient with VVI pacing. The first two events are native QRS complexes without pacing artifacts. They are followed by three QRS events with superimposed pacing artifacts but without deformation of the QRS, that is, pseudofusion, followed by a QRS of different morphology that is a fusion of native and paced events. The final three complexes are fully paced ventricular depolarizations.

consistently found within intrinsic P or QRS complexes, a triggered pacing mode (AAT or VVT) exists (Fig. 6–37).

It is usually not possible to determine from the ECG whether the pacemaker is operating in a bipolar or a unipolar configuration. With analog recording systems, it may be possible to assess the size of the pacemaker stimulus in an effort to determine polarity. If the pace-maker artifact is large, it is most likely of the unipolar configuration; if a very small pacemaker artifact is present, it is most likely of the bipolar configuration. With the more commonly used digital recording systems, which artificially simulate the pacemaker artifact, the size of pacing artifacts is meaningless. There may even be situations in which all cardiac activity is paced and no artifacts are visualized

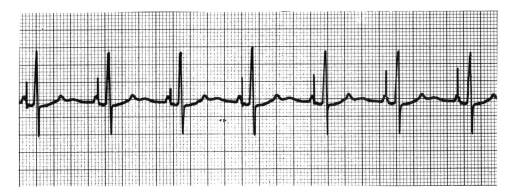

Fig. 6–37. Electrocardiographic tracing demonstrating normal sinus rhythm with pacing artifacts superimposed on every P wave. This is AAT pacing. (From Hayes DL: Pacemaker electrocardiography. *In* A Practice of Cardiac Pacing. Edited by S Furman, DL Hayes, DR Holmes Jr. Mount Kisco, NY, Futura Publishing Company, 1986, pp 305–331. By permission of the publisher.)

or artifacts are sometimes present and sometimes not even though all activity is paced.

Response to Magnet Application

Assessing the magnet response of the pacemaker provides additional information about pacemaker function and may be helpful in interpretation of the paced ECG. Magnet response may also help identify the pacing mode and often the specific pulse generator and is equally useful for single- and dual-chamber pacing.

Application of a magnet to a single-chamber pacemaker always results in single-chamber asynchronous pacing (Fig. 6–38). In dual-chamber pacemakers, magnet application usually but not always results in asynchronous pacing in both the atrial and the ventricular chambers (DOO mode) (Fig. 6–39). Exceptions exist. At least one older dual-chamber pulse generator did not have a magnet mode, and in others the magnet mode may be programmed "off." There have also been dual-chamber pacemakers available in which magnet application resulted in atrial asynchronous pacing with retention of ventricular sensing, and in another device, magnet application resulted in VOO pacing.

The pacing rate should be determined during magnet application. Is the magnet rate faster or slower than or the same as the programmed pacemaker rate? If the pacemaker is a single-chamber pacemaker, does it result in atrial or ventricular depolarization? Having determined what chamber is being paced, one can assess the pacemaker artifact and subsequent depolarization to assure proper capture. It should be remembered that pacemakers of different manufacturers respond differently to magnet application. Some continue to pace asynchronously for a specific number of beats after removal of the magnet and may do so at more than one rate. The magnet response of a particular pacemaker may vary depending on the programmed parameters, that is, the mode, of the pacemaker (Fig. 6–40). The individual specifics of magnet application must be known for each pacemaker to determine that behavior is normal during magnet application and after removal. For dual-chamber pacemakers operating in the DOO mode, the AV interval should be measured during magnet application.

When a single cardiac chamber is being paced, the effect of the paced chamber on the remaining chamber should be determined. For example, if an atrial

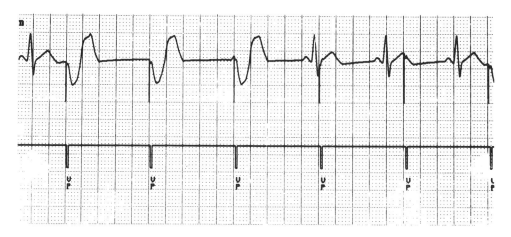

Fig. 6–38. Electrocardiographic tracing demonstrating VOO pacing. The pacing artifacts occur at a regular interval and are not "reset" by the native QRS complex. VP, ventricular pacing.

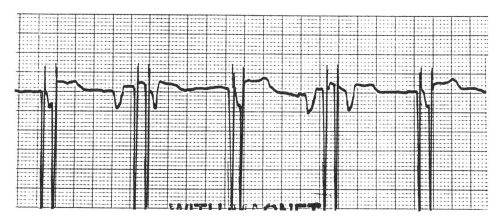

Fig. 6–39. Electrocardiographic tracing demonstrating DOO pacing. The pacing artifacts occur at a regular interval and are not "reset" by the native P or QRS events.

pacemaker is present, does atrial depolarization result in AV conduction and an intrinsic QRS complex, demonstrating intact AV conduction (Fig. 6–41)? Alternatively, if a ventricular pacemaker is present, is there retrograde activation of the atrium, resulting in retrograde P wave activity following the paced ventricular complex (Fig. 6–42)?

It is important that few assumptions be made about the details of the magnet mode of operation and that one be aware of the specifics of the magnet response in a particular unit; otherwise, an erroneous interpretation of inappropriate operation may be made. The magnet mode is usually (but not always) free of sensing any events and is often at a specific rate independent of the programmed rate and sensitivity settings. It allows determination, with a puzzling or unusual ECG, of whether the pulse generator is capable of operating normally.

Single-Chamber Pacemakers

By following the preceding steps, one will have determined whether a single- or dual-chamber pacemaker is present

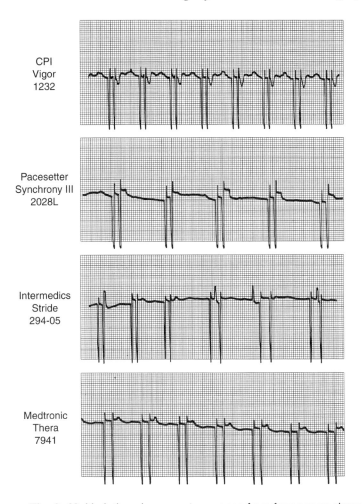

Fig. 6–40. Variations in magnet response from four pacemakers.

and whether the pacemaker stimuli result in atrial or ventricular depolarization (or both). If a single-chamber atrial pacemaker is present, if stimulation produces atrial capture, and if the pacemaker artifact is inhibited by intrinsic P waves, the pacemaker is in the atrial inhibited (AAI) mode (Fig. 6–34). In the AAI mode, paced ventricular activity is never seen, with or without magnet application, and with normal function, a pacemaker artifact never occurs within the intrinsic P waves. If a stimulus occurs that results in ventricular capture with inhibition by QRS complexes, the pacemaker is in the ventricular inhibited mode (VVI) (Fig. 6–36).

If the pacemaker is pacing asynchronously without sensing or capture of either the atrium or the ventricle, the mode cannot be determined. Similarly, with a single-chamber pacemaker, either atrial or ventricular, if intrinsic activity is never seen and every complex is paced, either the patient is pacemaker-dependent or the pacemaker has been programmed to be faster than the intrinsic cardiac rate.

If a single stimulus falls consistently into the spontaneous P wave or QRS complex, the mode is of the triggered variety (AAT/VVT) (Fig. 6–37). Although this mode of pacing is available in many multimodal programmable pacemakers,

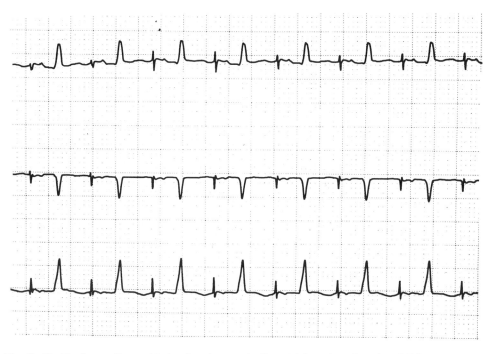

Fig. 6–41. Electrocardiographic tracing demonstrating atrial pacing. A native QRS at a consistent interval after each paced atrial event verifies intact atrioventricular nodal conduction.

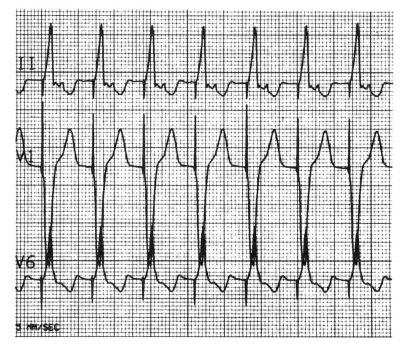

Fig. 6–42. Electrocardiographic tracing demonstrating VVI pacing with retrograde conduction. Consistent deformity of the T wave is compatible with retrograde P waves.

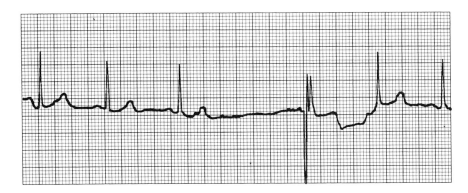

Fig. 6–43. Electrocardiographic tracing from a patient with a VVI pacemaker programmed to a lower rate of 60 ppm and a hysteresis rate of 40 ppm. The tracing begins with normal sinus rhythm, which is followed by an interval of 1,500 msec, 40 bpm, at which point a ventricular pacing artifact is delivered. A native QRS event then occurs at approximately 800 msec, 75 bpm, thus inhibiting the pacemaker, which would have emerged at 1,000 msec, or the lower rate of 60 bpm.

it rarely is used as a long-term pacing mode. Programming a pacemaker to the triggered mode is sometimes helpful to determine exactly where on the surface ECG sensing occurs.

An exception to the rule of the timing cycles in AAI and VVI pacing and a long-standing source of confusion is hysteresis. This programmable feature allows the escape interval for the initial paced beat to be at a longer cycle length than subsequent paced intervals (Fig. 6–43). For example, if a patient has sinus node dysfunction with episodes of sinus bradycardia or sinus arrest, the pacemaker can be programmed to pace continuously at an interval of 1,000 msec (rate of 60), but hysteresis takes place at a rate of 40, that is, 1,500 msec without a paced event is allowed before pacing is initiated. If one does not know that hysteresis is "on," the two different intervals may give the appearance of oversensing. However, if the intervals are repetitive and the longer interval always follows an intrinsic beat, hysteresis is the most likely explanation.

Dual-Chamber Pacemakers

If a dual-chamber pacemaker is present, the steps already outlined should be followed, including determination of the AVI and the status of AV and VA conduction.

The next step in interpretation of an ECG with dual-chamber pacing should be to determine the pacing mode. During the free-running (nonmagnet) pacemaker mode, it should be determined whether ventricular sensing, ventricular pacing, atrial pacing, or ventricular tracking of atrial activity occurs.

If P-wave activity is being sensed, does each P wave begin a pacemaker cycle? If each spontaneous P wave results in a paced ventricular complex at a consistent preset AV delay, the pacemaker is P-synchronous and may be in the DDD or VDD mode (Fig. 6–44). There are several ways to differentiate VDD from DDD pacing. Intermittent atrial pacing indicates DDD pacing; the absence of atrial activity followed by ventricular pacing at the lower rate or sensor-indicated rate is consistent with VDD pacing (Fig. 6–45). With magnet application, DDD pacemakers usually respond with DOO pacing and VDD pacemakers with VOO pacing.

If each sensed P wave inhibits pacemaker output but initiates synchronous ventricular pacing, the pacemaker is in

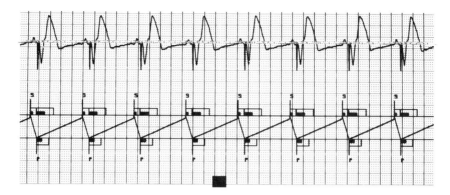

Fig. 6–44. Electrocardiographic tracing and ladder diagram compatible with P-synchronous pacing. The Marker Channel confirms atrial sensing (S) and ventricular pacing (P). It is impossible to say if the programmed pacing mode is VDD or DDD.

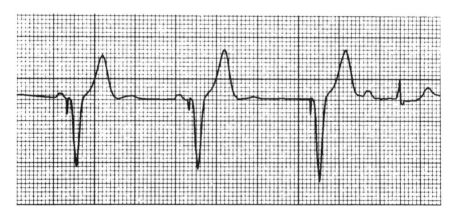

Fig. 6–45. Electrocardiographic tracing from a patient with VDD pacing. Two P-synchronous ventricular events are followed by a ventricular paced event without a preceding atrial event. In the absence of an intrinsic atrial event, the pacemaker "times out" with ventricular pacing at the programmed lower rate.

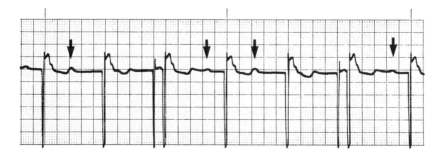

Fig. 6–46. Electrocardiographic tracing from a patient with a pacemaker programmed to the DDI pacing mode. When a P wave occurs outside the postventricular atrial refractory period (*arrows*), atrial output is inhibited, but ventricular pacing does not occur until the lower rate has "timed out."

the DDI mode (Fig. 6–46). Sensed atrial activity inhibits atrial output but does not result in a ventricular stimulus after the AV delay. AV sequential pacing at the programmed rate is provided if intrinsic activity is absent. Intrinsic ventricular activity occurring during the atrial escape interval or AV delay inhibits the pacemaker and resets the timing cycle.

Abnormalities of the Paced Electrocardiogram

Abnormalities of pacing that can be recognized electrocardiographically can be divided into the following broad categories.[27,29,30] More than one of these abnormalities may be present on a single tracing.

Electrocardiographic Manifestations of Pacemaker Malfunction

- Inappropriate lack of pacemaker artifacts (failure to output)
- Failure to capture
- Inappropriate pacemaker artifacts (undersensing)
- Inappropriate pacemaker rate

These abnormalities may apply to single- or dual-chamber pacemakers. Given the complexity of the timing cycles

of dual-chamber devices, it is sometimes difficult to determine from the surface ECG whether normal sensing and pacing are present. However, by approaching the ECG while keeping the timing cycle, potential abnormalities, and their differential diagnoses in mind, one should be able to determine whether a malfunction or pseudomalfunction exists.

Failure to Capture

If each pacemaker stimulus is not followed by a QRS or P-wave complex, failure to capture may exist (Fig. 6–47). When one determines the possible causes of failure to capture, both true malfunctions and pseudomalfunctions should be considered. The potential causes include

- High thresholds with an inadequately programmed output
- Partial conductor coil fracture
- Insulation defect
- Lead dislodgment or perforation
- Impending total battery depletion
- Functional noncapture
- Poor or incompatible connection at connector block
- Circuit failure
- Air in pocket (unipolar pacemaker)
- Increased thresholds due to drugs or metabolic abnormality

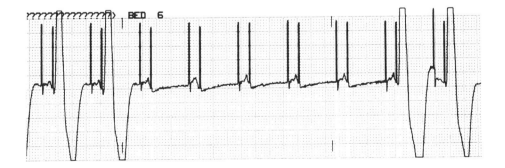

Fig. 6–47. Electrocardiographic tracing from a patient with a newly implanted DDD pacemaker. There is intermittent failure to capture the ventricle. (From Hayes.[2] By permission of Futura Publishing Company.)

It is sometimes difficult during magnet application to determine with certainty whether the myocardium is refractory at the time of the pacemaker artifact. (A pacemaker artifact that occurs relatively soon after an intrinsic beat may not result in capture because the myocardium is refractory. The appearance of failure to capture in this situation is best referred to as "functional failure to capture.") (Fig. 6–48). However, if a nonmagnet ECG is being evaluated, any failure to capture should be scrutinized carefully. If the pacemaker artifact is occurring early enough to raise the

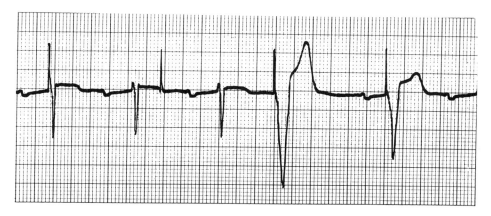

Fig. 6–48. Electrocardiographic tracing taken during magnet application from a patient with a VVI pacemaker. The first pacing artifact results in fusion with the native complex. The second pacing artifact does not result in ventricular capture. However, this is considered "functional failure to capture" because the ventricle is refractory from the native depolarization that occurred approximately 300 msec before the pacing artifact. The third pacing artifact results in ventricular depolarization, and the fourth artifact appears to result in pseudofusion.

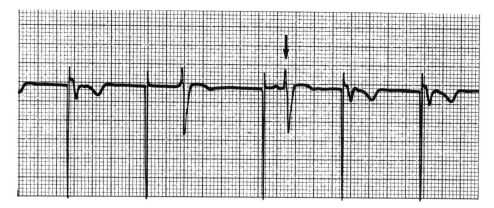

Fig. 6–49. Electrocardiographic tracing from a patient with a VVI pacemaker that has intermittent failure to capture and functional undersensing. Failure to capture is demonstrated by the second and third pacing artifacts. The intrinsic QRS that occurs after the second pacing artifact fails to capture is sensed normally and resets the timing cycle. The subsequent QRS is not sensed because it occurs at approximately 250 msec after the pacing artifact (*arrow*); it falls in the ventricular refractory period and is therefore not sensed.

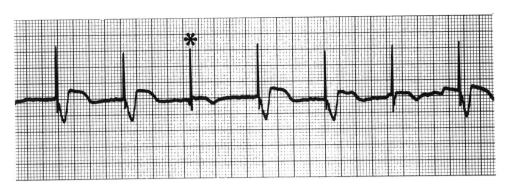

Fig. 6–50. Electrocardiographic tracing from a patient with a VVI pacemaker. The third pacemaker artifact (*) is probably a pseudofusion beat, and the sixth artifact results in a fusion beat. It is difficult to say with certainty that the third event is pseudofusion and not fusion in the absence of an intrinsic event without a pacemaker artifact present. (From Hayes DL: Pacemaker electrocardiography. *In* A Practice of Cardiac Pacing. Edited by S Furman, DL Hayes, DR Holmes Jr. Mount Kisco, NY, Futura Publishing Company, 1986, pp 305–331. By permission of the publisher.)

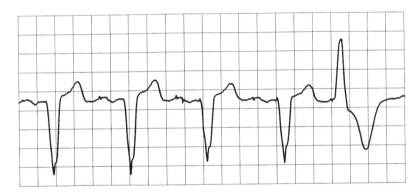

Fig. 6–51. Electrocardiographic tracing from a patient with a DDD pacemaker. All atrial and ventricular events are paced with the exception of the fifth ventricular event, which represents a premature ventricular contraction. An atrial pacing artifact immediately precedes the premature ventricular contraction and gives the appearance of ventricular pacing. The electrocardiographic finding of a pacing artifact from one chamber appearing to pace the other cardiac chamber is referred to as "pseudo-pseudofusion." (Courtesy of Sherman Kahan, M.D., Frederick, MD.)

question of myocardial refractoriness as the cause for noncapture, failure to sense may also be present (Fig. 6–49). If the surface QRS represents elements of two depolarizations, a fusion beat has occurred (Fig. 6–50). If the surface QRS is not altered by the pacing stimulus that is superimposed, the ECG finding is a pseudofusion beat. If a stimulus from one chamber occurs at the time of an intrinsic beat from the other chamber, giving the appearance of stimulation of the other chamber, the anomaly is referred to as "pseudo-pseudofusion" (Fig. 6–51).

Causes of Undersensing

The occurrence of pacemaker artifacts at an unexplained time suggests abnormal sensing. If the interval between the preceding QRS complex and the paced

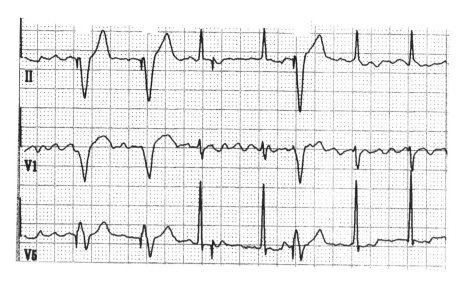

Fig. 6–52. Electrocardiographic tracing from a patient with a VVI pacemaker and underlying atrial fibrillation or flutter. Intermittent ventricular undersensing is noted after two intrinsic QRS complexes.

beat is shorter than the programmed paced cycle length, undersensing is likely (Fig. 6–52). Potential malfunctions, both true and false, that may result in undersensing include

- Morphology of intrinsic event different from that measured at implantation
- Lead dislodgment or poor lead positioning
- Lead insulation failure
- Circuit failure
- Magnet application
- Malfunction of reed switch
- Electromagnetic interference
- Battery depletion

Failure to sense is often seen in combination with failure to capture (Fig. 6–49), but the functions are separate and malfunctions may occur independently. The pacemaker senses the intracardiac electrogram. It is not possible to know from the surface ECG exactly where in relation to the ECG the intrinsic deflection, the maximum amplitude of the intracardiac electrogram, exists and thus where sensing occurs. The pacemaker artifact may fall within the QRS complex (Fig. 6–53).

This timing does not necessarily represent failure to sense. The stimulus may appear to be late when analyzed from the surface ECG, but it reflects only pacemaker sensing after the onset of the surface QRS complex or P wave. (A pacemaker stimulus occurring within the intrinsic event could also be due to a "triggered" pacing mode.)

It is not uncommon for an otherwise normally functioning pacing system to fail to sense premature ventricular contractions (PVC). The amplitude and frequency content of ventricular foci differ, and the pacemaker may not sense all possible foci (Fig. 6–54). When sensing thresholds are determined at the time of pacemaker implantation, they are based on sensing a normal QRS complex. Even though a PVC may appear much larger on the surface ECG, depending on the vector of the PVC in relation to the pacing electrode, it may have lower sensing characteristics than the normal QRS complex.

When interpreting ECGs of DDD pacemakers, all pacemaker intervals must be considered. A frequent source of confusion is the appearance of atrial undersensing caused by the occurrence of a P wave during the PVARP, so-called func-

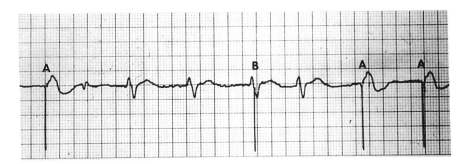

Fig. 6–53. Electrocardiographic tracing demonstrating intermittent ventricular capture (A) and a ventricular pacing artifact occurring within a native QRS (B). Although difficult to prove without an electrogram or Marker Channel, this event represents simultaneous occurrence of the native artifact and the release of the ventricular pacing artifact and does not indicate undersensing. Because there can be a significant variation between what is seen on the surface electrocardiogram and the actual timing of intracardiac events as documented by the electrogram, the surface tracing may suggest undersensing. (From Hayes.[2] By permission of Mayo Foundation.)

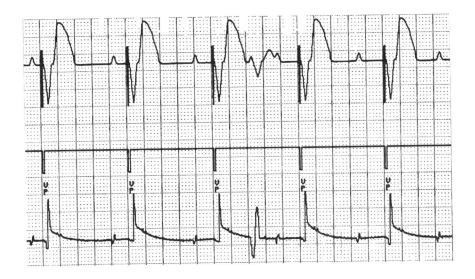

Fig. 6–54. Electrocardiographic tracing from a patient with a VVI pacemaker. There is failure to sense a premature ventricular contraction (PVC). Because PVCs arise from a different vector than native QRS complexes, intermittent undersensing of PVCs is not uncommon. Reprogramming the ventricular sensitivity is a reasonable measure to avoid PVC undersensing, but rarely would this necessitate lead repositioning. VP, ventricular pacing.

tional atrial undersensing.[31] When DDD pacemaker operation includes a PVARP that is extended after an event that the pacemaker identifies as a PVC, there is even more opportunity for P waves to occur in the extended PVARP. This possibility should be considered before it is concluded that there is true atrial undersensing (Fig. 6–55).

Failure to Output

In contrast to the ECG manifestation of undersensing, events may occur that result in inappropriately long intervals on the paced ECG. Although failure to output may be due to oversensing, other true malfunctions and pseudomalfunctions may result in failure to output.

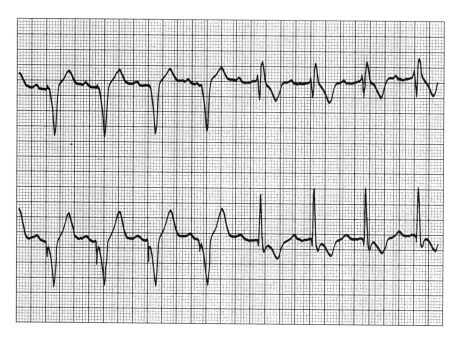

Fig. 6–55. Electrocardiographic tracing from a patient with a DDD pacemaker. The tracing begins with P-synchronous pacing with an atrioventricular interval (AVI) of approximately 160 msec. This is followed by sinus rhythm and then by intrinsic QRS complexes at an interval greater than the programmed AVI of 160 msec. The cause is functional undersensing. In this patient, Marker Channel documented intermittent T-wave oversensing that resulted in extension of the postventricular atrial refractory period (PVARP). PVARP extension perpetuated the inability to sense subsequent P waves.

These include

- Circuit failure
- Complete or intermittent conductor coil fracture
- Intermittently or permanently loose set screw
- Incompatible lead or header
- Total battery depletion
- Internal insulation failure (bipolar lead)
- Oversensing of any noncardiac activity
- Lack of anodal connector contact
- Crosstalk (Fig. 6–56)

Oversensing is the most common cause of failure to output. When oversensing occurs, the pacemaker interval is reset by inappropriate sensed events, so that the interval between the pacemaker stimulus or intrinsic QRS activity and the subsequent paced beat is greater than the programmed pacemaker cycle. T waves, P waves (Fig. 6–57), muscle activity or myopotentials (Fig. 6–58), electromagnetic interference, and, rarely, afterpotentials from pacemaker discharge may result in oversensing.

Ventricular activity may arise from different foci within the ventricle and appear with different configurations or even appear isoelectric on the surface ECG. An isoelectric QRS complex can cause an apparent "pause" that gives the impression of oversensing. Multichannel ECGs are helpful in evaluating that possibility, as it is unlikely that a QRS will be isoelectric in all leads (Fig. 6–59). Alternatively, if an isoelectric event occurs simultaneously with a pacemaker artifact, a fusion beat may result and may appear as failure to capture. Pacemaker capture can be confirmed by noting the T wave or

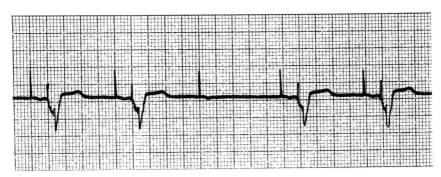

Fig. 6–56. Electrocardiographic tracing from a patient with a dual-chamber pacemaker. The third atrial pacing artifact results in atrial depolarization but is not followed by a ventricular pacing artifact. This "failure to output" is due to crosstalk, that is, the atrial pacing artifact was sensed on the ventricular sensing channel and ventricular output was inhibited.

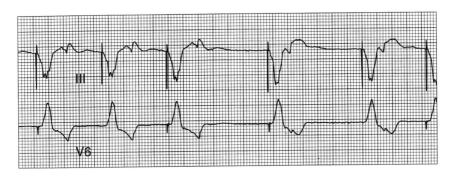

Fig. 6–57. Electrocardiographic tracing from a patient with a VVI pacemaker. There are two different VV intervals. The shorter interval of 857 msec is consistent with the programmed lower rate of 70 bpm. The longer interval of 1,340 msec occurs because there is oversensing of either the T wave or a retrograde P wave. Without an electrogram or Marker Channel, it is difficult to know precisely which is sensed. However, the point of sensing can be determined by measuring backward by 857 msec, the programmed lower rate, from the pacing artifact that follows the longer interval. (From Hayes DL: Programmability. *In* A Practice of Cardiac Pacing. Third edition. Edited by S Furman, DL Hayes, DR Holmes Jr. Mount Kisco, NY, Futura Publishing Company, 1993, pp 635–663. By permission of the publisher.)

Fig. 6–58. Electrocardiographic tracing from a patient with a VVI pacemaker. The lower rate is programmed to 70 bpm, 857 msec. There is pacemaker inhibition with an interval of approximately 2,000 msec, during which there is a considerable artifact effect in the baseline. This anomaly was reproducible and was due to myopotentials. The myopotentials were being sensed on the ventricular sensing circuit and inhibited ventricular output.

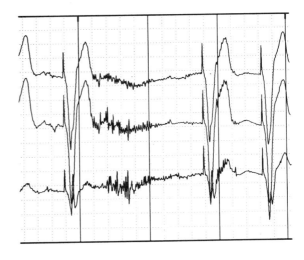

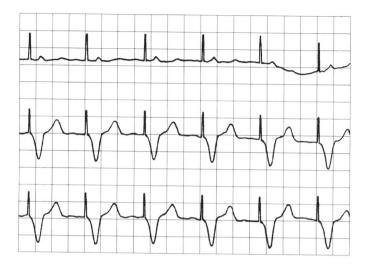

Fig. 6–59. Multichannel electrocardiographic tracing from a patient with a dual-chamber pacemaker. If the top tracing were reviewed in isolation, it would be possible to draw an erroneous conclusion of atrial pacing with ventricular output inhibition. However, simultaneous leads demonstrate definite ventricular activity. Although the intrinsic atrial activity is difficult to see, all ventricular activity is P-synchronous. (Courtesy of Sherman Kahan, M.D., Frederick, MD.)

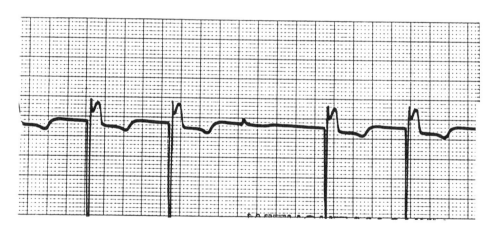

Fig. 6–60. Electrocardiographic tracing from a patient with a VVI pacemaker programmed to a lower rate of 70 bpm. A cursory glance may suggest pacemaker inhibition or oversensing. However, the small complex is a native QRS complex, and there is a subtle suggestion of a T wave following the native QRS complex. A multichannel recording would be helpful.

repolarization activity that follows the pacing artifact (Fig. 6–60).

As noted previously, digital recording systems may not always record pacing artifacts when they occur. Therefore, failure to capture could appear as oversensing if the pacing artifacts could not be seen (Fig. 6–61).

Altered Pacing Rate

As noted in the discussion of timing cycles, every pacing mode has a defined LRL, and dual-chamber pacemakers as well as rate-adaptive pacemakers also require a defined URL. One must be familiar with the timing cycle of a particular pac-

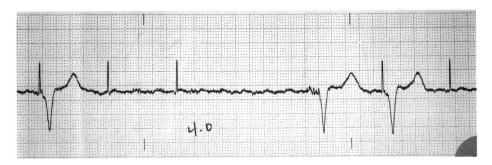

Fig. 6–61. Electrocardiographic tracing from a patient with a VVI pacemaker programmed to a lower rate of 60 bpm. A definite failure to capture is demonstrated by pacing artifacts without subsequent ventricular depolarization. It should also be noted that this patient is entirely pacemaker-dependent. The second QRS complex is identical to the other two shown, but no pacing artifact is seen, nor does a pacing artifact occur in the pause immediately preceding the second ventricular event; thus oversensing followed by a ventricular escape beat is suggested. Measuring from the beginning to the end of the tracing reveals consistent intervals. This tracing was taken from digital recording equipment. Pacemaker artifacts may not be consistently seen. This tracing is compatible with intermittent ventricular failure to capture only.

ing mode and with any idiosyncrasies of the specific pacemaker to determine whether the paced rate is appropriate. A paced rate that appears to differ from the programmed rate has multiple causes (see Chapter 9). These causes include

- Circuit failure
- Battery failure
- Magnet application
- Hysteresis
- Crosstalk
- Undocumented reprogramming of the pacemaker
- Oversensing
- Runaway
- Malfunction of the ECG recording equipment; alteration in paper speed

Atrioventricular Interval

The components and potential variations of the AVI have already been discussed. As the ECG is analyzed, the AVI should be assessed for any variations. The possible explanations for a variant AVI include

- Ventricular safety pacing

- Different AVI
- AVI hysteresis
- Rate-variable or rate-adaptive AVI

Upper Rate Behavior

Descriptions have already been provided for 1:1 P-synchronous pacing at the MTR, pseudo-Wenckebach, and 2:1 upper rate behavior (Fig. 6–62). Other variations are fallback and rate smoothing.

Rate Smoothing

Rate smoothing avoids abrupt changes in pacing rate, such as those that can occur during a sudden transition to pseudo-Wenckebach or 2:1 upper rate behavior, and may eliminate patient symptoms associated with sensed dysrhythmic events.[32]

Rate smoothing controls sudden changes in pacing rate by monitoring the interval between ventricular events (both paced and sensed) and storing the most recent RR interval in memory (Fig. 6–63). On the basis of this RR interval and the programmed rate-smoothing percentage,

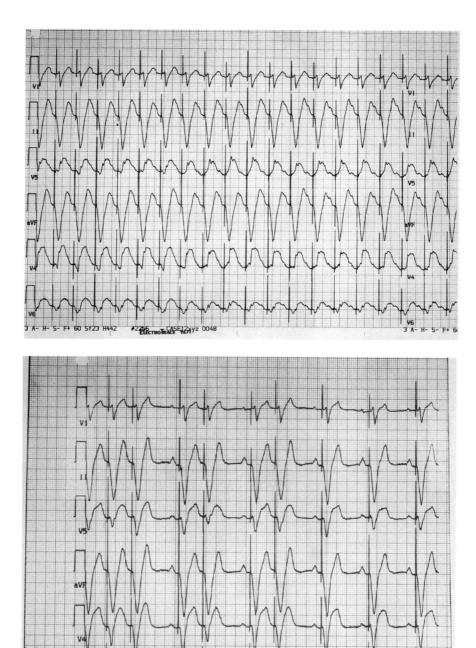

Fig. 6–62. *Upper panel,* 1:1 P-synchronous pacing during a treadmill exercise test. *Lower panel,* Pseudo-Wenckebach and 2:1 upper rate behavior as the same patient continues to exercise.

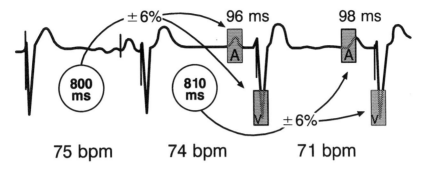

Fig. 6–63. Example of how two rate-smoothing synchronization windows are calculated. If the heart rate is 75 bpm (800 msec) and rate-smoothing is programmed "on" at 6%, the next cycle length may vary by 48 msec, a range from 752 to 848 msec. The subsequent cycle would be calculated as ± 6% of 752 or 848 msec, depending on whether the atrial rate was increasing or decreasing.

Without rate smoothing

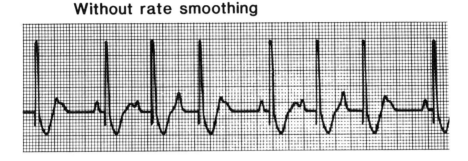

With rate smoothing (6%)

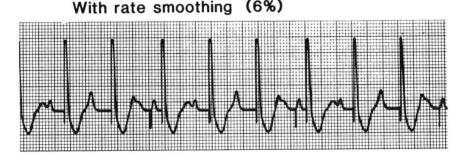

Fig. 6–64. Electrocardiogram demonstrating DDD pacing with true rate-smoothing capabilities (6% of the preceding RR interval). With true rate smoothing, the Wenckebach interval is allowed to lengthen only 36 msec over the preceding RR interval, at a maximum tracking rate of 100 ppm. (Reproduced with permission from Guidant-Cardiac Rhythm Management, Inc.)

the pulse generator sets up two rate-control windows for the next cycle—one for the atrium and one for the ventricle (Fig. 6–64). For example, if the monitored VV interval is 800 msec and 6% rate smoothing is programmed, the algorithm allows the upcoming ventricular rate of the cycle to increase or decrease a maximum of 6%, or ±48 msec (752 to 848 msec).

The rate-smoothing algorithm determines the atrial control window in a manner analogous to the basic ventricular timing cycle: VV = VA + AV. To determine the VA interval from this equation if the VV interval and AVI are known, one simply subtracts the AVI from the VV interval. Rate smoothing does likewise by subtracting the AVI value from the ventricular control window, and the result is a "rate-controlled VA interval." Extending the previous example, if the AVI is 150 msec, the atrial control window is also ±48 msec (602 to 698 msec). Atrial pacing is observed at the maximum calculated VA interval of 698 msec if no sensed event occurs before the end of the VA interval.

Fallback

While operating in the basic pseudo-Wenckebach or AV block upper rate mode, some DDD generators avoid marked variation in the RR interval during sinus or atrial tachycardia by use of a gradual fallback method.[8] Instead of blocking the atrial event or prolonging the AVI, rate fallback involves decoupling of atrial and ventricular events at the URL. The ventricular inhibited pacing rate then gradually decreases to a programmed lower or fallback rate over a programmable duration. When the fallback rate is reached, atrial synchrony is resumed. Although AV synchrony is lost temporarily, the gradual transition to a lower pacing rate may moderate the hemodynamic consequences of sudden shifts in RR intervals that can occur with the AV block mechanism.

Conclusion

Although the paced ECG may have infinite variations depending on the pacing mode, pacemaker model, combination of programmed parameters, and whether function is normal or abnormal, understanding basic timing cycles and a systematic approach to the ECG should allow successful interpretation. When difficulty in ECG interpretation persists despite a systematic approach, the technical manual or the manufacturer should be consulted for assistance.

References

1. Hayes DL, Levine PA: Pacemaker timing cycles. In Cardiac Pacing. Edited by KA Ellenbogen. Boston, Blackwell Scientific Publications, 1992, pp 263–308
2. Hayes DL: Pacemaker electrocardiography. In A Practice of Cardiac Pacing. Third edition. Edited by S Furman, DL Hayes, DR Holmes Jr. Mount Kisco, NY, Futura Publishing Company, 1993, pp 309–359
3. Barold SS, Douard H, Broustet JP, Clementy J: Irregular ventricular stimulation in the DDI mode of a dual chamber pacemaker with atrial-based lower rate timing. Pacing Clin Electrophysiol 22: 123–127, 1999
4. Levine PA, Lindenberg BS, Mace RC: Analysis of AV universal (DDD) pacemaker rhythms. Clin Prog Pacing Electrophysiol 2:54–70, 1984
5. Higano ST, Hayes DL: Quantitative analysis of Wenckebach behavior in DDD pacemakers. Pacing Clin Electrophysiol 13: 1456–1465, 1990
6. Janosik DL, Pearson AC, Buckingham TA, Labovitz AJ, Redd RM: The hemodynamic benefit of differential atrioventricular delay intervals for sensed and paced atrial events during physiologic pacing. J Am Coll Cardiol 14:499–507, 1989
7. Daubert C, Ritter P, Mabo P, Varin C, Leclercq C: AV delay optimization in DDD and DDDR pacing. In New Perspectives in Cardiac Pacing, 3. Edited by SS Barold, J Mugica. Mount Kisco, NY, Futura Publishing Company, 1993, pp 259–287
8. Rees M, Haennel RG, Black WR, Kappagoda T: Effect of rate-adapting atrioventricular delay on stroke volume and cardiac output during atrial synchronous pacing. Can J Cardiol 6:445–452, 1990
9. Daubert C, Ritter P, Mabo P, et al: Rate modulation of the AV delay in DDD pacing. In Progress in Clinical Pacing 1990. Edited by M Santini, M Pistolese, A Alliegro. New York, Elsevier Science Publishing Company, 1990, pp 415–430
10. Ritter P, Daubert C, Mabo P, Descaves C, Gouffault J: Haemodynamic benefit of a rate-adapted A-V delay in dual chamber pacing. Eur Heart J 10:637–646, 1989
11. Mayumi H, Kohno H, Yasui H, Kawachi Y, Tokunaga K: Use of automatic mode

change between DDD and AAI to facilitate native atrioventricular conduction in patients with sick sinus syndrome or transient atrioventricular block. Pacing Clin Electrophysiol 19:1740–1747, 1996

12. Stierle U, Kruger D, Vincent AM, Mitusch R, Giannitsis E, Wiegand U, Potratz J: An optimized AV delay algorithm for patients with intermittent atrioventricular conduction. Pacing Clin Electrophysiol 21:1035–1043, 1998

13. Barold SS: Ventricular- versus atrial-based lower rate timing in dual chamber pacemakers: does it really matter? Pacing Clin Electrophysiol 18:83–96, 1995

14. Barold SS, Fredman CS: Pure atrial-based lower rate timing of dual chamber pacemakers: implications for upper rate limitation. Pacing Clin Electrophysiol 18:391–400, 1995

15. Levine PA, Sholder JA: Interpretation of rate-modulated, dual-chamber rhythms: the effect of ventricular based and atrial based timing systems on DDD and DDDR rhythms, Pacesetter Systems, A Siemens Company, 1990

16. Hayes DL, Ketelson A, Levine PA, Markowitz HT, Sanders R, Schaney G: Understanding timing systems of current DDDR pacemakers. Eur J Cardiac Pacing Electrophysiol 3:70–86, 1993

17. Barold SS, Mond HG: Optimal antibradycardia pacing in patients with paroxysmal supraventricular tachyarrhythmias: role of fallback and automatic mode switching mechanisms. *In* New Perspectives in Cardiac Pacing, 3. Edited by SS Barold, J Mugica. Mount Kisco, NY, Futura Publishing Company, 1993, pp 483–518

18. Koglek W, Suntinger A, Wernisch M, Neuzner J, Sperzel J: Auto-Mode-Switch (AMS). Herzschrittmacherther Elektrophysiol 9:108–119, 1998

19. Lam CT, Lau CP, Leung SK, Tse HF, Ayers G: Improved efficacy of mode switching during atrial fibrillation using automatic atrial sensitivity adjustment. Pacing Clin Electrophysiol 22:17–25, 1999

20. Sutton R, Stack Z, Heaven D, Ingram A: Mode switching for atrial tachyarrhythmias. Am J Cardiol 83:202D-210D, 1999

21. Levine PA, Hayes DL, Wilkoff BL, Ohman AE: Electrocardiography of rate-modulated pacemaker rhythms. Sylmar, CA, Siemens-Pacesetter, 1990, pp 1–90

22. Hayes DL, Higano ST, Eisinger G: Electrocardiographic manifestations of a dual-chamber, rate-modulated (DDDR) pacemaker. Pacing Clin Electrophysiol 12:555–562, 1989

23. Furman S: Dual chamber pacemakers: upper rate behavior. Pacing Clin Electrophysiol 8:197–214, 1985

24. Higano ST, Hayes DL: Quantitative analysis of Wenckebach behavior in DDD pacemakers. Pacing Clin Electrophysiol 13:1456–1465, 1990

25. Higano ST, Hayes DL, Eisinger G: Sensor-driven rate smoothing in a DDDR pacemaker. Pacing Clin Electrophysiol 12:922–929, 1989

26. Higano ST, Hayes DL: P wave tracking above the maximum tracking rate in a DDDR pacemaker. Pacing Clin Electrophysiol 12:1044–1048, 1989

27. Hayes DL, Higano ST: DDR pacing: follow-up and complications. *In* New Perspectives in Cardiac Pacing. 2. Edited by SS Barold, J Mugica. Mount Kisco, NY, Futura Publishing Company, 1991, pp 473–491

28. Hayes DL: Endless-loop tachycardia: the problem has been solved? *In* New Perspectives in Cardiac Pacing. Edited by SS Barold, J Mugica. Mount Kisco, NY, Futura Publishing Company, 1988, pp 375–386

29. Levine PA: Differential diagnosis, evaluation, and management of pacing system malfunction. *In* Cardiac Pacing. Edited by KA Ellenbogen. Boston, Blackwell Scientific Publications, 1992, pp 309–382

30. Love CJ, Hayes DL: Evaluation of pacemaker malfunction. *In* Clinical Cardiac Pacing. Edited by KA Ellenbogen, GN Kay, BL Wilkoff. Philadelphia, WB Saunders Company, 1995, pp 656–683

31. Barold SS: Sustained inhibition of a DDD pacemaker at rates below the programmed lower rate during automatic PVARP extension. Pacing Clin Electrophysiol 22:521–524, 1999

32. van Mechelen R, Ruiter J, de Boer H, Hagemeijer F: Pacemaker electrocardiography of rate smoothing during DDD pacing. Pacing Clin Electrophysiol 8:684–690, 1985

7

Programming

Margaret A. Lloyd, M.D.,
David L. Hayes, M.D.,
Paul A. Friedman, M.D.

Pacemaker Programming

Programmability is defined as the ability to make noninvasive stable but reversible changes in pacemaker function. The pulse generator contains predetermined circuits from which one or several features or functions can be selected for variation within a restricted range. Using a "pacemaker programmer," one can change many aspects of pacemaker function. Although it is technologically possible to completely reprogram a pacemaker's software, there are no approved mechanisms by which this can be done at present.

The first modern programmable pacemakers were introduced in 1972. In this pacemaker, a magnetic code was introduced from an external programmer to manipulate four levels of output and six rates. Since 1972, innumerable changes have evolved in pacemaker programming capabilities. Radiofrequency signals are now exclusively used to communicate between the pacemaker and the programmer. The number of programmable features and the variability of each feature have also expanded greatly. By one calculation, potential programmable combinations with contemporary DDDR pacemakers exceed 4.3068×10^{48}.

All pacemakers implanted are programmable to some degree. The North American Society of Pacing and Electrophysiology/British Pacing and Electrophysiology Group (NASPE/BPG) code designates the degree of programmability and rate modulation in the fourth position.[1] In practice, only the designation "R" is used in this position. An "R" in the fourth position indicates that the pacemaker has a special sensor to control the rate independent of intrinsic electrical activity of the heart. Virtually all pacemakers with a sensor also have extensive telemetric and programmable capabilities. Designations of "O," "P," "M," and "C" are described but rarely used. "O" indicates that none of the parameters of the pacing system can be noninvasively altered. "P" is simple programmability; one or two parameters can be changed, but this code does not specify which ones. "M," multiparameter programmability, indicates that three or more parameters can be changed. "C" reflects the ability of the pacemaker to communicate with the programmer; namely, it has telemetry. By convention and in actual operation, it also means that the pacemaker has multi-parameter programmability.

The degree of programmability varies widely among pulse generators. The first determinant is whether the pacemaker paces a single chamber or has dual-chamber capabilities. Dual-chamber programmable parameters are discussed here, but additional information can be found in Chapters 6 and 8.

In this chapter, major programmable options (Table 7–1) are defined and the rationale for programming discussed (Table 7–2). Although an attempt is made to discuss programming generically, this is not always possible. Specific programmable variables may be protected by trademark and available from only one manufacturer. Therefore, it is necessary to refer to specific manufacturers at times.

A typical programming sequence is also referenced to demonstrate how various programmable options can be used at the time of pacemaker follow-up.

Mode Programming

Most programmable single-chamber pacemakers can be programmed to the inhibited, triggered, or asynchronous mode. The inhibited (AAI, VVI) mode is most commonly used for long-term pacing. The triggered (AAT, VVT) mode is helpful during follow-up to determine normal sensing (Fig. 7–1). The triggered mode cannot be inhibited (only partially true in at least one older pulse generator) and is therefore useful when noncompetitive pacing is associated with electromagnetic interference. The asynchronous (AOO, VOO) mode is rarely used for long-term pacing because it is potentially competitive with intrinsic activity.

If the single-chamber pacemaker is capable of rate adaptation, other programmable mode options are VVIR and VOOR for ventricular application and AAIR and AOOR for atrial application. (Not all single-chamber rate-adaptive pacemakers

---

Table 7–1.
Potential Programmable Values

Mode
Lower rate limit
Maximum pacing rate*†
Hysteresis
Atrioventricular delay*
Adaptive atrioventricular delay*
Atrial refractory period
Postventricular atrial refractory period*
Ventricular refractory period
Pulse width (atrial or ventricular, or both)
Pulse amplitude (atrial or ventricular, or both)
Sensitivity (atrial or ventricular, or both)
Blanking period*
Polarity
Rate adaptation (on or off)‡
Rate-adaptive sensor variables§

---

*Applicable to dual-chamber pacemakers only.

†In dual-chamber rate-adaptive pacemakers, the maximum pacing rate may be a single programmable value or there may be independently programmable maximum P-tracking and maximum sensor-driven rates.

‡Rate adaptation may be a function of the programmed mode; for example, the pacemaker may have DDDR as a programmable option. Or rate adaptation may require programming "on" in conjunction with the desired pacing mode; for example, programming the mode to DDD and rate adaptation "on" delivers DDDR pacing.

§Rate-adaptive sensor variables are not listed separately because they vary significantly from sensor to sensor.

Table 7–2.
Programmable Options for Pacemakers

Parameter	Description	Typical variables
Mode	Preset or programmed response from a pacemaker with or without intrinsic cardiac events.	VOO, AOO, VVI, AAI, VDD, DVI, DDD, DDI, DOO, VVT, AAT (all but AAT, VVT could also have "R," or rate-adaptive, capability)
Lower rate limit	Preset or programmed rate at which a pacemaker emits an output pulse without intrinsic cardiac activity.	30 to 150 bpm (options faster than 150 bpm available in some pulse generators)
Ventricular refractory period	An interval of the pacemaker timing cycle following a sensed or paced ventricular event during which the ventricular sensing channel is totally or partially unresponsive to incoming signals.	150 to 500 msec
Pulse width	Duration, in milliseconds, over which the output is delivered.	0.05 to 1.9 msec
Pulse amplitude	Magnitude of the voltage level reached during a pacemaker output pulse, usually expressed in volts.	0.5 to 8.1 V
Sensitivity	Ability to sense an intrinsic electrical signal, which depends on the amplitude, slew rate, and frequency of the signal.	Atrial: 0.18 to 8 mV Ventricular: 1.0 to 14 mV
Polarity	Stimulating electrode typically is the cathode, which has negative polarity relative to the indifferent electrode (anode).	Device may be programmable to only bipolar or unipolar; others may have more control by programming unipolar-bipolar pace-sense on either lead
Hysteresis	Extension of the escape interval after a sensed intrinsic event.	In single-chamber modes, commonly 40, 50, or 60 bpm or off
Circadian lower rate limit	Reduces the lower rate limit during sleeping hours.	Lower rates during sleep, programmable from 30 bpm as the slowest rate usually offered
Mode switch	Capability of a dual-chamber pacemaker to automatically switch from an atrial tracking (P-synchronous) mode to a non-atrial-tracking mode when an atrial rhythm occurs that the pacemaker determines to be pathologic. When the atrial rhythm meets the criteria for a physiologic rhythm, the mode switches back to an atrial-tracking mode.	On or off; if on, the detection rates are often programmable for rates 120 to 190 bpm
Fallback	An upper rate response in which the ventricular paced rate decelerates to, and is maintained at, a programmable fallback rate that is lower than the original programmed MTR. Fallback mechanisms vary among pacemakers.	May be programmable on or off; if on, the rate to which the fallback occurs may be fixed or programmable, i.e., 50 to 80 bpm

continues

Table 7–2. (*Continued*)
Programmable Options for Pacemakers

Parameter	Description	Typical variables
Rate smoothing	Prevents atrial or ventricular paced rate from changing by more than a programmed percentage from one cardiac cycle to the next. This prevents large cycle-to-cycle intervals that can be seen at the upper rate limit or during rapid acceleration of atrial rate.	On or off; may then have options of % smoothing, i.e., 9% to 25% change per cycle length allowed; may also have option of being on or off for rate increments or decrements, or both
Atrioventricular interval (AVI)	Period between the initiation of the paced or sensed atrial event and the delivery of a consecutive ventricular output pulse.	30 to 350 msec
Differential AVI	Feature that permits a longer AVI after a paced atrial event than after a sensed AVI. In some pacemakers, this differential is fixed; in others, it is programmable.	Offset from 0 to 200 msec
Rate-adaptive AVI	Shortens the AVI as the heart rate increases.	On or off only in some devices; in others, able to set the minimum AV delay to as short as 30 msec
Postventricular atrial refractory period (PVARP)	Period after a paced or sensed ventricular event during which the atrial channel is refractory.	150 to 500 msec; in some devices, auto-PVARP adjusts with cycle length
PVARP extension	Lengthening of the PVARP after a sensed premature ventricular contraction to prevent sensing of a retrograde P wave.	On or off in some; others may program length of extension to as long as ~ 500 msec
PMT algorithms	Manufacturer-specific algorithms to terminate pacemaker-mediated tachycardia (PMT)	On or off; in others, can choose how long the MTR must persist before detection criteria are met
Blanking period	Temporary disabling of pacemaker-sensing amplifiers after an output pulse.	Ventricular blanking: 20 to 50 msec Postventricular atrial blanking: 100 to 350 msec
Ventricular safety pacing	Delivery of a ventricular output pulse after atrial pacing if a signal is sensed by the ventricular channel during the crosstalk sensing portion of the AVI.	On or off
Maximum tracking rate (MTR)	The sum of the AVI and the PVARP.	80 to 180 bpm

offer rate adaptation in the asynchronous mode.)

(Reference is sometimes made to the SSI, SSIR, SST, or SOO mode. Manufacturers use "S" in both the first and the second positions of the pacemaker code to indicate that the device is capable of pacing a single cardiac chamber. Once the device is implanted and connected to a lead in either the atrium or the ventricle, "S" should be changed to either "A" or "V" in the clinical record to reflect the

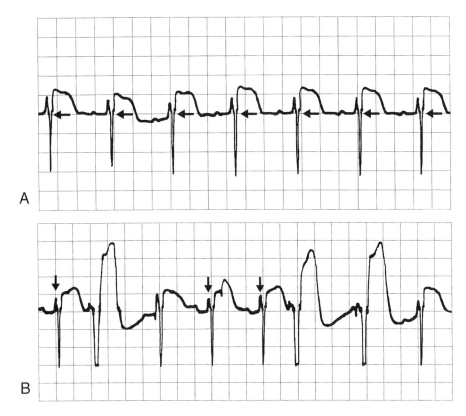

Fig. 7–1. Determination of ventricular sensing thresholds in the VVT mode. *A*, The pacemaker has been programmed to VVT, rate of 75 bpm, ventricular sensitivity of 5 mV. A pacemaker artifact (*arrows*) can be seen in each intrinsic QRS complex at the intrinsic ventricular rate of approximately 90 bpm. The triggered artifact within the intrinsic event indicates that the QRS is being sensed appropriately. *B*, Ventricular sensitivity has been programmed to 14 mV. *Arrows* indicate intrinsic ventricular events that are not sensed. The first intrinsic event is not sensed because it is followed by a paced event approximately 440 msec later. The event at the *second arrow* is not sensed, and a pacing artifact is delivered in the T wave of the event, but there is failure to capture because the ventricle is refractory. The next event (*third arrow*) is not sensed and is followed by a paced event approximately 360 msec later.

chamber in which pacing and sensing are occurring.)

In dual-chamber pacemakers, multiple single- and dual-chamber modes are usually available. Dual-chamber rate-adaptive pacemakers have many programmable modes, often including DDD, DDDR, DOO, DOOR, DDI, DDIR, DVI, DVIR, VDD, VDDR, VVI, VVIR, VVT, VOO, VOOR, AAI, AAIR, AAT, AOOR, and OOO (Table 7–3).

Rate Programmability

Rate programmability is the most frequently used programmable feature and is almost always used in routine pacemaker programming. During programming for pacemaker follow-up, if the patient's intrinsic rate is greater than the programmed rate, the pacing rate is increased to assess the threshold of stimulation. If pacing is at the programmed

Table 7–3.
Programmable Pacing Modes

VOO	Ventricular pacing; no sensing	DOO	Dual-chamber pacing; no sensing
VVI	Ventricular pacing; ventricular sensing and inhibition	DVI	Dual-chamber pacing; ventricular sensing and inhibition; no tracking of the atrium
VVT	Ventricular pacing; ventricular sensing and triggering	DVIR	Dual-chamber pacing; ventricular sensing and inhibition; no tracking of the atrium; AV sequential rate modulation
VVIR	Ventricular pacing; ventricular sensing with inhibition; rate-modulated pacing	DDI	Dual-chamber pacing; dual-chamber sensing and inhibition; no tracking of the atrium
VOOR	Ventricular pacing; no sensing; rate-modulated pacing	DDIR	Dual-chamber pacing; dual-chamber sensing and inhibition; no tracking of the atrium; AV sequential rate modulation
AOO	Atrial pacing; no sensing	VDD	Ventricular pacing; dual-chamber sensing; tracking of atrium with ventricular inhibition
AAI	Atrial pacing; atrial sensing and inhibition	VDDR*	Ventricular pacing; dual-chamber sensing; tracking of atrium with ventricular inhibition and ventricular rate modulation
AAT	Atrial pacing; atrial sensing and triggering	DDD	Dual-chamber pacing; dual-chamber sensing and inhibition; tracking of the atrium
AAIR	Atrial pacing; atrial sensing with inhibition; rate-modulated pacing	DDDR	Dual-chamber pacing; dual-chamber sensing and inhibition; tracking of the atrium; AV sequential rate modulation
AOOR	Atrial pacing; no sensing; rate modulation	DOOR	Dual-chamber pacing; insensitive; AV sequential rate modulation
		OOO	Pacemaker is programmed "off" (allows assessment of underlying rhythm)

AV, atrioventricular.
*VDDR is a misnomer by the North American Society of Pacing and Electrophysiology/British Pacing and Electrophysiology Group code for pacing modes. The "R" in this context would generally indicate the capability of dual-chamber, sensor-driven pacing. However, VDD by definition excludes atrial pacing. The designation VDDR is being used by manufacturers for a device that operates in a P-synchronous mode except when sensor-driven, when pacing may be VVIR or DDDR, depending on the specific device.

lower rate, the rate should be decreased to determine the status of the patient's underlying conduction (Fig. 7–2). It is necessary to know this before checking stimulation threshold; for example, if the patient is pacemaker-dependent and has no reliable ventricular escape rhythm, loss of capture during threshold determination could have severe clinical consequences.

The nominal rate of single-chamber pacemakers is frequently 60 bpm. Pro-gramming to a slower rate may be helpful in an attempt to allow a patient with rare episodes of bradycardia to remain in sinus rhythm rather than in paced rhythm. Programming a rate of 50 bpm or even one as low as 40 bpm may allow the patient's intrinsic rhythm to exist much of the time, with pacing only in the event of a more profound sinus bradycardia or asystole. Hysteresis (see below) may allow an even greater pro-

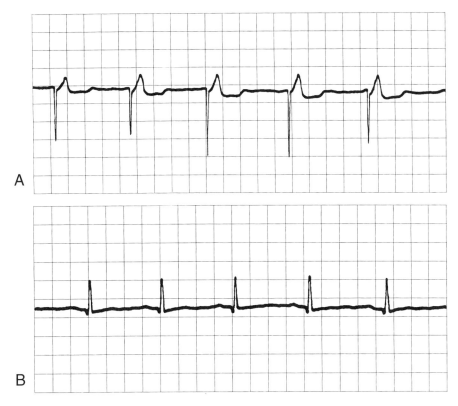

Fig. 7–2. Reprogramming the pacemaker from DDD mode (*A*), lower rate of 60 bpm, upper rate of 125 bpm, to VVI mode (*B*), rate of 60 bpm, allows the patient's intrinsic rhythm to predominate. The status of the underlying ventricular escape rhythm should be determined before determination of stimulation thresholds.

portion of time in intrinsic rhythm (Fig. 7–3).

More rapid pacing rates, that is, greater than 70 bpm, are used most commonly in pediatric patients and are sometimes useful when faster pacing rates may be necessary to enhance cardiac output, for example, postoperatively. In an occasional patient, a faster rate may be used to suppress an atrial or ventricular arrhythmia.

In dual-chamber devices capable of atrial tracking or rate adaptation, both lower and upper rates must be programmed. The programmed lower rate determines the lowest ventricular rate allowed. The lower rate is usually programmed in the range of 50 to 70 bpm, depending on the individual patient and other factors already discussed for determining the lower rate for single-chamber pacemakers.

The upper rate defines the fastest paced ventricular rate allowed. Determining the appropriate upper rate depends on the patient's exercise requirements and associated cardiac and other medical problems. The total atrial refractory period, which is the postventricular atrial refractory period plus the atrioventricular (AV) interval, effectively determines the maximum achievable tracking rate (see Chapter 6).

In dual-chamber rate-adaptive pacemakers, the upper rate limit may be a single programmable value, or independent programming of the maximum tracking rate and maximum sensor-driven rate may be required (see Chapter 6).

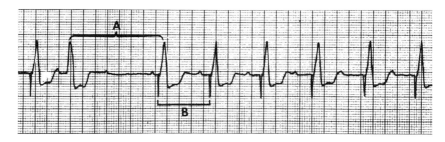

Fig. 7–3. Hysteresis in a VVI pacemaker programmed to a lower rate of 70 bpm (B), and hysteresis at 40 bpm (A). (From Hayes DL: Pacemaker electrocardiography. *In* A Practice of Cardiac Pacing. Edited by S Furman, DL Hayes, DR Holmes Jr. Mount Kisco, NY, Futura Publishing Company, 1986, pp 305–331. By permission of the publisher.)

An option for "circadian response," or "sleep rate," is available in many contemporary pacemakers[2] (Fig. 7–4). This feature allows a lower rate to be programmed for the approximate time during which the patient is sleeping. A separate, potentially faster lower rate limit may then be programmed for waking hours. (For example, the lower rate limit may be programmed to 70 bpm during waking hours and 50 bpm during sleeping hours.) In some pacemakers, this feature is tied to a "clock," and the usual waking and sleeping hours are programmed into the pacemaker. In other pacemakers, the sleep rate is also set on the basis of waking and sleeping hours, but verification by a sensor is required to allow rate changes to occur.

Hysteresis Programming

Programming of hysteresis permits prolongation of the first pacemaker escape interval after a sensed event. A pacemaker programmed at a cycle length of 1,000 msec (60 bpm) and a hysteresis of 1,200 msec (50 bpm) allows 200 msec more for another sensed QRS complex. Should another QRS complex not be recognized, the pacemaker stimulates continuously at the programmed rate of 60 bpm, an escape interval of 1,000 msec (Fig. 7–4), until a sensed event restarts the cycle. The advantage of hysteresis in a single-chamber pacing mode is the ability to maintain spontaneous AV synchrony as long as possible.[3] This may prevent symptomatic retrograde ventriculoatrial (VA) conduction. In patients with VVI pacing and pacemaker syndrome, hysteresis increases the potential for maintaining the patient's intrinsic rhythm.

Several types of hysteresis may be a programmable option in some dual-chamber pacemakers. Dual-chamber pacing with search hysteresis has been advocated for patients with carotid sinus hypersensitivity who require pacing for cardioinhibition but who also have a significant vasodepressor component. In conventional hysteresis, as described above, once pacing begins, it continues until a spontaneous event such as a premature ventricular beat or sinus rhythm inhibits the pacing sequence. In search hysteresis, after a specific number of timing cycles at the more rapid rate (the number of cycles may be fixed or programmable), the prolonged escape interval is permitted to allow a slower intrinsic rate to appear, that is, a rate greater than the programmed lower rate limit. If intrinsic rhythm at a rate exceeding the programmed lower rate is not present, stimulation resumes at the more rapid rate for a given number of cycles (Fig. 7–5).

Rate Drop Response (RDR) is a proprietary refinement of search hysteresis.[4] With this feature, if a significant decrease

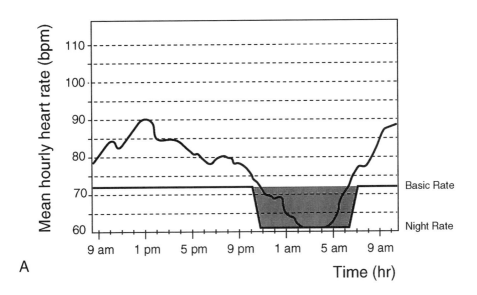

A

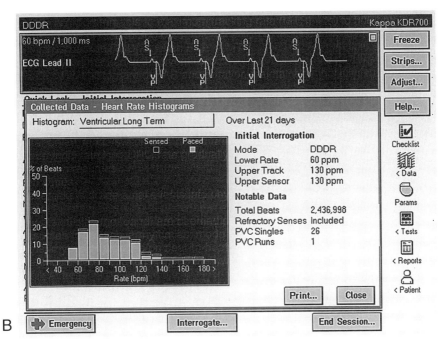

B

Fig. 7–4. *A,* Printout of telemetered data of patient's mean hourly heart rate. The pacemaker is programmed to a lower, or basic, rate of 72 bpm and to a sleep rate, or night rate, of approximately 60 bpm. The graph demonstrates the slower rates allowed during night hours, in this example from 10 P.M. to 7 A.M. *B,* Heart rate histogram from a patient with a DDDR pacemaker programmed to a lower rate of 60 bpm and an upper rate of 130 bpm. However, the histogram is compatible with approximately 7% of the rates being less than 60 bpm. This can be explained by a sleep rate programmed to 50 bpm.

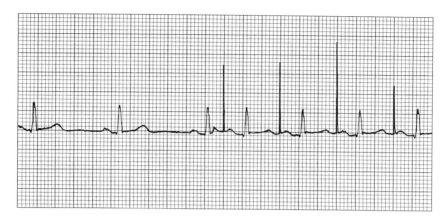

Fig. 7–5. Onset of pacing in a DDDR pacemaker programmed to a lower rate of 100 bpm, hysteresis at 65 bpm. After 256 cycles of pacing at 100 bpm, pacing is suspended for the pacemaker to "search" for the intrinsic lower rate. If the lower rate is greater than the hysteresis rate, pacing is inhibited until the rate again falls below the hysteresis rate.

in heart rate occurs, the pacemaker intervenes with pacing at an increased rate in both chambers for a specific, programmed duration (Fig. 7–6). At the conclusion of the programmed duration of more rapid pacing, the pacing rate gradually returns to the programmed lower rate. Two programmable detection algorithms are available in the most recent RDR. The first algorithm available was "drop detect," in which the pacemaker monitors a drop in heart rate that must meet two programmable requirements to trigger an intervention. It must satisfy the programmable degree of rate decrease, the number of beats the rate must fall, and the "detection window," which is the amount of time monitored for a rate drop (this is a programmable interval) (Fig. 7–7). The "nominal" values for RDR are not successful for

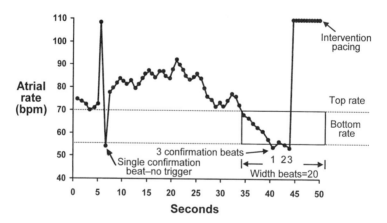

Fig. 7–6. Diagrammatic representation of Rate Drop Response. This algorithm requires that "top" and "bottom" rates be defined for rate drop detection, a specific number of beats, width over which the rate may drop, and the pacing rate that will result if criteria are met, that is, the intervention rate. Three confirmation beats below the bottom rate must occur before therapy is triggered. In the early portion of this diagram, a single beat falls below the bottom rate but fails to trigger intervention because confirmation is not met.

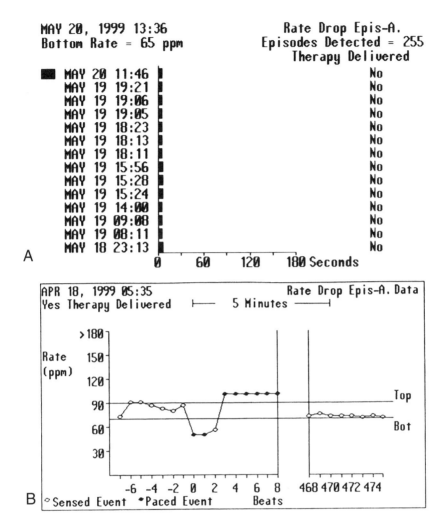

Fig. 7–7. *A,* The Rate Drop Response (RDR) counters indicate that the pacemaker had documented multiple episodes of sudden rate drop. However, "therapy," that is, a response to the sudden drop in rate with an increase in pacing rate for a programmed period, had not been initiated. *B,* With a pacemaker in place and RDR that had been programmed "on" but not initiated because of the programmed parameters, adjusting the RDR parameters would be reasonable. For this patient, the RDR criteria were programmed more sensitively. When the patient returned, the rate counter was again full, with 255 episodes detected and therapy delivered on two occasions. The second printout details the event on April 18 at 05:35 when therapy was delivered. The diagram documents a sudden drop in rate; RDR was met and therapy delivered.

everyone.[4,5] Table 7–4 includes programming considerations for RDR, taking into account the version of RDR available and whether pacing is for carotid sinus syndrome or vasovagal syncope.

In the "low rate detect" algorithm, therapy is triggered when pacing occurs at the programmed lower rate for the programmable consecutive number of "detection beats." This detection method can be used as a backup to the "drop detect" method if the sudden drop in rate varies between slow and fast[6] (Fig. 7–8).

Table 7–4.
Programming Considerations for Rate Drop Response (RDR)

Parameters	Thera-i DR		Kappa 400 & 700	
	CSS	VVS	CSS	VVS
Top rate, bpm	60	70		
Bottom rate, bpm	50	55		
Width beats	10–30	30–50		
Confirmation beats	2	2		
Drop detect			On	On
Low rate detect			On	On
Drop rate			50	60
Drop size			30	25
Detection window (Kappa 700 only)			30 sec	1 min
Detection beats			2	2
Lower rate			45	45
Intervention rate	40	50	45	45
Intervention duration	1	2	1	2

CSS, carotid sinus syndrome; VVS, vasovagal syncope.

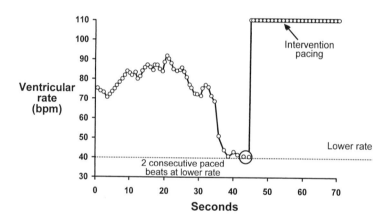

Fig. 7–8. Medtronic "Low Rate Detect." When pacing occurs at the programmed lower rate for the programmable consecutive number of detection beats, therapy is triggered. Low Rate Detect may be used as a backup to the Drop Detect Method if the sudden drop in rate varies between slow and fast.

Programming Output (Pulse Width and Voltage Amplitude)

Programming the energy output of the pacemaker is one of the most important programmable features and remains one of the most controversial. Programming output can be used to extend pulse generator life by reducing output or to solve the clinical problem of increased or increasing stimulation thresholds. Contemporary pulse generators provide significant flexibility in pulse width and voltage amplitude. Voltage amplitude is typically programmable from 0.5 to 7.5 V and pulse width from 0.05 to 1.9 msec.

With good implantation technique and low-threshold lead designs, for example, steroid elution, it is most common to program the voltage output to 2.5 V (the nominal voltage for many pacemakers). By programming the output at an efficient but safe level, the projected battery life can be increased significantly (Table 7–5). A decrease in energy output can also be used to eliminate extracardiac (diaphragmatic or pectoral muscle) stimulation.

Conversely, in some patients, thresholds may increase after implantation. Although a transient and mild increase in thresholds is not uncommon in the first 4 to 6 weeks after implantation, higher outputs can be programmed until thresholds return to a stable level. (This threshold evolution can largely be avoided with steroid-eluting leads.) These high thresholds may be transient or permanent (Fig. 7–9). Output programmability is useful in transient and permanent situations. In patients with a transient elevation, higher outputs can be used until thresholds return to a stable chronic level. In patients with chronically high thresholds, the pulse generator can be programmed to higher output to permit reliable pacing (albeit with reduced pulse generator longevity) (See Chapter 9).

The output function to be programmed for the most effective control of a rising threshold depends on the actual threshold.[7] Both pulse duration and output voltage (amplitude) are programmable in most pacemakers. Programming the

pulse duration to greater than 1.0 msec approaches rheobase—the lowest voltage threshold at an infinitely long pulse duration—does not provide much additional pacing margin of safety, and results in high current and energy drain.[8] If pulse duration programmability defines a threshold lasting more than 1.0 msec, increasing the output voltage is a better option.

Experts disagree about the optimal method to program the safety margin once the stimulation threshold has been established. Options include

- Double the voltage amplitude
- Triple the pulse width
- Determine the energy in microjoules required at threshold and program the voltage amplitude and pulse width to achieve three times the threshold in microjoules

In an effort to simplify programming and to be certain that an adequate safety margin is provided, some pacemakers plot the autothreshold values in a strength-duration curve and suggest values for optimal output programming (Fig. 7–10).

If the threshold is high, the rheobase may be above a specific voltage setting no matter how long the programmed pulse duration. If pulse duration threshold is high, output voltage is more useful. Conversely, if pulse duration threshold is

Table 7–5.
Output Variables for Calculations of Theoretical Battery Longevity

	Projected pacemaker longevity, mo								
	143	102	67	138	87	52	147	113	80
Ventricular output, V	1.0	2.5	4.0	1.0	2.5	4.0	1.0	2.5	4.0
Atrial output, V	1.0	2.5	4.0	1.0	2.5	4.0	1.0	2.5	4.0
Ventricular pulse width, msec	0.4	0.4	0.4	0.6	0.6	0.6	0.4	0.4	0.4
Atrial pulse width, msec	0.4	0.4	0.4	0.6	0.6	0.6	0.4	0.4	0.4
Ventricular lead impedance, Ω	500	500	500	500	500	500	700	700	700
Atrial lead impedance, Ω	500	500	500	500	500	500	700	700	700

Calculations assume 100% ventricular pacing, 60% atrial pacing, and rate of 60 bpm.

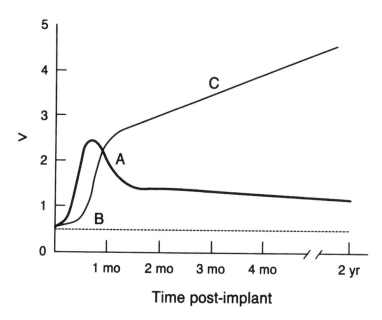

Fig. 7–9. At implantation, patients A, B, and C have similar thresholds of approximately 0.75 V at 0.5-msec pulse duration. Stimulation threshold evolutions for the three patients differ significantly. Threshold in patient A peaked at approximately 2.5 V at 2 to 3 weeks after implantation, with the chronic threshold approximately twice the acute threshold. Patient B, with a steroid (dexamethasone)-eluting lead, has a lower acute threshold of stimulation, and during follow-up, no significant increase in threshold occurs. Patient C has the least common threshold evolution seen. Initial thresholds are similar to those of patients A and B, but the threshold gradually continues to climb. This response may occur with "exit block." (Modified from Hayes DL: Programmability. *In* A Practice of Cardiac Pacing. Third edition. Edited by S Furman, DL Hayes, DR Holmes Jr. Mount Kisco, NY, Futura Publishing Company, 1993, pp 635–663. By permission of Mayo Foundation.)

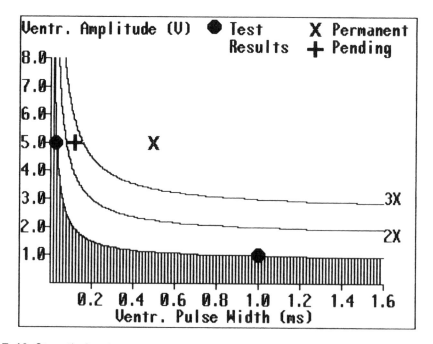

Fig. 7–10. Strength-duration curve generated by the pacemaker programmer. The (x) notes suggested output programming to achieve an optimal and efficient safety margin.

very low, that is, in the range of 0.05 to 0.1 msec at a given output voltage, reducing the voltage and modestly prolonging the pulse duration could be considered. It is possible to program output on the basis of delivered energy at threshold. Output programmability should not, at any time, be a substitute for proper lead placement.

Determination of the stimulation threshold should be a part of routine pacemaker follow-up. Determining stimulation threshold is now fairly easy with autothreshold measurements that are optional in many pacemakers and defibrillators. This is often accomplished by programming the output values—voltage amplitude and pulse width—at which the threshold determination is to begin and then observing the electrocardiogram during decrement of the output variables until capture is lost. The programmer for the specific device should provide clear directions on how to respond when capture is lost, for instance, move the programming head or release pressure from the programming screen (Fig. 7–11).

Thresholds can still be determined by manually reprogramming the output variables until the threshold is determined. In the non-pacemaker-dependent patient, our preferred method of manual ventricular threshold determination is as follows: the pacemaker is programmed to the VVI mode and the rate decreased until the patient's intrinsic rhythm is observed. In devices capable of "batch" programming—more than one programmable variable changed at one time—the pacing is increased to a rate exceeding the intrinsic ventricular rate simultaneously with a decrease in the voltage amplitude and pulse width. For example, with the pacemaker programmed to VVI at 40 bpm, if the intrinsic rate is 70, the next programming step could include VVI at 80 bpm, voltage amplitude of 1.0 V, and pulse width of 0.12 msec. If pacing is reestablished, the stimulation threshold is less than or equal to 1.0

V, 0.12 msec. In some pacemakers, even lower values are possible, but anything less than this provides little, if any, additional clinical information. If capture is not reestablished at 1.0 V and 0.12 msec, one of these two variables can be increased until stimulation occurs. Stimulation threshold should be considered the output settings at which capture is reestablished (Fig. 7–12). Whether one increases pulse width or voltage amplitude for determination of stimulation threshold is in large part personal bias, although some experts make a strong case for doing one or the other.

Other methods to provide some sense of stimulation threshold have also been used for many years. One manufacturer incorporates a Threshold Margin Test with magnet application.[9] With this technique, magnet application results in a rate of 100 bpm for three beats followed by asynchronous pacing at the programmed rate. The first and second pacing artifacts at a rate of 100 bpm are of normal, that is, programmed, pulse duration. The third pacing artifact at a rate of 100 bpm is at 75% of the programmed pulse duration. Loss of capture on the third beat indicates a narrow pacing margin of safety (Fig. 7–13). Another approach is a proprietary feature called "Vario."[10] This is a programmable option in multiprogrammable pacemakers from several manufacturers. In the Vario mode, magnet application results in 16 asynchronous beats at a magnet rate of 100 bpm followed by 16 asynchronous beats at a rate of 125 bpm. During the 16 beats at 125 bpm, the voltage output is reduced by 1/15 progressively until zero output is reached (Fig. 7–14). Removal of the magnet returns full output at the next stimulus. The Vario mode can be activated for the test procedure only or programmed "on" permanently.

If during the course of programming in a pacemaker-dependent patient the pacemaker is programmed to subthreshold output parameters, ventricular

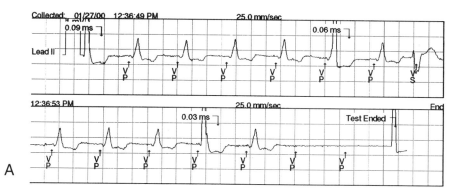

A

Date of implantation = 01/12/2000
Battery resistance   = 916 Ohms
Magnet rate   = 96.00 ppm
Beg. of life = 96 ppm -- E.R.I. = 80 ppm

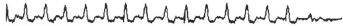

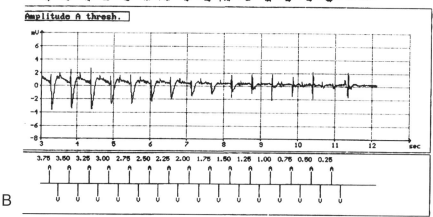

B

U. THRESHOLD UUI

Basic Rate   100   ppm
AVD Pace   -----   ms

                        Atr.   Ven.
Pulse Ampl   -----   3.6   V
Pulse Width   -----   0.40   ms
Polar Pace   -----   BIPL
Threshold   0.7   **U**

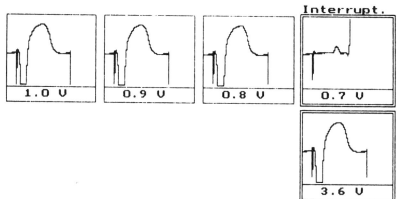

C

Fig. 7–11. Printouts from three different pacemaker programmers displaying autothreshold testing. *A,* Ventricular pulse width threshold; that is, voltage is held constant and pulse width is decreased in decrements. Capture is lost at 0.03 msec. *B,* Atrial voltage threshold with loss of capture at 2.5 V. *C,* Ventricular autothreshold in which voltage is decrementally decreased and capture is lost at 0.7 V.

asystole will occur. Every pacemaker is equipped with an emergency or "stat set" button that restores nominal pacing parameters if activated. However, there may be a delay between activation of the stat set parameters and actual restoration of nominal pacing parameters.[11] It is important that the health care professional performing the threshold determination be familiar with the specific programmer and the steps necessary to activate stat set or emergency back-up parameters.

Research to develop a pacemaker algorithm that would automatically adjust energy output began in 1973.[12] Such a feature would allow the pacemaker to adjust energy output to threshold alterations. This capability could conserve battery consumption and prolong device longevity as well as protect patients from increasing stimulation thresholds.

Automatic output adjustment and management is available in some pacemakers. The proprietary AutoCapture system confirms capture on a beat-by-beat basis by monitoring the "evoked response" (ER) associated with the ventricular pacing output.[7] To detect the ER signal, a bipolar low polarization pacing lead must be used. Each paced ventricular beat is assessed for capture by the system through monitoring of the ER signal. When no ER signal is detected, the AutoCapture system delivers a 4.5 backup safety pulse. This backup safety pulse functions as the "safety margin." After a 14-msec blanking period that follows the ventricular output, there is an ER detection window of 46 msec, for a total window of 60 msec before delivery of the backup safety pulse, if necessary. With two consecutive loss-of-capture events fol-

lowed by backup safety pulses, the AutoCapture system automatically increases the output of the primary pacing pulse until capture is regained from the primary pacing pulse (Fig. 7–15). At the beginning of this increment, the first paced event is increased by 0.25 V. If capture is not confirmed with this paced event, the pulse amplitude continues to increase in 0.125-V steps until capture is verified from the primary pacing pulse for two consecutive paced events. Once verification occurs, the pacemaker automatically initiates a threshold search. If capture for two consecutive events is not confirmed by the time the pacemaker output reaches 3.875 V, the pacemaker automatically reprograms to 4.5 V and 0.5 msec pulse width, or "high output mode" pacing.

A threshold search is initiated whenever the programmer head is placed over the pacemaker and then removed and, as noted above, when two consecutive loss-of-capture events result in an increase in the ventricular amplitude. When a threshold search begins, the pacemaker automatically decreases the pulse amplitude in 0.25-V steps until two consecutive loss-of-capture events occur, at which point the primary pacing pulse amplitude is increased by 0.125-V steps until two consecutive capture events are confirmed.

Another manufacturer uses Capture Management to provide monitoring of ventricular pacing thresholds and automatic adjustment of amplitude and pulse width to maintain capture.[13] This feature can be programmed to "monitor only" or "adaptive." In the monitor only mode, the pacemaker periodically delivers a pacing artifact and monitors the paces by changing first amplitude and then pulse width

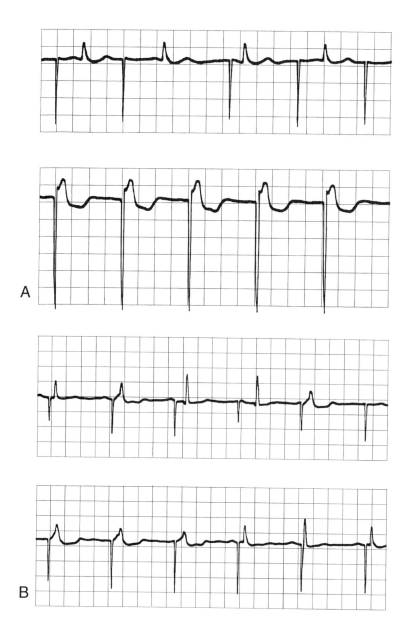

Fig. 7–12. Determination of ventricular stimulation threshold during routine pacemaker follow-up. *A,* The pacemaker is programmed VVI, rate of 75 ppm, voltage amplitude of 2.5 V, and pulse duration (PW) of 0.05 msec (*upper tracing*) and 0.1 msec (*lower tracing*). Capture is consistently lost at 0.05 msec but restored at 0.1 msec. The stimulation threshold is 2.5 V, 0.1 msec. *B,* In the *upper tracing,* the pacemaker is programmed VVI at 70 ppm, 2.5 V, and 0.1 msec pulse width. There is intermittent failure to capture. In the *lower tracing,* the pulse width has been increased to 0.3 and there is consistent failure to capture. However, one should not be confused by the variation in QRS morphology. The fourth and sixth beats represent fusion beats, and the fifth beat is a pseudofusion beat. *Continues.*

DVI
Atrial, 0.15 ms/2.7 V

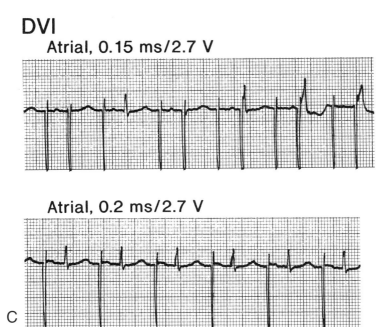

Atrial, 0.2 ms/2.7 V

C

Fig. 7–12 *continued. C,* Manual atrial threshold determination with the pacemaker programmed to the DVI pacing mode. In the *upper tracing,* the pacemaker is programmed to 80 ppm, 2.7 V, and 0.15 msec pulse width. There is complete failure to capture the atrium. In the *lower tracing,* the pulse width has been increased to 0.2 msec. There is consistent atrial capture, which can be determined not only by a consistent and uniform atrial depolarization but also by consistent intrinsic ventricular depolarization. (*A,* Modified from Hayes DL: Programmability. *In* A Practice of Cardiac Pacing. Third edition. Edited by S Furman, DL Hayes, DR Holmes Jr. Mount Kisco, NY, Futura Publishing Company, 1993, pp 635–663. By permission of Mayo Foundation.)

to find two points on the strength duration curve that define the boundary between settings that capture and those that do not. The frequency with which the search is done is programmable (Fig. 7–16). When programmed to "adaptive," the pacemaker responds to monitoring by adapting ventricular amplitude and pulse width through use of several programmable parameters (Fig. 7–17). An "amplitude margin and pulse width margin" refers to the programmable selected safety margin desired; the "minimum adapted amplitude and minimum adapted pulse width" defines the lower limit to which the voltage amplitude and pulse width can be set during adaptation; and the "acute phase days remaining" sets an initial interval during which the output settings are not de-

creased. (The final parameter is used during the lead maturation period.)

Because output adjustment is critical for both extremes, that is, for maintaining an adequate safety margin and for prolonging battery longevity, automatic regulation of output will certainly become a standard feature of future pacemakers.

Sensitivity Programmability

All pulse generators sense and filter the intracardiac electrogram delivered through the electrodes. For atrial and ventricular sensing (one or both), the R and P waves must be of significant amplitude (millivolts) and slew rate (dV/dt) for proper sensing to occur. The sensitiv-

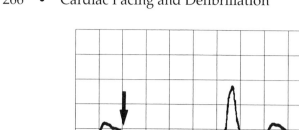

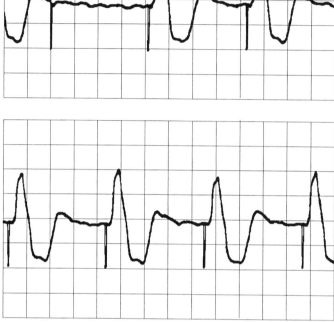

Fig. 7–13. Electrocardiographic tracings from a patient with a VVI Medtronic pacemaker programmed to a rate of 70 bpm and 5.0 V. The pacemaker is capable of a Threshold Margin Test (TMT) during magnet application. In the *upper panel,* the pulse duration is 0.5 msec. There is failure to capture with the first pacing artifact seen (*arrow*). This pacing artifact is the third of three asynchronous pulses at 100 bpm that occur with magnet application. As part of the Threshold Margin Test, the pulse duration of this pacemaker stimulus is 75% of the programmed pulse duration of 0.5 msec. A suprathreshold stimulus is at 0.5 msec, but at 75% of this output duration (equivalent to a pulse duration of 0.375 msec), failure to capture occurs. In the *lower panel,* the programmed pulse duration is 0.7 msec. The first pacing artifact is again the third of the three asynchronous pulses and is therefore at 75% of the programmed duration, or 0.525 msec, and capture is maintained. (Modified from Hayes DL: Programmability. *In* A Practice of Cardiac Pacing. Edited by S Furman, DL Hayes, DR Holmes Jr. Mount Kisco, NY, Futura Publishing Company, 1986, pp 219–251. By permission of the publisher.)

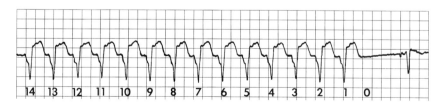

Fig. 7–14. "Vario" test of a pacemaker programmed to 5.0 V. Capture is maintained at 0.3 V, indicated here by "1," and appropriately there is no capture when output is 0 V.

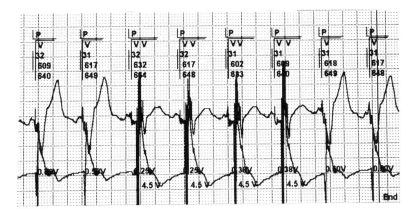

Fig. 7–15. AutoCapture demonstrating loss of capture at 0.25 and 0.38 V. Each failure to capture is followed by a second output pulse at a higher output, with successful capture. The output is subsequently increased to 0.5 V, and two consecutive successful captures occur.

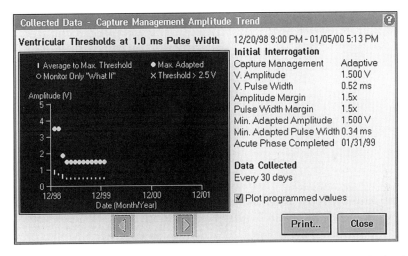

Fig. 7–16. Capture management amplitude trend demonstrating a stable ventricular threshold of approximately 0.5 V. The pacemaker output is maintained at 1.5 V and 0.52 msec.

ity of the pulse generator is the R (or P) wave of the lowest amplitude that the pacemaker recognizes as a ventricular (or atrial) depolarization. The pacemaker definition of whether it is an R or a P wave depends on the channel through which it is sensed. Events sensed through the atrial channel are defined as P waves, those through the ventricular channel as R waves. Nominal ventricular sensitivity is usually in the range of 1.2 to 2.5 mV, and nominal atrial sensitivity is usually in the range of 0.5 to

1.2 mV. Although the amplitude of the intracardiac R or P waves may be adequate at the time of implantation, it may change for a variety of reasons, including metabolic and drug effects and lead dislodgment. Each focus of intrinsic activity, be it atrial or ventricular, is not equally sensed, and some foci (conducted or ectopic) may not reach an adequate level of amplitude or slew rate to be sensed. Some extrasystoles may be sensed, whereas conducted beats may not be sensed, and vice versa.

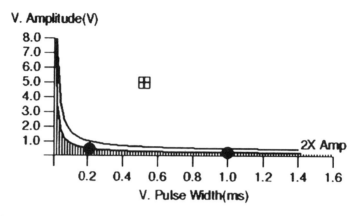

Clinical Status: 01/10/00 to 01/11/00

V. Capture Management - from 01/11/00 12:26 AM

Calculated Threshold: 0.375 V at 0.52 ms

● Threshold   ⊞ Adapted

V. Amplitude(V)

2X Amp

V. Pulse Width(ms)

Fig. 7–17. Telemetered data of ventricular capture management. The calculated threshold was 0.375 V at 0.52 msec. The adapted threshold was approximately 5.0 V and 0.5 msec. The adapted threshold depends in part on the programmed settings that define the safety margin desired.

Sensitivity programming can be accomplished by an increase in the sensitivity of the amplifier, that is, by decreasing the amplitude of the signal required to trigger the sensing circuit but maintaining the same frequency spectrum. (The terminology is confusing because the amplifier is made more sensitive as the number decreases, that is, 1.25 mV is more sensitive than 2.5 mV.)

The sensing threshold can be determined during routine pacemaker follow-up by programming the pacemaker to less sensitive values until there is failure to sense (Fig. 7–18). (Sensing thresholds could also be determined by altering sensing values during programming to a triggered pacing mode, that is, AAT or VVT [Fig. 7–1].)

Increased sensitivity is especially useful in atrial pacing, because the electrograms are usually far smaller than those obtained during ventricular pacing.

Decreasing sensitivity is useful in eliminating oversensing of nonphysiologic signals that result from electromagnetic interference or of such physiologic signals as pectoral muscle artifacts (Fig. 7–19).

Automatic sensitivity adjustment is available in a limited number of pacemakers. Autosensing adjusts sensitivity on the basis of amplitude of the intrinsic waveform. In one of the first pacemakers with an autosensing feature, the autosensing feature ensures a 2:1 margin for sensing intracardiac activity.[14] The purpose of automatic sensitivity is to prevent or minimize episodes of both oversensing and undersensing. Although not as critical clinically as automatic output management, automatic sensing has potential merit.

Polarity Programmability

Polarity programmability is available on most pacemakers with bipolar

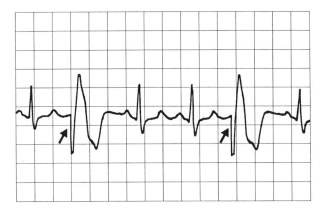

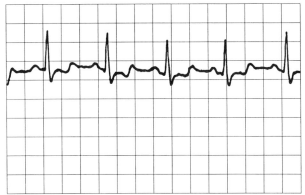

Fig. 7–18. Determination of sensing threshold in a VVI pacemaker programmed to a rate of 60 bpm. In the *upper panel,* the sensitivity is programmed to 2.5 mV, and there is failure to sense (*arrows*). In the *lower panel,* the sensitivity has been reprogrammed to 1.25 mV, and there is normal sensing. (Modified from Hayes DL: Programmability. *In* A Practice of Cardiac Pacing. Edited by S Furman, DL Hayes, DR Holmes Jr. Mount Kisco, NY, Futura Publishing Company, 1986, pp 219–251. By permission of the publisher.)

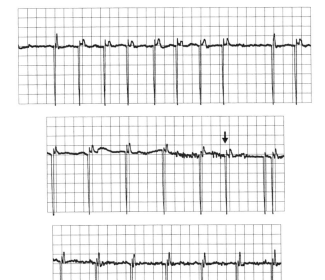

Fig. 7–19. In P-synchronous pacemakers, VDD or DDD, oversensing of myopotentials on the atrial lead may result in inappropriately fast rates because of ventricular tracking of the false signals. In this example from a patient with a unipolar DDD pacemaker, isometrics were performed at various atrial sensitivity values to determine the potential for tracking of myopotential interference. *Top panel,* Atrial sensitivity is most sensitive at 0.4 mV, and there is irregular rapid ventricular pacing as myopotentials are tracked. *Middle panel,* Atrial sensitivity at 1.2 mV results in less myopotential interference, but it is not completely eliminated (*arrow*). *Bottom panel,* At an atrial sensitivity of 2.0 mV, there is no myopotential interference. (Modified from Hayes DL: Programmability. *In* A Practice of Cardiac Pacing. Edited by S Furman, DL Hayes, DR Holmes Jr. Mount Kisco, NY, Futura Publishing Company, 1986, pp 219–251. By permission of the publisher.)

configuration. It allows programming from unipolar to bipolar functions. (In some dual-chamber pacemakers, the polarities of the atrial and ventricular channels are independently programmable; in others, they are not.) This feature is helpful in patients who have myopotential or electromagnetic inhibition in the unipolar mode but not in the bipolar mode. Unipolar and bipolar electrograms have distinctly different characteristics, and programming from one polarity to the other may eliminate the sensing of an unwanted electrogram or interfering signal. It is possible but improbable that sensing in one polarity configuration will be superior to that in the other.

Polarity programmability may be helpful in a patient with a lead fracture by converting from bipolar to unipolar configuration, that is, by eliminating the fractured portion of the lead, normal pacing may be restored through the remaining intact pole of the pacing lead (Fig. 7–20). This alternative should usually be considered a temporary measure, because whatever force resulted in one fractured conductor may eventually lead to fracture of the second. In an increasing number of pulse generators, a change from bipolar to unipolar pacing configuration may be triggered automatically if a sudden change in impedance is detected during bipolar pacing[15] (Fig. 7–21).

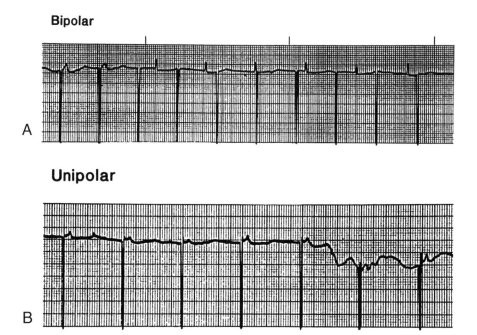

Bipolar

A

Unipolar

B

Fig. 7–20. Electrocardiographic tracings from a patient with a VVI pacemaker. *A*, In the bipolar configuration, there is intermittent failure to capture. Capture is demonstrated only with the first two pacing stimuli. *B*, Programmed to the unipolar configuration at the same pulse duration and voltage, the pacemaker demonstrates consistent capture. (From Hayes DL: Programmability. *In* A Practice of Cardiac Pacing. Third edition. Edited by S Furman, DL Hayes, DR Holmes Jr. Mount Kisco, NY, Futura Publishing Company, 1993, pp 635–663. By permission of Mayo Foundation.)

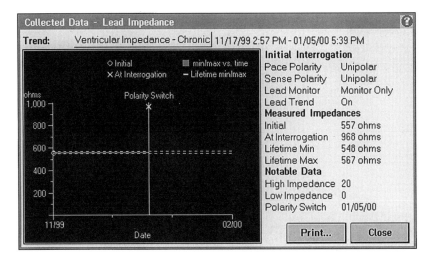

Fig. 7–21. Telemetered data of lead impedance. The graph displays impedance measurements that the pacemaker performs every 3 hours. By this display, the impedance is stable at approximately 560 Ω. However, there is a notation that a polarity switch has occurred. The polarity switch occurred because of "high" impedance measured on a beat-to-beat measurement. The "Notable Data" section states that 20 episodes of high impedance occurred. There were no instances of low impedance.

Refractory and Blanking Periods

Single-Chamber Pacemakers

A refractory period can be defined as an interval during which a given sensing circuit does not respond to sensed events. This is in contrast to a blanking period, which is an interval during which a given sensing circuit is disabled.

Refractory period programming may be necessary in a variety of clinical circumstances. In the VVI mode, the ventricular refractory period (VRP) is the interval during which the ventricular sensing circuit does not respond to sensed events. The first portion of the VRP is usually a nonprogrammable ventricular blanking period in which ventricular sensing is disabled after paced, sensed, and refractory sensed ventricular events. Depending on the pacemaker, the ventricular blanking period may be fixed, programmable, or dynamic, that is, vary on the basis of strength and duration of the ventricular event. Refractory period programming in single-chamber pacing is not commonly required but can be advantageous in some situations. Lengthening of the VRP may help prevent sensing of afterpotential depolarizations, T waves, or premature ventricular contractions (Fig. 7–22). If the refractory period is so long that some ventricular electrograms are not sensed, the subsequent pacemaker stimulus could potentially fall on the T wave of the unsensed beat. In this circumstance, shortening of the VRP would be appropriate.

If a single-chamber pacemaker is used for atrial pacing, a longer refractory period, the atrial refractory period (ARP), is desirable to avoid sensing of the QRS electrogram (far-field R waves) (Fig. 7–23).

Dual-Chamber Pacemakers

Refractory periods in dual-chamber, dual-sensing units are much more complex than in single-chamber units because the events and timing cycles in one channel

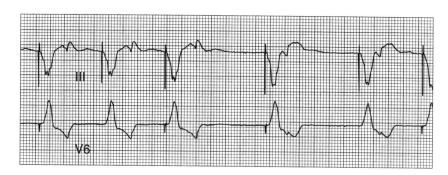

Fig. 7–22. Electrocardiographic tracing from a patient with a VVI pacemaker programmed to a rate of 70 bpm. The ventricular refractory period (VRP) is programmed to 400 msec. After the third and fourth paced ventricular events, something is sensed after the VRP and resets the timing cycle. Retrograde P waves are present. However, without a marker channel or electrogram, it is not possible to determine whether the T wave or retrograde P wave is being sensed. (From Hayes DL: Programmability. *In* A Practice of Cardiac Pacing. Third edition. Edited by S Furman, DL Hayes, DR Holmes Jr. Mount Kisco, NY, Futura Publishing Company, 1993, pp 635–663. By permission of Mayo Foundation.)

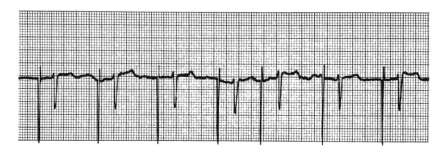

Fig. 7–23. Electrocardiographic tracing from a patient with an AAI pacemaker programmed to a rate of 90 bpm (667 msec). There are AA cycles longer than 667 msec. The only correct interval is between the fourth and fifth atrial pacing artifacts. Measuring back 667 msec from the atrial pacing artifacts following the longer cycles determines that the QRS has been sensed and atrial pacing reset. (From Hayes DL: Programmability. *In* A Practice of Cardiac Pacing. Third edition. Edited by S Furman, DL Hayes, DR Holmes Jr. Mount Kisco, NY, Futura Publishing Company, 1993, pp 635–663. By permission of Mayo Foundation.)

affect those in the other. With programming to a dual-chamber sensing mode, refractory periods exist for each sensing channel. The refractory period for the ventricular channel behaves the same as that for single-chamber sensing. The operation of the refractory period on the atrial channel is quite different. After an atrial stimulus or a sensed atrial event, the initial portion of the atrioventricular interval (AVI) is the atrial blanking period. During this interval, atrial sensing cannot take place. Depending on the pacemaker, the atrial blanking period is fixed, programmable, or dynamic, that is, varying in relation to the strength and duration of the atrial event.

A ventricular blanking period is also initiated with a sensed or paced atrial event. The intent of this interval is to avoid sensing the electronic event of one channel in the opposite channel. The blanking period is usually programmable. It may be desirable to prolong the blanking period to prevent crosstalk (Fig. 7–24). It may be necessary to shorten the blanking period if ventricular extrasystoles are sensed dur-

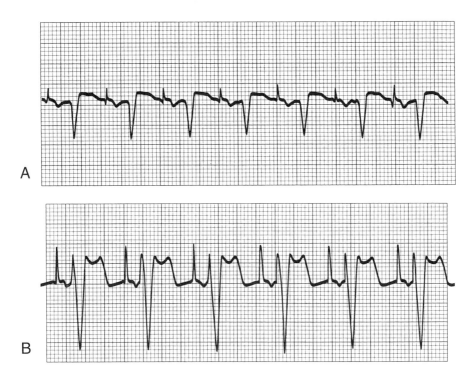

Fig. 7–24. *A,* Electrocardiogram from a patient with a DDI pacemaker programmed to a rate of 86 bpm, atrioventricular (AV) interval of 165 msec, and a blanking period of 13 msec. The interval from the atrial pacing stimulus to the intrinsic QRS complex is actually 220 msec. This abnormality occurs because the atrial output is sensed on the ventricular sensing circuit and inhibits ventricular output. AV nodal conduction is intact with a first-degree AV block. *B,* When the blanking period is lengthened to 45 msec, crosstalk is prevented. A ventricular pacing stimulus occurs 165 msec after the atrial pacing stimulus, that is, at the programmed AV interval. (From Hayes DL: Programmability. *In* A Practice of Cardiac Pacing. Third edition. Edited by S Furman, DL Hayes, DR Holmes Jr. Mount Kisco, NY, Futura Publishing Company, 1993, pp 635–663. By permission of Mayo Foundation.)

ing this period, because the result could be pacing during the early portion of ventricular repolarization (Fig. 7–25). Shortening the blanking period should diminish the likelihood of the QRS occurring within the blanking period.

The atrial sensing amplifier remains refractory for the remainder of the AVI plus the programmed atrial refractory interval after the ventricular event, the postventricular atrial refractory period (PVARP). (The total atrial refractory period [TARP] is the sum of the AVI and the PVARP.)

The first portion of the PVARP disables atrial sensing after paced, sensed, and refractory sensed ventricular events. Once again, this interval may be fixed or programmable, depending on the pacemaker.

Programmable flexibility of the PVARP is especially important because of its role in preventing endless-loop tachycardia (ELT)[16] (Fig. 7–26). Because ELT can occur only when the ARP is shorter than the retrograde (VA) conduction time, this is an especially important interval. Not all patients, however, have intact VA conduction, and some have short retrograde conduction times. Programmable options other than a prolonged PVARP can avoid ELT. Algo-

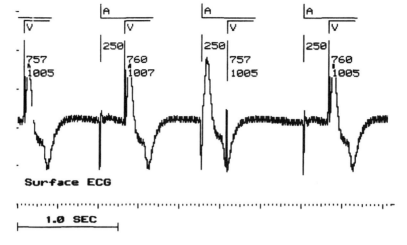

Surface ECG

|··········|··········|··········|··········|··········|··········|··········|··········|··········|··········|··········|··········|·· ‾
|—————| 1.0 SEC

Fig. 7–25. Electrocardiographic tracing obtained by the programmer from a dual-chamber pacemaker. An intrinsic ventricular event, the third ventricular depolarization, occurs in the blanking period. Because it was not sensed, the subsequent ventricular pacing artifact is released at the programmed atrioventricular interval of 220 msec. The result is that the ventricular pacing artifact occurs in the T wave of the intrinsic ventricular event.

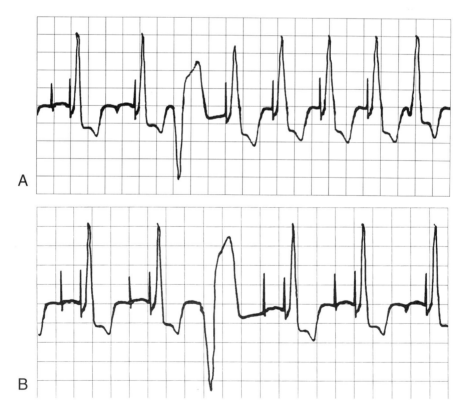

A

B

Fig. 7–26. Programming the postventricular atrial refractory period (PVARP) to manage prolonged retrograde conduction. A, After two cycles of atrioventricular sequential pacing, a premature ventricular contraction occurs with retrograde conduction, which initiates an endless-loop tachycardia. B, After lengthening of the PVARP, endless-loop tachycardia is not initiated after a premature ventricular contraction.

rithms to detect and interrupt ELT have been incorporated in many DDD pacemakers. Some DDD pacemakers use algorithms that automatically alter the PVARP or the AVI, or both. Prevention of ELT with available algorithms has been quite successful (Fig. 7–27).

The pacemaker may have a programmable option of "PVARP extension." If this feature is enabled, the PVARP is lengthened a defined duration if a premature ventricular contraction (PVC) is sensed. In actuality, the pacemaker cannot differentiate a PVC from any other ventricular beat. The most common mechanism for designating a ventricular depolarization as a PVC is sensing by the pacemaker of two ventricular events without an intervening atrial event. Should this happen, the PVARP is extended in an effort to avoid sensing of the potential retrograde atrial activation that occurs as a result of the PVC. PVARP extension may result in confusing electrocardiographic presentations. If the extended PVARP encompasses the subsequent atrial or ventricular event, the appearance of undersensing results. This is considered "functional undersensing," because it is a function of the extended PVARP (Fig. 7–28).

With shorter RR or VV cycles that may occur with atrial tracking or with sensor-driven pacemakers, it would seem log-ical for the PVARP to shorten in proportion to the entire cycle length. Automatic regulation of the PVARP has been introduced in DDDR pacemakers to prevent tracking of pathologic atrial rhythms[17] (Fig. 7–29). If a P wave falls in the PVARP (the PVARP automatically decreases as the sensor-driven interval decreases), the next atrial stimulus is omitted, and if the next P wave occurs before the subsequent ventricular output, it will not initiate an AV delay. In effect, the pacemaker is operating in the VVIR mode. This sequence continues until the P-to-P interval is longer than the adapted PVARP. When P waves no longer fall within the adapted PVARP, AV synchrony is restored.

Mode Switching

One of the main disadvantages of DDD pacing is its tendency to track atrial tachyarrhythmias, which are common in patients with pacemakers. Pacing in patients with paroxysmal atrial arrhythmias can be done with "conventional" dual-chamber pacemakers programmed in various modes or responses to cope with the atrial arrhythmias. In DDD pacemakers, any programming options other than the DDD pacing mode have in common some compromise of AV synchrony or maximal achievable paced rate

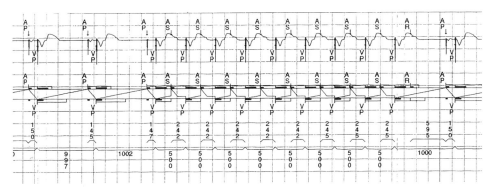

Fig. 7–27. Electrocardiographic tracing from a patient with pacemaker-mediated (endless-loop) tachycardia (PMT). The PMT is occurring at the upper rate limit of 120 bpm. The PMT algorithm suspends atrial sensing for one beat, terminating the PMT.

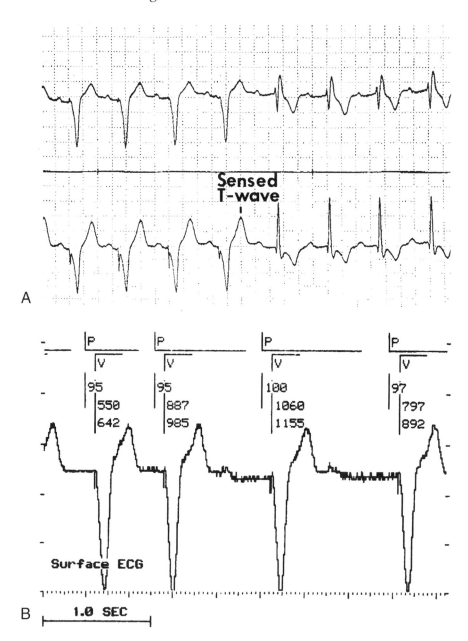

during exercise. Most contemporary pacemakers have algorithms that are designed to detect and respond efficiently to atrial tachyarrhythmias.

Mode switching refers to the ability of the pacemaker to automatically change from one mode to another in response to an inappropriately rapid atrial rhythm.[18] With the early forms of mode switching, when the pacemaker was functioning in the DDDR mode, the algorithm automatically reprogrammed the pacemaker to the VVIR mode if specific criteria were met for what was considered to be a pathologic atrial rhythm. Mode switching is particularly useful for patients with paroxysmal supraventricular rhythm disturbances. In the DDD or DDDR pacing

Fig. 7–28. *A*, Electrocardiogram (ECG) from a patient with a DDD pacemaker with extension of the postventricular atrial refractory period (PVARP). The upper and lower tracings occur simultaneously. The T wave that follows the fourth paced ventricular complex is oversensed. Because the pacemaker senses two consecutive events that are thought to represent ventricular activity—the paced QRS complex and the T wave—without sensing an intervening atrial event, the PVARP extension occurs. PVARP is extended to 480 msec. The subsequent P wave falls into the extended PVARP and is therefore not sensed. The next native QRS complex is sensed, and because there has been no sensed atrial activity, the PVARP extension is continued. This appearance of atrial failure to sense with first-degree atrioventricular block is functional undersensing due to the PVARP extension. *B*, Programmer printout of the surface ECG and markers from a patient with a DDD pacemaker. The pacemaker is sensing intrinsic atrial activity (noted as "P" in the markers). The intrinsic atrial activity is not apparent on the surface ECG at the point where the Ps are noted. However, there are definite P waves after the second and third paced ventricular events that are not tracked, that is, do not result in a paced ventricular event. The horizontal lines on the marker channel represent the refractory periods. The upper horizontal line indicates the PVARP, and the lower horizontal line associated with marker "V" represents the ventricular refractory period. There is a suggestion of a sensing abnormality because of the sensed P where no obvious intrinsic atrial activity exists. However, what appears to be definite failure to sense the obvious P waves is functional undersensing. These P waves occur in an extended PVARP represented by the upper horizontal line. Although not noted on the marker channel, the T waves are intermittently sensed and result in PVARP extension. (*A*, From Hayes DL: Pacemaker electrocardiography. *In* A Practice of Cardiac Pacing. Third edition. Edited by S Furman, DL Hayes, DR Holmes Jr. Mount Kisco, NY Futura Publishing Company, 1993, pp 309–359. By permission of Mayo Foundation.)

Fixed PVARP

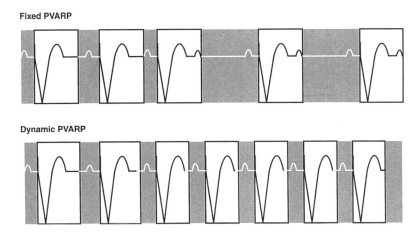

Dynamic PVARP

Fig. 7–29. Diagram of automatic alteration of the postventricular atrial refractory period (PVARP). The *upper tracing* demonstrates pacing at the lower rate limit at the programmed PVARP. The *lower tracing* demonstrates shortening of the PVARP when the ventricular rate increases.

mode, if a supraventricular rhythm disturbance occurs and the pathologic atrial rhythm is sensed by the pacemaker, rapid ventricular pacing may occur (Fig. 7–30). Any pacing mode that eliminates tracking of the pathologic rhythm, that is, DDI, DDIR, DVI, or DVIR, also eliminates the ability to track normal sinus rhythm, which is usually the predominant rhythm. Mode switching avoids this limitation. The non-atrial-sensing mode (VVI, VVIR, DDI, DDIR, etc.) to which the device is automatically programmed is specific to an individual pacemaker.

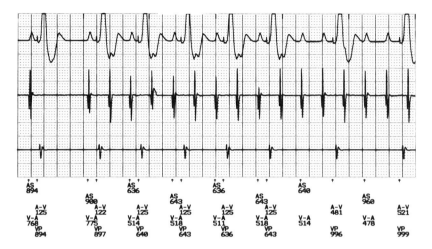

Fig. 7–30. Printout from a pacemaker demonstrating a supraventricular rhythm disturbance that results in mode switching. The tracings are the surface electrocardiogram (*top*), the atrial electrogram (*middle*), and the annotated event channel (*bottom*).

The rate at which mode switching occurs is usually programmable.

Currently available mode-switching algorithms are highly effective. Multiple manufacturer-specific algorithms are available to determine whether a pathologic atrial rhythm is present and subsequently switch to a non-atrial-sensing pacing mode (Table 7–6).

Many pacemakers have "counters" that provide the clinician with information on the frequency of mode switching. However, depending on the mode-switching algorithm in use, inappropriate mode switching may occur. With newer, more specific algorithms, it is less frequent. In some pacemakers, the appropriateness of mode switching can be verified by stored electrograms (Fig. 7–30).

Atrioventricular Interval

In dual-chamber pacemakers, an AVI must be programmed. Optimal programming of the AVI is discussed in Chapter 2. The AVI is no longer a single programmable value in many dual-chamber pacemakers. The AVI and its programmable variations are described and illustrated in Chapter 6.

Although there are many considerations in programming the AVI, the status of the patient's intrinsic AV conduction is important to determine. If the patient has normal or near-normal AV nodal conduction, it may be desirable to program a longer AVI or positive AVI hysteresis to allow intrinsic conduction. This can be considered in a routine programming sequence by gradually prolonging the AVI and determining at what interval intrinsic AV nodal conduction occurs, that is, the AR interval (Fig. 7–31).

Programming Rate-Adaptive Variables

Parameters that determine rate adaptation in a sensor-driven pacemaker vary considerably depending on the sensor incorporated. Programming rate-adaptive parameters is discussed in Chapter 8.

Unexpected Programming

There may be times when interrogation reveals something other than the expected programmed parameters. In early programmable devices before programming was accomplished exclusively by radiofrequency, faulty transmission of

Table 7–6.
Mode-Switching Algorithms

THERA DR
- Mean atrial rate (MAR) monitored continuously
- Mode switch to DDIR at MAR > 190 bpm
- Ventricular rate gradually reduced to sensor-indicated rate
- Return to DDD(R) when MAR < 190 bpm or 5 consecutive atrial paced events occur
- Gradual return to intrinsic atrial rate, lower rate limit (LRL), or sensor-indicated rate
- No protection for atrial tachyarrhythmias < 190 bpm

VIGOR DR/DDD
- Atrial tachycardia response (ATR)
- Counts AA intervals > URL (upper rate limit)
- Eight short intervals start ATR duration
- ATR duration programmable
- When duration met, mode switch to VVIR
- Programmable fallback to LRL or sensor-indicated rate
- Eight AA intervals < URL reverts to DDDR
- Complex algorithm and ECG manifestations

TRILOGY DR
- Digitally filtered atrial rate (FAR) is computed each pacing cycle
- Mode switch occurs when FAR > ATDR (atrial tachycardia detection rate)
- DDDR switches to DDIR; DDD to DDI
- ATDR is programmable to maximum tracking rate (MTR) +20 to 300 bpm or maximum sensing rate of +20 to 300 bpm
- Switches back to DDD(R) when FAR < MTR
- Mode switch marked in the event record
- Mode switch histogram of FAR and duration maintained

ChorusRM
- Program to change from DDD to VVI, DDD to VVIR, or DDDR to VVIR
- Program the delay before mode switching (10, 30, 50 . . . cycles)
- Atrial rates in Wenckebach zone begin delay count
- After delay, mode switch occurs and rate gradually decreases to sensor rate or basic rate
- Once atrial rate is < URL, rate gradually increases to meet sinus rate and dual-chamber operation resumes

Vitatron series
- Pacemakers divide atrial events into physiologic or pathologic with a physiologic rate band
- Events outside the "band" are deemed pathologic, and rates > the URL of the band are assumed to be tachyarrhythmias; mode switching occurs
- Atrial rhythm interpreted on beat-to-beat basis
- Ventricular rate variations limited by flywheel rate or sensor rate

Biotronik Actros
- Measures PP intervals; if a PP interval is shorter than the atrial refractory period (ARP), mode switch occurs
- Atrial sensed event during ARP restarts the ARP, and this continues until either LRL is reached, so that an atrial paced event occurs, or a sensed atrial beat occurs outside the ARP and is tracked
- Once the PP interval lengthens to longer than the ARP, mode is switched back to programmed mode

Biotronik Inos
- Monitors length of preceding 8 atrial intervals; if 5 of 8 are shorter than the programmed tachycardia interval or intervention rate, pacemaker switches mode to VDI
- After mode switch, ventricular rate decreases at rate of 1 pulse per minute or interval until lower rate reached

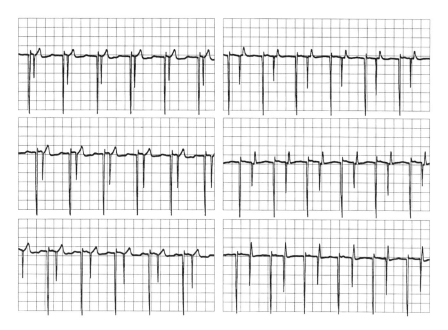

Fig. 7–31. Sequence of electrocardiographic tracings with alteration of the atrioventricular interval (AVI). In the *top left tracing,* the AVI is approximately 140 msec. The paced morphology remains similar in all three tracings on the left. In the *top right tracing,* the AVI is approximately 220 msec and there is a change in morphology suggesting fusion. In the *bottom right tracing,* the QRS complex is narrow and probably represents pseudofusion, although this determination cannot be made with certainty because an intrinsic ventricular event without a pacing artifact is not seen. In the *bottom right tracing,* the AVI is approximately 300 msec. This programming sequence is helpful in establishing the status of the patient's intrinsic atrioventricular nodal conduction. (Modified from Hayes DL: Programmability. *In* A Practice of Cardiac Pacing. Edited by S Furman, DL Hayes, DR Holmes Jr. Mount Kisco, NY, Futura Publishing Company, 1986, pp 219–251. By permission of the publisher.)

signals between programmer and pacemaker would occasionally result in abnormal programming. With contemporary devices, unexpected programming most likely occurs either because someone has reprogrammed the device and failed to document the changes or the pacemaker has been exposed to electromagnetic interference (Fig. 7–32).

Sources and management of electromagnetic interference are discussed in Chapter 12.

Programming During Routine Follow-up

The importance and usefulness of noninvasive programmability during routine follow-up and troubleshooting cannot

be overstated. Potential improvements in automaticity may eventually minimize the need for rigorous programming.[19] At the present, however, a definite approach to programming should be adopted to be certain that the pacemaker is thoroughly evaluated and to optimize pacemaker function. The following programming sequence for a rate-adaptive dual-chamber pacemaker (DDDR) can be adapted for other pacing modes.

1. If other than the initial programming session, interrogate the pacemaker and print out stored data.
2. Assess magnet response.
3. Determine the status of the underlying rhythm.
   • If pacing is occurring, program

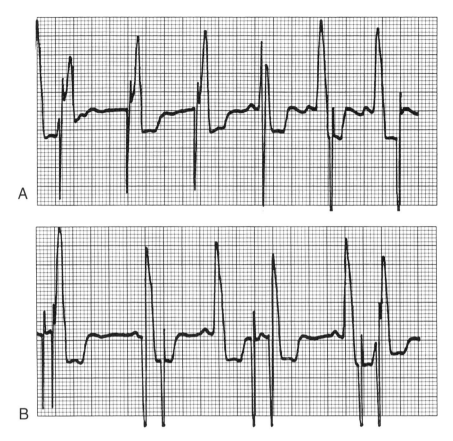

Fig. 7–32. *A*, Transtelephonic electrocardiographic (ECG) tracing from a patient with a pacemaker programmed to the DDD pacing mode. The transmission reveals VOO pacing instead of the expected DOO response. *B*, ECG tracing obtained after reprogramming in the pacemaker clinic to the DDD mode; there is appropriate DOO pacing. When a history was obtained from the patient, it was discovered that she had undergone magnetic resonance imaging (MRI) of the head. The MRI had reprogrammed the pacemaker to the backup mode, that is, VVI at a rate of 65 bpm.

the rate of the pacemaker to the lowest programmable value, 30 or 40 bpm.

4. Determine the ventricular stimulation threshold.
   - Program the pacemaker to the VVI mode.
   - Decrease the voltage amplitude to the lowest programmable value.
   - If capture is maintained, decrease the pulse width until capture is lost, and then increase the pulse width until capture is regained.
   - Increase the pulse width as needed to restore capture, and record the

voltage and pulse duration threshold parameters.
   - If the patient has no ventricular escape rhythm, manual determination of the ventricular stimulation threshold poses some risk to the patient. Risk can be minimized by automatic threshold determination.

5. Determine the atrial stimulation threshold.
   - If the patient has intact AV nodal conduction, program the pacemaker to the AAI mode.
   - Proceed as described for the ven-

tricular stimulation threshold by decreasing the voltage and then the pulse duration until loss of capture occurs.

- Regain atrial capture, and record the threshold parameters.
- If AV nodal conduction is not intact, program to DVI or DDD at a rate fast enough to override the intrinsic atrial rate.

6. Determine the sensing thresholds.
   - Beginning with ventricular sensing, program to VVI and decrease sensitivity until there is failure to sense, and record the value at which sensing was last maintained. Alternatively, program to VVT and do the same.
   - In the AAI, DVI, or DDD mode, depending on the status of AV nodal conduction, determine the atrial sensing thresholds. The AAT mode can also be used and is often helpful because intrinsic P waves may be very difficult to appreciate on a single-lead monitoring system.

7. Determine the appropriate upper rate limit by considering
   - Patient's age.
   - Physical requirements.
   - Associated medical conditions.

8. Determine the atrioventricular interval.
   - Determine the patient's AV conduction status.
   - In the patient with normal AV conduction and normal left ventricular function, consider a longer AVI to allow intrinsic conduction. This could also be accomplished with positive AVI hysteresis.
   - In the patient with AV conduction disease and normal left ventricular function, program "on" the differential AVI and rate-adaptive AVI. The actual values for paced and sensed AVI are somewhat empirical. Nominal values for many pacemakers are "paced

AVI" of 150 to 175 msec and "sensed AVI" of 125 to 140 msec.
   - In the patient with AV conduction disease and significant left ventricular dysfunction, consider AVI optimization by Doppler echocardiography or impedance plethysmography.

9. Program rate-adaptive parameters.
   - Assess exercise, either formally or informally (see Chapter 8).

10. Evaluate other parameters.
    - In most patients, activate the pacemaker-mediated tachycardia algorithm.
    - In most patients, program PVARP extension "on."
    - Review features available for the individual pacemaker, and program "on" other desirable features.

11. Review programmable telemetry options, and program as desired. (These features are discussed in Chapter 13.)

Defibrillator Programming and Algorithms

Like pacemakers, implantable defibrillators incorporate many programmable parameters that enable device function to be tailored to an individual's cardiac disease. Indeed, many of the programmable features discussed in the pacemaker section of this chapter—pacing modes, programmable pacing output, mode switch, pacing rate smoothing algorithms, and others—are currently available in defibrillators. However, in addition to providing sophisticated antibradycardia support, implantable defibrillators must be able to detect low-amplitude ventricular fibrillation (VF) electrograms, to differentiate ventricular tachyarrhythmias from supraventricular tachycardias, and to deliver overdrive pacing and high energy shocks to treat tachyarrhythmias. These demands have resulted in additional programmable features and algorithms that must be understood for optimal use of the devices. This chapter focuses on the operation and programming of these features and is divided into the following sections:

- Implantable cardioverter-defibrillator (ICD) sensing
- ICD single-chamber detection
- Single-chamber detection enhancements
- Dual-chamber detection
- Atrial detection and therapies
- Low-energy ventricular therapies (antitachycardia pacing)
- High-energy ventricular therapies (cardioversion and defibrillation)

Implantable Cardioverter-Defibrillator Sensing

Sensing of ventricular or atrial depolarization refers to the determination of the presence of an electrical event by a device. Detection, on the other hand, is the analysis of a sequence of sensed events by the defibrillator using an algorithm to detect an arrhythmia. Oversensing occurs when non-QRS potentials are greater than the reference threshold voltage and are considered sensed events. Oversensing may arise from T-wave voltage or noncardiac electrical noise exceeding the reference threshold (Fig. 7–33), leading the defibrillator to determine that cardiac events are present when in fact they are not. In contrast, undersensing occurs when the electrical signals of interest, whether QRS complexes or the electrograms of fibrillation, do not reach the threshold voltage to be sensed as an event (Fig. 7–34). Because the number of sensed events is either too high (oversensing) or too low (undersensing), the actual rhythm may be misinterpreted by the defibrillator's algorithm, resulting in inappropriate device action.[20,21]

Generally, if the measured R wave at implantation is at least 5 mV, appropriate sensing occurs during VF with normal settings. During implant testing, it is useful to assess detection at the least sensitive setting. This determines the safety margin for sensing should a reduction in programmed sensitivity be required in the future (due to oversensing, for example). However, if intervening changes in medication or clinical status have occurred since implantation, induction of arrhythmia to reassess VF detection should be performed before sensitivity is reprogrammed. Assessment of sensing after a failed defibrillation shock is useful if VF sensing is borderline, as it tests the worst possible case.

Determination of the intracardiac ventricular rate requires appropriate sensing of QRS complexes of relatively large amplitude and avoiding detection of the subsequent midsized T wave (which would result in double counting of a single contraction) while maintaining adequate sensitivity to detect fibrillatory electrograms of small amplitude.[22] Because the amplitude of VF is small, ICDs must amplify electrograms 10 times more than bradycardia pacemakers. The need to sense signals of markedly different amplitude has been addressed by a dynamic gain or sensitivity threshold. In many devices, this effectively increases the sensitivity throughout the cardiac cycle until the next QRS occurs, at which point sensitivity is diminished[22,23] (Fig. 7–35). Consequently, oversensing of noncardiac signals is most likely to occur during slow heart rates, late in diastole, when sensitivity is greatest. This is particularly true in some devices after paced events, after which the attack rate (rate of increase in sensitivity or gain) is greatest.

The manner in which dynamic sensing is applied differs among manufacturers, and the actual maximum and minimum sensing floor for each setting varies, as shown in Table 7–7. In the Guidant devices, the gain is dynamically adjusted while a constant sensing threshold is maintained (Fig. 7–35). Sensitivity is programmed to one of three values: "nominal," "less," and "least." Templates with

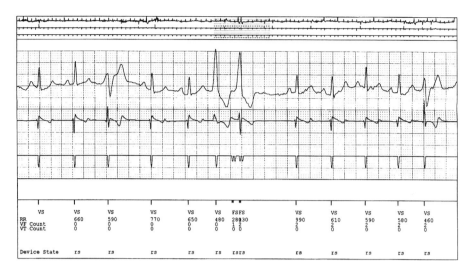

Fig. 7–33. Oversensing. A recording from an implantable cardioverter-defibrillator is shown with surface electrocardiogram (*top*), electrogram (*middle*), and marker (*bottom*). Below are shown the markers again, annotated with cycle length and ventricular fibrillation (VF) and ventricular tachycardia (VT) counter values. During the ventricular couplet, the T wave exceeds the voltage threshold for sensing and is oversensed.

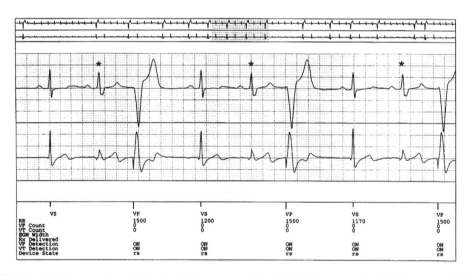

Fig. 7–34. Undersensing. An implantable cardioverter-defibrillator recording is shown, as in the preceding figure. The QRS complexes marked with an asterisk have an RBBB morphology due to intermittent bundle branch block and are not sensed. Note that the marked complexes appear smaller on the electrogram (*bottom tracing*) and are not sensed (no marker) and that a pacing pulse is inappropriately delivered shortly after the undersensed event (VP).

unique attack rates for pacing, normal rate sensing, and tachycardia sensing are applied (Fig. 7–36). In pacemaker-dependent patients with slow pacing rates, a sensitivity of "less" (in Ventak AV series, which is the same as "nominal" in the Prizm series) may be preferable to avoid diaphragmatic oversensing, assuming that adequate VF detection has been assessed.

In Medtronic devices, the concept is similar, but rather than adjustment of the gain throughout the cardiac cycle, the threshold for sensing is altered (Fig. 7–35). A sensitivity level is programmed

Table 7–7.
Sensitivity Values for Defibrillators*

Manufacturer	Programmed sensitivity	Sensitivity floor, mV	
		Minimum	Maximum
Guidant, Ventak AV family	Nominal	Sensing: 0.18 Paced: 0.36	Sensing: 1.08 Paced: 2.3
	Less	Sensing: 0.24 Paced: 0.49	Sensing: 1.44 Paced: 2.9
	Least	Sensing: 0.29 Paced: 0.58	Sensing: 1.74 Paced: 0.58
Medtronic, Gem AF†	0.15 mV	0.15	1.2
	0.3 mV (nominal)	0.3	2.4
	0.45 mV	0.45	3.6
	0.6 mV	0.6	4.8
	0.9 mV	0.9	7.2
	1.2 mV	1.2	9.6
St. Jude, Cadet, Contour,	AGC = 7	0.2	‡
Angstrom	AGC = 6	0.3	‡

AGC, automatic gain control.
*This table is not comprehensive but illustrates ranges of sensitivity in implantable defibrillators.
†Postpacing sensitivity is 4.5 times the programmed sensitivity value with the same decay constant.
‡The maximum sensitivity floor is independently programmable.

by selection of the smallest signal that can be detected during the time in the cardiac cycle that sensitivity is maximum, nominally 0.3 mV in the ventricle (Fig. 7–37).

In St. Jude defibrillators, on the other hand, the gain is fixed within a given cardiac cycle but can change with each ventricular complex (Fig. 7–38). However, a more dynamic approach will be used in upcoming models.

Implantable Cardioverter-Defibrillator Detection

Single-Chamber Defibrillators

The detection of a ventricular arrhythmia is based primarily on two rhythm characteristics—heart rate and arrhythmia duration (typically 1 to 3 seconds)—which are programmable to meet the needs of the patient.[24] The rate criterion distinguishes between a tachyarrhythmia and a normal rhythm, and the duration requirement prevents detection of nonsustained episodes. Thus, all defibrillators use heart rate zones (Fig. 7–39) as the first step in classifying a rhythm. Different types of therapies and detection enhancements can be applied to tachyarrhythmias of different rates by further division into "slow VT (ventricular tachycardia)," "fast VT," and "VF" zones[25,26] (Fig. 7–39 B). In programming detection and therapy zones, two general principles apply: 1. Programming for detection of unstable (fast) VT and VF must be highly sensitive and therapies highly effective. The cost of this sensitivity is some inappropriate treatment of rapid supraventricular tachycardias (SVTs). 2. Programming should be more specific for hemodynamically tolerated (i.e., usually slower) VT, and therapies should be better tolerated (i.e., antitachycardia pacing should generally be used). This improved specificity may come at the cost of some delay in detection, and the application of painless therapies (antitachycardia pacing) at the cost of *initial* therapeutic efficacy.[27]

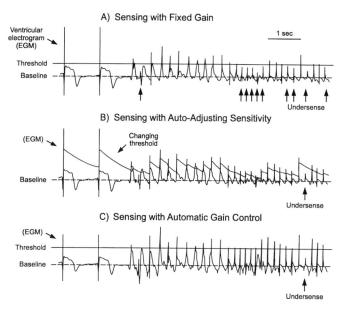

Fig. 7–35. Implantable cardioverter-defibrillator sensing systems. *A,* Fixed gain (and sensitivity) requires that the sensed potential exceed a fixed threshold. Because of the highly variable amplitude during ventricular fibrillation, undersensing occurs (*arrows*). If the threshold is lowered, T-wave oversensing may occur (note that the threshold is just above the T-wave amplitude during sinus rhythm, first two complexes). *B,* Autoadjusting sensitivity. The gain is fixed, but the threshold for sensing changes throughout the cardiac cycle. Undersensing is diminished. *C,* Automatic gain control. The threshold for sensing is fixed, but the gain is adjusted throughout the cardiac cycle, so that very small electrograms are at a higher gain to increase the likelihood that they will exceed the sensing threshold. Undersensing is diminished. (Modified from Olson WH: Tachyarrhythmia sensing and detection. *In* Implantable Cardioverter-Defibrillator. Edited by I Singer. Armonk, NY, Futura Publishing Company, 1994, pp 71–107. By permission of the publisher.)

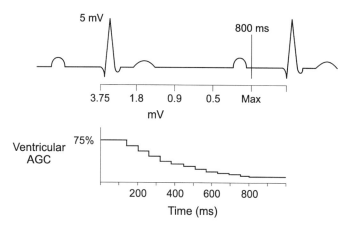

Fig. 7–36. Automatic gain control (AGC) (Guidant defibrillators). Templates with unique attack rates (rate of change in gain) for pacing, normal rate sensing, and tachycardia sensing are applied. During normal sinus rhythm sensing in the ventricle (shown), after a sensed event the sensing floor decreases to 75% of the R-wave amplitude, and the attack range becomes twice as sensitive every 200 msec, achieving maximum sensitivity 800 msec after an intrinsic R wave. During pacing, on the other hand (not shown), with the sensitivity programmed to "nominal," the automatic gain control uses different values (2.3 to 0.28 mV in the ventricle), with maximum sensitivity reached 200 msec before the next paced interval to maximize sensing of ventricular arrhythmias before another paced event. Thus, both the duration of gain adjustment and the maximum and minimum gain values change dynamically under varying conditions, resulting in dynamic sensing.

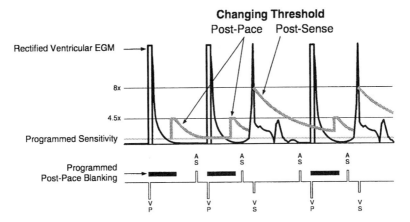

Fig. 7–37. Autoadjusting sensitivity (Medtronic defibrillators). A sensitivity level is programmed by selection of the smallest signal that can be detected during the time in the cardiac cycle that sensitivity is maximum. This value can range from 0.15 to 1.2 mV and is nominally programmed to 0.3 mV. After a sensed R wave, the sensitivity decreases to 75% of R-wave amplitude (to a maximum of eight times the programmed value) and then decays with a time constant of 450 msec to the programmed maximum sensitivity, as shown. After a paced event, the sensitivity decreases to 1.8 mV (maximum of 4.5 times the programmed value); the decay constant is not changed on the basis of heart rate. Similar dynamic sensing is applied in the atrium in dual-chamber devices. Note the absence of blanking in the atrial channel after a ventricular sensed event. This diminishes atrial undersensing during tachyarrhythmias. However, far-field R waves may be sensed; this is handled by a far-field R-wave oversensing algorithm.

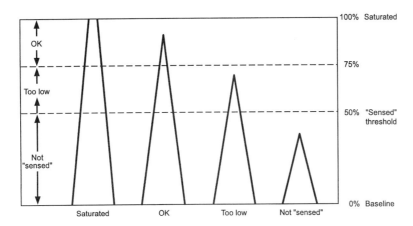

Fig. 7–38. Beat-to-beat adjustment of sensing (St. Jude defibrillators). Eight gain settings (labeled 0 to 7) are used. The pulse generator chooses the appropriate gain on the basis of the amplitude of the previous electrogram signals. Signals that are too low lead to an increased gain, whereas saturated signals lead to a lower gain. Since gain is evaluated with each ventricular complex, gain adjustment occurs more rapidly with fast heart rhythms. If there are no sensed events during bradycardia pacing, the gain is increased one step with each paced event (two steps in some models). Thus, the gain is fixed within a given cardiac cycle but can change with each ventricular complex. The maximum and minimum gain values may be programmed to prevent oversensing (by not allowing maximum sensitivity) or to avoid undersensing (by not permitting adjustment to the least sensitive setting after a premature ventricular contraction, for example).

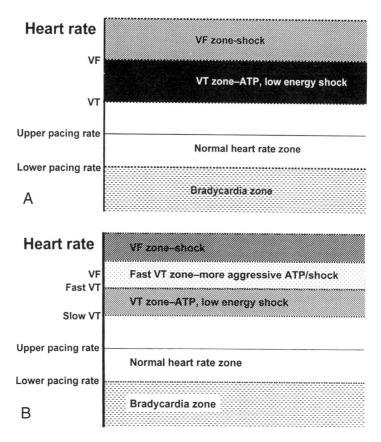

Fig. 7–39. Heart rate zones used to classify arrhythmias. *A,* The defibrillator permits heart rates above the lower pacing rate and below the ventricular tachycardia (VT) rate. Tachycardias in the VT zone (usually programmed for heart rates in the 150 to 180 bpm range) are more likely to be hemodynamically stable. Thus, detection enhancements may be applied to improve specificity, and better tolerated but less effective therapies such as antitachycardia pacing (ATP) and low energy shocks are delivered. Very fast VTs and ventricular fibrillation (VF) will be detected in the VF zone. In the VF zone, detection enhancements are typically not applied (to err on the side of overtreatment of these faster tachyarrhythmias), and high-energy shocks are the first therapy delivered. *B,* In most defibrillators, the tachycardia zones can be further subdivided into fast and slow VT zones to permit greater tailoring of therapies based on ventricular rate.

Arrhythmia detection begins with each ventricular event. After each sensed or paced event, the time interval to the next sensed ventricular event determines its classification (Fig. 7–40). A sequence of classified ventricular events is accumulated in VT and VF counters until criteria for arrhythmia detection are met. The type of counting used varies between detection zones and among manufacturers. Because of highly variable electro-gram amplitude during VF, some signal dropout may occur despite dynamic sensing. Therefore, to enhance sensitivity, initial detection occurs when a certain percentage (usually 70% to 80%) of sensed events within a continuously rolling detection window fall within the VF zone (Fig. 7–41). In many defibrillators, this X of Y counting is also used for detection in VT zones[27] (Fig. 7–42). During ongoing detection with more than

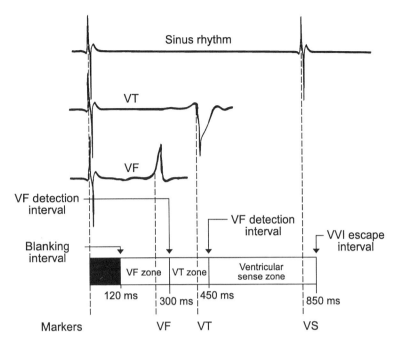

Fig. 7–40. Classification of each ventricular complex on the basis of cycle length. After each sensed or paced event, the time interval to the next sensed ventricular event determines its classification. If another ventricular event is sensed after the blanking period but within the programmed ventricular fibrillation (VF) detection interval (typically 300 to 320 msec), the event is classified as a VF complex, regardless of the actual cause of the ventricular depolarization. A delay greater than the programmed VF interval but shorter than the maximum VT cycle length results in a ventricular tachycardia (VT) event. If the time between ventricular depolarizations exceeds the programmed length of the VT detection cycle, the event is sensed without classification as a tachyarrhythmia ("VS," for ventricular sensed event). If no event is sensed and the pacing rate interval is reached, a pacing impulse is generated. This example includes only two tachycardia zones (VF and VT). In most defibrillators, up to three tachycardia detection zones may be programmed to allow progressively more aggressive delivery of therapy for faster VTs. (From Olson WH: Tachyarrhythmia sensing and detection. *In* Implantable Cardioverter-Defibrillator. Edited by I Singer. Armonk, NY, Futura Publishing Company, 1994, pp 71–107. By permission of the publisher.)

one programmed zone, the higher zone (i.e., VF) takes priority over the lower zone (i.e., VT) (Fig. 7–42). Once the X of Y counter is satisfied in some defibrillators (Guidant), a programmable duration for which the arrhythmia must persist is required before therapy delivery. For unstable VTs and VF, this duration is kept short (1 second). The duration in slower VT zones is independently programmable, so that longer intervals (2.5 seconds and occasionally longer) can be programmed to avoid detection of slower nonsustained episodes. Generally, the VT cutoff rate is programmed for 10 to 20 bpm slower than the slowest known VT.

In some defibrillators (Medtronic), X of Y counting is used for VF detection (Fig. 7–41), but consecutive interval counting is used for VT detection. Consecutive interval counting requires that a programmable number of consecutive intervals shorter (faster) than the VT cycle length be present for VT detection to occur; a single long (slow) interval resets the VT counter to zero (Fig. 7–43). This method increases specificity by avoiding detection of atrial fibrillation (AF) with-

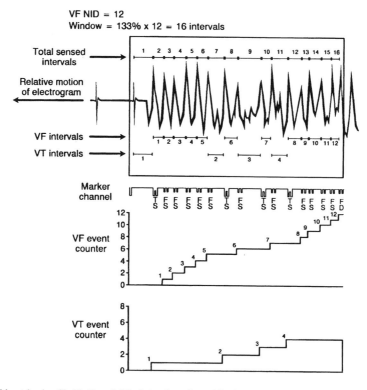

Fig. 7–41. Ventricular fibrillation (VF) detection (in a Medtronic implantable cardioverter-defibrillator). The box at the top shows the moving window during ventricular fibrillation (VF) detection. Twelve of the 16 intervals in the moving window must be shorter than the fibrillation detection interval for VF detection to occur. The marker channel demonstrates whether events are sensed as VF ("FS") or ventricular tachycardia (VT) ("TS"). The VF and VT counters below the markers show that VT counting is not reset by VF sensed events. The VF counter is never suddenly reset to zero under any circumstances, since, contrary to VT detection, a moving window is always used for VF detection. VF NID, number of intervals to detect ventricular fibrillation. (From Friedman and Stanton.[22] By permission of Futura Publishing Company.)

out compromising VT sensitivity.[27] AF with a mean cycle length shorter than the tachycardia detection interval may escape inappropriate detection if periodic intervals longer than the cutoff rate reset the tachycardia counter to zero (Fig. 7–43). For patients with known VT, a detection zone 30 msec longer than the slowest VT cycle length is typically used, with the VT counter set nominally to 16. In patients with recurrent runs of nonsustained VT, a higher VT counter value is used, and shocks are programmed for noncommitted delivery (discussed below). Conversely, rapid and poorly tolerated VT that is nonetheless responsive to antitachycardia pacing warrants a shorter

detection count or, alternatively, use of three tachycardia zones.[22]

To avoid delayed detection when a tachyarrhythmia straddles the VT and VF zones, a combined counter that is incrementally activated by VT or VF events is used. When the sum of the VT and VF counters reaches a threshold (nominally 21), VF is detected unless eight or more of the preceding events were in the VT zone, in which case VT is detected (Fig. 7–44).

Since in Medtronic devices different counting methods are used in the VT and VF zones, when a third tachycardia zone (fast VT [FVT] zone) is added, the physician may choose whether to use VT-type consecutive interval or VF-type X of Y in-

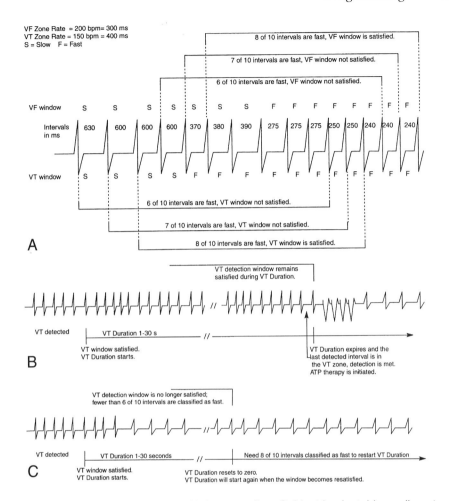

Fig. 7–42. Use of X of Y counting in multiple zones (in a Guidant implantable cardioverter-defibrillator). *A,* For each zone, the detection heart rate and tachycardia duration are programmed independently. Each zone has a detection window composed of the 10 most recent RR intervals. As each new interval is measured, it is defined as either fast—above the programmed rate threshold for the window—or slow. A window is satisfied when 8 of the 10 most recent RR intervals are fast and remains satisfied as long as 6 of 10 intervals in the moving window are fast. *B,* Once a detection window is satisfied, a programmable duration timer is started, nominally 2.5 seconds for ventricular tachycardia (VT) and 1 second for ventricular fibrillation (VF). If after the duration timer expires the last detected interval is in the zone of the timer, detection is met and therapy is delivered (unless a detection enhancement is programmed; see text). When multiple zones are programmed "on," the higher zone takes priority over the lower zone. Up to three tachycardia zones (VT-1, VT, and VF) with independently programmable criteria and therapies may be used to enhance detection and specificity of therapy. *C,* If the VT detection window does not remain satisfied until the end of the VT duration window, VT duration resets to zero, and timing will resume when the window becomes resatisfied. ATP, antitachycardia pacing. (Modified from Guidant ICD reference manual.)

terval counting. If the FVT zone is programmed via VF, events in the VF or FVT zone are added to the VF counter and detection follows VF rules. Once detection is met, if all the preceding eight events were in the FVT zone, FVT therapy is delivered; otherwise, VF therapy is delivered. Conversely, if the FVT zone is programmed via the VT zone, events in the FVT zone are added to the VT counter

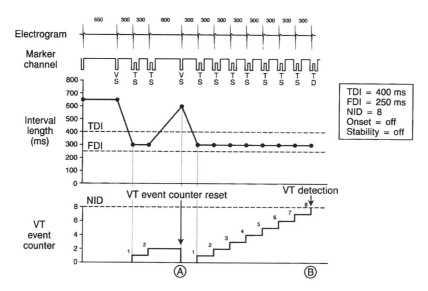

Fig. 7–43. Consecutive interval counting ventricular tachycardia (VT) detection (Medtronic). At the top is the ventricular electrogram with the individual intervals labeled in milliseconds. Beneath the electrograms are the corresponding markers for each sensed event. Next is a graph of the individual intervals, with dashed lines delineating the tachycardia detection interval (TDI) and fibrillation detection interval (FDI). At the bottom, the graph displays how each sensed event affects the VT event counter. The dashed line denotes the programmed number of intervals needed to detect VT (NID). In this figure, the third electrogram occurs at a cycle length of 300 msec, which is less than the programmed TDI of 400 msec; the VT counter increases to 1. Note that the marker channel displays a VT sense. At point "A," the VT counter is reset to zero by a sensed interval of 600 msec, which is longer than the TDI. At point "B," VT detection occurs, as the counter reaches the programmed NID of 8. Depending on the type of therapy programmed, antitachycardia pacing or charging of the capacitors would begin at this point. (From Friedman and Stanton.[22] By permission of Futura Publishing Company.)

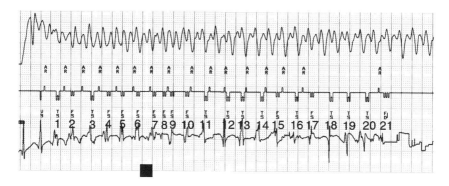

Fig. 7–44. Combined counter to avoid detection delay when a tachyarrhythmia straddles the ventricular tachycardia (VT) and ventricular fibrillation (VF) zones. Detection occurs after 21 complexes even though neither the VT nor the VF counters were satisfied. Events present in the VF zone (e.g., complex 17 and 15) result in detection as VF.

and detection follows VT rules. Once detection is met, if any of the preceding eight events were in the FVT zone, FVT therapy is delivered (Fig. 7–45).

St. Jude defibrillators can also use up to three distinct rate-detection zones, called "fibrillation," "Tach B," and "Tach A," with separate counters and independently programmable criteria for each of the zones. For detection to occur in any zone, a programmable number of intervals must be classified and counted in that zone. In contrast to other devices, the classification of a sensed event depends on both the current interval and the average of the current interval and the previous three intervals (Table 7–8). The sinus counter is reset to zero whenever any interval is classified in a tachycardia zone.

When the sinus rhythm counter reaches a programmable value, sinus rhythm is detected and all counters are reset to zero. To prevent detection of bigeminy with average rates in a tachycardia zone, more tachyarrhythmia intervals than sinus intervals are required by an additional bigeminy detection algorithm, which withholds therapy if bigeminy is present.

Committed and Noncommitted Shocks.

All early defibrillators delivered committed shocks; once a tachyarrhythmia was detected and capacitor charging initiated, a shock was committed to follow, irrespective of arrhythmia termination. Most late-generation devices can be programmed to deliver noncommitted

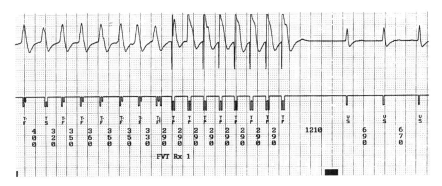

Fig. 7–45. Fast ventricular tachycardia (FVT) detection via ventricular tachycardia (VT). In this example, the FVT zone overlaps the upper (faster) end of the VT zone. The second complex (interval, 400 msec) is detected as VT ("TS" for tachycardia sense). The next interval (320 msec) is detected as FVT ("TF"). Once the VT counter is satisfied (at the "TF|" marker), the arrhythmia is classified as FVT, since at least one of the previous eight events was in the FVT zone. The first FVT therapy, in this case antitachycardia pacing, is delivered.

Table 7–8.
Classification of Ventricular Events in St. Jude Defibrillators*

Interval	Average for interval	Bin
Fibrillation	Tach A	Fibrillation
Tach A	Tach B	Tach B
Fibrillation	Sinus	Not placed
Sinus	Sinus	Sinus

*This classification is used when an interval and its average are not the same.

therapy; after detection and capacitor charging, the pulse generator confirms continuing tachyarrhythmia before delivery of a shock. If the arrhythmia has ended, the capacitors remain charged but therapy is withheld, and the device continues to monitor the rhythm (Fig. 7–46). For a given episode, typically only the first shock can be programmed as noncommitted; in redetected arrhythmia, shocks are committed.

Detection Enhancements. Since early implantable defibrillator use, it has been apparent that a supraventricular rhythm with a rapid ventricular response could lead to inappropriate therapies. This phenomenon was found in up to 30% of patients with defibrillators once electrograms of treated episodes became available, permitting diagnosis of arrhythmia.[28–31] Inappropriate shocks may limit quality of life, utilize medical resources, and result in proarrhythmia. Consequently, detection enhancements have been added to defibrillators to improve specificity. When programmed "on," detection enhancements prevent delivery of therapy despite a heart rate in the tachycardia zone if other factors (e.g., a narrow QRS complex) suggest a supraventricular mechanism. Since the overlap in heart rate between ventricular and supraventricular arrhythmias occurs predominantly in the "slower" tachycardia zones, and since the very fast rhythms detected in the VF zone (usually > 185 to 200 bpm) are more likely to be hemodynamically unstable and require immediate therapy, detection enhancements are usually applied only in the VT zone (Fig. 7–39).

Single-chamber defibrillators must use QRS morphology or rhythm patterns such as rate of onset or regularity to enhance rhythm diagnosis; in contrast, dual-chamber defibrillators (discussed in the next section) can also compare and analyze atrial and ventricular rates and patterns. A summary of single-chamber detection enhancements and their operation is provided in Table 7–9. The general principles guiding optimal programming of single-chamber detection enhancements are as follows: 1. Specificity enhancements should be applied to slower, hemodynamically tolerated VT zones, in which a modest delay in therapy is tolerable. 2. Dis-

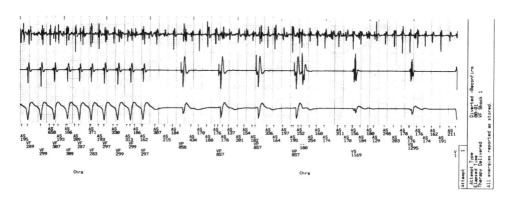

Fig. 7–46. Noncommitted shocks. Stored episode on a nonsustained ventricular tachycardia (VT) in a noncommitted device. From top to bottom are atrial electrogram, near-field ventricular electrogram, and far-field ventricular electrogram. Continuing atrial fibrillation is present. During capacitor charge, the VT terminates. Slow sensed events ("VS") after charge completion (at the second "Chrg" marker) indicate arrhythmia termination, so that the shock is withheld ("Diverted-Reconfirm" in the box at far right). Note that during the charge, pacing support ("VP") is provided.

Table 7–9.
Single-Chamber Detection Enhancements

Detection enhancement	Function
Stability (inhibit therapy if ventricular rate is unstable; or in some devices, accelerate therapy if unstable)	• Main use: differentiate atrial fibrillation (irregular, unstable intervals) from ventricular tachycardia (regular, stable intervals) • In Guidant devices, can also be used to accelerate therapy (e.g., to avoid antitachycardia pacing in patient with known polymorphic ventricular tachycardia, which is irregular and unstable)
Onset (inhibit therapy if gradual onset)	• Main use: differentiate sinus tachycardia (gradual onset) from ventricular tachycardia (sudden onset)
Electrogram width (inhibit therapy if narrow complex)	• Main use: differentiate supraventricular (narrow) from ventricular (wide) arrhythmias • Distinguishes between narrow complex and wide complex arrhythmias by determining width of the far-field intracardiac electrogram
Morphology discrimination (inhibit therapy if intracardiac morphology matches normal sinus rhythm)	• Main use: differentiate ventricular (do not match template) from supraventricular (match template) arrhythmias • A template of the bipolar near-field electrogram is made during sinus rhythm • During tachycardia, the tachycardia template is compared with the baseline template
Sustained rate duration (override inhibitor if fast rate persistent)	• Main use: limit the length of time inhibitor can withhold therapy during a high-ventricular-rate episode • Overrides therapy inhibitors after duration timer expires • Many devices also have timers to limit the total duration of antitachycardia pacing therapies; after the programmed time elapses, the device delivers a shock, even if pacing therapies remain

crimination algorithms that continuously reassess the rhythm during tachycardia (such as "stability") are preferable and should generally be used in patients with known SVTs or AF. 3. Discrimination algorithms that perform a single classification based on a limited number of ventricular events (such as "onset") should be used more judiciously or in conjunction with sustained duration timers (that deliver therapy irrespective of classification if the tachycardia duration exceeds a programmable time limit).

Stability Enhancement.—This detection enhancement is used to differentiate AF from VT. When programmed "on," the stability algorithm withholds therapy despite ventricular rates in the tachycar-

dia zone if the cycle length is irregular (Fig. 7–47 and 7–48). The rationale for this approach is that VTs have a relatively stable heart rate with little variation in cycle length, whereas AF with a rapid ventricular response is characterized by variability in cycle length. In one study, for example, the average stability (i.e., RR variability) during VT episodes was 16 ± 15 msec, compared with 49 ± 15 msec during AF.[32] The stability enhancement prevents inappropriate detection of AF in up to 95% of AF episodes, with only a minimal or no decrease in VT sensitivity[32–34] (Table 7–10). Atrial flutter may be fairly regular and difficult to differentiate from VT in single-chamber devices.

In patients with a history of paroxys-

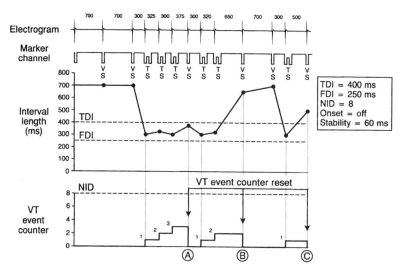

Fig. 7–47. Stability criterion (as implemented by Medtronic). Ventricular tachycardia (VT) counting commences with the first 300-msec interval. At point "A," the VT counter is reset to zero, since the cycle length of 375 msec, although less than the tachycardia detection interval (TDI), is more than 60 msec greater than the preceding interval, and the stability criterion is not met. Note that the marker channel registers a normal sensed event at that point even though the interval is less than the TDI. The stability criterion is not applied until after the VT counter reaches 3. At points "B" and "C," the VT counter is reset by intervals greater than the TDI. This pattern would be consistent with atrial fibrillation. FDI, fibrillation detection interval; NID, number of intervals needed to detect ventricular tachycardia. (From Friedman and Stanton.[22] By permission of Futura Publishing Company.)

mal AF, stability should be programmed "on." The value used depends on the specific defibrillator, since stability algorithms differ among manufacturers. In Medtronic devices, for example, the typical programmed value is 40 msec (Table 7–10). Since stability is continuously reassessed once the heart rate exceeds the VT detection rate, should the ventricular rhythm become regular (suggesting the development of VT), therapy is delivered. In patients who have poorly tolerated VT, it may be useful to program three zones. Stability is applied in the slowest zone, more aggressive therapies without specificity enhancements are programmed in the middle zone, and VF detection and therapies are applied in the fastest zone.

The recommended stability value in Guidant devices is 24 to 40 msec (Table 7–10). The additional use of a programmed, sustained rate duration to override the stability inhibitor and deliver

therapy if the ventricular rate remains elevated for 30 to 60 seconds maintains a very high sensitivity (100%) for VT[32] (Table 7–10). Sustained rate duration is typically programmed for 30 seconds and increased as needed in patients who receive or are susceptible to inappropriate therapies for AF. When sustained rate duration is programmed to longer values, using three zones may be preferable so that potentially long delays in therapy occur only in the slowest (VT-1) zone, often limited to heart rates under 150 to 160 bpm. The measured stability for all stored episodes—regardless of whether the stability feature is programmed "on" or "off"—is recorded in the episode header and in the printed episode summary (Fig. 7–48 B). This information is very useful in tailoring the stability parameter to an individual's arrhythmia profile.[38] Of note, in addition to acting as a therapy inhibitor, stability can be used as a therapy accelerator in Guidant defibrillators. In patients with anticipated polymorphic VT, stability as an accelerator causes the pulse generator to bypass antitachycardia pacing for irregular rhythms and instead proceed to a shock. However, stability cannot be used as an inhibitor and an accelerator in the same zone.

Onset Enhancement.—This enhancement differentiates VT from sinus tachycardia because most VTs have a sudden onset, whereas sinus tachycardia begins gradually (Table 7–10 and Fig. 7–49). The onset criterion rejects inappropriate detection of 64% to 98% of sinus tachycardias with heart rates in the VT zone but results in underdetection of 0.5% to 5% of VTs.[32–34] Unlike stability, which continuously reevaluates the rhythm diagnosis during tachycardia, onset is determined only once. Moreover, since ectopy preceding VT may seem gradual in onset to the algorithm, this enhancement is best limited to slow VT zones (heart rate < 140 to 150), where the risk for overlap with sinus tachycardia is greatest, to avoid underdetection of faster VT.[38] Additionally, when available, sustained rate duration is often used with the onset algorithm, as many cardiac patients are unable to maintain prolonged sinus tachycardia. In patients prone to sinus tachycardia and slow VTs, use of β-blockers and digitalis, which improve survival and reduce symptoms, respectively, is also helpful. Dual-chamber devices may prove particularly useful in patients with very slow VTs, although confirmation is required.

Electrogram Width.—This algorithm uses digital signal processing to measure the electrogram width and define a rhythm as narrow complex or wide complex on the basis of its intracardiac morphology. The choice of intracardiac source is programmable, although the far-field electrogram is preferred. The beginning and end of the intracardiac QRS complex are determined by a programmable slew rate[37] (Fig. 7–50). The QRS width threshold is then programmed at the maximum QRS width during supraventricular rhythm plus 4 to 8 msec. This detection enhancement may be programmed "off," "on," or "passive." In the passive mode, the device reports how the rhythm would have been classified by the algorithm without actually applying the results to withhold therapy. When programmed "on," narrow-complex tachycardias with heart rates in the VT zone are not treated. This criterion should be used cautiously or avoided in patients with preexisting bundle branch block or surface QRS exceeding 100 msec. Additionally, because the width of the intracardiac electrogram changes with exercise and with system maturation, some investigators program this feature to the passive mode for the first 6 months or, preferentially, until it is shown to be effective during spontaneous or induced ventricular arrhythmias. Despite these limitations, this algorithm increases the specificity of detection of VT, particularly when used in conjunction with other algorithms.[35,37,41–43]

Morphology Discrimination.—This algorithm is based on acquisition by the defibrillator of a patient-specific, near-field bipolar electrogram template during sinus rhythm. The morphology of complexes during tachycardia is compared with the template, on the assumption that supraventricular rhythms have the same morphology as the sinus rhythm template. In contrast to the electrogram width criterion, the entire morphology (as opposed to a calculated width) is analyzed (Fig. 7–51). The degree of match between the tachycardia morphology and the stored supraventricular morphology is calculated by the algorithm as a percentage for each sensed event. The percent match with the template required to determine that a sensed complex is supraventricular is programmable, as is the number of beats in the rolling detection window, which must be supraventricular to diagnose the rhythm as SVT. Thorough evaluation of the performance of that algorithm is not yet

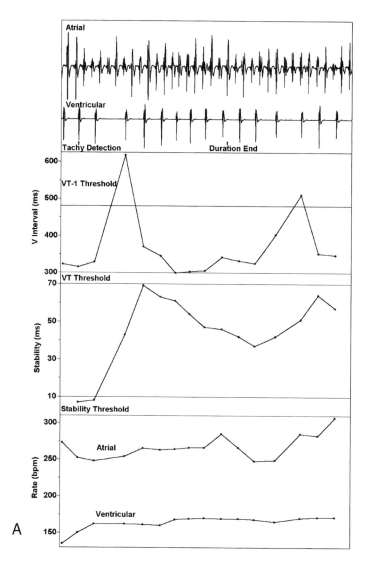

Fig. 7–48. The stability criterion (as implemented by Guidant). *A,* From top to bottom are the atrial and ventricular electrograms, ventricular interval, calculated stability, and atrial and ventricular rates. Atrial fibrillation with a rapid ventricular response is present. The ventricular interval drops below the ventricular tachycardia (VT) detection rate (475 msec in this example, shown as a line on the "V Interval" plot). Despite tachyarrhythmia detection and satisfaction of duration, therapy is withheld since the stability threshold (programmed to 30 msec in this example) is exceeded. *Continued.*

available, but very preliminary results seem promising (Table 7–10).

Dual-Chamber Detection

In addition to providing dual-chamber pacing functionality, dual-chamber defibrillators use the information acquired simultaneously from the atrial and the ventricular leads in an effort to enhance arrhythmia diagnosis.[44-47] Although different manufacturers have adopted very different approaches, the algorithms share many common principles:

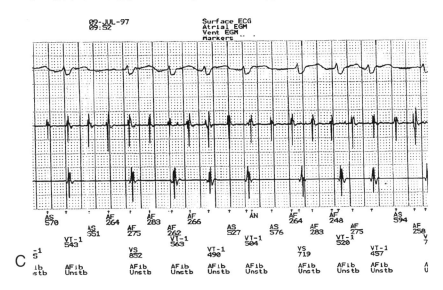

Guidant								VENTAK PRIZM DR
Patient								14-OCT-99 14:29
Institution								
Model		1851		RAM Version		2901	Programmer	
Serial				1.2		2844	Software	1.1

Quick Notes Report

Tachy Mode	Monitor+Therapy

Therapy History: 28-SEP-99 to 14-OCT-99

Episode and Attempt #	Date/Time and Elapsed Time m:s	Stb ms	Ons	V > A	AF ib	A/V Pre bpm	Therapy	A/V Post bpm
12	13-OCT-99 17:27	--	--	-	-	202/ 84	ATR 00:48 m:s	--/ --
11	13-OCT-99 16:46	37	56%	F	T	--/ --	Nonsustained	--/ --
10 1	06-OCT-99 14:53 00:03	3	56%	T	F	70/171	VT ATP1x1 Burst	/ 70
9	04-OCT-99 08:25	--	--	-	-	202/ 67	ATR >9:59 h:m	--/ --
8	30-SEP-99 16:26	--	--	-	-	270/ 67	ATR 02:00 m:s	--/ --

B

O = OFF, T = TRUE, F = FALSE, "-" = Not Applicable/Recorded

Fig. 7–48 *continued. B,* The therapy history summarizes the stability (Stb), onset (Ons), V > A, detection of atrial fibrillation (AFib), and atrial and ventricular rates for each episode, irrespective of whether the detection enhancements were actually programmed "on" or not. This is very useful in tailoring detection enhancements to an individual's specific arrhythmia history. ATR, atrial tracking rate. *C,* Real-time recording with surface electrocardiogram (ECG), atrial electrogram (EGM), and ventricular electrogram, from top to bottom. VT therapy is withheld because of unstable ventricular intervals. The atrial electrogram confirms the presence of atrial fibrillation. (Courtesy of Dr. Michael Glikson, Heart Institute, Sheba Medical Center, Tel Hashomer, Israel.)

Table 7–10.
Summary of Studies Assessing Single-Chamber Detection Enhancements*

Study	Manufacturer	Detection enhancement	Results, main findings
Swerdlow et al.[33]	Medtronic	Stability, 40 msec; onset, 87%	Delay in detection > 5 sec in 1.9% (13/677) of episodes; 0.6% VTs not detected (correctable with reprogramming).
Swerdlow et al.[34]	Medtronic	Stability, 40 msec; onset, 87%	Stability: AF detection decreased 95%; all VTs detected. Onset: sinus acceleration rejected (98%); 0.5% VTs underdetected.
Barold et al.[35]	Medtronic	Stability, 40 msec; onset, 91% (initially); EGM width	Stability prevented 88% of AF episodes from being detected. Onset prevented 64% of episodes from being detected. EGM width changed over time in 59% patients but was stable at 6 months.
Brachmann et al.[36]	Medtronic	EGM width	Sensitivity, 96%. Specificity, 76%.
Klingenheben et al.[37]	Medtronic	EGM width	EGM width changes with exercise should be considered in program, either with an exercise test or by adding 8 msec to QRS width.
Brugada et al.[32]	Guidant	Stability, 40 msec; onset, > 9%	Specificity 96% (stability), 97% (onset). Sensitivity for VT detection, 90%. With use of SRD, VT sensitivity increased to 100%, but specificity decreased 96% to 83%.
Schaumann et al.[38]	Guidant	Stability and onset individualized; SRD, 30 sec	Stability programmed to 22 msec had sensitivity of 95%, to 30 msec had sensitivity of 99%. Onset at 9% may result in underdetection of 5% of VTs; best limited to slow VT zone (< 150 bpm) and used with SRD.
Higgins et al.[39]	Guidant	Stability	Applied to heart rates < 220. Sensitivity, 100% for all settings (8–55 msec). Specificity, 100% for all settings ≤ 47 msec and 91% for stability to 55 msec.

continues

Table 7–10. (*Continued*)
Summary of Studies Assessing Single-Chamber Detection Enhancements*

Study	Manufacturer	Detection enhancement	Results, main findings
Neuzner et al.[40]	Guidant	Stability, onset	Measured recorded stability and onset values for spontaneous arrhythmias:
St. Jude PMA	St. Jude	Morphology discrimination	Sensitivity (VT only), 97.8%; (VT + VF), 99.4%. Specificity (adjusted), 75.6%; (unadjusted), 78.7%.

For Neuzner et al. results:

	Onset	Stability, msec
Sinus, tachycardia	0%	2.2 ± 0.9
Atrial, tachyarrhythmias	8.5% ± 9.5%	41 ± 24
VT,	30% ± 12%	7.8 ± 6

AF, atrial fibrillation; EGM, electrogram; SRD, sustained rate duration; VF, ventricular fibrillation; VT, ventricular tachycardia.
*Listed by manufacturer, since algorithms vary with manufacturer.

- The identification of AV dissociation is characteristic of VT, especially when the ventricular rate exceeds the atrial rate.
- The identification of N:1 AV association is characteristic of supraventricular rhythms (with the exception of VT with 1:1 retrograde conduction).[48,49]
- The assessment of ventricular cycle length regularity (stability algorithm) is done only when fibrillation is diagnosed in the atria.

Overall, dual-chamber enhancements have been shown to improve discrimination and to decrease inappropriate therapies by correctly diagnosing 60% to 95% of supraventricular arrhythmia episodes without missing VT episodes.[44–46] These results are similar to[33,34] or somewhat better than[32,35] those previously published for traditional single-chamber enhancement criteria. Data supporting the advantage of dual-chamber algorithms over algorithms in appropriately programmed single-chamber defibrillators are limited, largely because the introduction of dual-chamber devices is fairly recent. It is clear that any advantage of dual-chamber devices over single-chamber devices for rhythm detection is very device- and algorithm-specific and that studies directly comparing single- and dual-chamber algorithms will be required to determine relative specificity.[47,50,51] Additionally, most studies have compared dual-chamber algorithms with single-chamber rate detection alone, whereas the more appropriate comparison would be with single-chamber devices using detection enhancements. Given the marked differences in approach to dual-chamber detection taken by manufacturers, each manufacturer is considered separately. For each, the basics of operation and available performance data are reviewed.

Atrial View Enhanced Onset and Stability (Guidant).

The Guidant Ventak AV and Prizm dual-chamber defibrillators add two programmable detection enhancements that use the atrial lead to enhance specificity: V Rate > A Rate and Afib Rate

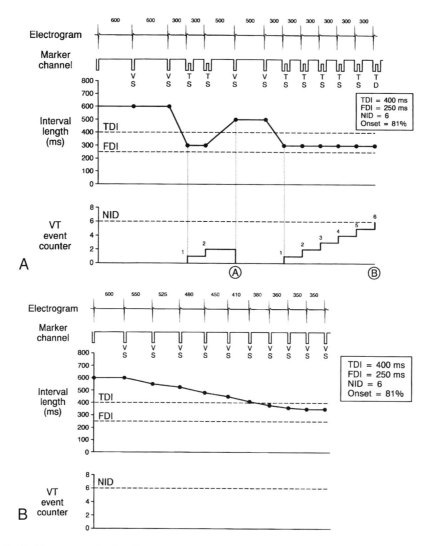

Fig. 7–49. The onset criterion (as implemented by Medtronic). *A,* The first 300-msec interval is less than the tachycardia detection interval (TDI) and 81% of the average of the preceding four intervals; thus, onset is satisfied and the ventricular tachycardia (VT) counter incremented. At point "A," an interval greater than the TDI resets the VT counter to zero. Onset is again met with the next interval, and VT counting resumes anew, culminating in detection at point "B." *B,* Onset is programmed to 81%. The heart rate increases gradually (as in sinus tachycardia), so that despite cycle lengths that are less than the TDI (last four intervals), VT is not detected, since no interval is 81% of the average of the preceding four intervals. Note that the marker channel continues to show normal sensing (not VT sensing) and that the VT event counter is not incremented. In newer single-chamber Medtronic defibrillators, onset is replaced by other algorithms (electrogram width). FDI, fibrillation detection interval; NID, number of intervals needed to detect ventricular tachycardia. (From Friedman and Stanton.[22] By permission of Futura Publishing Company.)

Fig. 7–50. Electrogram width criterion (Medtronic). *A,* Episode data from a patient who had a supraventricular tachycardia inappropriately detected as ventricular tachycardia (VT). Note that all of the eight complexes preceding detection were narrow. Since the device was programmed in the passive mode, the electrogram (EGM) width result is reported, but therapy is not affected. This patient subsequently had the criteria reprogrammed from "passive" to "on" to prevent further inappropriate detections. *B,* The eight complexes and how they were defined (all narrow in this case). Determination of the beginning and end of a complex is a function of the slew, which is programmable. *C,* Electrogram of the onset of the arrhythmia, which matches the sinus rhythm electrogram (not shown), confirming a supraventricular mechanism.

ICD Model: Gem 7227
Serial Number: PIP101752H

Apr 26, 1999 08:48:28
9962 Software Version 2.0
Copyright (c) Medtronic, Inc. 1997

VT VF Episode #15 Report   Page 3

EGM Width Measurements Prior to Detection (ms)

-8. 84   Narrow
-7. 84   Narrow
-6. 84   Narrow
-5. 88   Narrow
-4. 88   Narrow
-3. 84   Narrow
-2. 80   Narrow
-1. 84   Narrow
 0. Detection

EGM Width Result: Narrow, but passive mode

Parameter Settings

VF	On	320 ms (188 bpm)
FVT	Off	
VT	On	400 ms (150 bpm)

Sensitivity

V. Sensitivity	0.3 mV

A

ICD Model: Gem 7227
Serial Number: PIP101752H

Apr 26, 1999 08:49:03
9962 Software Version 2.0
Copyright (c) Medtronic, Inc. 1997

VT VF Episode #15 Report   Page 1

ID#	Date/Time	Type	V. Cycle	Last Rx	Success	Duration
15	Apr 25 10:29:05	VT	390 ms	VF Rx 3	Yes	48 sec

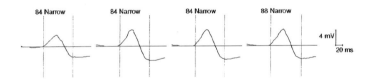

84 Narrow   84 Narrow   84 Narrow   88 Narrow   4 mV
                                                          20 ms

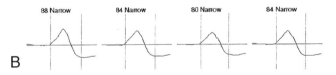

88 Narrow   84 Narrow   80 Narrow   84 Narrow

B

Episode #15 - VT
Chart speed: 25.0 mm/sec

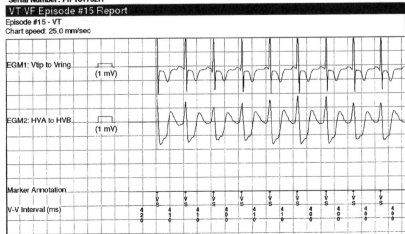

EGM1: Vtip to Vring
(1 mV)

EGM2: HVA to HVB
(1 mV)

Marker Annotation

V-V Interval (ms)

C

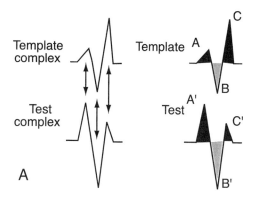

Fig. 7–51. Morphology discrimination (St. Jude). *A*, An electrogram template is made during sinus rhythm, unique for each patient. During a tachyarrhythmia, each tachycardia complex ("test complex") is compared with the template. A morphology score is derived from the sum of the differences of aligned test complex and template. The % Match score is a function of the difference between the areas under the aligned complexes (i.e., [area A − area A'] + [area B − area B'] + [area C − area C']). The % Match score required to consider a supraventricular complex is programmable. *B*, Example of ventricular tachycardia with nonmatching morphology scores (electrograms depicted with an "x" below).

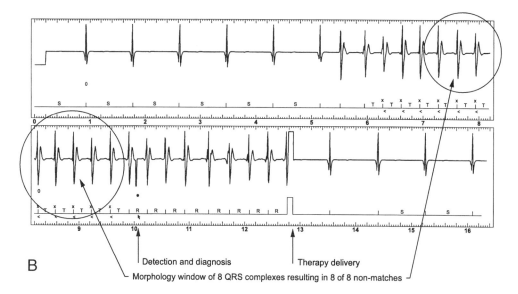

Detection and diagnosis | Therapy delivery

B   Morphology window of 8 QRS complexes resulting in 8 of 8 non-matches

Threshold. These two additional features work in conjunction with the ventricular-based detection enhancements, described above (stability and onset) and are thus applied only in VT zones. The V Rate > A Rate feature utilizes the fact that a ventricular rate greater than an atrial rate is pathognomonic for VT. When V Rate > A Rate (ventricular rate greater than atrial rate) is "on," therapy inhibitors (onset or stability, or both) are bypassed and therapy is immediately delivered to tachycardias with a ventricular rate greater than the atrial rate by 10 bpm (Fig. 7–52). If the ventricular rate is not greater than the atrial rate (which is indicated as false on

the episode detail report), therapy continues to be inhibited. In that case, the V Rate > A Rate analysis continues until the ventricular rate exceeds the atrial rate or other enhancements indicate that therapy is warranted, at which time treatment is delivered.

The Afib Rate Threshold aims to increase specificity by withholding therapy for unstable (irregular) ventricular rhythms only when the atrial lead confirms AF. If an unstable (irregular) ventricular rhythm is in the tachycardia zone but the atrial lead does not confirm fibrillation, therapy is delivered. If fibrillation is present in the atrium, the ventricular rate

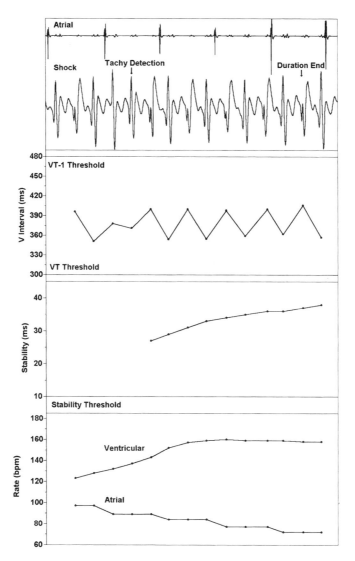

Fig. 7–52. Use of V rate > A rate (ventricular rate greater than atrial rate) to bypass therapy inhibitors. From top to bottom are the atrial and ventricular electrograms, the V intervals, the calculated stability, and the atrial and ventricular rates. The 10 most recent PP intervals and RR intervals are used to assess the rate in each chamber. An irregular ventricular tachycardia (VT) is present. The VT has a shorter interval (is faster) than the slow VT (VT-1) cutoff threshold. Thus, VT detection and duration are both satisfied (*top box*). Because the RR intervals are variable, the stability threshold is above the programmed value (in this case, 24 msec; not shown on graph). This inhibits therapy in a single-chamber device. However, since the ventricular rate is greater than the atrial rate, the stability inhibitor is bypassed and appropriate therapy delivered.

is unstable, and Afib Rate Threshold is "on," therapy is withheld until the atrial rate drops below the Afib Rate Threshold, the ventricular rhythm becomes stable, or the sustained rate duration timer expires. A comparison of single-chamber and dual-chamber detection algorithms in Guidant devices is shown in Figure 7–53.

Several reports have assessed the performance of this algorithm. In a study comparing 39 patients with the Ventak AV and 55 patients with the Ventak Mini, Kühlkamp et al.[47] found that inappropriate therapies were applied to 4% of atrial flutter or AF episodes in the dual-chamber devices with V > A and Afib Rate

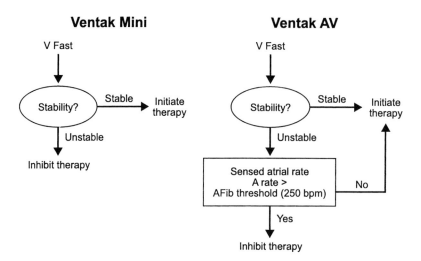

Fig. 7–53. Comparison of single-chamber and dual-chamber detection enhancements in Guidant defibrillators. Dual-chamber defibrillators use atrial lead information to bypass single-chamber-based inhibitors if atrial fibrillation is present or if the ventricular rate exceeds the atrial rate (by > 10 bpm). Atrial fibrillation is diagnosed when 6 of the last 10 atrial intervals are faster than the afibrillation rate threshold, and the atrial window remains satisfied as long as 4 of 10 intervals remain fast. Although in early Ventak AV devices (Model 1810) the rate threshold was set at 250, in subsequent versions it has been programmable from 200 to 400 bpm or "off." Further details in the text. (From Kühlkamp et al.[47] By permission of Futura Publishing Company.)

Threshold "on," compared with 24% of the episodes in the single-chamber devices with the stability enhancement "on" ($P < 0.001$). The increased rate of inappropriate therapies in dual-chamber devices was in large measure due to atrial undersensing in the early Ventak AV models, resulting in the false appearance of V > A rates. In contrast, initial results from the ASTRID study reported a significant reduction in inappropriate therapies with rigidly defined use of dual-chamber enhancements (11% inappropriate therapies compared with 26% for the control group; $P < 0.002$), but the control group consisted of rate only detection without use of single-chamber detection enhancements.[52]

PARAD Atrioventricular Sequence Analysis (ELA). The ELA Defender uses a dual-chamber algorithm that sequentially analyzes interval stability, AV association, and (for 1:1 arrhythmias) the chamber of onset to differentiate supra-

ventricular from ventricular arrhythmias for heart rates in the VT zone (Fig. 7–54). As with other defibrillators, VF and VT zones are programmed on the basis of heart rate. Although many other parameters within the algorithm are programmable (discussed below), the preponderance of clinical data have been collected using nominal values, so that in most cases only the desired rate cutoffs need to be programmed. In the PARAD algorithm, each new RR interval is classified by whether it is in the VF, VT, or sinus heart rate zone. When 75% (programmable, 63% to 100%) of the last eight RR intervals fall into the VF or sinus rhythm zone, the rhythm is classified accordingly; for VF, shock is immediately delivered, and for sinus rhythm, no therapy is offered. In contrast, if the initial classification is to the VT zone, analysis continues to further differentiate ventricular from supraventricular arrhythmias. Of note, the initial intervals of a tachycardia (programmable, 0 to 8; nominal, 0) can be

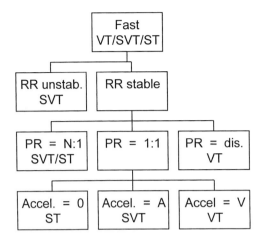

Fig. 7–54. PARAD algorithm (ELA). Tachyarrhythmias in the ventricular tachycardia (VT) zone are sequentially analyzed for RR interval stability, P:R relationship, and acceleration at onset for classification. Further details in text. dis., dissociation; ST, sinus tachycardia; SVT, supraventricular tachycardia.

excluded from analysis to allow the rhythm to stabilize.

For tachycardias in the VT zone, the first step in the algorithm is determination of RR interval stability (Fig. 7–54). If the rhythm is classified as unstable and diagnosed as AF, no therapy is delivered. In contrast, if the rhythm is determined to be stable, the algorithm next assesses AV association. A stable rhythm with AV dissociation is classified as VT and treated (Fig. 7–55). A stable rhythm with N:1 association is classified as SVT, and therapy is withheld (Fig. 7–56). A rhythm with 1:1

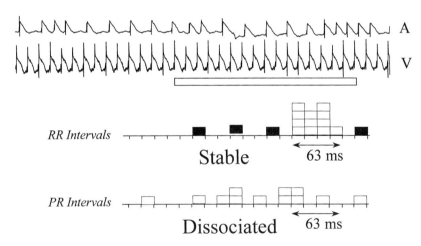

Fig. 7–55. Detection of ventricular tachycardia with atrioventricular (AV) dissociation by the PARAD algorithm (ELA). From top to bottom are atrial and ventricular electrograms, RR interval histogram, and PR interval histogram. The histogram of the RR intervals is created in a correlation window with four bins that are nominally 63 msec wide, with the window positioned to maximize the number of RR intervals in it. If fewer than 75% (nominally) of the RR intervals fall into the window, the rhythm is classified as unstable and diagnosed as atrial fibrillation, and no therapy is delivered. In contrast, if the rhythm is determined to be stable (as in the present example, in which nearly all intervals fall into the same bin), the algorithm proceeds to assess AV association. The widely scattered PR intervals in this case are consistent with AV dissociation. This stable rhythm with AV dissociation is classified as ventricular tachycardia and treated.

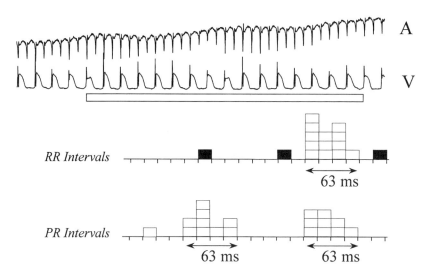

Fig. 7–56. Detection of atrial flutter by the PARAD algorithm (ELA). The format is that of the preceding figure. Atrial flutter with 2:1 conduction to the ventricles is present. The histogram of RR intervals defines the rhythm as stable, since nearly all the intervals fall into one bin. Therefore, analysis proceeds to A:V association classification. Atrioventricular association is determined in a manner analogous to stability determination; PR interval histograms are created by use of up to five PR intervals from each RR interval. A correlation window is positioned to maximize the number of PR intervals in the window, and the rhythm is deemed associated if the number of stable PR intervals is at least 75% (nominally) of the number of stable RR intervals found in the RR histogram. In this example, the PR intervals fall into two bins, consistent with a 2:1 conduction pattern. This stable rhythm with N:1 association is classified as supraventricular tachycardia, and therapy is withheld.

association is further analyzed to determine whether acceleration was present at the onset of arrhythmia and whether it was atrial or ventricular in origin (Fig. 7–54). Acceleration is defined by an RR interval at onset that is shorter than the previous reference RR interval by 25% (nominal). If acceleration is absent or atrial, the arrhythmia is classified as SVT, and therapy is withheld. If acceleration is present and ventricular (RR intervals accelerated without antecedent PR intervals), the arrhythmia is classified as VT, and therapy is delivered.

Several early reports that included up to 50 patients described the performance of this algorithm.[46,50,53] VF sensitivity and specificity were both 100%, with detection times of 2.1 ± 0.4 seconds. VT sensitivity was 96% (85 of 88 episodes), with one VT missed for each of the following: unstable RR intervals, low VT rate limit, and oversensing an artifact. On the basis of data from the Food and Drug Administration PMA submission, global sensitivity for VT and VF is 99% and specificity is 90%. This algorithm is unique in that it permits the bradycardia pacing upper rate limit to exceed the slowest VT zone. This capability may prove useful in treating patients with very slow VTs that overlap the sinus rate, although data are lacking.

PR Logic Pattern and Rate Analysis (Medtronic). The algorithm used in Medtronic defibrillators is fundamentally based on the ventricular-rate-only detection used in Medtronic devices, with subsequent additional analysis for arrhythmias that also fall into an independently programmable SVT zone. Additionally, the same stability criterion used in single-chamber devices is retained in dual-chamber defibrillators (Fig. 7–57). Thus, if a

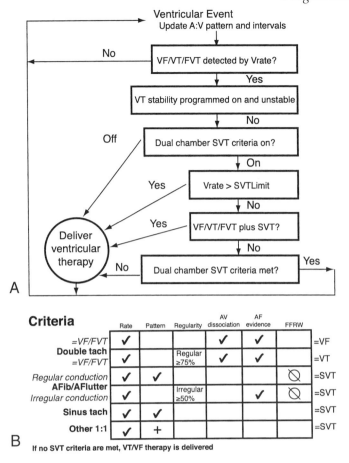

Fig. 7–57. Detection process in PR Logic (Medtronic). *A,* With each sensed event, ventricular rate detection, as found in single-chamber implantable cardioverter-defibrillators, is applied. If rate detection criteria are met in the ventricular tachycardia (VT) zone, the stability algorithm (identical to that in single-chamber defibrillators) is applied if programmed "on." If the rhythm is not unstable, the algorithm proceeds to see whether the dual-chamber supraventricular tachycardia (SVT) criteria are programmed "on" and whether the ventricular rate exceeds the SVT limit. The next step screens for dual tachycardia (simultaneous atrial and ventricular tachycardia); if it is present, ventricular therapy is delivered. If dual tachycardia is absent, the presence of an SVT ("AFib/AFlutter," "Sinus Tach," or "Other 1:1" SVT) is assessed by use of the dual-chamber SVT criteria. If an SVT is not positively identified, ventricular therapy is delivered. *B,* Dual-chamber SVT criteria. The column headings are the six elements used for arrhythmia classification; the table indicates the elements required for diagnosis of each arrhythmia by PR Logic. AF, atrial fibrillation; AV, atrioventricular; FFRW, far-field R waves; FVT, fast ventricular tachycardia; VF, ventricular fibrillation.

tachycardia meets ventricular tachyarrhythmia rate detection criteria (as described for single-chamber ICDs, above), the stability enhancement is applied if the rate is in the VT zone and stability is programmed "on." If stability is "off" or stability fails to inhibit therapy and the arrhythmia falls in the SVT zone, PR Logic is applied to further categorize the arrhythmia. Of note, in contrast to stability, which is applied only in the VT zones, the SVT zone to which PR Logic is applied is independently programmable and can overlap with VT and VF zones (Fig. 7–58). Thus, tachycardias with ventricular rates in a VT or VF zone not inhibited by stability and in the SVT zone are further analyzed by the PR Logic algorithm.

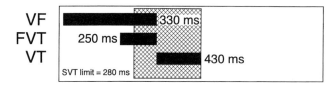

Fig. 7–58. Independently programmable supraventricular tachycardia (SVT) limit in PR Logic (Medtronic). In contrast to Medtronic single-chamber defibrillators, in which detection enhancements are applied only in the ventricular tachycardia (VT) zone, the dual-chamber defibrillators have an independently programmable SVT limit that can be applied over part or all of one or more zones.

Aside from the SVT limit, the PR Logic algorithm has three programmable parameters, each of which is programmed either "on" or "off": A fib/A flutter, sinus tachycardia, and other 1:1 SVTs. When programmed "on," positive identification of one of these arrhythmias is required to withhold ventricular therapies.[24] As shown in Figure 7–57, the algorithm initially seeks to determine whether a dual tachycardia (simultaneous atrial and ventricular tachycardias) is present. If so, ventricular therapy is delivered; if not, positive identification of each of the independently programmable supraventricular arrhythmias (AF, sinus tachycardia, and 1:1 SVTs) is sought. The algorithm relies on six elements in making this identification: rate (atrial and ventricular), pattern, regularity, AV dissociation, far-field R wave, and AF evidence. These six elements are then used to analyze the rhythm to arrive at a classification (Fig. 7–57 B). Each of the elements used by PR Logic is discussed briefly below.

Rate.—The median PP and the median RR intervals for the preceding 12 respective intervals are updated after each ventricular event and used for analysis.

PR Pattern.—The number and position of P waves relative to R waves are analyzed for each of the two preceding RR intervals. On the basis of the number of atrial events and the location relative to R waves, one of 19 codes is assigned to the intervals (Fig. 7–59). Any cardiac rhythm generates a string of code letters, and these are compared with sequences known to

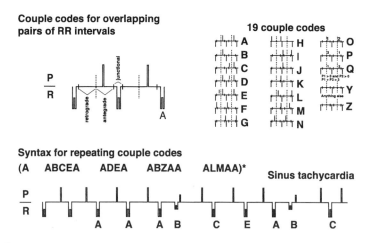

Fig. 7–59. Couple code syntax analysis in PR Logic. The PR pattern code is one of six elements used by PR Logic for arrhythmia classification. Details in text. (From Olson.[24] By permission of Futura Publishing Company.)

occur during specific rhythms, such as sinus tachycardia or sinus tachycardia with PVCs. This pattern-matching is continuous, analogous to a word processing spelling checker analyzing a stream of new text by comparing it with known catalogs of text.[24] When the pattern changes and fails to match a known SVT, the algorithm, to avoid inappropriate VT detection during the transition between different types of SVTs, does not immediately stop recognizing the SVT. As noted in Figure 7–57, pattern analysis is used not alone but in conjunction with the other elements of the algorithm (rate, regularity, AV dissociation, far-field R wave, and AF evidence) to make a rhythm classification.

Regularity.—This element measures the variability in RR cycle length. Importantly, although conceptually similar to the stability inhibitor, the regularity counter is part of PR Logic and is independent of and not related to the stability algorithm (Fig. 7–60).

AV Dissociation.—The mean of the most recent eight PR intervals is computed, and an individual PR interval is considered dissociated if its absolute difference from the mean is greater than 40 msec. If four of the last eight intervals in a rhythm are dissociated, the rhythm is declared dissociated.

Far-field R Wave.—To avoid undersensing of P waves, the algorithm does not include cross-chamber blanking in the atrium after sensed ventricular events and has short (30 msec) atrial blanking after a paced ventricular event. Consequently, far-field R waves are not uncommonly sensed on the atrial channel (depending on atrial lead position). This subalgorithm determines whether sensed events in the atrial channel are likely to be due to far-field R waves, the result of which is then incorporated into rhythm analysis (Fig. 7–61). As a practical matter, if far-field R-wave oversensing is consistently present or consistently absent, the

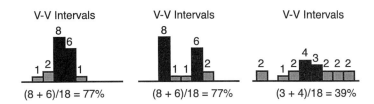

Fig. 7–60. Regularity assessment in PR Logic. The regularity counter (also called the "modesum") analyzes the last 18 RR intervals by placing them into a histogram with 10-msec bins and comparing the sum of the number of intervals in the two largest bins to the total number of intervals to determine regularity.

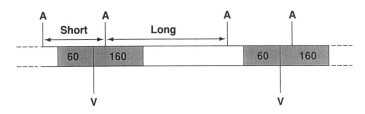

Fig. 7–61. Far-field R-wave oversensing. This subalgorithm determines whether sensed events on the atrial channel are due to atrial events or sensing of the far-field R wave. If each RR interval has exactly two atrial events and PP intervals alternate in a consistent manner, far-field R-wave oversensing can be diagnosed. The criteria must be met for 10 of the last 12 RR intervals to have atrial events rejected as far-field R waves. Further details in the text.

algorithm functions effectively. Intermittent sensing of far-field R waves prevents their appropriate identification by the defibrillator and may lead to arrhythmia misclassification. Atrial sensitivity should be adjusted so that R waves are either consistently absent or consistently sensed on the atrial channel. This should be considered at the time of atrial lead implantation and in programming atrial sensitivity.

AF Evidence.—An up-down atrial event counter is used to evaluate atrial tachyarrhythmias. When two or more atrial events occur during an RR interval, the counter is augmented by one. If the preceding RR interval had two or more atrial events but the most recent RR interval had zero or one atrial event, the counter is unchanged. If both the present and the preceding RR intervals had zero or one atrial event, the counter total is decreased. A value of six or more on this counter is evidence for AF, since P and R relationships during AF do not have reliable pattern information.[24]

In summary, the PR Logic algorithm uses the six elements described to classify tachyarrhythmias, as shown in the flow diagram and table in Figure 7–57. In clinical evaluation, including preliminary reports on 80 patients with 383 spontaneous episodes, sensitivity for sustained VT or VF (>20 beats) was 100%.[24,45,54] Inappropriate detection of SVT occurred in 12% (47) of episodes, compared with inappropriate detection in 29% (127 of 444) of spontaneous episodes in 95 patients with single-chamber ICDs that used the same kind of rate-only detection. The causes of inappropriate detections were as follows: in 64%, sinus rhythm with first-degree AV block (because of the long PR interval, P waves occurred immediately after the preceding QRS, leading the algorithm to interpret the rhythm as VT with retrograde conduction); in 17%, SVT cycle length shorter than the programmed minimum SVT cycle length

(so that the algorithm was not applied by the device); in 13%, atrial sensing errors detected as PR dissociation; and in 6%, rapid and regular AF detected as double tachycardia.[24,54]

Many experts routinely program A fib/A flutter and sinus rhythm enhancements "on." In the first month, 1:1 SVTs are not programmed "on," since an atrial lead dislodgment into the ventricle may result in the inappropriate classification of VT as SVT. Additionally, in the rare patient with atrioventricular nodal reentrant tachycardia or orthodromic tachycardia (both typically 1:1 SVTs), ventricular antitachycardia pacing usually terminates the SVT, so that an intentional decision to deliver therapy may be appropriate.

Atrial Defibrillators: Detection and Therapies

In contrast to dedicated ventricular defibrillators, which seek to diagnose atrial arrhythmias so that therapies can be withheld, atrial defibrillators diagnose atrial arrhythmias to enable delivery of specific atrial therapies. At the time of this writing, the only atrial device available is the Medtronic Jewel AF, an atrial and ventricular defibrillator. In addition to standard ventricular therapies (antitachycardia pacing, cardioversion, and defibrillation, all discussed later in this chapter), this device includes atrial prevention and termination therapies (Table 7–11 and Fig. 7–62). The dual-chamber detection algorithm has two steps: (1) Detection based on PR Logic (described above) is used to diagnose ventricular arrhythmias and to prevent ventricular therapies for atrial arrhythmias, and (2) a separate detection algorithm is used to manage active therapy for atrial arrhythmias. Thus, it is important to note that a supraventricular arrhythmia with a rate in the VT zone may result in inhibition of ventricular therapy by PR Logic but may not result in

Table 7–11.
Atrial Prevention and Termination Therapies in the
Jewel AF Atrial and Ventricular Defibrillator*

Therapies	Comments
Prevention of atrial fibrillation	
High-rate overdrive DDI pacing (switchback delay)	Goal: prevent early recurrence of atrial arrhythmias after episode termination
	Function: provide a high rate of atrial pacing immediately after termination of atrial tachyarrhythmia episode for a programmable duration
Atrial rate stabilization	Goal: prevent onset of atrial arrhythmia
	Function: prevent long pauses after premature atrial contractions by pacing with a gradually prolonging interval back to the intrinsic or programmed rate (Fig. 7–62)
Termination of atrial tachyarrhythmia	
Atrial antitachycardia pacing	Provides autodecremental bursts at rates typically 10% to 20% faster than the atrial rate to terminate the atrial tachyarrhythmia
Atrial 50-Hz high-frequency burst	Delivers AOO pacing pulses every 20 msec for a programmed duration to interrupt faster atrial arrhythmias
Atrial shock	Delivers a shock over independently programmable electrodes with independently programmable energies to treat atrial tachyarrhythmias

*Ventricular therapies are similar to those in other ventricular defibrillators and include antitachycardia pacing, cardioversion, and defibrillation.

atrial therapy delivery by the independently programmable atrial algorithm. Moreover, since atrial arrhythmias are not immediately life-threatening (in contrast to ventricular arrhythmias), atrial therapies can be restricted to certain times of the day or limited in the number of therapies per day to enhance patient acceptance, as discussed below. There is one important dictum to guide optimal programming of atrial therapies: unlike ventricular arrhythmias, which are treated because they are immediately life-threatening, atrial arrhythmias are treated to improve quality of life and reduce symptoms.

Atrial Detection

Atrial arrhythmias can be classified as atrial tachycardia (AT) or AF, depending on atrial cycle length and regularity (Fig. 7–63). Different therapies are independently programmable for the AT and AF zones. The AT/AF evidence counter is an up-down counter that is augmented when there are two or more P waves in an RR interval and decreased after the second RR interval that has zero or one P wave associated with it. Importantly, detection is specific for greater than 1:1 tachycardias, so that ATs with 1:1 conduction are not detected. The PP median cycle length is used to define the arrhythmia as AT or AF (Fig. 7–63). Episodes are considered terminated with any of the following: (1) The sinus rhythm criterion is satisfied (five consecutive beats with PR pattern of sinus rhythm; AT/AF evidence counter is then reset to zero), (2) the rhythm has not been positively classified as AF or AT for 3 minutes, and (3) a ventricular arrhythmia is detected.

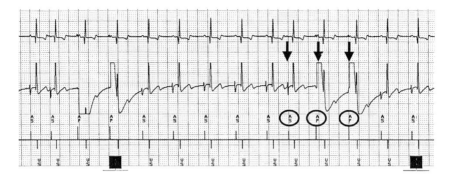

Fig. 7–62. Atrial rate stabilization is designed to prevent atrial fibrillation onset by eliminating pauses after premature atrial complexes (PACs). From top to bottom are shown the surface electrocardiogram, intracardiac electrogram, and markers. A PAC is present and sensed (*first arrow,* circled "AS" on marker channel). To prevent a long pause, two paced beats at gradually prolonging intervals are delivered (circled "AP" markers) until sinus rhythm returns ("AS" following the last "AP").

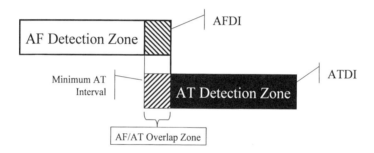

Fig. 7–63. Atrial fibrillation (AF) and atrial tachycardia (AT) detection in the Medtronic 7250 atrial and ventricular defibrillator. AF and AT detection zones are independently programmable, and overlap is permitted. If the median atrial cycle length is in the AF zone and detection achieved (the counter reaches 32), AF is detected; if the median atrial cycle length is in the AT zone when the counter reaches detection, AT is detected. If the median atrial rate is in the overlap zone between AT and AF when the AT/AF evidence counter reaches detection, the device determines whether the episode is AT or AF by the regularity of recent PP intervals (regular PP intervals define AT). AFDI, atrial fibrillation detection interval; ATDI, atrial tachycardia detection interval.

Atrial Therapies

Atrial therapies are independently programmed for AT and AF zones. They include atrial antitachycardia pacing, high-frequency burst pacing, and atrial defibrillation. Antitachycardia pacing (ATP) is available as a burst+ or ramp. Burst+ is a train of pulses delivered at a fixed cycle length that is a percentage of the rate of atrial arrhythmia (e.g., 88%) followed by two premature extrastimuli at the end of the sequence. Ramp begins with a pacing pulse delivered at a coupling interval that is a percentage of the atrial arrhythmia cycle and is followed by a sequence with cycle length decrement within the pulse train. High-frequency burst pacing, on the other hand, delivers a burst of AOO pulses for a programmable duration at very short intervals (20 msec) independent of the arrhythmia cycle length (Fig. 7–64). The rationale for the high-frequency burst is that fast atrial arrhyth-

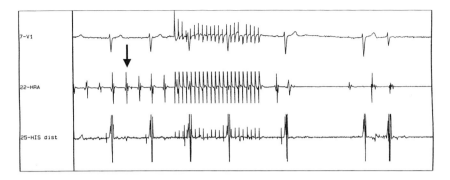

Fig. 7–64. High-frequency burst to terminate intra-atrial arrhythmias. This tracing is from a catheter electrophysiologic study. From top to bottom are surface electrocardiogram lead V_1, intracardiac high-right atrial electrogram (HRA), and His bundle electrogram (HIS dist). An atypical atrial flutter is present (*arrow*). Subsequent to high-frequency burst delivery, sinus rhythm is restored.

mias, such as AF and atypical flutter, may have a small excitable gap (i.e., a short period between tachycardia wave fronts during which the myocardium is excitable), so that pacing at a very high rate may be able to penetrate the gap and terminate the arrhythmia (Fig. 7–65).

Atrial shocks can be delivered by independently programmable pathways, so that electrodes within the lead system

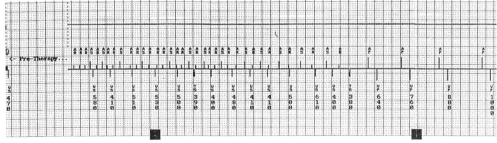

Fig. 7–65. Stored episode from a patient with hypertrophic cardiomyopathy, highly symptomatic atrial fibrillation, and an atrial and ventricular defibrillator (Medtronic 7250). From top to bottom are the electrogram, markers, and intervals. The initial rhythm is atrial fibrillation (top strip; upgoing "FD" marker is atrial fibrillation detect). Subsequent to the delivery of a high-frequency burst (not shown), AV sequential pacing ("AP" and "VP" markers) ensues after several seconds of atrial fibrillation that persisted immediately after the burst.

other than those for ventricular defibrillation can be used. For example, in a given patient, ventricular defibrillation may be programmed to occur between the distal right ventricular coil and the pulse generator can, whereas atrial defibrillation may occur between the proximal right ventricular lead coil and the can. The defibrillation pathways are software-controlled so that they can be modified noninvasively after implantation.

Since, in contrast to VT and VF, atrial fibrillation is not immediately life-threatening, the timing and mode of therapy delivery are highly programmable to tailor therapy to patient and physician preference. Shocks may be automatically delivered by the device or self-administered by the patient by means of a handheld activator. During symptoms, the activator is placed over the pulse generator and a button pressed; if the defibrillator confirms the presence of an atrial arrhythmia, an atrial shock is delivered. Automatic atrial shocks may be restricted by the required arrhythmia duration before shock delivery (to avoid treating short-lived episodes), the time of day during which shocks are available, the total number of shocks de-liverable in a given day or window, and the time at which all atrial therapies are stopped (to prevent late cardioversion of AF with risk of thromboembolism) (Fig. 7–66). Additionally, atrial shocks are restricted from delivery during a user-definable ventricular refractory period (programmable from 350 to 600 msec) to prevent shock on T-wave proarrhythmia.

The clinical performance of the Jewel AF for the treatment of ventricular arrhythmias is similar to that of the Medtronic Gem DR. Only limited data are available on the effectiveness of atrial therapies. In a preliminary study, we analyzed the performance of the atrial therapies in 60 patients who were randomized to have atrial prevention and treatment therapies "on" or "off" for 3 months with subsequent crossover to the opposite arm.[55] All patients had a ventricular ICD indication, and 75% of patients also had a history of atrial arrhythmias. The study end point was atrial tachyarrhythmia burden, which could be accurately determined by the device and which was defined as (total time in AT/AF) ÷ (time with AT/AF therapies "on" or "off"). With prevention and ter-

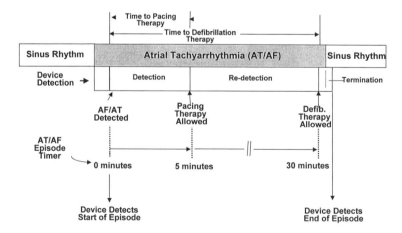

Fig. 7–66. Anatomy of an atrial episode. Once an atrial arrhythmia is detected, the time until therapy is allowed is independently programmable for pacing therapies and for initial pacing therapy or defibrillation. Further programmable restrictions can be applied to shock therapy, such as time of day and total number of shocks per day. Further details in the text.

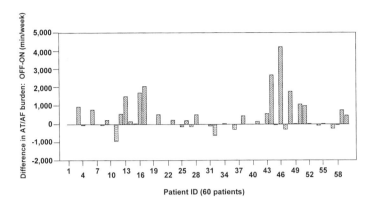

Fig. 7–67. Atrial tachycardia (AT) and atrial fibrillation (AF) burden by individual patient. The abscissa shows the individual patient number, the ordinate the difference in AT/AF burden with atrial prevention and termination therapies "on" and "off." Patients with upgoing bars had a greater atrial arrhythmia burden while therapies were "off" than when they were "on." Patients with downgoing bars had an episode while therapies were programmed "on"; high-frequency burst failed, but no shocks were programmed, so the arrhythmia persisted. Further details in the text.

mination therapies "on," patients had an arrhythmia burden of 115 ± 212 min/week, compared with 436 ± 874 min/week with therapies "off" ($P = 0.05$). The subset of patients who had an increased burden with therapies turned on had their devices programmed to deliver atrial pacing therapies (which failed) without subsequent shocks, so that the episode persisted (Fig. 7–67). Interestingly, painless pacing therapies were

successful for 52% of episodes in this population (Fig. 7–68).

When device therapy is used to treat atrial arrhythmias, the following general principles guide optimal programming. 1. Atrial pacing therapies should be used liberally. Even if efficacy is less than that of shocks, the main treatment goal is improvement in arrhythmia symptoms and quality of life. 2. Shock energies should be programmed to make the first shock

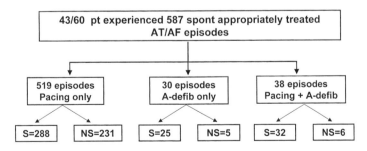

- **Pacing therapy success = 288/(519+38) = 288/557 = 52%**

- A-defib therapy success = (32+25)/(38+30) = 57/68 = 84%

Fig. 7–68. Effectiveness of atrial therapies. The success of arrhythmia termination with atrial therapies was 52%, suggesting that patients were spared shocks for these episodes. NS, not successful; S, successful.

work. In the clinically effective range, pain is more closely correlated with the number of shocks than with the shock strength.[56] 3. Patient preference is critical for effective programming. Some patients may prefer to self-administer pacing therapies (ATP or burst, or both) for treating atrial arrhythmias, typically with no or only brief delay after onset of arrhythmia. Atrial defibrillation is offered after detailed discussion and the option of receiving a test shock in the hospital. The specific approach used for shock delivery depends on the degree of symptoms experienced during arrhythmia and patient comfort with activator use.

Ventricular Therapies

Antitachycardia Pacing

Antitachycardia (overdrive) pacing consists of short bursts of pacing impulses at rates 10% to 20% greater than the tachycardia. It terminates 60% to 90% of arrhythmia episodes, eliminating the need for shocks.[25,57–59] By pacing the ventricle at a rate greater than the tachycardia, some of the pacing impulses may enter the tachycardia circuit and render it refractory, so that the returning tachycardia wave front does not find excitable tissue[60] (further discussed in Chapter 1). Overdrive pacing can be delivered as bursts (all pulses in a sequence at the same rate), as ramps (sequential pulses within a burst delivered at a progressively faster rate), or as a combination, although no scheme has been shown clearly superior to another.[26] In about 10% of patients, ATP may accelerate the arrhythmia,[25,57] which may necessitate proceeding to a more aggressive therapy. Overall, ATP is a very effective and well-tolerated mode of therapy for patients with recurrent stable or semistable monomorphic VT.

Traditionally, noninvasive induction of VT through the defibrillator has been used to tailor ATP therapies, assure that VT is responsive to ATP, and exclude arrhythmia acceleration. However, the need for this testing has never been well supported, and several recent studies have cast doubt upon its usefulness. In assessing the utility of routine VT inductions in the first year after follow-up in 153 recipients of ICD, we found that in patients who did not have inducible VT at baseline electrophysiologic study, the yield of routine additional inductions approximated 0%.[61] In a study of 200 patients, Schaumann et al.[26] compared the use of tested ATP (54 patients) with empirical ATP (146 patients, in 128 of whom monomorphic VT could not be induced). All ATPs were programmed to three scans of an autodecremental ramp with 8 to 10 pulses, 8-msec decrement within burst, cycle length 81% of the detected tachycardia, and minimum pacing interval of 200 msec. ATP was effective in both groups, successfully terminating 95% (4,845 of 5,165) of episodes in the tested group and 90% (1,205 of 1,346) in the empirical group. Although statistically different, the clinically minimal 5% improvement found with testing suggests that empirical therapy is very effective, even in patients without inducible VT. Acceleration after VT was infrequent in both groups: 2.4% in the tested group and 5% in the empirical group. These data suggest that empirical ATP can be safely programmed in most patients without routine testing. Nonetheless, testing should be performed in specific clinical situations (Table 7–12).

Defibrillation

Defibrillation is the mainstay of therapy for VF and rapid VT. Its efficacy in VF termination exceeds 98%.[62,63] Current-generation defibrillators deliver up to between four and eight shocks per episode to ensure arrhythmia termination. Available maximal shock energies

Table 7–12.
Clinical Situations Favoring Inductions of Ventricular Tachycardia
for Defibrillator Testing of Antitachycardia Pacing

- Initiation of or change in antiarrhythmic drug therapy
- Significant change in patient clinical status (myocardial infarction, marked worsening of heart failure)
- Observed proarrhythmia after antitachycardia pacing
- Frequent failure of antitachycardia pacing
- Patient with separate pacemaker and defibrillator
- Significant change in pacing threshold

range from 25 to 42 J in current devices, enough for defibrillation in most patients through an endocardial approach with biphasic waveforms and modern leads. Indeed, the mean energy required for successful defibrillation in current devices is approximately 10 J.[64–66]

To ensure effective defibrillation, the system must be tested at implantation and found to reproducibly terminate induced fibrillation with an energy that is at least 10 J less than the maximal device output.[67,68] If two shocks with a 10-J safety margin are effective, the defibrillator can safely be programmed to deliver maximal output shocks without further testing. Alternatively, if a step-down-to-failure defibrillation threshold is found, the initial shock energy may be programmed to the threshold plus 10 J.[69] This approach has the potential advantage of shorter time to first shock. If defibrillation with a 10-J safety margin cannot be achieved, changes in lead configuration, repositioning of electrodes, or addition of defibrillating elements is required to achieve an acceptable defibrillation threshold.[70] With biphasic waveforms, this approach is infrequently required (3.7% of implantations).[71] Defibrillation threshold testing, safety margins, and waveforms are covered in extensive detail in Chapter 1.

Low-Energy Cardioversion

Many monomorphic VTs are susceptible to low-energy shocks, even if they fail to respond to overdrive pacing. Therefore, for regular tachycardia, particularly with heart rate under 200 bpm, a synchronized shock with energy of 1 to 5 J is often programmed after ATP to spare the patient high-energy (less well tolerated) shocks after failed ATP.[72] Low-energy cardioversion should always be backed up by successive high-energy shocks, because arrhythmia occasionally accelerates.[25,57]

Interactions of Antibradycardia Pacing With Tachycardia Programming

The pacing and tachycardia functions of some defibrillators have interactions that put constraints on available parameters. The most commonly encountered one is related to maximum pacing rates and the slowest tachycardia zone to allow an adequate window for sensing. This interaction is discussed in Chapter 4.

Conclusion

Implantable defibrillators have undergone enormous technical advances since their initial implantation in a human in 1980. With the introduction of many new features, a large number of programmable parameters have been introduced to enable the caregiver to tailor device function to an individual's clinical arrhythmia. With a thorough understanding of defibrillator function, the device can indeed be optimized to provide life-prolonging therapy with minimal morbidity.

References

1. Bernstein AD, Camm AJ, Fletcher RD, Gold RD, Rickards AF, Smyth NP, Spielman SR, Sutton R: The NASPE/BPEG generic pacemaker code for antibradyarrhythmia and adaptive-rate pacing and antitachyarrhythmia devices. Pacing Clin Electrophysiol 10:794–799, 1987
2. Lee MT, Baker R: Circadian rate variation in rate-adaptive pacing systems. Pacing Clin Electrophysiol 13:1797–1801, 1990
3. Rosenqvist M, Vallin HO, Edhag KO: Rate hysteresis pacing: how valuable is it? A comparison of the stimulation rates of 70 and 50 beats per minute and rate hysteresis in patients with sinus node disease. Pacing Clin Electrophysiol 7:332–340, 1984
4. Benditt DG, Sutton R, Gammage MD, Markowitz T, Gorski J, Nygaard GA, Fetter J: Clinical experience with Thera DR rate-drop response pacing algorithm in carotid sinus syndrome and vasovagal syncope. The International Rate-Drop Investigators Group. Pacing Clin Electrophysiol 20:832–839, 1997
5. Gammage MD: Rate-drop response programming. Pacing Clin Electrophysiol 20:841–843, 1997
6. Erickson M, Jensen N: Rate drop response in Medtronic Kappa™ 400 and 700 pacemakers, Medtronic, Inc., 1999
7. Clarke M, Liu B, Schuller H, Binner L, Kennergren C, Guerola M, Weinmann P, Ohm OJ: Automatic adjustment of pacemaker stimulation output correlated with continuously monitored capture thresholds: a multicenter study. European Microny Study Group. Pacing Clin Electrophysiol 21:1567–1575, 1998
8. Hynes JK, Holmes DR Jr, Merideth J, Trusty JM: An evaluation of long-term stimulation thresholds by measurement of chronic strength duration curve. Pacing Clin Electrophysiol 4:376–379, 1981
9. Mond HG: The Cardiac Pacemaker: Function and Malfunction. New York, Grune & Stratton, 1983, p 176
10. Roy PR, Sowton E: Clinical experience with the Elema Vario pacemaker. Br Med J 4:637–640, 1974
11. Sweesy MW, Batey RL, Forney RC: Activation times for "emergency back-up"

12. Preston TA, Bowers DL: The automatic threshold tracking pacemaker. Med Instrum 8:322–325, 1974
13. O'Hara GE, Kristensson B-E, Lundstrom R Jr, Kempen K, Soucy B, Lynn T, on behalf of the worldwide Kappa 700 Investigators: First clinical experience with a new pacemaker with ventricular Capture Management™ feature (abstract). Pacing Clin Electrophysiol 21:892, 1998
14. Lazarus A, Cazeau S, Ritter P, Gras D, Mugica J: Reliability of an automatic sensing test with beat-to-beat display of the signal amplitude. Pacing Clin Electrophysiol 21:1881–1884, 1998
15. Felices Nieto A, Picon Intantes R, Diaz Ortuno F, Gimenez Raurell J, Herrera Rojas D, Lopez Cuervo JF: Loss of integrity of bipolar cardiac stimulation and its automatic correction. Report of 2 cases [Spanish]. Rev Esp Cardiol 47:407–409, 1994
16. Hayes DL: Endless loop tachycardia—the problem has been solved? In New Perspectives in Cardiac Pacing. Edited by SS Barold, J Mugica. Mount Kisco, NY, Futura Publishing Company, 1988, pp 375–386
17. Kutalek SP, Schuster MM, Hessen SE, Sheppard R, Maquilan M, Nydegger C: Clinical experience with a new multiprogrammable dual chamber pacemaker. Pacing Clin Electrophysiol 15:1830–1835, 1992
18. Israel CW, Lemke B: Modern concepts of automatic mode switching. Herz 10 Suppl 1:I/1-I/80, 1999
19. Jones BR, Kim J, Zhu Q, Nelson JP, KenKnight BH, Lang DJ, Warren JA: Future of bradyarrhythmia therapy systems: automaticity. Am J Cardiol 83:192D–201D, 1999
20. Frazier DW, Stanton MS: Pseudo-oversensing of the T wave by an implantable cardioverter defibrillator: a nonclinical problem. Pacing Clin Electrophysiol 17:1311–1315, 1994
21. Perry GY, Kosar EM: Problems in managing patients with long QT syndrome and implantable cardioverter defibrillators: a report of two cases. Pacing Clin Electrophysiol 19:863–867, 1996
22. Friedman PA, Stanton MS: The pacer-cardioverter-defibrillator: function and clinical experience. J Cardiovasc Electrophysiol 6:48–68, 1995
23. Brady PA, Friedman PA, Stanton MS: Effect of failed defibrillation shocks on electrogram amplitude in a nonintegrated

transvenous defibrillation lead system. Am J Cardiol 76:580–584, 1995

24. Olson WH: Dual chamber sensing and detection for implantable cardioverter-defibrillators. *In* Nonpharmacological Therapy of Arrhythmias for the 21st Century: The State of the Art. Edited by I Singer, SS Barold, AJ Camm. Armonk, NY, Futura Publishing Company, 1998, pp 385–421

25. Hammill SC, Packer DL, Stanton MS, Fetter J: Termination and acceleration of ventricular tachycardia with autodecremental pacing, burst pacing, and cardioversion in patients with an implantable cardioverter defibrillator. Multicenter PCD Investigator Group. Pacing Clin Electrophysiol 18:3–10, 1995

26. Schaumann A, von zur Muhlen F, Herse B, Gonska BD, Kreuzer H: Empirical versus tested antitachycardia pacing in implantable cardioverter defibrillators: a prospective study including 200 patients. Circulation 97:66–74, 1998

27. Wood MA, Swerdlow C, Olson WH: Sensing and arrhythmia detection by implantable devices. *In* Clinical Cardiac Pacing and Defibrillation. Second edition. Edited by KA Ellenbogen, GN Kay, BL Wilkoff. Philadelphia, WB Saunders Company, 2000, pp 68–126

28. Grimm W, Flores BF, Marchlinski FE: Electrocardiographically documented unnecessary, spontaneous shocks in 241 patients with implantable cardioverter defibrillators. Pacing Clin Electrophysiol 15:1667–1673, 1992

29. Winkle RA, Mead RH, Ruder MA, Gaudiani VA, Smith NA, Buch WS, Schmidt P, Shipman T: Long-term outcome with the automatic implantable cardioverter-defibrillator. J Am Coll Cardiol 13:1353–1361, 1989

30. Kelly PA, Cannom DS, Garan H, Mirabal GS, Harthorne JW, Hurvitz RJ, Vlahakes GJ, Jacobs ML, Ilvento JP, Buckley MJ, Ruskin JN: The automatic implantable cardioverter-defibrillator: efficacy, complications and survival in patients with malignant ventricular arrhythmias. J Am Coll Cardiol 11:1278–1286, 1988

31. Schmitt C, Montero M, Melichercik J: Significance of supraventricular tachyarrhythmias in patients with implanted pacing cardioverter defibrillators. Pacing Clin Electrophysiol 17:295–302, 1994

32. Brugada J, Mont L, Figueiredo M, Valentino M, Matas M, Navarro-Lopez F: Enhanced detection criteria in implantable defibrilla-

tors. J Cardiovasc Electrophysiol 9:261–268, 1998

33. Swerdlow CD, Ahern T, Chen PS, Hwang C, Gang E, Mandel W, Kass RM, Peter CT: Underdetection of ventricular tachycardia by algorithms to enhance specificity in a tiered-therapy cardioverter-defibrillator. J Am Coll Cardiol 24:416–424, 1994

34. Swerdlow CD, Chen PS, Kass RM, Allard JR, Peter CT: Discrimination of ventricular tachycardia from sinus tachycardia and atrial fibrillation in a tiered-therapy cardioverter-defibrillator. J Am Coll Cardiol 23:1342–1355, 1994

35. Barold HS, Newby KH, Tomassoni G, Kearney M, Brandon J, Natale A: Prospective evaluation of new and old criteria to discriminate between supraventricular and ventricular tachycardia in implantable defibrillators. Pacing Clin Electrophysiol 21:1347–1355, 1998

36. Brachmann J, Swerdlow CD, Mitchell BL, Miller T, van Veen BK, for the Worldwide 7218 KD investigators: Worldwide experience with the electrogram width feature for improved detection in an implantable pacer-cardioverter-defibrillator (abstract). J Am Coll Cardiol 29 (Suppl A):115A, 1997

37. Klingenheben T, Sticherling C, Skupin M, Hohnloser SH: Intracardiac QRS electrogram width—an arrhythmia detection feature for implantable cardioverter defibrillators: exercise induced variation as a base for device programming. Pacing Clin Electrophysiol 21:1609–1617, 1998

38. Schaumann A, von zur Muhlen F, Gonska BD, Kreuzer H: Enhanced detection criteria in implantable cardioverter-defibrillators to avoid inappropriate therapy. Am J Cardiol 78:42–50, 1996

39. Higgins SL, Lee RS, Kramer RL: Stability: an ICD detection criterion for discriminating atrial fibrillation from ventricular tachycardia. J Cardiovasc Electrophysiol 6:1081–1088, 1995

40. Neuzner J, Pitschner HF, Schlepper M: Programmable VT detection enhancements in implantable cardioverter defibrillator therapy. Pacing Clin Electrophysiol 18:539–547, 1995

41. Gillberg JM, Olson WH, Bardy GH, Mader SJ: Electrogram width algorithm for discrimination of supraventricular rhythm from ventricular tachycardia (abstract). Pacing Clin Electrophysiol 17:866, 1994

42. Brachmann J, Seidl K, Hauer B, Hilbel T, Lighezan D, Schoels W, Beyer T, Ruf-Richter J, Schwink N, Senges J, Kübler W:

Intracardiac electrogram width measurement for improved tachycardia discrimination: initial results of a new implantable cardioverter-defibrillator (ICD) (abstract). J Am Coll Cardiol 27:96A, 1996

43. Duru F, Schonbeck M, Luscher TF, Candinas R: The potential for inappropriate ventricular tachycardia confirmation using the Intracardiac Electrogram (EGM) Width Criterion. Pacing Clin Electrophysiol 22:1039–1046, 1999

44. Wilkoff BL, Kühlkamp V, Gillberg JM, Brown AB, Cuijpers A, DeSouza CM, and the 7271 GEM DR Worldwide Investigators: Performance of a dual chamber detection algorithm (PR Logic™) based on the worldwide Gem DR clinical results (abstract). Pacing Clin Electrophysiol 22:720, 1999

45. Swerdlow CD, Gunderson BD, Gillberg JM, Pietersen AH, Volosin KJ, Stadler RW, Olson WH, for the Worldwide Gem DR™ Investigators: Discrimination of concurrent atrial and ventricular tachyarrhythmias from rapidly-conducted atrial arrhythmias by a dual-chamber ICD (abstract). Pacing Clin Electrophysiol 22:775, 1999

46. Lavergne T, Daubert JC, Chauvin M, Dolla E, Kacet S, Leenhardt A, Mabo P, Ritter P, Sadoul N, Saoudi N, Henry C, Nitzsche R, Ripart A, Murgatroyd F: Preliminary clinical experience with the first dual chamber pacemaker defibrillator. Pacing Clin Electrophysiol 20:182–188, 1997

47. Kühlkamp V, Dörnberger V, Mewis C, Suchalla R, Bosch RF, Seipel L: Clinical experience with the new detection algorithms for atrial fibrillation of a defibrillator with dual chamber sensing and pacing. J Cardiovasc Electrophysiol 10:905–915, 1999

48. Li HG, Thakur RK, Yee R, Klein GJ: Ventriculoatrial conduction in patients with implantable cardioverter defibrillators: implications for tachycardia discrimination by dual chamber sensing. Pacing Clin Electrophysiol 17:2304–2306, 1994

49. Militianu A, Salacata A, Meissner MD, Grill C, Mahmud R, Palti AJ, Ben David J, Mosteller R, Lessmeier TJ, Baga JJ, Pires LA, Schuger CD, Steinman RT, Lehmann MH: Ventriculoatrial conduction capability and prevalence of 1:1 retrograde conduction during inducible sustained monomorphic ventricular tachycardia in 305 implantable cardioverter defibrillator recipients. Pacing Clin Electrophysiol 20:2378–2384, 1997

50. Nair M, Saoudi N, Kroiss D, Letac B: Automatic arrhythmia identification using analysis of the atrioventricular association. Application to a new generation of implantable defibrillators. Participating Centers of the Automatic Recognition of Arrhythmia Study Group. Circulation 95:967–973, 1997

51. Swerdlow CD, Sheth NV, Olson WH, for the Worldwide Jewel AF Investigators: Clinical performance of a pattern-based, dual-chamber algorithm for discrimination of ventricular from supraventricular arrhythmias (abstract). Pacing Clin Electrophysiol 21:800, 1998

52. Dorian P, Newman D, Thibault B, Philippon F, Kimber S: A randomized clinical trial of a standardized protocol for the prevention of inappropriate therapy using a dual chamber implantable cardioverter defibrillator (abstract). Circulation 100 Suppl I:I-786, 1999

53. Korte T, Jung W, Wolpert C, Spehl S, Schumacher B, Esmailzadeh B, Luderitz B: A new classification algorithm for discrimination of ventricular from supraventricular tachycardia in a dual chamber implantable cardioverter defibrillator. J Cardiovasc Electrophysiol 9:70–73, 1998

54. Swerdlow C, Sheth N, Olson W: Clinical performance of a pattern-based, dual chamber algorithm for discrimination of ventricular from supraventricular arrhythmias. Pacing Clin Electrophysiol (in press)

55. Friedman PA, Stein KM, Wharton JM, Hammill SC: Reduced atrial fibrillation burden with prompt treatment by an implantable arrhythmia management device: evidence of reverse remodelling? (Abstract.) Circulation 100 Suppl I:I-69, 1999

56. Jung J, Heisel A, Fries R, Kollner V: Tolerability of internal low-energy shock strengths currently needed for endocardial atrial cardioversion. Am J Cardiol 80:1489–1490, 1997

57. Bardy GH, Poole JE, Kudenchuk PJ, Dolack GL, Kelso D, Mitchell R: A prospective randomized repeat-crossover comparison of antitachycardia pacing with low-energy cardioversion. Circulation 87:1889–1896, 1993

58. Calkins H, el-Atassi R, Kalbfleisch S, Langberg J, Morady F: Comparison of fixed burst versus decremental burst pacing for termination of ventricular tachycardia. Pacing Clin Electrophysiol 16:26–32, 1993

59. Wietholt D, Block M, Isbruch F, Bocker D, Borggrefe M, Shenasa M, Breithardt G: Clinical experience with antitachycardia pacing and improved detection algorithms

in a new implantable cardioverter-defibrillator. J Am Coll Cardiol 21:885–894, 1993

60. Josephson ME: Clinical Cardiac Electrophysiology: Techniques and Interpretation. Second edition. Philadelphia, Lea & Febiger, 1993, pp 417–615

61. Glikson M, Luria D, Friedman PA, Trusty JM, Benderly M, Hammill SC, Stanton MS: Are routine arrhythmia inductions necessary in patients with pectoral implantable cardioverter defibrillators? J Cardiovasc Electrophysiol 11:127–135, 2000

62. Pacifico A, Johnson JW, Stanton MS, Steinhaus DM, Gabler R, Church T, Henry PD: Comparison of results in two implantable defibrillators. Jewel 7219D Investigators. Am J Cardiol 82:875–880, 1998

63. Hoffmann E, Steinbeck G: Experience with pectoral versus abdominal implantation of a small defibrillator. A multicenter comparison in 778 patients. European Jewel Investigators. Eur Heart J 19:1085–1098, 1998

64. Sticherling C, Klingenheben T, Cameron D, Hohnloser SH: Worldwide clinical experience with a down-sized active can implantable cardioverter defibrillator in 162 consecutive patients. Worldwide 7221 ICD Investigators. Pacing Clin Electrophysiol 21:1778–1783, 1998

65. Mehdirad AA, Love CJ, Stanton MS, Strickberger SA, Duncan JL, Kroll MW: Preliminary clinical results of a biphasic waveform and an RV lead system. Pacing Clin Electrophysiol 22:594–599, 1999

66. Boriani G, Frabetti L, Biffi M, Sallusti L: Clinical experience with downsized lower energy output implantable cardioverter defibrillators. Ventak Mini II Clinical Investigators. Int J Cardiol 66:261–266, 1998

67. Neuzner J, Liebrich A, Jung J, Himmrich E, Pitschner HF, Winter J, Vester EG, Michel U, Nisam S, Heisel A: Safety and efficacy of implantable defibrillator therapy with programmed shock energy at twice the augmented step-down defibrillation threshold: results of the prospective, randomized, multicenter Low-Energy Endotak Trial. Am J Cardiol 83:34D–39D, 1999

68. Fotuhi PC, Epstein AE, Ideker RE: Energy levels for defibrillation: what is of real clinical importance? Am J Cardiol 83:24D–33D, 1999

69. Strickberger SA, Daoud EG, Davidson T, Weiss R, Bogun F, Knight BP, Bahu M, Goyal R, Man KC, Morady F: Probability of successful defibrillation at multiples of the defibrillation energy requirement in patients with an implantable defibrillator. Circulation 96:1217–1223, 1997

70. Friedman PA, Rasmussen MJ, Grice S, Trusty J, Glikson M, Stanton MS: Defibrillation thresholds are increased by right-sided implantation of totally transvenous implantable cardioverter defibrillators. Pacing Clin Electrophysiol 22:1186–1192, 1999

71. Trusty JM, Hayes DL, Stanton MS, Friedman PA: Factors affecting the frequency of subcutaneous lead usage in implantable defibrillators. Pacing Clin Electrophysiol 23:842–846, 2000

72. Ammer R, Alt E, Ayers G, Lehmann G, Schmitt C, Pasquantonio J, Putter K, Schmidt M, Schomig A: Pain threshold for low energy intracardiac cardioversion of atrial fibrillation with low or no sedation. Pacing Clin Electrophysiol 20:230–236, 1997

8

Rate-Adaptive Pacing

David L. Hayes, M.D.

When rate-adaptive pacing was introduced in the mid-1980s, it was rapidly embraced by clinicians. In the United States, it is estimated that more than 70% of pacemakers currently implanted have rate-adaptive pacing capability.

In the early single-chamber rate-adaptive (AAIR, VVIR) pacemaker era, investigators were quick to demonstrate hemodynamic advantages of rate-adaptive modes, that is, VVIR versus VVI and AAIR versus AAI.[1] Similarly, when dual-chamber rate-adaptive pacing was introduced later in the 1980s, literature emerged demonstrating hemodynamic superiority of DDDR over DDD in the chronotropically incompetent patient. Although there are other benefits of rate-adaptive pacing, correcting the chronotropic response remains the most important.

Indications for Rate-Adaptive Pacing

The indications for rate-adaptive pacing are relatively straightforward (also reviewed in Chapter 3). VVIR pacing is indicated primarily for the patient with chronic atrial fibrillation and a slow ventricular response that requires bradycardia support. AAIR, not widely used, is appropriate for the patient with sinus node dysfunction and intact atrioventricular (AV) node conduction. Even though a significant number of patients require permanent pacing for sinus node dysfunction, many clinicians remain uncomfortable with a system that does not provide ventricular pacing support.

Chronotropic incompetence also remains the primary indication for DDDR pacing. However, DDDR can be considered for any patient requiring dual-chamber pacing because it provides clinical flexibility. For example, should atrial fibrillation develop in a patient with a DDDR pacemaker, the pacemaker can be programmed to VVIR. In addition, if the patient has symptoms with traditional DDD upper rate response, that is, symptomatic 2:1 AV block, optimal programming of sensor response in a DDDR pacemaker may provide "sensor-driven rate-smoothing."[2]

In a review of our practice, we found that of all patients receiving pacemakers capable of DDDR pacing, only half were being dismissed from the hospital with a rate-adaptive pacing mode in effect. During follow-up, however, 18% of the patients required programming to a different pacing mode, and the DDDR pacemaker provided the necessary programmable flexibility to meet the patients' changing clinical needs.

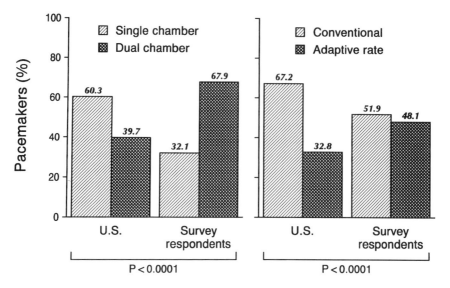

Fig. 8–1. United States use of rate-adaptive and non-rate-adaptive (conventional) pacemakers, 1998 data. The bars labeled "U.S." represent industry-based data on total pacemakers distributed in 1998. Industry estimates of the type of pacemaker used differ significantly from those of physicians responding to the survey. (From Bernstein and Parsonnet.[3] By permission of Excerpta Medica.)

Prescribing practices for rate-adaptive pacemakers appear to vary with the level of the implanter's experience. Utilization of rate-adaptive pacemakers is shown in Figure 8–1. This figure, from a survey of U.S. pacing practices by Bernstein and Parsonnet,[3] contrasts two sources of information. Industry estimates of rate-adaptive pacemaker utilization are less than those of survey respondents. This suggests that survey respondents, generally thought to have a greater interest and level of experience in cardiac pacing, tended to use rate-adaptive pacemakers more frequently.

Sensors Available for Rate-Adaptive Pacing

In an effort to classify sensors on the basis of their response to physiologic variables, Rossi[4] divided sensors into five orders (Table 8–1). Sensors can also be classified as open- or closed-loop (Fig. 8–2). All commercially available sensors are open-loop sensors in that the parameter being sensed requires input externally to optimize sensor response, and the sensor is unable to react appropriately to stimuli that do not affect the specific sensor. Conversely, a closed-loop system ideally does not require external input or manipulation because intrinsic feedback to the sensor self-regulates its response. The ideal closed-loop sensor responds to emotional as well as physical stress. Rate-adaptive sensors that respond to noncardiac signals generally have minimal response to emotional or psychologic stress. Characteristics of the ideal sensor are listed in Table 8–2.

A variety of sensors appropriate for rate-adaptive pacing have been developed; they are displayed in Figure 8–3 as end points of some physiologic response. Some of these sensors are clinically available, others are undergoing clinical in-

Table 8–1.
Classification of Sensors by Response to Physiologic Variables

Order	Description	Physiologic variable
First	A sensor that directly measures oxygen consumption or energy expenditure	Oxygen uptake
Second	A sensor with a linear relationship to sensors of the first order	Cardiac output, minute ventilation,* atrioventricular oxygen difference
Third	A sensor with a linear relationship to sensors of the second order	Heart rate,* stroke volume,† mixed oxygen saturation,† respiratory rate,* tidal volume
Fourth	A sensor that relies on changes in sympathetic activity and circulating catecholamines	QT interval,* right ventricular dP/dt,† preejection interval,† ventricular depolarization gradient†
Fifth	A sensor that responds to physiologic feedback from metabolic activity or receptor reflexes	Central venous pH, central venous temperature,* right atrial pressure,† mixed venous lactate and bicarbonate levels

*Available clinically in the United States or Europe.
†Under investigation.
Data from Rossi.[4]

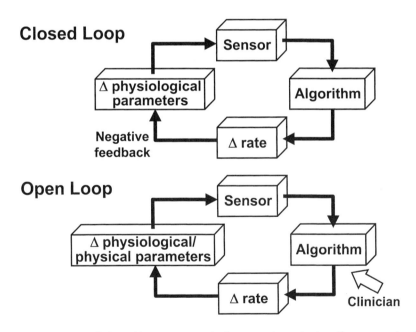

Fig. 8–2. Open-loop and closed-loop sensors. In the open-loop design, the parameter detected by the sensor is translated to a change in rate by use of an algorithm. Altering or optimizing the sensor requires input by the clinician. The rate change that results from the sensor activation does not have any negative feedback effect on the parameter that is being sensed. In the closed-loop design, the physiologic parameter detected by the sensor is translated to a change in rate by use of an algorithm. However, the rate change resulting from sensor activation results in a change in the physiologic parameter in the opposite direction, that is, a negative feedback loop. For a true closed-loop sensor, clinician input should not be necessary; that is, the ideal physiologic parameter that responds proportionally to all forms of stress should not need external input or manipulation by the clinician.

Table 8–2.
Characteristics of the Ideal Rate-Adaptive Sensor

- *Proportional* to the level of metabolic demand
- *Speed of response* is appropriate to the onset and offset of metabolic demand
- *Sensitive* enough to detect both exercise and nonexercise (emotional) needs for rate increase
- *Specific* enough not to be influenced by signals not representing metabolic demand
- *Standard pacing lead* supports the rate-adaptive pacing system
- *Stability* of sensor in the long term
- *Easy* to program

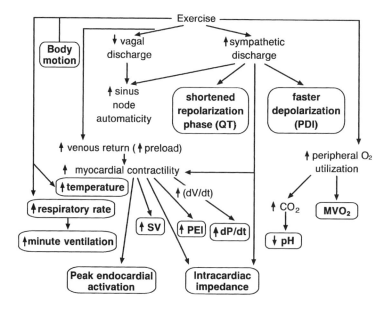

Fig. 8–3. Physiologic responses that have been investigated or clinically used for rate adaptation of permanent pacemakers. The boxed terms represent the end points used for rate adaptation. PDI, paced depolarization integral; PEI, preejection interval; MVO_2, myocardial oxygen consumption; SV, stroke volume.

vestigation or are available outside the United States, and others have previously been investigated and subsequently abandoned. Even though some sensors may never have been clinically released as single-sensor rate-adaptive pacing systems, for example, ventricular depolarization gradient and dP/dt, they may eventually be used as part of a multisensor pacing system.

Three varieties of sensors account for most rate-adaptive pacing systems worldwide. Activity sensing and minute ventilation have been the primary rate-adaptive pacing systems in the United States and have also been widely used throughout the world. In Europe, stimulus-T, or QT, sensing pacemakers have been used extensively as well.

Activity Sensors

Activity-controlled pacing with vibration detection (piezoelectric crystal or accelerometer) is currently the most widely used form of rate adaptation because it is simple, easy to apply clinically, and rapid in onset of rate response (Fig. 8–4).

The main difference between the piezoelectric crystal sensor and the accelerometer is that the crystal senses vibration from up-and-down motion and the accelerometer senses in addition anterior and posterior motion. Accelerometer-based systems may respond more appropriately to specific activities, such as cycling. For example, the typical cyclist may not generate much vibratory sensation above the trunk level. Therefore, a rate-adaptive pacemaker based on a piezoelectric crystal may have a limited response in the patient riding a bicycle. However, since the accelerometer senses anterior and posterior motion, it may be more responsive to such an activity.

Other than for a specific activity such as cycling, the debate continues about whether, in general, accelerometer-based activity sensing has any significant and demonstrable advantage over sensing based on the piezoelectric crystal. On balance, the literature suggests a slight advantage for accelerometer-based activity sensing.[5–7] The accelerometer has two main potential advantages. The first is improvement of the specificity of sensor response, that is, in avoiding inappropriate responses. The second is a tendency to a more physiologic heart rate response and lesser response to local pressure and tapping. Rhythmic body motion such as that produced by walking or bicycle riding is typically in the range of 1 to 8 Hz.[8] Non-exercise-related vibrations that arise from such sources as riding in a car or from nonspecific skeletal muscle noise are often greater than 10 Hz. The accelerometer, which limits analysis of signals to the 1- to 10-Hz range, should be more specific in its response to activity.

Although there have been subsequent variations of activity sensors, including a

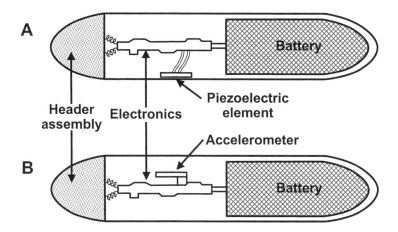

Fig. 8–4. Schematic drawings of how activity sensors are positioned within the pulse generator. *A,* The piezoelectric sensor is bonded to the inside surface of the pacemaker can and senses tissue vibration from mechanical forces transmitted by the surrounding tissues. *B,* An accelerometer is mounted on the hybrid circuitry of the pacemaker and is structurally insulated from the pacemaker can, that is, independent of the mechanical forces of the surrounding tissue but dependent on patient motion. Signals can be processed by "peak counting" or acceleration integration. Acceleration integration achieved with the accelerometer allows all signals to be used to determine the level of rate response, because there is no amplitude threshold that must be exceeded. (From Millerhagen JO, Combs WJ: Activity sensing and accelerometer-based pacemakers. *In* Clinical Cardiac Pacing and Defibrillation. Second edition. Edited by KA Ellenbogen, GN Kay, BL Wilkoff. Philadelphia, WB Saunders Company, 2000, pp 249–270. By permission of the publisher.)

gravitational sensor able to discriminate changes in vertical gravitational acceleration and a moving magnetic ball that measures electrical signals, none has had the clinical success of the piezoelectric crystal and accelerometer.

Minute-Ventilation Sensors

Minute volume (respiratory rate times tidal volume) has an excellent correlation with metabolic demand. In a rate-adaptive pacing system, measurement of minute volume is accomplished by emission of a small charge of known current (1 mA every 15 msec) from the pacemaker and measurement of the resulting voltage at the lead tip[9] (Fig. 8–5). When both current and voltage are known, transthoracic impedance can be measured between the ring electrode and the pacemaker can. Because transthoracic impedance varies with respiration and its amplitude varies with tidal volume, the impedance measurement can be used to determine respiratory rate and tidal volume, which in turn can be used to alter pacing rate. Long-term reliability of the minute-volume sensor has been excellent.

Stimulus-T, or QT, Sensing Pacemaker

The interval from the onset of a paced QRS complex to the end of the T wave has been used for rate adaptation for many years. Autonomic activity and heart rate affect this stimulus-T interval[10] (Fig. 8–6). Because of this relationship, measurement of the stimulus-T interval can be used for rate adaptation. The QT-

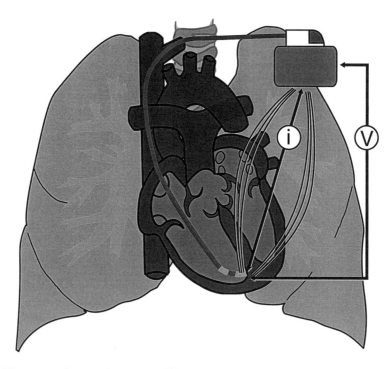

Fig. 8–5. The pacemaker sends a current (i) between the ring electrode and the pacemaker can. The sensor detects voltage (V) modulations between the tip electrode and the indifferent electrode on the pacemaker header that occur as a result of changes in transthoracic impedance.

At Rest   During Exercise

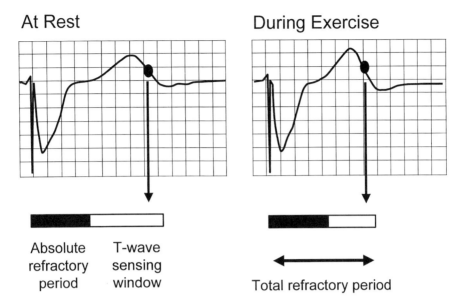

| Absolute refractory period | T-wave sensing window |

Total refractory period

Fig. 8–6. The QT sensor, or stimulus-T sensor, depends on evoked endocardial T-wave sensing. The maximum slope of the evoked T wave is sensed, T-wave sensing ends, and QRS sensing is initiated after a short interval, approximately 25 msec. During exercise, the stimulus-T interval shortens. Stimuli other than exercise may also affect the stimulus-T duration. The changes in stimulus-T duration can be used to drive an algorithm to adapt the pacing rate. (From Connelly and Rickards.[10] By permission of WB Saunders Company.)

sensing rate-adaptive pacing system has been very successful clinically.

Temperature Sensors

Because central venous temperature increases with exercise, it is reasonable to consider this factor as the basis for a physiologic sensor. The increase in temperature can be measured by a thermistor contained within the right ventricular portion of the pacing lead. At the onset of exercise, core body temperature decreases as cooler peripheral blood is returned to the central circulation.

Temperature-sensing rate-adaptive pacemakers have been available for many years but have never gained widespread acceptance, in part because a special pacing lead is required but also because the relatively slow response of central venous temperature as a variable results in

a less adequate rate response at low workloads.

Other Sensors

Several intracardiac impedance-based indicators can be used as rate-adaptive sensors.[11] The *preejection interval* is the systolic interval from the onset of electrical ventricular depolarization to the onset of ventricular ejection (Fig. 8–7). For ventricular pacing, the preejection interval is the interval between a right ventricular pacing stimulus and the onset of contraction determined by an impedance catheter. The preejection interval shortens as exercise workload increases, and this effect can be used as a signal to increase the pacing rate. An increase in heart rate does not appreciably affect the preejection interval; that is, no significant positive feedback occurs. *Stroke volume*, also measured by an

INTRACARDIAC SENSOR SIGNAL

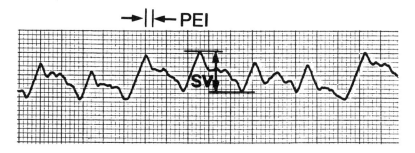

Fig. 8–7. Waveform obtained from a rate-adaptive pacemaker that utilized a sensor to measure preejection interval (PEI) and stroke volume (SV). PEI is defined as a right heart analogue of the preejection period, which also includes a portion of the ejection time. The SV was calculated as the relative difference between end-diastolic and end-systolic volumes.

impedance catheter in the right ventricle, can be used for rate-adaptive pacing by incorporation of a pacing algorithm that alters the pacing rate to keep the right ventricular stroke volume relatively constant and within physiologic values.

Change in right ventricular pressure, dP/dt, has been used for rate-adaptive pacing. This change is measured by a pressure transducer incorporated in the right ventricular portion of the pacing lead.[12] In clinical investigations and in follow-up, the sensor has performed very well.

In healthy persons, the autonomic nervous system adjusts cardiac output to meet hemodynamic and metabolic requirements. Even in persons with chronotropic insufficiency, the autonomic nervous system controls the performance of the heart through changes in myocardial contractility. One rate-adaptive pacing system evaluates changes in myocardial contractility to restore chronotropic competence in an attempt to reestablish closed-loop cardiovascular regulation (Fig. 8–8). This sensor technology measures the unipo-lar intracardiac impedance signal to assess wall motion in the vicinity of the electrode tip located in the ventricle. Changes in myocardial contractility are thus mapped to the time course of the impedance signal as a shift of the intracardiac impedance signal and are used to derive a rate-control parameter that assesses the beat-by-beat changes in contraction dynamics to reestablish a normal chronotropic response. The control parameter derived with use of this sensor principle has been shown to correlate very well with established measures of myocardial contractility.[13]

Mixed venous oxygen saturation, measured by hemoreflectance oximetry, varies with physical activity and changes rapidly with the onset of exercise[14] (Fig. 8–9). For a rate-adaptive pacing system, the oximeter is incorporated in the right ventricular portion of the pacing lead. There is concern about long-term reliability of the sensor.[15]

Paced depolarization integral refers to the vector integral of the paced QRS, or ventricular depolarization gradient (VDG).[16] During fixed-rate ventricular pacing, exercise and the effect of circulating catecholamines decrease the VDG. An increase in pacing rate increases the VDG. In a normal heart, therefore, the VDG should remain relatively unchanged during exercise and other forms of stress, representing a closed-loop rate-adaptive pacing system.

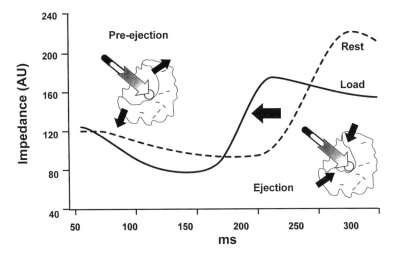

Fig. 8–8. Schematic representation of how changes in myocardial contractility are mapped to the time course of an impedance signal as a shift of the intracardiac impedance signal and used to derive a rate control parameter to assess the beat-by-beat changes in cardiac contraction. ms, milliseconds; a.u., arbitrary units for impedance. (Reproduced with permission from Biotronik.)

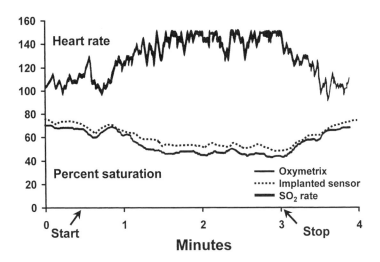

Fig. 8–9. Effect of exercise on right ventricular oxygen saturation measured by a permanently implanted rate-adaptive pacing system recording myocardial oxygen consumption in a canine. (Reproduced with permission from St. Jude Medical.)

Newer Sensors

Of significant interest is monitoring of autonomic activity and use of this information as the basis for a rate-adaptive pacing system. Some aspects of autonomic monitoring are a part of stimulus-T sensing pacemakers and pacemakers incorporating paced depolarization integral (VDG), both of which have been previously described.

Another newer rate-adaptive pacing system, *peak endocardial acceleration,* incorporates a microaccelerometer in the tip of a normal endocardial pacing lead.[17] Peak endocardial acceleration can be correlated with maximum dP/dt and should therefore represent the heart's contractile function (Fig. 8–10 and 8–11). As a potential indicator of the initial increase in sympathetic activity that is believed to precede symptomatic hypotension in patients with malignant neurocardiogenic syncope, peak endocardial acceleration could theoretically allow earlier pacing intervention[18] (Fig. 8–12).

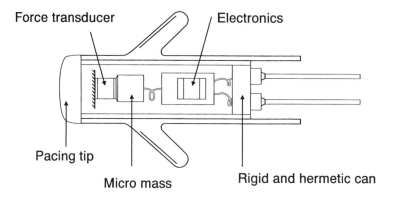

Fig. 8–10. Peak endocardial acceleration pacing system. The sensor is a microaccelerometer housed inside a rigid, perfectly hermetic capsule within the distal portion of the lead. An associated electronic circuit preprocesses the signal to ensure its correct transmission through the catheter. The rigidity of the capsule allegedly makes the sensor totally insensitive to ventricular pressures and to fibrosis on the lead tip, so that the sensor is sensitive only to the inertial forces generated by myocardial movement.

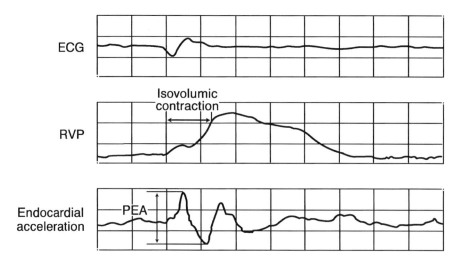

Fig. 8–11. Simultaneous electrocardiogram (ECG), right ventricular pressure (RVP) curve, and peak endocardial acceleration (PEA) waveform. The PEA is represented by the peak-to-peak value of the endocardial acceleration signal measured inside a time window containing the isovolumic contraction phase. (Reproduced with permission from Sorin Biomedica.)

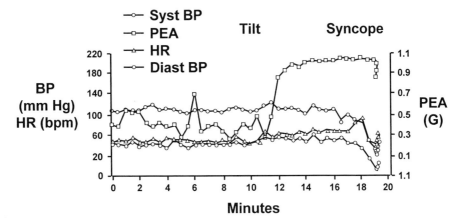

Fig. 8–12. Blood pressure (BP), heart rate (HR), and peak endocardial acceleration (PEA) measurements from a patient undergoing tilt testing for presumed neurocardiogenic syncope. The PEA increases dramatically at approximately 11 minutes. The patient subsequently has typical symptoms accompanied by a decrease in BP and HR approximately 7 minutes later. Reacting to the earlier increase in PEA has been shown in some patients to prevent or minimize the subsequent vasodepression. (Modified from Deharo et al.[18] By permission of Futura Publishing Company.)

Dual-Sensor Rate-Adaptive Pacing

The overall performance of market-approved single-sensor rate-adaptive systems has been excellent. However, the perfect sensor would mimic the response of the normal sinus node at all levels of activity and during emotional stress and would be resistant to nonphysiologic stimuli. Although some closed-loop physiologic sensors could potentially be at or near 100% specificity, none is available clinically.

A multisensor rate-adaptive pacing system could improve specificity by having one sensor verify or cross-check the other.[19,20] For example, a dual-sensor pacemaker could be designed so that if sensor 1 indicated a rate response to a given stimulus but sensor 2 indicated that a rate increase was inappropriate, no rate increase would occur. Both sensors would have to indicate a rate increase before it would be allowed (Fig. 8–13).

Because some sensors perform in a more physiologic manner at low levels of exercise and others perform in a more physiologic manner at high levels of exercise, a combination of two or more sensors could better simulate the normal sinus node response. A multisensor study, well ahead of its time, was performed by Stangl et al.[21] Seven different sensors were compared in 12 control patients with normal sinus rhythm. The system was designed as a transvenous temporary pacing system, and the patients exercised using bicycle ergometry. Several potential sensor combinations were used after rate response was analyzed at low and high workloads to find complementary combinations that could mimic normal sinus rhythm better than any single sensor.

When more than one sensor is available, the programming must remain relatively simple. Although there should be options for choosing one sensor or both, if both sensors are used, the pacemaker must be capable of blending or mixing

QT interval

		Rate ↑	Rate ↓
Activity	**Rate ↑**	Exercise confirmed Increase pacing rate	Exercise NOT confirmed False-positive activity sensing Ignore activity sensor
	Rate ↓	Emotional or isometric stress confirmed Limited increase in pacing rate	Recovery confirmed Decrease pacing rate

Fig. 8–13. Diagram demonstrating the logic involved in sensor cross-checking. Sensors must be in agreement on the appropriateness of a rate increase for any change in the paced rate to occur. (Modified and reproduced with permission from Vitatron.)

their responses (Fig. 8–14). Current pacemakers with dual sensors are listed in Table 8–3. At this time, dual-sensor technology is not an option in implantable cardioverter-defibrillators.

During initial clinical evaluation of single-sensor rate-adaptive pacemakers, the clinical advantages of rate adaptation over fixed-rate pacing in the chronotropically incompetent patient were easily and repeatedly demonstrated. To date, the clinical superiority of dual-sensor rate-adaptive pacing systems is less well proven.

What can be stated definitively about dual-sensor rate-adaptive pacing systems?

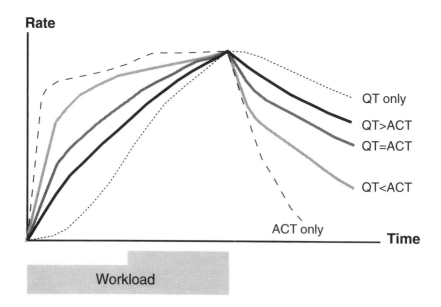

Fig. 8–14. Effects of sensor blending on the rate response of a Vitatron dual-sensor (QT and activity [ACT]) pacemaker. (Reproduced with permission from Vitatron.)

Table 8–3.
Pacemakers With Dual Sensors

Sensors	Company	Modes
Minute ventilation and activity (piezoelectric crystal)	Medtronic	DDDR, DVIR, DDIR, VDIR, VVIR, AAIR, ADIR
QT interval and activity (piezoelectric crystal)	Vitatron	DDDR, DDIR, VDDR, VVIR, AAIR
Gravitational accelerometer and microaccelerometer (PEA)	Sorin Biomedica	DDDR, VDDR, DDIR, DVIR, VVIR, VVTR, AAIR, AATR
PDI and minute ventilation	Telectronics*	VVIR

PDI, paced depolarization integral; PEA, peak endocardial acceleration.

*This device is not currently available; whether it will be further investigated or marketed in the future is not clear.

It seems clear that sensor cross-checking will prevent inappropriate false-positive rate response if complementary sensors are used. It also seems likely that a dual-sensor pacemaker will be more expensive than a single-sensor pacemaker. Another disadvantage is that increased current drain probably needed for dual-sensor activities may compromise battery longevity.

Improving Sensor Automaticity

With the earliest activity-sensing pacemakers, the sensor at times needed to be reprogrammed at a later date because the pocket matured and the patient's exercise capabilities improved after chronotropic response was restored. Minute-ventilation sensor-driven pacemakers also required reprogramming in some patients as conditioning improved.

In the current generation of rate-adaptive pacemakers, both single- and dual-sensor systems, an increasing degree of automaticity assists in programming and optimization of sensor function.[22,23]

Many rate-adaptive pacemakers provide histograms of achieved sensor-driven paced rates to assist in reprogramming of the sensor variables in an effort to optimize chronotropic response[24] (Fig. 8–15

and 8–16). Some pacemakers display sinus-achieved heart rates as well as raw or passive sensor data, that is, how the sensor would have responded had it been activated (Fig. 8–17). Still others provide autocalibration of the sensor, adjusting sensor activity against patient activity levels as determined by maximum and minimum sensor values over a given time (Fig. 8–18).

Programming and Practical Clinical Considerations

As sensor technology has matured, programming has become much simpler. However, one basic tenet persists: *Every patient with a pacemaker programmed to a rate-adaptive pacing mode MUST be functionally assessed, in some way, to determine that the functional response to the sensor is appropriate.* Despite autocalibration or autoprogramming of the sensor, there must be a clinical determination that the sensor response is appropriate, or perhaps more importantly, that the sensor response is not inappropriate. For example, there have been multiple reports of patients who had anginal symptoms unmasked by restoration of chronotropic competence. Such a clinical response to rate-adaptive pacing should ideally be detected before the patient is sent home. Therefore, after programming to a rate-adaptive pacing

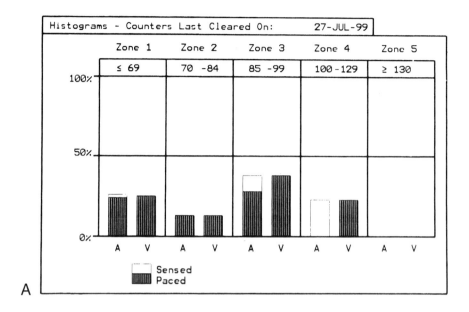

A

Counters Last Cleared On:						
	Totals	Zone 1 ≤69	Zone 2 70-84	Zone 3 85-99	Zone 4 100-129	Zone 5 ≥130
ATRIUM						
Paced	3.2M	2.6M	484.9K	111.1K	1.6K	1.6K
	81%	66%	12%	3%	0%	0%
Sensed	776.0K	491.9K	236.4K	41.3K	5.4K	1.1K
	19%	12%	6%	1%	0%	0%
VENTRICLE						
Paced	4.0M	3.1M	728.2K	156.5K	16.9K	0
	99%	77%	18%	4%	0%	0%
Sensed	25.6K	881	8.0K	5.4K	9.9K	1.5K
	1%	0%	0%	0%	0%	0%

Lifetime Counters						
	Totals	Zone 1 ≤69	Zone 2 70-84	Zone 3 85-99	Zone 4 100-129	Zone 5 ≥130
ATRIUM						
Paced	3.2M	2.6M	484.9K	111.1K	1.6K	1.6K
	81%	66%	12%	3%	0%	0%
Sensed	776.0K	491.9K	236.4K	41.3K	5.4K	1.1K
	19%	12%	6%	1%	0%	0%
VENTRICLE						
Paced	4.0M	3.1M	728.2K	156.5K	16.9K	0
	99%	77%	18%	4%	0%	0%
Sensed	25.6K	881	8.0K	5.4K	9.9K	1.5K
	1%	0%	0%	0%	0%	0%

B

Fig. 8–15. Rate histograms from a DDDR pacemaker. *A,* Presentation as a bar diagram. The histogram displays rates achieved since the counters were last cleared and the percentage of time the atrium (A) and ventricle (V) were paced or sensed in each of the rate bins. In this example, rates were primarily sensor-driven, that is, atrially placed, in all rate bins except the highest rate bin of 100 to 129 bpm. In this bin, only atrial sensing occurred. *B,* Presentation in a tabular format. The pacemaker provides not only data since the time the counters were last cleared but also "lifetime counters" data. In this example, the data from both halves of the chart are identical because this was the first interrogation after implantation.

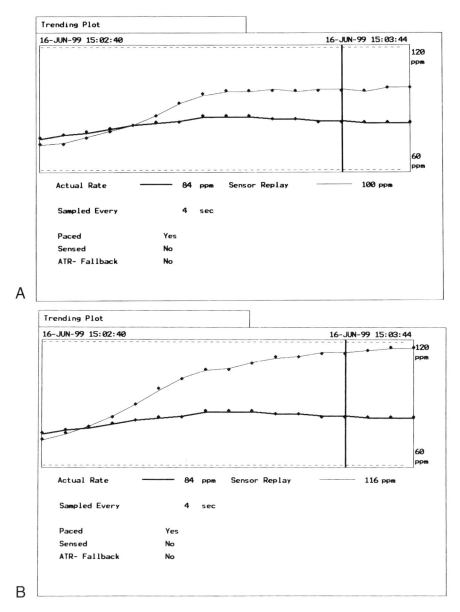

Fig. 8–16. Trending plots from a DDDR pacemaker. *A,* With a brisk walk, the patient achieved a maximal rate of 84 bpm, as shown by the darker line. Different sensor variables can be entered, and the rate trend is redrawn to depict what rates would have been achieved with the new sensor settings. In this example, a rate of 100 bpm would have been achieved. *B,* In the same patient, a higher rate response was desired with a brisk walk. When the trending plot was redrawn with more aggressive rate-adaptive programming, the projected maximal rate was 120 bpm.

Sensor Indicated Rate Histogram

Sensor	Passive
Base Rate	60 ppm
Max Sensor Rate	110 ppm
Slope	8 Normal
Threshold	2.0
Measured Average Sensor	2.6
Reaction Time	Fast
Recovery Time	Medium

Date Read:	Mar 25 1999 10:03 am
Total Time Sampled:	203d 1h 35m 31s
Sampling Rate	1.6s

Note: The above values were obtained when the histogram was interrogated.

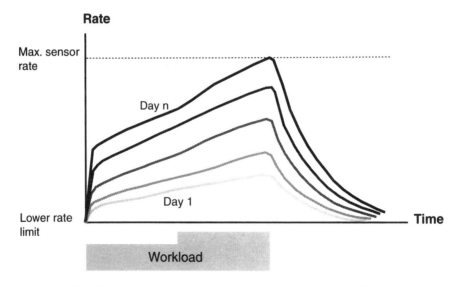

Bin Number	Range (ppm)	Time	Sample Counts
1	45-61	135d 13h 46m 13 s	7,208,353
2	61-67	23d 3h 3m 11s	1,229,656
3	67-73	27d 16h 58m 18s	1,473,168
4	73-79	12d 10h 21m 9s	660,966
5	79-86	3d 0h 21m 9s	159,708
6	86-92	0d 20h 15m 57s	44,897
7	92-98	0d 3h 54m 50s	8,671
8	98-104	0d 3h 34m 31s	7,921
9	104-110	0d 1h 35m 54s	3,541
		Total:	10,796,881

Fig. 8–17. Sensor-indicated rate histogram with the sensor "passive." The data, collected over a period of 203 days, indicate that the sensor would have resulted in rates primarily in the range of 45 to 61 bpm, and 95% of the rates would have been 86 bpm or lower. This sensor-driven rate response would have been markedly inadequate had the patient been "active" rather than "passive" and dependent on sensor-driven pacing for a rate response.

Fig. 8–18. Automatic adjustment of the sensor response is depicted in this figure as the "daily learning" process in a Vitatron dual-sensor pacemaker. The QT interval and activity slopes are automatically adjusted at the lower and upper rate limits by this process. Once activated, the pacemaker requires approximately 14 days for the slopes to be optimized, and after this time only minor variations occur. (Reproduced with permission from Vitatron.)

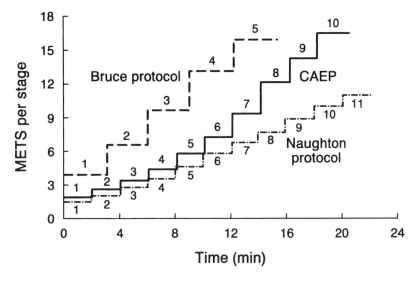

Fig. 8–19. Comparison of three exercise protocols: Bruce, Naughton, and CAEP (chronotropic assessment exercise protocol). METS, metabolic equivalents

mode, some form of exercise should be performed.

Our approach is relatively simple. If the patient, regardless of age, performs at a very high functional aerobic capacity, a standard stress test that pushes the patient to a high level of exertion is reasonable to be certain that the sensor responds appropriately. If a treadmill test is performed, the chronotropic assessment exercise protocol[25] is probably the most appropriate exercise protocol (Fig. 8–19). It allows for a gradual increase in speed and grade and thus mimics more levels of exercise likely to occur during activities of daily living (Table 8–4). Also, if the pacemaker incorporates an activity sensor, specifically a piezoelectric crystal, the patient should be encouraged to walk on the treadmill without holding on, that is, allowing the arms to swing naturally at the sides. Gripping the treadmill tightly may blunt the sensor's activity response.

Many pacemaker recipients do not routinely reach high levels of exertion, and it may be more important to be certain

Table 8–4.
Chronotropic Assessment Exercise Protocol

Stage	m/hour	Grade, %	Time, min	Cumulative time, min	Metabolic equivalents
Warm-up	1.0	0	. . .	. . .	1.5
1	1.0	2	2.0	2.0	2.0
2	1.5	3	2.0	4.0	2.8
3	2.0	4	2.0	6.0	3.6
4	2.5	5	2.0	8.0	4.6
5	3.0	6	2.0	10.0	5.8
6	3.5	8	2.0	12.0	7.5
7	4.0	10	2.0	14.0	9.6
8	5.0	10	2.0	16.0	12.1
9	6.0	10	2.0	18.0	14.3
10	7.0	10	2.0	20.0	16.5
11	7.0	15	2.0	22.0	19.0

that rate response is appropriate during an exertional range that corresponds to their activities of daily living. For these patients, casual exercise assessment is performed. If the patient is to be dismissed from the hospital in a rate-adaptive pacing mode, the assessment is performed in the hospital the morning after implantation. The rate response is reassessed in the outpatient clinic at approximately 3 months and yearly thereafter. Whether monitored by hospital telemetry or a strip-chart recorder in the pacemaker clinic, the patient is asked to walk at a casual pace in the corridor for approximately 2 minutes.[26] The rate is assessed during the walk or immediately afterward. Any patient capable of walking at a faster pace is asked to repeat the walk at a brisk pace. We use the values shown in Figure 8–20 as a guideline for appropriate rates during casual and brisk walks (Fig. 8–21).

Reassessment of sensor response should be considered if the patient has complaints of exertional fatigue or sudden changes in heart rate (Fig. 8–22). Rate histograms can be invaluable in determining whether rate response is appropriate. For example, Figure 8–23 displays a histogram in which the rates remain in the lowermost "bins," suggesting that the sensor is not programmed aggressively enough. Conversely, a histogram in which there is a significant amount of time at faster sensor-driven rates may suggest that the sensor is programmed too aggressively, especially if there are associated symptoms (Fig. 8–23).

If rate response is inadequate, whether determined by histograms or by exercise, the following inspections should be considered:

• Determine whether the sensor needs to be programmed more sensitively.
• Be certain that the sensor is definitely programmed correctly. Terminology for sensor settings is not uniform among manufacturers. Be certain that in an attempt to obtain more rate response, the sensor is not inadvertently being made even less sensitive.

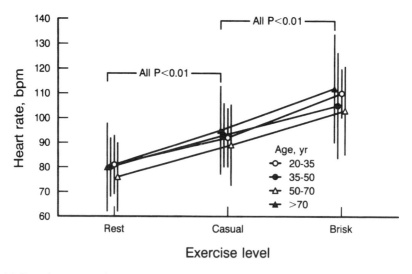

Fig. 8–20. Data from an early study to assess rates achieved during informal exercise. Patients walked at cadences determined as casual and brisk. Most patients achieved heart rates of 85 to 90 bpm with a casual walk and 100 to 110 bpm with a brisk walk.

A Total Time Sampled: 0d, 0h, 1m, 57s
    Sampling Rate: 1.6 seconds

Bin Number	Range (ppm)		Sample Counts
1	60	— 71	13
2	71	— 82	26
3	82	— 94	35
4	94	— 105	0
5	105	— 116	0
6	116	— 127	0
7	127	— 139	0
8	139	— 150	0
		Total:	74

B Total Time Sampled: 0d, 0h, 2m, 31s
    Sampling Rate: 1.6 seconds

Bin Number	Range (ppm)		Sample Counts
1	60	— 71	14
2	71	— 82	3
3	82	— 94	1
4	94	— 105	3
5	105	— 116	57
6	116	— 127	8
7	127	— 139	9
8	139	— 150	0
		Total:	95

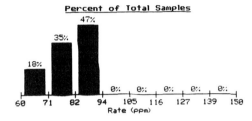

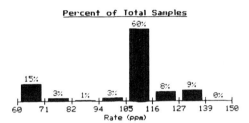

Fig. 8–21. Sensor histograms obtained after a patient exercises. *A,* After a casual walk of approximately 2 minutes, there is an acceptable rate response, with peak rates in rate bin 3, 82 to 94 bpm. On the basis of data from Figure 8–20, this should be a reasonable response. *B,* After a brisk walk, rates are achieved in rate bin 7, 127 to 139 bpm, with the greatest number of cycles falling in rate bin 5, 105 to 116 bpm. Once again, this appears reasonable on the basis of the previously described data.

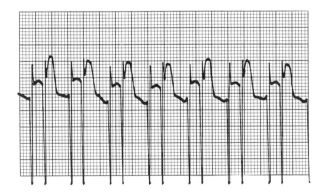

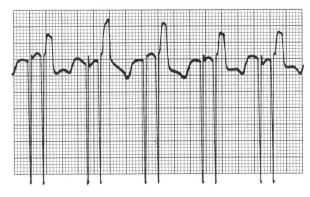

Fig. 8–22. Electrocardiographic tracings obtained during casual walking from a 70-year-old patient with a DDDR pacemaker. The patient had returned to the pacemaker clinic because of exertional dyspnea and palpitations. *Top,* The rate response is excessive, with a sensor-driven rate of approximately 120 bpm with a casual walk. *Bottom,* After reprogramming, a sensor-driven rate of approximately 85 bpm is obtained. This rate is more appropriate for an elderly patient during casual exercise.

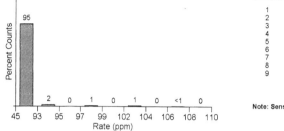

Sensor Indicated Rate Histogram

Sensor	On		
Base Rate	90	ppm	
Max Sensor Rate	110	ppm	
Slope	8 Normal		
Threshold	2.0		
Measured Average Sensor	2.1		
Reaction Time	Fast		
Recovery Time	Medium		

Date Read:	9 Jan 2000 11:57
Total Time Sampled:	5d 1h 37m 11s
Sampling Rate	1.6 s

Note: The above values were obtained when the histogram was interrogated.

Bin Number	Range (ppm)	Time	Sample Counts
1	45 - 93	4d 19h 33m 57s	256,023
2	93 - 95	0d 2h 34m 45s	5,714
3	95 - 97	0d 0h 0m 0s	0
4	97 - 99	0d 1h 21m 0s	2,991
5	99 - 102	0d 0h 0m 0s	0
6	102 - 104	0d 1h 32m 6s	3,401
7	104 - 106	0d 0h 0m 0s	0
8	106 - 108	0d 0h 35m 22s	1,306
9	108 - 110	0d 0h 0m 0s	0
		Total:	269,435

Note: Sensor Param. changed since Histogram was cleared.

Fig. 8–23. Sensor-indicated rate histogram from a patient with a DDDR pacemaker implanted 5 days earlier after an atrioventricular node ablation. The pacemaker is programmed to a lower rate of 90 ppm as part of the protocol following ablation. In 5 days, however, 95% of the sensor-indicated rates have been at or near the programmed lower rate of 90 ppm despite the patient's usual activity. Even though the sensor response was limited to a narrow range of 90 to 110 ppm, this sensor-driven rate is suboptimal.

- Be certain that the sensor is programmed to the active mode (not all pacemakers have this option).
- For piezoelectric crystal sensors, determine whether the pacemaker is implanted correctly. For the sensor to adequately sense vibrations, the pulse generator must be implanted with the "writing" up, which in turn places the piezoelectric crystal on the surface closest to the pectoral muscle.

Upgrade to Rate-Adaptive Pacing

When battery depletion indicators are reached in a patient with a non-rate-adaptive pacemaker, that is, VVI or DDD, should the pacemaker be upgraded to one with rate-adaptive capability? As a practical consideration, if the existing leads were to remain in site, a rate-adaptive pacemaker compatible with a standard lead would be required, that is, piezoelectric crystal, accelerometer, minute ventilation, or QT.

We strongly consider an upgrade in any patient with chronotropic incompetence. This can be assessed by exercise, formal or informal, or ambulatory monitoring, or both. A sense of the patient's chronotropic response can be gained at times by a review of transtelephonic strips. If this review reveals that pacing is always occurring at the lower rate limit on nonmagnet tracings, chronotropic incompetence may be present.

Again, if the pacemaker is upgraded, some exercise assessment must be performed after implantation to be certain that the patient tolerates the new chronotropic response and that the rate response is appropriate.

References

1. Nordlander R, Hedman A, Pehrsson SK: Rate responsive pacing and exercise

capacity—a comment (editorial). Pacing Clin Electrophysiol 12:749–751, 1989

2. Higano ST, Hayes DL, Eisinger G: Sensor-driven rate smoothing in a DDDR pacemaker. Pacing Clin Electrophysiol 12:922–929, 1989

3. Bernstein AD, Parsonnet V: Survey of cardiac pacing and defibrillation in the United States in 1993. Am J Cardiol 78: 187–196, 1996

4. Rossi P: Rate-responsive pacing: biosensor reliability and physiological sensitivity. Pacing Clin Electrophysiol 10:454–466, 1987

5. Alt E, Millerhagen JO, Heemels J-P: Accelerometers. *In* Clinical Cardiac Pacing. Edited by KA Ellenbogen, GN Kay, BL Wilkoff. Philadelphia, WB Saunders Company, 1995, pp 267–276

6. Benditt DG, Duncan JL: Activity-sensing, rate-adaptive pacemakers. *In* Clinical Cardiac Pacing. Edited by KA Ellenbogen, GN Kay, BL Wilkoff. Philadelphia, WB Saunders Company, 1995, pp 167–186

7. Alt E, Combs W, Willhaus R, Condie C, Bambl E, Fotuhi P, Pache J, Schomig A: A comparative study of activity and dual sensor: activity and minute ventilation pacing responses to ascending and descending stairs. Pacing Clin Electrophysiol 21:1862–1868, 1998

8. Alt E, Matula M, Theres H, Heinz M, Baker R: The basis for activity controlled rate variable cardiac pacemakers: an analysis of mechanical forces on the human body induced by exercise and environment. Pacing Clin Electrophysiol 12: 1667–1680, 1989

9. Nappholtz T, Valenta H, Maloney J, Simmons T: Electrode configurations for a respiratory impedance measurement suitable for rate responsive pacing. Pacing Clin Electrophysiol 9:960–964, 1986

10. Connelly DT, Rickards AF: The evoked QT interval. *In* Clinical Cardiac Pacing. Edited by KA Ellenbogen, GN Kay, BL Wilkoff. Philadelphia, WB Saunders Company, 1995, pp 250–257

11. Salo R, O'Donoghue S, Platia EV: The use of intracardiac impedance-based indicators to optimize pacing rate. *In* Clinical Cardiac Pacing. Edited by KA Ellenbogen, GN Kay, BL Wilkoff. Philadelphia, WB Saunders Company, 1995, pp 234–249

12. Yee R, Bennett TD: Rate-adaptive pacing controlled by dynamic right ventricular pressure (dP/dtmax). *In* Clinical Cardiac Pacing. Edited by KA Ellenbogen, GN

Kay, BL Wilkoff. Philadelphia, WB Saunders Company, 1995, pp 212–218

13. Osswald S, Grädel Ch, Cron T, Lippert M, Schaldach M, Buser P, Pfisterer M: New sensor technology: correlation of intracardiac impedance and right ventricular contractility during dobutamine stress test (abstract). Pacing Clin Electrophysiol 21: 895, 1998

14. Kay GN, Bornzin GA: Rate-modulated pacing controlled by mixed venous oxygen saturation. *In* Clinical Cardiac Pacing. Edited by KA Ellenbogen, GN Kay, BL Wilkoff. Philadelphia, WB Saunders Company, 1995, pp 187–200

15. Windecker S, Bubien RS, Halperin L, Moore A, Kay GN: Two-year experience with rate-modulated pacing controlled by mixed venous oxygen saturation. Pacing Clin Electrophysiol 21:1396–1404, 1998

16. Singer I, Callaghan FJ: Evoked potentials as a sensor for rate-adaptive pacing. *In* Clinical Cardiac Pacing. Edited by KA Ellenbogen, GN Kay, BL Wilkoff. Philadelphia, WB Saunders Company, 1995, pp 258–266

17. Langenfeld H, Krein A, Kirstein M, Binner L, for the European PEA Clinical Investigation Group: Peak endocardial acceleration-based clinical testing of the "BEST" DDDR pacemaker. Pacing Clin Electrophysiol 21:2187–2191, 1998

18. Deharo JC, Peyre JP, Ritter PH, Chalvidan T, Berland Y, Djiane P: A sensor-based evaluation of heart contractility in patients with head-up tilt-induced syncope. Pacing Clin Electrophysiol 21:223–226, 1998

19. Lau C-P: Rate Adaptive Cardiac Pacing: Single and Dual Chamber. Mount Kisco, NY, Futura Publishing Company, 1993, pp 213–227

20. Clementy J, Barold SS, Garrigue S, Shah DC, Jais P, Le Metayer P, Haissaguerre M: Clinical significance of multiple sensor options: rate response optimization, sensor blending, and trending. Am J Cardiol 83:166D–171D, 1999

21. Stangl K, Wirtzfeld A, Heinze R, Laule M, Seitz K, Gobl G: A new multisensor pacing system using stroke volume, respiratory rate, mixed venous oxygen saturation, and temperature, right atrial pressure, right ventricular pressure, and dP/dt. Pacing Clin Electrophysiol 11:712–724, 1988

22. Lau CP, Leung SK, Guerola M, Crijns HJ: Comparison of continuously recorded sensor and sinus rates during daily life activities and standardized exercise testing: efficacy of automatically optimized rate adaptive dual sensor pacing to simulate

sinus rhythm. Pacing Clin Electrophysiol 19:1672–1677, 1996

23. Cazeau S, Ritter P, Lazarus A, Garrigue S, Gras D, Henry L, Podeur H, Abastado M, Mugica J: Diagnostic functions in implantable cardiac pacemakers. *In* Prevention of Tachyarrhythmias With Cardiac Pacing. Edited by JC Daubert, EN Prystowsky, A Ripart. Armonk, NY, Futura Publishing Company, 1997, pp 179–188

24. Levine PA, Sanders R, Markowitz HT: Pacemaker diagnostics: measured data, event marker, electrogram, and event counter telemetry. *In* Clinical Cardiac Pacing. Edited by KA Ellenbogen, GN Kay, BL Wilkoff. Philadelphia, WB Saunders Company, 1995, pp 639–655

25. Wilkoff BL, Corey J, Blackburn G: A mathematical model of the cardiac chronotropic response to exercise. J Electrophysiol 3: 176–180, 1989

26. Hayes DL, Von Feldt L, Higano ST: Standardized informal exercise testing for programming rate adaptive pacemakers. Pacing Clin Electrophysiol 14:1772–1776, 1991

9

Troubleshooting

Margaret A. Lloyd, M.D.,
David L. Hayes, M.D.,
Paul A. Friedman, M.D.

Pacemaker Troubleshooting

The increasing sophistication of pacing devices has made troubleshooting a more complex endeavor. Knowledge of the device capabilities and the clinical situation of the patient is key to successful troubleshooting. Whether a patient has a clinical episode that suggests system malfunction or is having routine follow-up, evaluation should be performed in an orderly fashion so that potential malfunction is not overlooked. Some instances of device "malfunction" are not malfunctions at all but rather are the result of an inappropriately programmed device functioning as programmed or unrecognized appropriate function, that is, pseudomalfunction. In some instances, early component failure is intermittent, and even meticulous evaluation of the system may not initially reveal a problem.

Successful troubleshooting requires a systematic approach[1,2] (Table 9–1). It should initially be noninvasive and involve careful evaluation of any events experienced by the patient, the indication for pacing, the electrocardiographic tracings, the function and appearance of the lead system, and the information obtained by telemetry from the pulse generator. If possible, noninvasive diagnosis and correction of the problem are preferable to operative management. Before invasive troubleshooting, one should take advantage of every possible source of assistance, including careful review of the technical manual of the device and contacting the manufacturer for help. If noninvasive evaluation is unrewarding, operative assessment may be necessary.

In addition to having a systematic approach to troubleshooting and a differential diagnosis for each category, it is helpful to understand the most common problems encountered in a pacemaker clinic and the most likely causes of these problems.

In an older abstract, Parsonnet et al.[3] assessed records of 615 patients in a 6-year period to identify the frequency and character of problems encountered, causes confirmed, and action taken to correct the problems. They identified the following most commonly encountered problems:

Problem	Means of identification	Percent of all interventions performed	Years to diagnosis
Failure to sense	Clinic	15.9	2.0
Failure to capture	Clinic	13.9	1.6
Change in magnet rate	Transtelephonic	6.1	6.9
Suboptimal cardiac output	Referring M.D.	5.8	1.4
Syncope or near-syncope	Patient	5.7	3.4
Altered rate, slower than programmed	Transtelephonic	5.6	5.9
Failure to output	Transtelephonic	4.5	4.9

They identified the following causes as the most common sources of the clinical problems:

Cause	Percent of all causes found	Percent of interventions performed	Years to diagnosis
High threshold	18.2	13.2	1.4
Battery depletion	13.8	10.0	7.4
Atrial fibrillation	8.8	6.3	2.0
Change in underlying rhythm	6.0	4.4	2.1
Conductor fracture	3.7	2.7	2.3
Inappropriate programmed pacing rate	3.4	2.5	0.6

An awareness of data such as these and keeping personal experience in mind are helpful as one approaches a new troubleshooting challenge.

Clinical Assessment

Knowing the patient well (Table 9–2) and taking a careful history are very important in evaluating any pacing system, especially if malfunction is suspected.[1] Clinical assessment should include the original indication for pacing (if known), whether or not the patient is pacemaker-dependent, activity immediately preceding the clinical event, symptoms experienced by the patient during the event, observations of any bystanders, and duration of the event. Symptoms of pacing system malfunction may be subtle and include fatigue, weakness, confusion, neck pulsations, or activity intolerance. During routine evaluations, the patient should be asked about symptoms potentially related to pacemaker complications, such as fever, chills, night sweats, palpitations, and slow, fast, or irregular pulse. It is important to obtain information from the operative report if at all possible, including device model, lead models, acute intraoperative pacing and sensing thresholds and impedance values, and any difficulty encountered during implantation. Some newer devices allow recording and storing of information on lead

Table 9–1.
Troubleshooting Steps

Clinical assessment
  Indication for pacing
  Focused history and physical
    examination
  Review of operative report
Electrocardiography
  Rate
  Pacing and sensing
  QRS axis
  Magnet response
Chest radiograph
  Device type and location
  Proper contact between lead pins and
    setscrews
  Lead integrity
  Lead position
Pacemaker interrogation
  Sensing threshold(s)
  Pacing threshold(s)
  Lead impedance
  Battery status
  Special features
  Histograms
  Trend data
  Counters
Programing
Review technical manual for other "clues" to
    perceived malfunction
Contact the manufacturer for assistance
Operative assessment
  Appearance of pocket
  Assessment of lead connection(s)
  Visual inspection of lead(s)
  Electrical assessment of lead(s)
  Patency of venous system

Table 9–2.
Knowing the Patient and the Pacing System

Know the patient
- Cardiac diagnoses
- Noncardiac diagnoses
- Exposure to electromagnetic interference, e.g., workplace, hobbies, medical procedures
- Any physical trauma since prior evaluation
- Any reprogramming at other institutions since prior evaluation

Know the pacemaker
- Manufacturer
- Model number
- Serial number
- Medical advisory or recall that may apply
- Previously programmed values
- Previous battery status
- Device idiosyncracies

Know the lead or leads
- Manufacturer
- Model number
- Serial number
- Medical advisory or recall that may apply
- Connector type
- Polarity
- Insulation material
- Fixation mechanism
- Normal radiographic appearance

Modified from Love and Hayes.[1] By permission of WB Saunders Company.

models, acute threshold data, clinical information (e.g., medication regimen), name of institution where the device was implanted, and name of the implanting physician. All manufacturers have toll-free numbers that may be used to obtain implant information (generally kept by the manufacturer of the pulse generator), such as device model and lead models (Table 9–3). The manufacturers can also provide technical information about device and lead performance. It is also very useful (but sometimes difficult) to obtain the chest radiograph taken immediately

after implantation for comparison with current radiographs.

Electrocardiographic Tracings

The pacemaker should first be interrogated to determine the device settings. Is it a single- or dual-chamber device (see Chapter 6)? What is the programmed pacing mode? What are the lower and (if applicable) upper rate limits? This information should be compared with that on the electrocardiographic strips, especially if one is fortunate enough to capture tracings during a clinical event.

Strips should be evaluated to determine (in both chambers, if applicable) whether sensing and pacing are appropri-

Table 9–3.
Toll-free, 24-Hour Telephone Numbers of
Manufacturers*

• Biotronik	1-800-547-0394
• CPI/Guidant	1-800-CARDIAC
• ELA	1-800-352-6466
• Medtronic	1-800-328-2518
• St. Jude/Pacesetter	1-800-722-3774
• Vitatron	1-800-VITATRON

*As of January 2000.

ate, capture is consistent, pacing rate is appropriate, and there is any loss of output.

Lead Integrity

The lead system is the most vulnerable component of the pacing system and the most frequent site of system failure. The rate of failure has been higher than expected in a number of leads, and they have been placed on advisory. Several lead model failures were attributed to a specific type of polyurethane, Pellethane 80A, although failures of Pellethane 55D have also occurred.[4] In patients with a ventricular lead on advisory and a clinical event suggestive of pacemaker failure, serious consideration should be given to lead replacement regardless of the results of noninvasive or invasive evaluation.

The coaxial design of many transvenous bipolar pacing leads makes them more susceptible than unipolar leads to lead failure. Initial damage is usually to the outer insulation or coil and may be manifested by sensing problems when programmed in a bipolar sensing mode; sometimes programming the device to unipolar sensing restores appropriate sensing.[5] Although such programming temporarily corrects the problem, lead replacement should be considered, especially if the lead is ventricular and the patient is pacemaker-dependent.

The chest radiograph is a valuable

component in lead evaluation. The lead should be inspected in its entirety, from the contact of the pin with the setscrew to the position of the lead within its cardiac chamber. Unfortunately, deterioration of the lead insulation is not visible on the chest radiograph, and fractures of the coil are not always obvious. A frequent site of lead damage is the region between the first rib and the clavicle; this site should be carefully inspected for coil fracture ("subclavian crush syndrome").[6,7] The risk of subclavian crush becomes higher if multiple leads are in place. If an old chest radiograph is available for comparison, it can be determined whether or not gross lead dislodgment has occurred. Abandoned leads in contact with the electrode portion of an active lead may cause an artifact, which can be interpreted by the pacemaker as a cardiac event and cause inappropriate inhibition. Although findings on the chest radiograph suggestive of lead fracture, dislodgment, or poor connection between the lead pin and generator setscrew are helpful in identifying lead problems, a negative radiographic result does not exclude lead failure. (For detailed information on the radiographic appearance of pacing systems, see Chapter 11.)

A special note should be made about patients with Telectronics (Englewood, CO) Accufix and Encor atrial leads. These leads, which have preformed J-shaped retention wires in the distal portion to maintain the J shape of the lead, are on advisory because of reports of retention wire fracture, extrusion, and perforation of critical cardiac structures.[8,9] Fracture of the retention wire frequently does not result in any pacing abnormalities. Therefore, in a patient with one of these leads who has chest pain, unexplained pericardial effusion, or hemodynamic collapse, the lead should be carefully scrutinized with digital fluoroscopy to determine the status of the retention wire. Occasionally, a fractured or extruded retention wire can be seen on the chest radiograph.

Lead evaluation should also include telemetered data on lead impedance from the pacemaker (Fig. 9–1). All leads have a characteristic range of lead impedance; an unusually high impedance (for most leads, above 1,000 Ω) may represent fracture of the conductor coil, and a low impedance (generally below 300 Ω) may indicate insulation failure. (Note: some new "high-impedance" leads have much higher impedance values than those previously seen, typically with a range of 800 to 2,000 Ω.) Some newer pacemakers periodically measure and store impedance values, making it easier to compare implantation and current values (Fig. 9–2). Even if a measured value is within the "normal" range for that particular lead, a notable change in impedance from previous values should raise suspicion. Some contemporary devices respond to a sudden change in impedance by automatically reprogramming the pacemaker from bipolar to unipolar pacing and sensing configuration (Fig. 9–3).

Daily Measurement - Data Table

Date	Atrial Amplitude (mV)	Atrial Impedance (Ω)	Ventricular Amplitude (mV)	Ventricular Impedance (Ω)
26-DEC-99	1.1	200	>9.0	1150
25-DEC-99	1.0	SENSED	PACED	1180
24-DEC-99	1.0	240	>9.0	1220
23-DEC-99	0.6	SENSED	>9.0	1140
22-DEC-99	PACED	240	>9.0	1160
21-DEC-99	1.1	220	>9.0	SENSED
20-DEC-99	1.0	190	>9.0	1140
20-DEC-99	0.9	190	>9.0	SENSED
13-DEC-99	PACED	220	>9.0	1140
06-DEC-99	1.1	200	>9.0	1140
29-NOV-99	0.9	240	PACED	1140
22-NOV-99	0.9	240	>9.0	1140
15-NOV-99	0.9	SENSED	>9.0	1150
08-NOV-99	0.6	200	PACED	1140
01-NOV-99	PACED	220	>9.0	1140
25-OCT-99	0.6	190	>9.0	1120
18-OCT-99	0.6	190	>9.0	SENSED
11-OCT-99	0.6	200	>9.0	1140
04-OCT-99	PACED	SENSED	>9.0	1140
27-SEP-99	1.0	190	PACED	SENSED
20-SEP-99	1.6	380	>9.0	1140
13-SEP-99	1.8	480	>9.0	1130
06-SEP-99	2.4	580	>9.0	1100
30-AUG-99	PACED	700	>9.0	SENSED
23-AUG-99	2.8	670	PACED	1090
16-AUG-99	2.8	670	>9.0	1120
09-AUG-99	2.8	660	>9.0	1100
02-AUG-99	2.8	SENSED	>9.0	1120
26-JUL-99	PACED	640	>9.0	1140
19-JUL-99	2.8	660	>9.0	1150
12-JUL-99	3.1	660	PACED	1150
05-JUL-99	3.3	650	>9.0	1140
28-JUN-99	3.3	660	>9.0	SENSED
21-JUN-99	3.4	680	>9.0	1130
14-JUN-99	PACED	700	>9.0	1100
07-JUN-99	>3.5	SENSED	>9.0	1080
31-MAY-99	3.4	740	PACED	1100
24-MAY-99	3.3	760	>9.0	1090
17-MAY-99	>3.5	730	>9.0	SENSED
10-MAY-99	>3.5	770	>9.0	1100
03-MAY-99	3.4	770	PACED	1100
26-APR-99	PACED	780	PACED	1090
19-APR-99	3.4	SENSED	>9.0	1120
12-APR-99	3.3	SENSED	>9.0	1090
05-APR-99	3.3	760	>9.0	1080
29-MAR-99	3.4	730	PACED	SENSED
22-MAR-99	3.3	740	>9.0	1060
15-MAR-99	3.3	760	>9.0	SENSED
08-MAR-99	PACED	780	>9.0	1080
01-MAR-99	PACED	800	>9.0	1070
22-FEB-99	3.3	820	>9.0	1070
15-FEB-99	3.3	800	>9.0	1080
08-FEB-99	3.3	840	PACED	SENSED
01-FEB-99	PACED	830	>9.0	1090
25-JAN-99	>3.5	SENSED	>9.0	1090
18-JAN-99	>3.5	860	>9.0	1080
11-JAN-99	>3.5	890	>9.0	1070
04-JAN-99	PACED	SENSED	>9.0	1080
28-DEC-98	>3.5	900	>9.0	1090

Fig. 9–1. Programmer printout of pacemaker telemetry noting lead impedance. In this patient, the onset of a low atrial lead impedance suggests an atrial insulation defect.

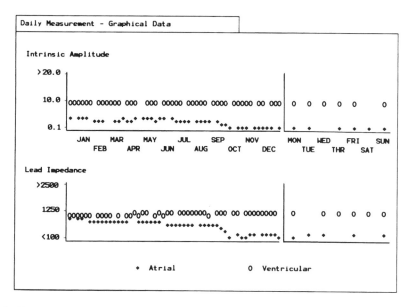

Fig. 9–2. Programmer printout of lead impedance trend. A change in lead impedance, either gradual or sudden, may be helpful in troubleshooting. In this example, there is a decrease in atrial lead impedance.

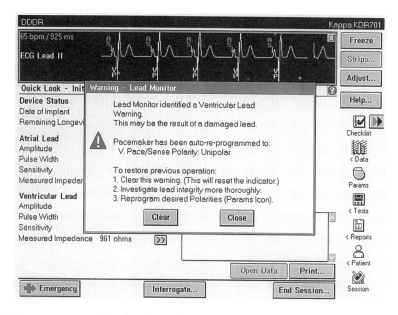

Fig. 9–3. Programmer warning that there has been a significant change detected in lead impedance, with automatic reprogramming to a unipolar pacing configuration.

Pulse Generators

The number of programmable features available in pacemakers has increased greatly over the past decades. Al-

though these options have increased our ability to provide optimal pacing therapy to patients, they can make troubleshooting a complex endeavor. Detailed understanding of the correct function of these devices is necessary to provide comprehensive evaluation; technical manuals and company representatives can provide additional assistance.

Pacing and Sensing Threshold Evaluation

An initial step in troubleshooting is to determine the patient's native rhythm.[1,2] This may require turning down the rate of the pacemaker or programming it to a nontracking ventricular mode, or both. Whether a spontaneous rhythm is pres-ent, the type of rhythm, and the length of time it takes to initiate it should be noted. If the patient is found to have no underlying rhythm, care should be taken to ensure that the patient does not become asystolic for any significant length of time during the troubleshooting session.

Pacing thresholds should then be evaluated. Many devices allow semiautomatic evaluation of pacing thresholds; the output is incrementally decreased until loss of capture occurs, and termination of the test results in immediate pacing at pretest values[10,11] (Fig. 9–4). This feature is especially useful in pacemaker-dependent

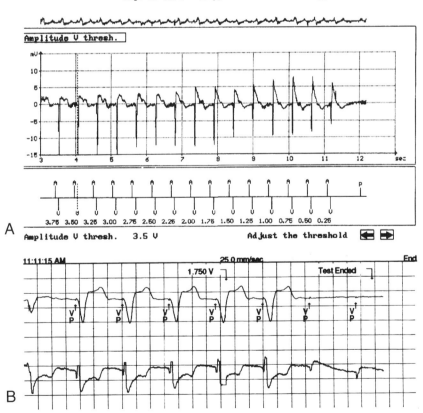

Fig. 9–4. Two examples of autothreshold determination by the programmer. Autothreshold determination allows ventricular thresholds to be determined in the pacemaker-dependent patient, with minimal risk of clinically significant asystole. *A*, Ventricular capture is maintained to the lowest value of 0.25 V. *B*, Ventricular capture is lost at 1.75 V.

patients. In many devices, pacing thresholds need to be obtained manually, and the operator should be familiar with the programmer emergency pacing feature should it become necessary. After determination of the pacing threshold or thresholds, the chronically programmed output parameters, that is, voltage amplitude and pulse width, should be reassessed to be certain that the patient has an adequate safety margin. There are several ways to program output parameters to assure an adequate safety margin. These are described in detail in Chapter 7. During the evaluation of pacing thresholds, the presence or absence of ventriculoatrial conduction should be noted, and the patient should be questioned about symptoms of pacemaker syndrome, especially if it is suspected on the basis of the clinical findings.

Threshold values should be compared with those at implantation, if possible, keeping three things in mind: thresholds temporarily increase in the initial months after implantation, active-fixation leads generally have higher thresholds than passive-fixation leads, and leads with steroid-eluting tips generally have lower

| Table 9–4. |
| Effect of Drugs on Pacing Thresholds |

Increase in threshold
  Bretylium
  Encainide*
  Flecainide
  Moricizine*
  Procainamide†
  Propafenone
  Sotalol
Decrease in threshold
  Atropine
  Epinephrine
  Isoproterenol
  Corticosteroids

*Off market in the United States.
†At supratherapeutic levels.

thresholds than those with non-steroid-eluting tips. The development of exit block, administration of drugs that potentially affect pacing thresholds, and occurrence of new myocardial infarction may also affect pacing thresholds (Table 9–4).

Specific devices now offer some type of periodic assessment of pacing threshold in the ventricle, with resetting of the energy output to maintain capture but minimize energy levels[11] (Fig. 9–5). In these de-

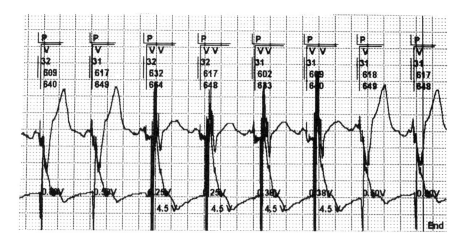

Fig. 9–5. Electrocardiographic tracing demonstrating proprietary Autocapture threshold determination. In this example, capture is lost at 0.25 V and the output is automatically increased to 0.38 V, which fails to capture, and the device again increases output, to 0.5 V, and confirms capture for two consecutive beats.

vices, the output on the ventricular channel may be different at the time of interrogation from that initially programmed because of self-adjustment of the device. Additionally, electrocardiographic monitoring during a periodic threshold check may suggest device malfunction if one is not familiar with this feature.

The sensitivity of each lead should be assessed. Some newer devices automatically measure the native atrial and ventricular electrograms, whereas in older devices, measurement must be manual. The measured sensitivity should be compared with the programmed value to ensure that the chronically programmed value is adequate.

Assessing the Pacing Rate

An understanding of basic pacemaker timing cycles is mandatory (explained in detail in Chapter 6). Many abnormal-appearing electrocardiograms actually represent normal device function when it is understood how the device is programmed.

To know whether the pacing rate is appropriate, it is first necessary to determine the pacing mode and programmed lower and (if applicable) upper rate limits. Under certain circumstances, the rate may be outside programmed values. The upper rate limit may be overridden by the spontaneous sinus rhythm, atrial or ventricular tachyarrhythmias, or, in rare instances, runaway pacemaker (see below).

Several optional features allow rates below the lower rate limit under certain circumstances. Some devices have a nocturnal or sleep function. During sleep time, the pacemaker allows programming of the lower rate limit to a rate generally 10 or 15 bpm less than that during wake time, replicating the natural circadian sleep-wake cycle and helping to conserve battery life.[12] If it is not known that a "sleep rate" is programmed "on," confu-

sion may arise when the patient's paced rate decreases at a certain time.

Hysteresis features allow the natural heart rate to decrease to a programmed rate below the lower rate limit before pacing begins at the programmed lower rate. Although useful in patients whose native rate approximates that of the lower rate limit to allow native conduction as much as possible, hysteresis has been a source of confusion for many years. Unless it is realized that hysteresis is programmed "on" and the mechanism of this feature is understood, the uninformed often interpret this electrocardiographic finding as "oversensing," since the cycle length is intermittently longer than the recognized programmed lower rate limit.

Most current dual-chamber devices offer multiple variations in the atrioventricular (AV) interval. Independently programmable paced and sensed AV intervals allow for more consistent mechanical AV activation in patients with interatrial and intra-atrial conduction delay but can cause confusion when electrocardiographic strips are interpreted. This effect may also cause minor variations in the paced lower and upper rates. Rate-adaptive AV delay is also available in most contemporary dual-chamber pacemakers. Because the rate-adaptive AV interval affects the total atrial refractory period and therefore the achievable upper rate limit, confusion may arise (see Chapter 6).

Another classic source of confusion during assessment of pacing rates and alterations in cycle length is rate smoothing.[13] Rate smoothing avoids abrupt changes in pacing rate, such as those that can occur during a sudden transition to pseudo-Wenckebach or 2:1 upper rate behavior, and may eliminate symptoms associated with sensed dysrhythmic events. Rate smoothing controls sudden changes in pacing rate by monitoring the interval between ventricular events (both paced and sensed) and storing the most recent RR interval in memory (Fig. 9–6). On the

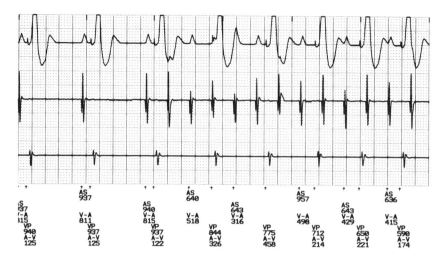

Fig. 9–6. Rate smoothing can confound electrocardiographic interpretation if one is not familiar with it or aware that it is programmed "on." In this tracing, normal sinus rhythm is replaced by an atrial tachyarrhythmia. Rather than an abrupt increase in the paced ventricular rate in response to the atrial tachyarrhythmia, there is gradual shortening of the VV cycle length. The cycle length is regulated by rate smoothing and is allowed to change by the programmed smoothing factor; in this example, the smoothing factor is 9%. AS, atrial sensing; V-A, interval from ventricular sensed or paced event to atrial paced event; VP, ventricular pacing.

basis of this RR interval and the programmed rate-smoothing percentage, the pulse generator sets up two rate-control windows for the next cycle—one for the atrium and one for the ventricle. For example, if the monitored VV interval is 800 msec and 6% rate smoothing is programmed, the algorithm allows the upcoming ventricular rate of the cycle to increase or decrease a maximum of 6%, or ± 48 msec (752 to 848 msec).

Some current devices also offer a specific feature used if a neurocardiogenic event is detected.[14] Medtronic, Inc. (Minneapolis, MN) offers a feature called "rate drop," which is triggered when the native heart rate decreases through a programmed rate-drop window, after which the device paces at a faster programmed rate (generally 90 to 100 ppm) until spontaneous rhythm is detected. Other devices offer some type of search hysteresis, by which the device paces for a programmed number of cycles at an accelerated rate (again, usually 90 to 100 pulses/min) when the native rate drops below the

lower rate limit. Hysteresis can lead to misinterpretation of the electrocardiogram if the feature is not well understood or if the health care professional interpreting the electrocardiogram is unaware that the feature is programmed "on" (Fig. 9–7).

Rate-adaptive sensors can also cause confusion. Some sensors are based on physiologic stimuli, such as thoracic impedance or QT interval, and therefore may drive the rate even when the patient is not physically active (as with activity-based sensors). The sensor-driven rates may therefore cause confusion because the rates seem inappropriate for a given time (Fig. 9–8). Patients may experience symptoms of fatigue or effort intolerance if the sensor is not programmed aggressively enough and symptoms of palpitations or tachycardia if it is programmed too aggressively.

Diagnostic Features

Many current devices offer sophisticated diagnostic options that can help ret-

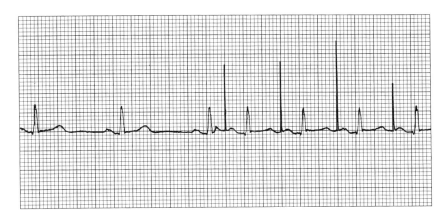

Fig. 9–7. Electrocardiographic example of sudden change in paced rate caused by hysteresis. In this example, the intrinsic rate falls to slightly less than 65 bpm, the hysteresis rate, and the pacing rate increases to the programmed lower rate of 100 bpm. This feature has proven successful in minimizing symptoms of neurocardiogenic syncope, but the sudden change in paced rate may confuse electrocardiographic interpretation.

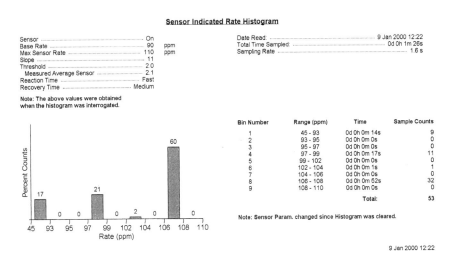

Fig. 9–8. Inappropriate sensor response is determined from the "Sensor Indicated Rate Histogram." During a casual walk of 1 min 26 sec, the patient's heart rate varied from the lowest rate bin to a point near the maximum sensor rate of 110. Sixty percent of the counts were in the 106 to 108 bpm rate bin. The patient complained of dyspnea during the casual walk. With reprogramming to less aggressive rate-adaptive parameters, the walk was well tolerated.

rospectively determine potential causes of clinical events and aid in optimal programming and detection of potential problems before symptoms develop.[1,2,15–17] Such diagnostic features include number of mode-switching events (Fig. 9–9), number of high-rate atrial events (Fig. 9–10), number of ventricular high-rate episodes (Fig. 9–11), number of ectopic events, percentage of time paced and sensed in all chambers (Fig. 9–12 and 9–13), electrograms (Fig. 9–14), and trending of such values as lead impedance (Fig. 9–2).

Most pacemakers provide diagnostic interpretation channels. An electrocardiographic recorder from the programmer is

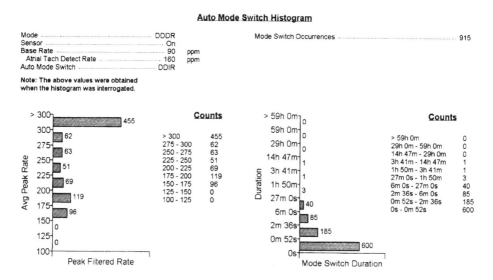

Auto Mode Switch Histogram

Mode .... DDDR
Sensor .... On
Base Rate .... 90 ppm
   Atrial Tach Detect Rate .... 160 ppm
Auto Mode Switch .... DDIR

Note: The above values were obtained
when the histogram was interrogated.

Mode Switch Occurrences 915

Counts

> 300	455
275 - 300	62
250 - 275	63
225 - 250	51
200 - 225	69
175 - 200	119
150 - 175	96
125 - 150	0
100 - 125	0

Avg Peak Rate — Peak Filtered Rate

Counts

> 59h 0m	0
29h 0m - 59h 0m	0
14h 47m - 29h 0m	0
3h 41m - 14h 47m	1
1h 50m - 3h 41m	1
27m 0s - 1h 50m	3
6m 0s - 27m 0s	40
2m 36s - 6m 0s	85
0m 52s - 2m 36s	185
0s - 0m 52s	600

Duration — Mode Switch Duration

Fig. 9–9. Data telemetered from the pacemaker have been collected over 44 hours. The mode-switch counter indicates that there have been 915 mode-switch episodes. This information does not verify that all mode-switch events were appropriate. Assuming that all the mode-switch events were appropriate, the telemetered data also provide information on the average peak rate and mode-switch duration. In this patient, the average peak rate varied greatly, usually exceeding 300 bpm, consistent with atrial fibrillation. Most of the mode-switch episodes were less than 52 msec in length.

Data Collection Period: 08/26/99 3:01 PM - 10/07/99 1:09 PM (Over Last 42 days)

Detection Rate	180 ppm		Mode	DDIR
Detection Duration	5 sec		Lower Rate	70 ppm
Termination Beats	5 beats		Upper Sensor Rate	130 ppm
Episodes Detected	353			
Episodes Recorded	16		Percent of Total Duration	1%
PAC Runs	28,082			

Date/Time	Duration hh:mm:ss		Max Atrial Rate (bpm)
08/27/99 8:20 AM	:15	First	218
10/01/99 5:01 AM	12:01:12	Longest...	362
10/02/99 4:32 PM	:10		191
10/02/99 4:32 PM	:11		196
10/02/99 6:42 PM	:36		196
10/03/99 8:42 PM	:27		206
10/03/99 8:44 PM	:29		201
10/03/99 8:45 PM	:28		206
10/03/99 8:50 PM	:26		201
10/03/99 10:59 PM	:59		196
10/05/99 6:42 PM	:09		196
10/05/99 7:04 PM	:16		191
10/05/99 7:17 PM	:30		201
10/05/99 9:53 PM	:06		196
10/05/99 9:54 PM	:14		196
10/05/99 10:04 PM	:21	Last	201

A

Fig. 9–10. *A,* Telemetered information of "atrial high rate" events detected in a 42-day period. The pacemaker has detected 353 episodes and recorded 16 of them. The detection rate was set at 180 ppm. *Continues.*

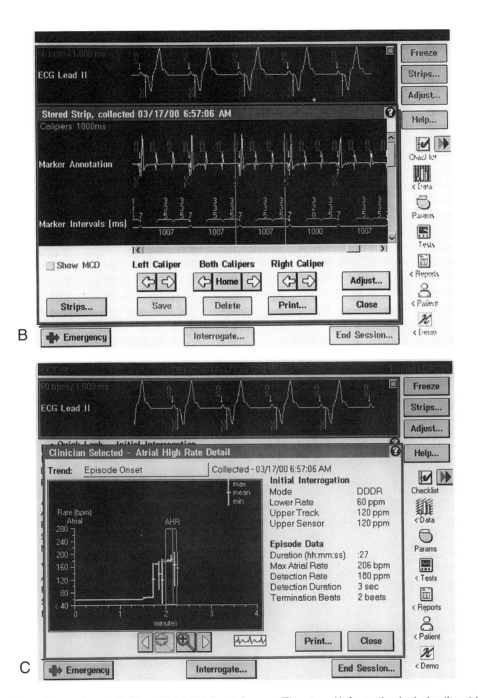

Fig. 9–10 *continued. B,* Stored "atrial high rate" event. The stored information includes the atrial electrogram with markers as well as measured intervals. *C,* Another display of an "atrial high rate" event. This episode lasted 27 seconds with a maximum atrial rate of 206 bpm.

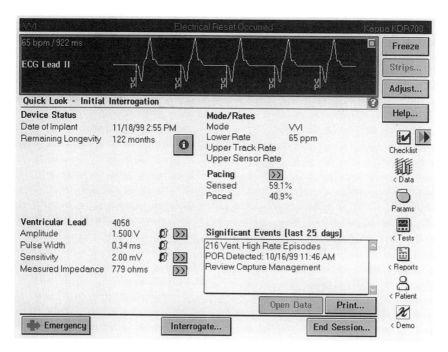

Fig. 9–11. Telemetered data with notation of several "significant events" (*boxed area, lower right*). Since the last interrogation, there have been 216 events that met criteria for a ventricular high-rate episode. In addition, a "power-on-reset" (POR) has occurred, reprogramming the device to VVI, rate 65 ppm.

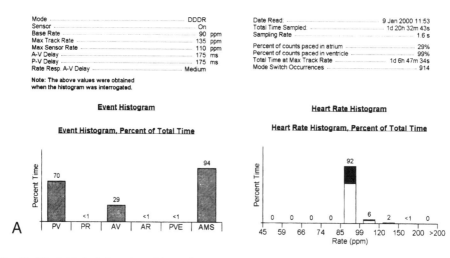

Fig. 9–12. *A,* Data telemetered from the pacemaker have been collected over 44 hours. This indicates the percentage of time that the patient has pacing or sensing in the atrium and ventricle. In this patient, 70% of cycles were P-synchronous pacing (PV) and 29% were AV sequential (AV). Of the total duration of time monitored, 94% was in mode switch. In the right panel, the heart rate histogram reveals that 92% of the time monitored, the heart rate was between 85 and 99 bpm, with the white portion of the bar indicating PV pacing and the black portion AV pacing. *Continues.*

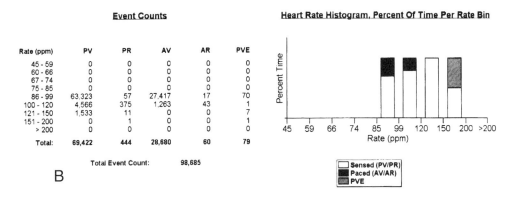

Fig. 9–12 *continued. B,* Specific event counts are also available, as shown in the table at the left. A normalized heart rate histogram is shown on the right. PVE, premature ventricular extrasystole.

applied to the patient, and telemetry is established with the pacemaker. When the marker channel feature is turned on, real-time, simultaneous electrocardiographic signals and markers denoting paced and sensed events in each channel are recorded. This feature is especially helpful in attempting to determine whether the device is undersensing or oversensing or if "functional" sensing abnormalities exist (Fig. 9–15).

In patients who are not pacemaker-dependent, who have experienced a clinical event suggesting possible failure of some component of the pacing system, and who do not have any source of failure revealed by a thorough noninvasive evaluation, Holter monitoring, an event recorder, or an implantable loop recorder may be considered[18,19] (Fig. 9–16).

One of the most important data that can be obtained from the pulse generator is the battery voltage. Battery depletion, although expected, is still the most common cause of pacemaker failure. Some devices provide a telemetered numerical battery voltage, which should generally be above 2.4 V in lithium-based batteries, and others give a "gas-gauge" representation of battery status (Fig. 9–17). Another way to determine battery voltage is to assess the magnet rate. All pacemakers have a characteristic magnet rate that changes predictably as the battery voltage decreases. Unfortunately, each manufacturer uses a different magnet rate, necessitating knowledge of or access to that information to ascertain battery status. Assessment of the magnet rate is a key component in transtelephonic pacemaker monitoring. As the battery approaches end of life, most devices reset to a "backup" mode. Backup mode is usually fixed-rate ventricular pacing at maximal output. Most devices also lose telemetry function and programmability when the battery nears imminent failure.

Unexpected Device Failure

Contemporary pacemakers and implantable cardioverter-defibrillators (ICDs) have achieved an extraordinary level of reliability. However, rare random component failures have been reported.[20]

If a true malfunction of the device is suspected, the manufacturer should be

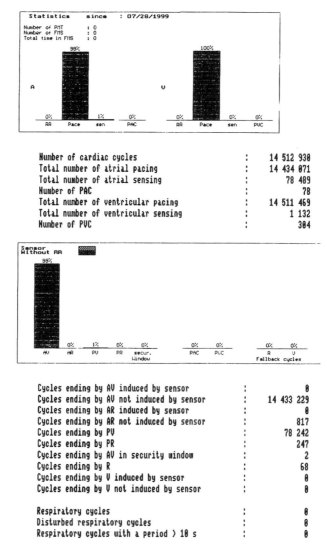

Fig. 9–13. Telemetered data representing percentage of beats paced and sensed. Also provided are specific counts of cardiac cycles and description and percentage of types of events counted, for example, 247 cycles ending in PR.

asked whether similar problems have been reported. Other sources of information also exist. No comprehensive database of pulse generators and leads is available at this time in the United States. Such registries are available in other countries.[21] A database is operational for the purpose of documenting hardware, lead, and pacemaker and ICD failures.[22] Because only failures are reported, the database does not provide an incidence with which specific failures might occur, but it may alert one to a potential problem or allow a search to see if others have reported a similar problem. This site, *www.pacerandicdregistry.com*, can be searched by model, manufacturer, or type of failure. This site is proving to be an excellent resource. Practitioners are encouraged to register their own device failures.

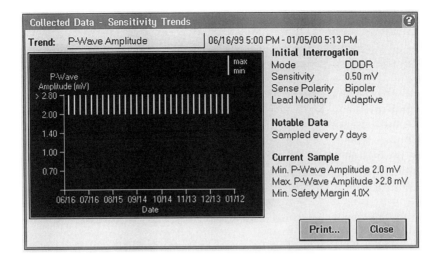

Fig. 9–14. Programmer screen depicting atrial sensitivity trends. In this example, the P-wave amplitude varied between 2.00 mV and > 2.80 mV for the period monitored.

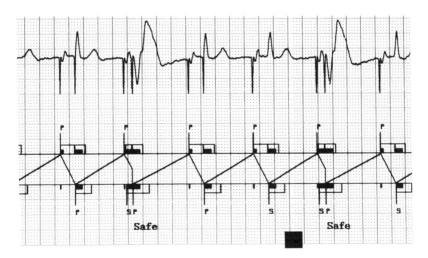

Fig. 9–15. Diagnostic interpretation channel provides markers of all cardiac events. In this example, there is evidence of atrial and ventricular capture, ventricular sensing, ventricular pseudofusion, and safety pacing. Paced ventricular events are identified by "P" and sensed events by "S." Ventricular safety pacing is appreciated on the surface electrocardiographic tracing by the abbreviated atrioventricular interval of approximately 100 msec and is verified on the ladder diagram by "Safe." Because the morphology of an intrinsic ventricular event is documented, it is possible to say that the first and third pacing artifacts result in pseudofusion and not fusion, because the ventricular morphology is not altered.

Operative Evaluation of Pacing Systems

Sometimes the status of a pacing system is impossible to determine noninvasively. If intermittent system failure is strongly suspected clinically and comprehensive noninvasive evaluation has been unrewarding, operative assessment may be in order (Table 9–5). This approach should be strongly considered if the patient is pacemaker-dependent and has ex-

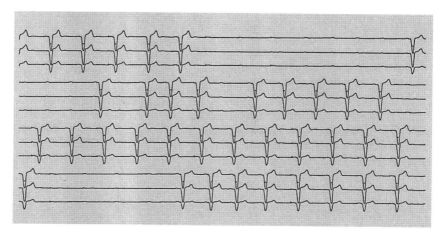

Fig. 9–16. Electrocardiographic recording from a pacemaker-dependent patient with recurrent symptoms after pacemaker implantation. The pacemaker was programmed to the DDD pacing mode. Despite thorough pacemaker clinic evaluation, no abnormalities had been documented. This tracing reveals long pauses that correlated with the patient's symptoms. (Pacemaker artifacts are difficult to appreciate, but all ventricular activity is paced.)

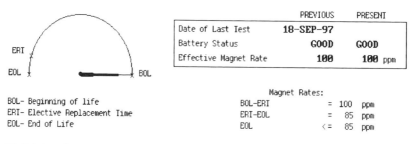

	PREVIOUS	PRESENT
Date of Last Test	18-SEP-97	
Battery Status	GOOD	GOOD
Effective Magnet Rate	100	100 ppm

BOL– Beginning of life
ERI– Elective Replacement Time
EOL– End of Life

Magnet Rates:
BOL-ERI = 100 ppm
ERI-EOL = 85 ppm
EOL < = 85 ppm

Fig. 9–17. Printout from the pacemaker programmer demonstrating remaining battery voltage. The "gas gauge" indicates that this pacemaker is near BOL (beginning of life).

perienced a clinical event, such as syncope or presyncope, that is thought to be rhythm-related.

Invasive troubleshooting should begin with pulse generator manipulation in the open pocket while the electrocardiogram is observed for abnormalities in pacing or sensing. After delivery of the generator from the pocket, the connection between the pins and the setscrews should be inspected. The lead or leads should then be disconnected from the pulse generator, and thresholds, current, and impedance should be directly measured by the pacing system analyzer before any further manipulation of the leads. Normally, only minor variation exists between the

Table 9–5.
Intraoperative Analysis of Pacing Systems

Visual inspection
 • Connector
 • Setscrews
 • Lead insulation
 • Conductor coil
 • Suturing sleeve
 • Pacemaker insulation and coating
Capture threshold
Sensing threshold
Impedance
Intracardiac electrogram
Manipulation of lead or patient (or both)

Modified from Love and Hayes.[1] By permission of WB Saunders Company.

values obtained by telemetry and those obtained by direct measurement; gross differences suggest lead abnormalities. One of the most important measurements obtained at the time of intraoperative troubleshooting is lead impedance. After the electrical integrity of the lead is assessed, the leads should be carefully dissected away from any fibrous tissue and visually inspected. Any obvious breaks in the insulation or fractures in the coil should be noted, especially in the area under any anchoring or purse-string sutures. Blood in the lead is de facto evidence of a breach in the insulation. Unfortunately, only that portion of the lead that is extravascular can be visually inspected. We believe that any breach of lead integrity warrants lead replacement rather than repair. Lead repair should rarely be attempted and only by someone with considerable experience.

One is sometimes left, however, with a clinical situation strongly suggestive of pacing system malfunction and no obvious point of failure. In that case, careful consideration could be given to empirically placing a new lead, especially the ventricular lead in a pacemaker-dependent patient. However, empirical replacement of any portion of the pacing system should be considered only as a last resort.

Focused Troubleshooting

Now that the broader issues that should be considered during troubleshooting have been discussed, the issue is next approached in a focused manner, that is, by the presenting clinical problem. Most problems can be categorized by electrocardiographic abnormalities:

- Failure to capture
- Failure to output
- Undersensing
- Alteration of pacing rate

Or by patient symptoms:

- Syncope or near-syncope
- Palpitations
- Fatigue

Each category is discussed after a differential diagnosis has been provided. Some problems occur more commonly early after implantation, that is, within the first few weeks after implantation, some at a much later date, and some completely independent of time. An attempt is made to classify each abnormality by whether it is most likely to occur early, late, or at any time after implantation.

Failure to Capture

The different reasons for failure to capture (Fig. 9–18) and the most likely time of appearance for the abnormality are as follows:

- Lead dislodgment — Early
- Damage at the electrode-myo-cardium interface — At any time
- Exit block — After the first 4 to 6 weeks
- Perforation — Acutely
- Lead fracture — Usually late
- Lead insulation failure — At any time
- Loose setscrew — Usually early
- Battery failure — Usually late
- Circuit failure — At any time
- Air in pocket (unipolar) — Acutely
- Pseudomalfunction — At any time
- Metabolic or drug effect — At any time

Lead dislodgment usually occurs relatively soon after implantation. It may be microdislodgment or macrodislodgment. Macrodislodgment implies that the problem is radiographically evident. Microdislodgment implies that the clinical situation is consistent with dislodgment but that there is no radiographic evidence that the lead has moved.

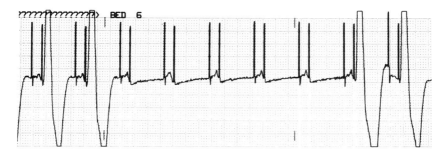

Fig. 9–18. Electrocardiographic tracing of a dual-chamber pacemaker. There is intermittent ventricular failure to capture. This tracing was obtained a few hours after pacemaker implantation. The most likely diagnosis is ventricular lead dislodgment. (From Hayes DL: Pacemaker electrocardiography. *In* A Practice of Cardiac Pacing. Third edition. Edited by S Furman, DL Hayes, DR Holmes Jr. Mount Kisco, NY, Futura Publishing Company, 1993, pp 309–359. By permission of Mayo Foundation.)

With lead dislodgment, failure to capture may be intermittent or persistent. It is often, but not always, accompanied by sensing abnormalities (Fig. 9–19). If macrodislodgment is confirmed, the lead should be repositioned. The diagnosis of microdislodgment should be entertained and the lead repositioned only if other causes of failure to capture have been excluded.

In Figure 9–20, atrial lead dislodgment leads to cross-stimulation. "Cross-stimulation" is defined as stimulation of a cardiac chamber different from the one to which the stimulus is directed.[23,24] This may result from atrial lead dislodgment into the ventricle or from atrial lead stimulation near the tricuspid valve or in the coronary sinus. Cross-stimulation as a reversal of lead connection could also occur but is uncommonly reported.

Elevated thresholds may be due to a variety of causes, including lead dislodgment, loss of lead integrity (e.g., fracture or insulation defect), damage at the electrode-myocardium interface, and meta-

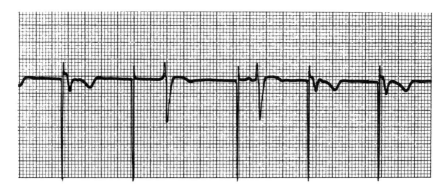

Fig. 9–19. Electrocardiographic tracing from a patient with a VVI pacemaker. The pacemaker is programmed to a rate of 70 bpm. There is intermittent failure to capture, with second and third pacing artifacts. Sensing is intermittent because the first intrinsic ventricular event resets the VV timing cycle but the second intrinsic ventricular event does not. (From Hayes DL: Pacemaker electrocardiography. *In* A Practice of Cardiac Pacing. Third edition. Edited by S Furman, DL Hayes, DR Holmes Jr. Mount Kisco, NY, Futura Publishing Company, 1993, pp 309–359. By permission of Mayo Foundation.)

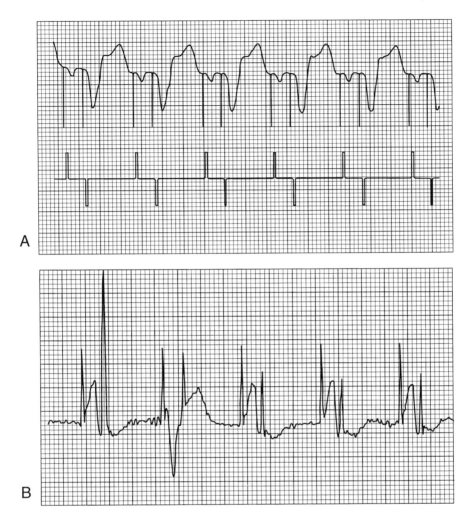

Fig. 9–20. *A,* Electrocardiographic tracing shortly after the implantation of a dual-chamber pacemaker. The tracing confirms atrial and ventricular capture. *B,* Electrocardiographic tracing from the same patient at a 4-week follow-up examination. The atrial pacing artifact results in ventricular stimulation, and the ventricular artifact occurs at the same atrioventricular interval but falls after the ventricular depolarization. Chest radiography confirmed that the atrial lead had dislodged into the ventricular lead. Because the intrinsic deflection of the ventricular depolarization was consistently falling within the blanking period, the atrioventricular interval was not disturbed. (Courtesy of Lisa Anderson, R.N., Wheeling, Illinois.)

bolic, electrolyte, or drug changes (Fig. 9–21). If threshold elevation is due to lead dislodgment, it may be possible, depending on the degree of dislodgment, to reestablish capture by increasing output parameters.

Damage at the electrode-myocardium interface may occur from several causes. Myocardial infarction, an infiltrative car-diomyopathic process, or localized damage secondary to cardioversion or defibrillation could damage the myocardium at the site of the electrode.[25] With an infiltrative process, the alteration in pacing or sensing threshold may be permanent. With myocardial infarction and after cardioversion or defibrillation, the changes may be transient or permanent.

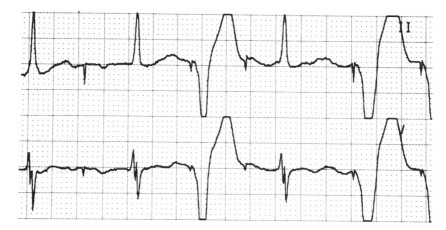

Fig. 9–21. Electrocardiographic tracing from a patient with a DDD pacemaker. The underlying rhythm was atrial fibrillation, and there was erratic ventricular tracking of the fibrillatory waves. Intermittently, loss of ventricular capture was noted. Output parameters were increased, and consistent capture was obtained. Lead impedance was normal, as was the radiographic appearance. The elevated thresholds were thought to be secondary to a transient electrolyte abnormality.

Altered pacing-sensing thresholds after cardioversion-defibrillation occur if the electrical current is transmitted through the lead and results in a circumscribed burn at the electrode-myocardium interface[25] (Fig. 9–22). The threshold alteration is usually transient, minutes or hours.

Exit block, by definition, is manifested by increased thresholds. Exit block is defined as chronically elevated thresholds, presumably due to excessive fibrosis or some other problem at the electrode-myocardium interface.[26] True exit block is uncommon, and the cause is not well understood. Steroid-eluting leads generally, but not always, prevent exit block. The diagnostic problem is trying to differentiate exit block from microdislodgment. If microdislodgment is the presumed diagnosis, the lead is repositioned, and thresholds improve, the problem remains unsolved. If exit block is the real problem, the thresholds will again rise. If this occurs with steroid-eluting leads, the only

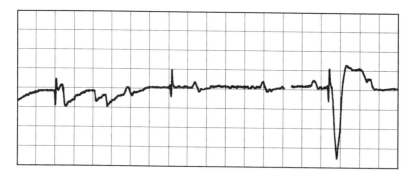

Fig. 9–22. Electrocardiographic tracing from a patient with a dual-chamber pacemaker programmed to the VVI pacing mode. Immediately after cardioversion, ventricular failure to capture occurs with the first two pacing artifacts and capture with the third. This is compatible with cardioversion-related damage at the electrode-myocardium interface.

option is to program the pacing output to levels that allow consistent pacing and potentially an adequate safety margin. Most contemporary pacemakers can be programmed to maximum outputs of 7.5 V and 1.5 msec. If capture cannot be maintained at these levels, a "high-output" generator could be considered. One manufacturer, Biotronik, Inc., makes pulse generators capable of 8.4 V. This voltage may provide the additional output necessary to maintain capture in some patients.

The use of systemic steroids to treat high outputs is often contemplated. Large doses of systemic steroids usually result in a decrement in pacing thresholds.[26,27] However, when administration is discontinued, the thresholds generally increase again. Long-term use of these steroids is obviously not desirable because of the systemic side effects.

Perforation may cause elevated thresholds. The effect of perforation on pacing thresholds depends on the extent and location of the perforation.[28] Perforation is often accompanied by other symptoms (see below), but increased thresholds can occur in isolation. When this diagnosis is considered, other symptoms and signs should be looked for, including extracardiac stimulation, pericardial pain, pericardial rub, and hemodynamic compromise. Electrocardiographic findings (Fig. 9–23), echocardiography, and cine computed tomography may all be helpful in making the diagnosis.

Metabolic and drug alterations may also affect thresholds and result in failure to capture.[29–38] Drugs that may affect pacing thresholds are listed in Table 9–4. Two comments should be made about drug therapy. Class IC antiarrhythmic agents are the most likely drugs to affect pacing thresholds. If a pacemaker-dependent patient is beginning to receive a Class IC agent, administration should be done cautiously and the patient's course followed carefully. This class of drugs may also affect sensing thresholds[28–31] (Fig. 9–24).

A common misconception is that amiodarone raises pacing thresholds. Amiodarone does increase defibrillation thresholds.[32] Amiodarone can raise pacing thresholds in patients with hypothyroidism.[33] In the euthyroid patient, amiodarone rarely if ever can be blamed for an increase in pacing thresholds.

Most severe metabolic disturbances can affect pacing and sensing thresholds.[34–38] Hyperkalemia is the most commonly encountered metabolic disturbance to do so. The most common clinical occurrence is in the patient with a pacemaker who is undergoing dialysis. Although programming output or sensing variables may help in the short term, the definitive treatment is to lower the potassium levels and avoid subsequent episodes of hyperkalemia.

Older studies have documented sensing and pacing threshold variations with such everyday activities as sleeping and eating.[34–38] Although well documented, the threshold variations are minimal. In addition, with the low achievable pacing thresholds and outstanding sensing thresholds available with contemporary pacing systems, the issue becomes even less significant.

Loose setscrew may cause failure to capture. Although this is usually detected in the early postimplantation period, a setscrew that has not been effectively tightened may not work loose for months. The clinical presentation of a loose setscrew depends on the degree of contact between the connector pin and the header. If the header and pin are completely disconnected, complete failure to output occurs because of the circuit interruption. If failure of contact is intermittent, failure to output is also intermittent (Fig. 9–25). This is probably the most common presentation. At other times, minimal contact between pin and header may allow transmission of a pacing artifact, but inadequate energy is transmitted to result in capture.

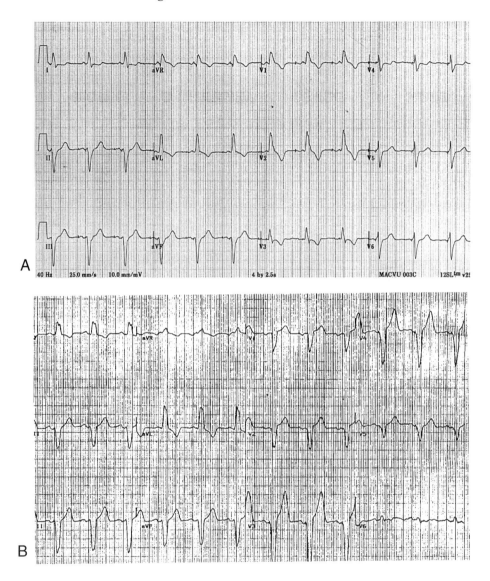

Fig. 9–23. *A*, Electrocardiographic tracing from a patient with a dual-chamber pacemaker. The paced ventricular events have an RBBB configuration, suggesting that pacing is from the left ventricle. In this patient, the right ventricular lead had been passed across a patent foramen ovale into the left atrium and then to the left ventricle. *B*, Electrocardiographic tracing after repositioning of the ventricular lead in the right ventricular apex. A more typical paced QRS morphology is now present. (Courtesy of Dr. John D. Symanski, Sanger Clinic, Charlotte, NC.)

Conductor coil fracture may produce failure to capture, failure to output, and sensing abnormalities (Fig. 9–26). In complete fracture, the electrocardiographic findings are persistent. In "make-or-break" fracture, the electrocardiographic abnormalities are intermittent. If the fracture is complete, that is, the circuit is interrupted, failure to output occurs. If the break is incomplete, that is, only a portion of the output pulse is transmitted to the heart, failure to capture is seen. Often,

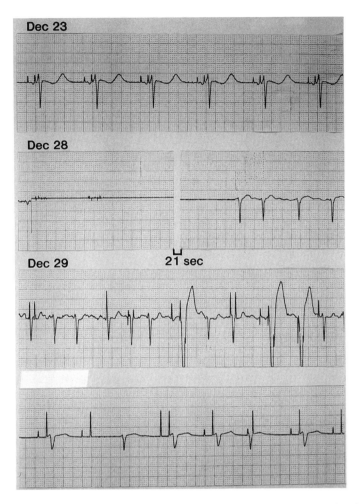

Fig. 9–24. Series of electrocardiographic tracings from a patient who received a dual-chamber pacemaker for tachycardia-bradycardia syndrome. The *top tracing* reveals dual-chamber pacing with atrial capture and ventricular fusion or pseudofusion. (Without an intrinsic ventricular event, it is impossible to state with certainty whether any degree of fusion exists.) The *second tracing* demonstrates a flat line that suggests an artifact. In fact, a monitoring electrode had fallen off, resulting in 21 seconds of artifactual recording. The *third tracing* reveals intermittent ventricular failure to sense and capture. The underlying rhythm appears to be atrial fibrillation. The *bottom tracing* suggests intermittent failure to capture and sense in both chambers. Administration of propafenone had been started for treatment of tachyarrhythmias. The drug resulted in significant elevation of both pacing and sensing thresholds.

both manifestations are present. Escaping current at the "break" may also cause sensing abnormalities.

Although programming a bipolar lead to a unipolar pacing and sensing configuration may restore normal pacing, this "fix" should be considered temporary

(Fig. 9–27). Whatever mechanism fractured the outer coil of a coaxial lead could eventually affect the inner coil as well.

Insulation break also can produce a variety of clinical manifestations. Insulation defects may involve the outer insulation or, in a bipolar lead, the insulation

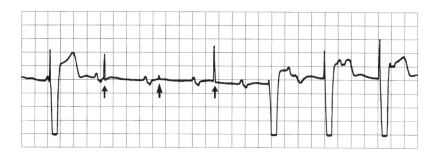

Fig. 9–25. Electrocardiographic tracing from a patient with a DDD pacemaker and recurrent near-syncope. This tracing was obtained during pocket manipulation. The pause occurs because of failure to capture due to a loose setscrew. With a loose setscrew and intermittent contact, the electrocardiogram may reveal intermittent capture, no output, or output with failure to capture.

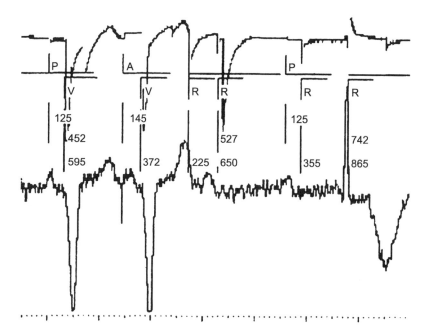

Fig. 9–26. Electrocardiographic tracing obtained by the programmer in a patient with a ventricular lead fracture. The electrogram identifies intrinsic ventricular events (R) where none occur, because escaping current is sensed by the pacemaker and identified as a ventricular event. There is also evidence of failure to capture, identified by a paced ventricular output (V) without a corresponding paced ventricular event on the surface electrocardiogram (*lower tracing*). The electrogram (*upper tracing*) is erratic because of the lead fracture. *P*, intrinsic atrial event; *A*, paced atrial event.

between conductors (Fig. 9–28). Sensing abnormalities are the most common electrocardiographic manifestation.[39] Failure to capture and failure to output, intermittent or persistent, may also be seen (Fig. 9–29 and 9–30).

As with conductor coil fracture, programming a bipolar lead to unipolar

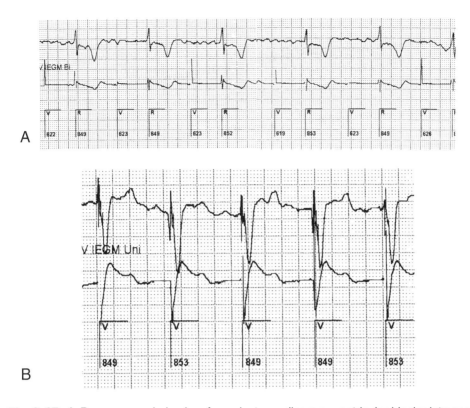

Fig. 9–27. *A,* Programmer-derived surface electrocardiogram, ventricular bipolar intracardiac electrogram, and markers demonstrating VVI pacing at 70 bpm with failure to capture. Telemetered ventricular impedance was > 9,999 Ω. *B,* Reprogrammed to the unipolar pacing configuration at the same output settings, ventricular capture is now consistent and the lead impedance is within normal range.

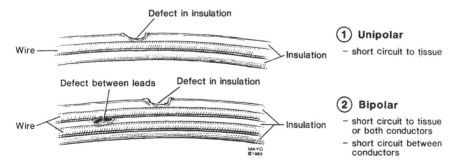

Fig. 9–28. *Top,* Insulation defect of a unipolar lead allows a short circuit to the tissue. *Bottom,* A bipolar lead can have an insulation defect that short-circuits to the tissue or between conductors. (From Furman S: Troubleshooting implanted cardiac pacemakers. *In* A Practice of Cardiac Pacing. Edited by S Furman, DL Hayes, DR Holmes Jr. Mount Kisco, NY, Futura Publishing Company, 1986, pp 273–303. By permission of Mayo Foundation.)

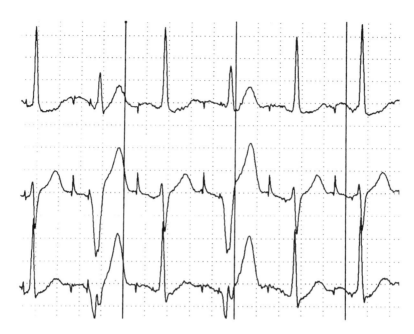

Fig. 9–29. Electrocardiographic tracing obtained from a patient with a ventricular polyurethane pacing lead on advisory. There is intermittent ventricular failure to capture. The finding is relatively subtle. The second and fourth ventricular events are paced. The other ventricular events are intrinsic. The ventricular pacing artifact precedes the intrinsic ventricular events but fails to capture. Interrogation revealed a lead impedance of < 250 Ω.

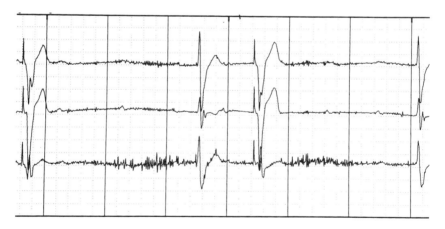

Fig. 9–30. Electrocardiographic tracing obtained from a patient with a ventricular polyurethane pacing lead on advisory. In this example, there are two pauses. The intervals are not exact multiples of the paced VV cycle (the distance from the second to third ventricular event). Without marker channel or intracardiac electrograms, it is not possible to say whether this is an example of oversensing or whether there is an undetected paced ventricular artifact with failure to capture. However, with the lead advisory, the possibility of a defective lead is difficult to ignore.

pacing and sensing configuration may restore normal pacing and sensing. In contrast to the situation with a conductor coil fracture, reprogramming to a unipolar configuration might be an acceptable longer-term solution. If the insulation defect is in a ventricular lead in a pacemaker-dependent patient, even if programming to a unipolar configuration restores normal function, the lead should be replaced.

Battery failure is an expected late complication. Fortunately, battery depletion is almost always a predictable phenomenon, one that is readily detected as part of a regular follow-up program.[20] Some pacemaker and ICD models have had battery depletion patterns that were unpredictable or earlier than projected. If a pacemaker or ICD is known to have unpredictable or sudden battery failure, the device should be prophylactically replaced.

Air in the pocket may result in a pacing failure if the pacemaker is functioning in a unipolar pacing configuration. Since a pacemaker in the unipolar pacing configuration must make tissue contact to "complete the circuit," air can insulate the pacemaker and prevent tissue contact. Failure to capture and failure to output may occur (Fig. 9–31).

This clinical problem is uncommon and usually occurs only if an older larger pacemaker is replaced with a smaller unipolar-configured pacemaker. If tissue contact is reestablished, the pacing abnormalities resolve immediately. Usually, simple pressure on the pacemaker pocket solves the problem.

Circuit or component failure is rare. Contemporary pacemakers and ICDs have achieved an extraordinary level of reliability. If a circuit or component failure occurs, the clinical manifestation is usually not predictable and almost any electrocardiographic abnormality is possible.[20]

For patients who are not pacemaker-dependent, who have experienced a clinical event that suggests failure of some component of the pacing system, and who do not have any source of failure revealed by a thorough noninvasive evaluation, Holter monitoring, an event recorder, or an implantable loop recorder may be considered. If a true malfunction of the device is suspected, the manufacturer should be asked whether similar problems have been reported (see above).

Several *pseudomalfunctions* may suggest failure to capture. *Functional failure to capture* occurs if a pacing artifact is deliv-

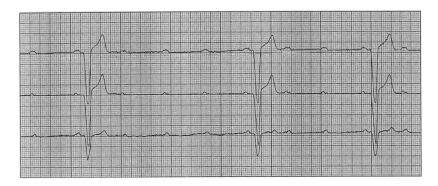

Fig. 9–31. Electrocardiographic tracing shortly after replacement of a dual-chamber pacemaker. The tracing demonstrates ventricular failure to pace (output) with ventricular asystole. The pacemaker was unipolar and had replaced a significantly larger unipolar device. "Air in the pocket" was thought to be the cause of the abnormality, and pressure on the pocket restored normal function.

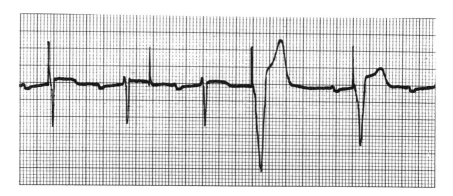

Fig. 9–32. Magnet application in a patient with a VVI pacemaker. When asynchronous pacing artifacts occur early after an intrinsic event, there is no capture. This is considered functional failure to capture because it is a function of the refractory state of the myocardium due to the immediately preceding intrinsic depolarization.

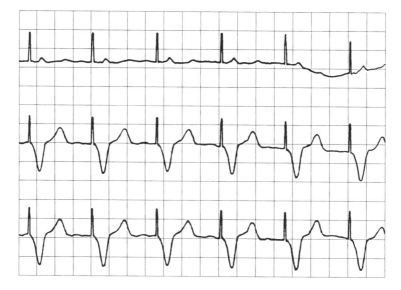

Fig. 9–33. Three-channel electrocardiographic tracing from a patient with P-synchronous pacing. If the top tracing is viewed in isolation, it is difficult to tell which chamber is paced and if there is capture. However, a clue in the top recording is that there appears to be ventricular repolarization, that is, a T wave; therefore, there must have been depolarization, even if the QRS is difficult to identify.

ered when the ventricle is functionally refractory. For example, during magnet application and asynchronous pacing, a pacing artifact that occurs early after an intrinsic event will not capture the myocardium (Fig. 9–32).

Isoelectric atrial or ventricular depolarization may suggest failure to capture; that is, a pacing artifact is recorded but there is minimal, if any, electrocardio-graphic evidence of depolarization. Confirmation can be obtained by a multichannel recording (Fig. 9–33).

Failure to Pace (No Output)

- Battery failure
- Circuit failure

- Lead fracture
- Insulation failure
- Oversensing
- Loose setscrew
- Crosstalk
- Incompatible lead and header
    Unipolar lead with a bipolar
        device
    Bipolar lead with a unipolar
        device
- Pseudomalfunction
    Small bipolar pacing artifacts
    Circadian function
    Mode switching
    Isoelectric intrinsic rhythm

Battery failure (Fig. 9–34), circuit or component failure, lead fracture, insulation defect, and loose setscrew have all been discussed as potential causes of failure to output.

The most common cause of failure to pace or output is probably oversensing. Oversensing implies that something is sensed other than an intrinsic atrial or ventricular depolarization and therefore the timing cycle is reset and the pacing output inhibited (Fig. 9–35). As previously noted, oversensing may be a manifestation of lead failure, either conductor coil fracture or insulation defect (Fig. 9–36).

Crosstalk occurs when an atrial pacing output is sensed on the ventricular sensing channel and inhibits ventricular output[40] (Fig. 9–37 and 9–38). Mechanisms that contribute to crosstalk include high atrial output, ventricular sensitivity programmed to a very sensitive value, and positioning of atrial and ventricular leads in close proximity. Crosstalk is less common with bipolar sensing configuration.

In an effort to prevent crosstalk, pacemakers incorporate a ventricular blanking period. The blanking period is the initial portion of the AV interval. During this period, decay of the atrial pacing output is maximal and the atrial output has the greatest potential for being sensed on the ventricular channel. If something is sensed immediately after the blanking period, it is not possible to distinguish between crosstalk and an intrinsic event. As a safety measure, dual-chamber pacemakers deliver a ventricular pacing artifact at a foreshortened AV interval if something is sensed in the interval after the blanking period. This portion of the AV interval has been dubbed the "crosstalk sensing window." If atrial afterpolarization is sensed, ventricular safety pacing results in effective ventricular capture at a short AV interval, usually 100 to 110 msec, and prevents ventricular asystole[40] (Fig. 9–39). If an intrinsic ventricular event, for example, a premature ventricular contraction, is sensed, the ventricular safety pacing artifact is delivered within the intrinsic event or shortly after and not during ventricular repolarization (T wave).

When ventricular events are sensed on the atrial sensing channel and reset the timing cycle, the most appropriate description for this abnormality is *far-field sensing* (Fig. 9–40). The longer intervals are equal to the AR or AV interval plus the programmed AA interval; for example, if the AR interval is 200 msec and the programmed lower rate limit is 60 bpm, or 1,000 msec, the interval lengthened as a result of far-field sensing is 200 plus 1,000, or 1,200 msec. This effect can usually be eliminated by lengthening the atrial refractory period so that the intrinsic ventricular event is ignored or by programming the atrial channel to a less sensitive value.

Oversensing can be caused by many things, which can be classified as

- Biologic sources of interference, for example, retrograde P-wave, T-wave myopotentials[41–44]
- Paced ventricular afterdepolarization
- Nonbiologic sources of electromagnetic interference (see Chapter 12)

If myopotential inhibition is suspected, a series of maneuvers should be

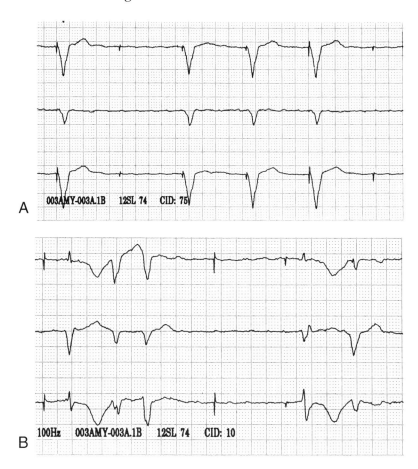

Fig. 9–34. *A,* Electrocardiographic tracing from a patient with a ventricular pacemaker and recurrent near-syncope. The patient had not had her pacemaker checked in several years. The electrocardiogram reveals intermittent failure to capture, and troubleshooting results were consistent with nearly total battery depletion. *B,* The patient was admitted to the hospital, and a subsequent tracing demonstrated complete failure to capture and ventricular rhythm disturbances secondary to the bradycardia. At the time of pulse generator replacement, lead function was normal.

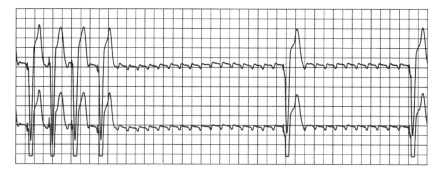

Fig. 9–35. Electrocardiographic tracing from a patient with a single-chamber pacemaker. The patient is exposed to an external source of electromagnetic interference, which profoundly inhibits ventricular output, that is, ventricular oversensing.

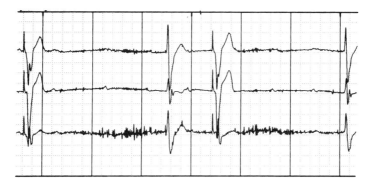

Fig. 9–36. Electrocardiographic tracing from a patient with a VVI pacemaker and a polyurethane ventricular lead on medical advisory. The patient presents with recurrent near-syncope, and the tracing reveals oversensing. Lead impedance is compatible with an insulation failure.

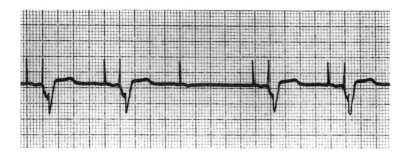

Fig. 9–37. Electrocardiographic tracing from a patient with a dual-chamber pacemaker and failure of ventricular output after the third atrial pacing artifact. Crosstalk is the most likely explanation, but without verification by intracardiac electrograms or a diagnostic interpretation channel, other explanations of oversensing should be considered.

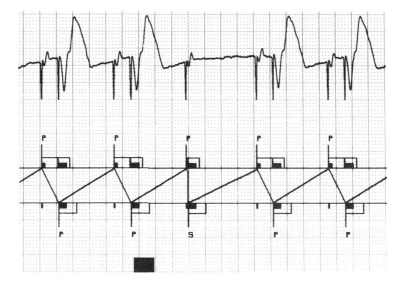

Fig. 9–38. Electrocardiographic example of "crosstalk." Although crosstalk appears to be the most likely cause of ventricular failure to output when the surface electrocardiogram is assessed, it is confirmed by the telemetered "ladder diagram." The ladder diagram confirms that the atrial output was detected almost simultaneously on the ventricular sensing channel and that ventricular output was inhibited. P, paced; S, sensed.

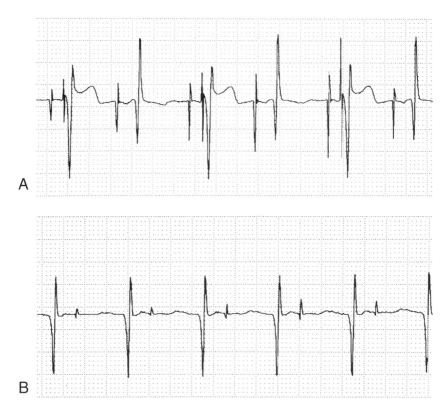

Fig. 9–39. *A*, Electrocardiographic tracing from a pediatric patient with a dual-chamber pacemaker after surgical correction of a congenital cardiac anomaly. Every other ventricular event is paced at an abbreviated atrioventricular interval consistent with ventricular safety pacing. The atrial lead was programmed to excessively high outputs. *B*, Tracing after reprogramming of the atrial output to values that allowed for an adequate safety margin but no longer resulted in ventricular safety pacing.

performed in an effort to document this cause. In our pacemaker clinic, a series of isometric maneuvers is accomplished while the electrocardiogram is monitored. These include

- Hands clasped, pulling against each other
- Palms of hands together, pushing against each other
- Reaching with right arm across left shoulder
- Reaching with left arm across right shoulder
- Pocket manipulation (although not specifically to bring out myopotential inhibition but instead to assess for integrity of the lead or leads and integrity of the lead-connector block connection, this procedure is done in concert with the other maneuvers)

If maneuvers induce myopotential inhibition, the programmed sensitivity is made less sensitive and the maneuvers are repeated in an effort to find a sensitivity value at which significant myopotential inhibition no longer occurs but sensing of intracardiac events is still intact (Fig. 9–41).

When an interval longer than the programmed lower rate is observed, the point of sensing can be determined by measuring backward from the pacing artifact that terminates the longer interval (Fig. 9–42). For example, if a VVI pace-

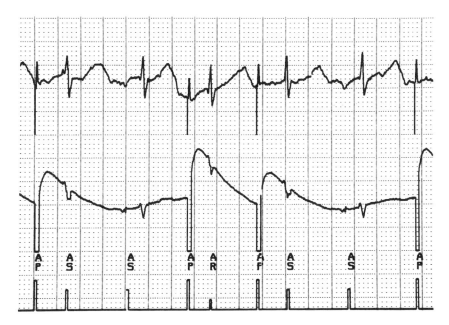

Fig. 9–40. Electrocardiographic example obtained from a patient with an AAI pacemaker. The programmed AA cycle length is 95 bpm, 630 msec. However, some AR intervals are greater than 630 msec. This occurs because there is far-field sensing; that is, the ventricular event is sensed on the atrial sensing channel and resets the timing cycle. This is verified on the simultaneous marker channel. Three ventricular events—first, third, and fourth—are sensed as atrial events. AP, atrial paced event; AR, atrial event occurring in the refractory period; AS, atrial sensed event.

maker is programmed to 60 bpm, 1,000 msec, and an interval of 1,500 msec is observed, measuring back 1,000 msec from the pacing artifact that ends the 1,500-msec interval marks the point of sensing, that is, the point at which the timing cycle is reset.

An *incompatible lead-header* combination is a clinical possibility but is rarely seen. Lead design and compatibility are discussed in Chapter 4. Any incompatibility of the lead and header should be readily apparent at the time they are connected. To be certain that an adequate connection has been established at the time of implantation if pacing output is not observed, a magnet should be applied to confirm output and capture.

With international standard (IS)-1 lead-header designs, unipolar and bipolar leads are of the same dimensions. If a unipolar IS-1 lead is connected to a bipolar pacemaker that is programmed to a bipolar configuration, no pacing will occur. Some contemporary pacemakers detect the incompatibility and prevent the programming combination, allowing the pacemaker to be programmed only to a unipolar configuration.

Pseudomalfunctions may also suggest failure to output. Small bipolar pacing artifacts may not be visible on the electrocardiogram and raise the question of failure to output or of oversensing.

Digital recording systems may also give the appearance of failure to output.[45] Digital recording systems, the type of electrocardiographic recording system used by most hospitals and offices today, artificially create the pacing artifact (Fig. 9–43). As a function of the system, pacing artifacts may not always be seen. A clue to this abnormality is that the ventricular depolarizations with and without pacing artifacts are of the same morphology. In Figure 9–44, this pseudomalfunction is

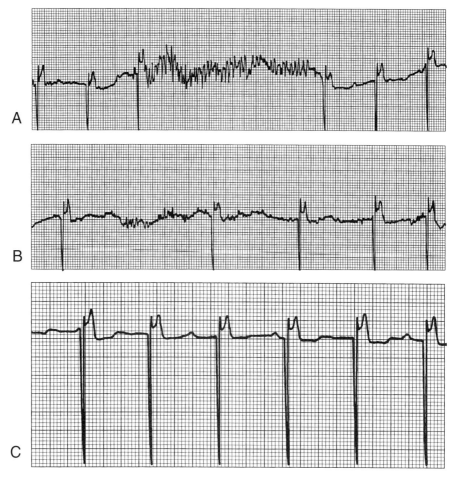

Fig. 9–41. Series of electrocardiographic tracings obtained during provocative maneuvers to induce myopotential inhibition in a patient with a pacemaker programmed to the VVI mode. There is significant inhibition at programming to 1 mV (*A*) sensitivity. Inhibition decreases at 2.0 mV (*B*) and is absent at 4.0 mV (*C*).

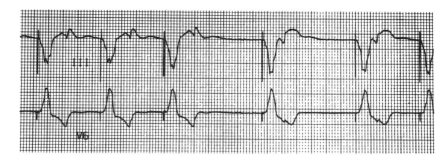

Fig. 9–42. Electrocardiographic tracing from a patient with a VVI pacemaker. The programmed rate of the pacemaker is 70 bpm, 857 msec, but there are longer intervals. Measuring 857 msec backward from the ventricular pacing artifact that ends the longer intervals determines that the point of sensing is either a retrograde P wave or a T wave. Without electrograms or a diagnostic interpretation channel, one cannot be certain which event was oversensed. (From Hayes DL, Zipes DP: Cardiac pacemakers and cardioverter-defibrillators. *In* Heart Disease: A Textbook of Cardiovascular Medicine. Sixth edition. Edited by E Braunwald, DP Zipes, P Libby. Philadelphia, WB Saunders Company [in press]. By permission of the publisher.

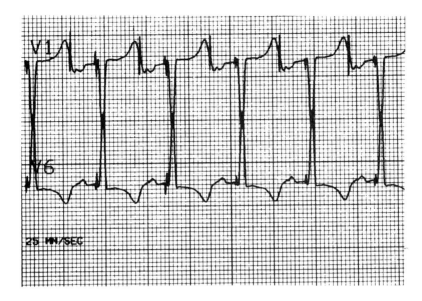

Fig. 9–43. Two-channel electrocardiographic recording from a digital recording system. In the *upper tracing,* the atrial pacing artifact is large (approximately 8 to 9 mm). In the *lower tracing,* the atrial pacing artifact cannot be appreciated at all.

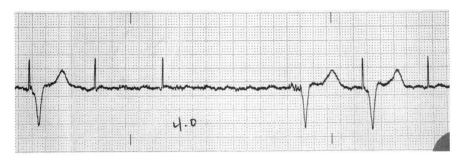

Fig. 9–44. Electrocardiographic tracing from a patient with a pacemaker programmed to the VVIR pacing mode. The lower rate of the pacemaker is programmed to 60 bpm. The tracing demonstrates intermittent failure to capture and a long pause without evidence of pacing artifacts, a suggestion of oversensing. Careful inspection of the second ventricular depolarization reveals the lack of a pacing artifact. This patient was pacemaker-dependent, and all ventricular activity was paced. Pacing artifacts occur during the interval that appears to be a pause without any pacing activity. This finding was proven by intracardiac electrograms. It can also be suspected from the surface electrocardiogram, because the pause is an even multiple of the programmed lower rate interval. If this were oversensing, a pause that was an exact multiple of the pacing rate would be unlikely. The inability to detect pacing artifacts is not uncommon with digital recording systems.

associated with true failure to capture in a patient with exit block. In this situation, another clue is that all the pauses are a multiple of the programmed lower rate.

Although not a pseudomalfunction, a common error is diagnosis of oversensing because a near-isoelectric event is overlooked. If an event is truly isoelectric, an intracardiac electrogram or a diagnostic interpretation channel is necessary to make the diagnosis. Figures 9–45, 9–46, and 9–47 show examples of near-isoelectric events. A basic tenet to remember in troubleshooting is that even without a

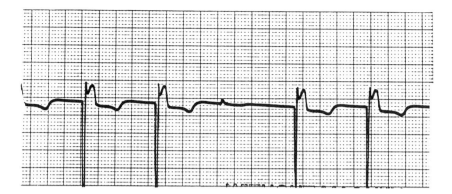

Fig. 9–45. Transtelephonic tracing with an intrinsic ventricular event of very small amplitude after the second paced ventricular event. The repolarization, that is, T wave, of the intrinsic event is not appreciated. If reviewed in a cursory fashion, this tracing would be easy to mistake as an example of oversensing.

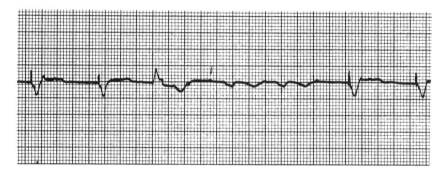

Fig. 9–46. Electrocardiographic tracing from a patient with a VVI pacemaker. After the third ventricular event, there appears to be some baseline activity but no clearcut cardiac activity. However, measuring backward from the subsequent paced ventricular event by the interval equal to the programmed pacing rate appears to indicate that the activity in the baseline is two intrinsic ventricular events and T waves.

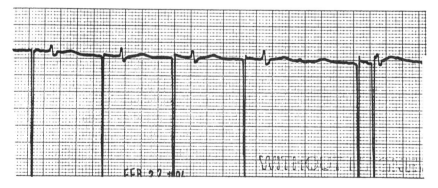

Fig. 9–47. Transtelephonic tracing from a patient with a dual-chamber pacemaker. Measuring back from the final ventricular paced event by an interval equal to the AA interval shows that a small-amplitude complex representing an intrinsic ventricular event is present. (The AA interval is used for measurement because only one paced ventricular event occurs. If there is no alteration of the AV or AR interval, the AA interval should generally be equivalent to the VV interval.)

recognizable depolarization, a subsequent repolarization, that is, a T wave, affirms a preceding depolarization.

Undersensing

- Change in intrinsic complex, e.g., bundle branch block, ventricular fibrillation, ventricular tachycardia, atrial fibrillation
- Myocardial infarction
- Lead dislodgment or poor positioning (Fig. 9–48)
- Lead insulation failure
- Magnet application
- Battery depletion
- Component failure (Fig. 9–49)
- Metabolic or drug effect
- Functional undersensing

Any event that results in an intrinsic complex that differs from the intrinsic complex that was present and measured at the time of pacemaker implantation may cause undersensing. For example, a premature ventricular contraction, which may actually appear larger than the normally conducted ventricular event on the surface electrocardiogram, may not be sensed (Fig. 9–50). Making the ventricular sensing channel more sensitive may allow normal sensing of premature ventricular contractions. However, if the undersensing is only intermittent, the premature ventricular contractions occur rarely, and the normally conducted beats are appropriately sensed, it may not be necessary to take any additional action.

Undersensing in either chamber is theoretically troublesome because of the potential for competitive pacing. Specifically, the concern is one of pacing in a vulnerable portion of the cardiac cycle, that is, during repolarization. Pacing on a T wave could initiate ventricular fibrillation or ventricular tachycardia, and pacing during atrial repolarization could initiate atrial fibrillation. Both have been documented, but both are uncommon. This conclusion is supported by the fact that although magnet application results in competitive pacing, as a routine part of transtelephonic follow-up it is rarely identified as inducing a tachyarrhythmia.

As noted above, any event that damages the myocardium at the electrode-myocardium interface could alter sensing thresholds. Undersensing may be a manifestation of conductor coil fracture and insulation break. In fact, sensing abnormalities are the most common electrocardiographic manifestation of loss of insulation integrity.

Also noted previously, metabolic disturbances and drugs can affect sensing thresholds. Class IC antiarrhythmic agents are the most likely to alter sensing thresholds, and hyperkalemia is the most common metabolic disturbance to result in undersensing.

If the pacemaker battery reaches the very low voltage level, undersensing may occur.

Functional undersensing occurs when an intrinsic event falls within a blanking period or refractory period and is not sensed as a function of the pacemaker programming.[2] This can cause confusion in electrocardiographic interpretation unless electrograms or a Marker Channel is available. Figure 9–51 demonstrates functional undersensing as a result of extension of the postventricular atrial refractory period. Because the postventricular atrial refractory period is extended in consecutive cycles, the P waves are consecutively within this period and therefore not tracked. The appearance is of true undersensing, but function is normal.

When undersensing occurs (Fig. 9–52), the approach should be as follows:

- Determine the cause of the undersensing.
- Assess the amplitude of the undersensed event by telemetered electrograms, if available. Compare the measured amplitude with the programmed sensitivity.

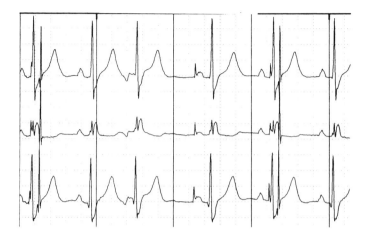

Fig. 9–48. Tracing from an ambulatory monitor shows intermittent atrial failure to sense. This is best seen at the fifth ventricular complex. A P wave precedes the intrinsic ventricular event, but this is not sensed, and an atrial pacing artifact occurs immediately before the intrinsic ventricular complex. The ventricular complex is sensed in the crosstalk sensing window. As a result, the ventricular pacing artifact is delivered early after the intrinsic ventricular event, that is, ventricular safety pacing.

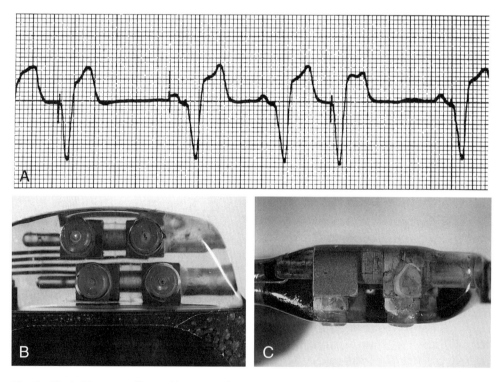

Fig. 9–49. *A*, Electrocardiographic tracing from a patient with a dual-chamber pacemaker and intermittent atrial failure to sense. Despite reprogramming, the intermittent undersensing of atrial sensitivity persisted for years. *B* (side view of pulse generator) and *C* (top view), At the time of pulse generator replacement, inspection revealed an area of corrosion at the site of one of the atrial grommets. After pulse generator replacement, no further atrial undersensing was noted.

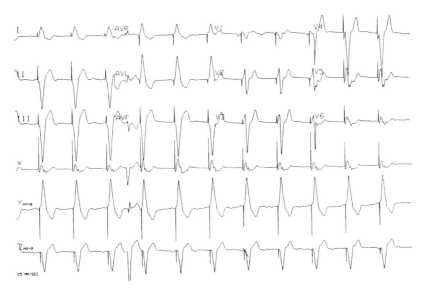

Fig. 9–50. Electrocardiographic tracing in which a single premature ventricular contraction is not sensed.

- If possible, correct whatever change has resulted in undersensing.
- If the cause of the undersensing cannot be corrected or if immediate resolution is required, reprogram the sensitivity to a more sensitive value.

Alteration in Programmed Pacing Rate

- Circuit failure
- Battery failure
- Magnet application
- Hysteresis
- Crosstalk
- Undocumented reprogramming
- Oversensing
- Runaway pacemaker
- Malfunction of electrocardiographic recording equipment; alteration in paper speed

Undocumented reprogramming is probably the most common cause of an alteration in the programmed pacing rate; that is, another health care professional has reprogrammed the pacing rate and failed to document the change. To avoid this, a system should be in place whereby any reprogramming requires that the pacemaker be interrogated, the programmed values printed out and left in a central area, the data retrieved, and the programming change recorded in the pacemaker clinic records.

Hysteresis, crosstalk, far-field sensing, and oversensing alter pacing rate, as previously described. If hysteresis is the cause of the altered rate, obviously no action need be taken, since the hysteresis is presumably desirable. If oversensing of any type is causing the altered pacing rate, steps should be taken to correct or remove the source that is being oversensed (see above).

Circuit or component failure could alter the programmed rate in an unpredictable fashion. *Runaway pacemaker* is a manifestation of a component failure. It is most likely to occur if a pacemaker is in the field of therapeutic radiation.[46,47] Therapeutic radiation can cause failure of the complementary oxide semiconductor. The failure is unpredictable by both time of exposure and total radiation. Runaway pacemaker constitutes an emergency. If the patient is hemodynamically compromised, the pacemaker must be urgently disconnected. If time allows, the pacing lead can be properly released

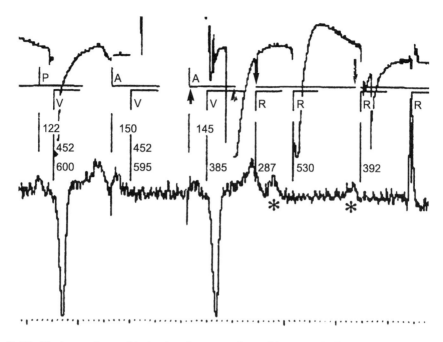

Fig. 9–51. Electrocardiographic tracing from a patient with a ventricular "make-or-break" fracture. At times it appears that there is failure to sense atrial events on the surface electrocardiogram. However, the electrogram and diagnostic interpretation channel demonstrate extension of the postventricular atrial refractory period (PVARP), which masks the intrinsic P waves. (*Short arrows* pointing up note onset and offset of the PVARP. *Longer arrows* pointing down note onset and offset of an extended PVARP. Several P waves occur in the extended PVARP [*] and are not sensed.) This is functional undersensing, that is, a function of the extended PVARP. The PVARP was extended whenever two consecutive ventricular events occurred without an intervening atrial event, because escaping current from the ventricular lead fracture was sensed as ventricular activity. A, paced atrial event; P, sensed atrial event; V, paced ventricular event; R, sensed ventricular event.

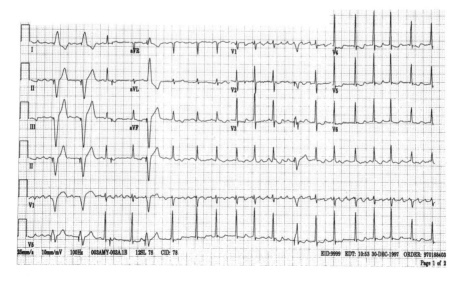

Fig. 9–52. Electrocardiographic tracing demonstrating VVI pacing with intermittent failure to sense.

from the pacemaker. If hemodynamic failure does not allow the extra time required to properly release the lead, the lead should be transected and temporary pacing should be available if necessary.

Confusion may arise if there is *malfunction of the electrocardiographic recording equipment;* for example, the paper sticks or the speed is not constant. This defect can give the appearance that the pacing rate is different from the programmed rate or erratic. The clinical approach to an alteration in pacing rate depends entirely on the cause.

New Symptoms After Pacemaker Implantation

As initially discussed, some of the most frequently encountered new complaints after pacemaker placement are recurrent syncope or presyncope, fatigue, and palpitations. Many potential causes of recurrent syncope or presyncope have already been mentioned. In addition, they are discussed in detail in Chapter 10. In the data from Parsonnet et al.[3] discussed earlier in this chapter, "suboptimal cardiac output" was included as a frequently encountered problem. This designation had been made by the referring physician, since patient complaints of fatigue or malaise are obviously very nonspecific. However, several pacemaker-specific causes should be considered in the paced patient complaining of these symptoms.

- Pacemaker syndrome (Fig. 9–53)
- Failure to capture
- Reversion to backup mode (Fig. 9–11)

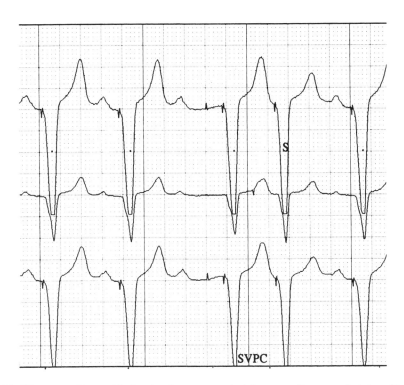

Fig. 9–53. Electrocardiographic tracing from an ambulatory monitor reveals intermittent atrial failure to capture. (It is possible that the atrium is still refractory from the preceding P wave that was not "tracked.") A retrograde P wave is sensed and results in a single echo beat. Longer episodes of atrial failure to capture correlated with the patient's symptoms of fatigue and malaise, that is, intermittent pacemaker syndrome. The ambulatory monitor has incorrectly designated a paced ventricular event as a supraventricular premature contraction (SVPC).

- Inappropriate programmed rate or sensor
- Symptomatic upper rate response
- Primary myocardial abnormality or ventricular rhythm disturbance

Pacemaker syndrome should be suspected if the paced patient complains of general malaise and fatigue. This diagnosis is discussed in Chapter 10. Symptoms may include

- General malaise and fatigue
- Chest discomfort
- Cough
- Symptomatic cannon a waves
- Presyncope or syncope
- Confusion
- Dyspnea on exertion

As part of the troubleshooting process, orthostatic blood pressure readings should be obtained, with and without pacing if the patient is not pacemaker-dependent. It must be remembered that pacemaker syndrome can occur with any pacing mode if AV synchrony is uncoupled (Fig. 9–54).

Failure to capture or output may result in relative bradycardia and symptoms compatible with low cardiac output. Failure to adequately restore rate response, that is, persistent chronotropic incompetence, may also be accompanied by symptoms compatible with low cardiac output.

Exposure of the pacemaker to electromagnetic interference could potentially cause reversion to a back-up mode. Because most backup pacing modes are non-rate-responsive and often single-chamber, patients may experience symptoms of pacemaker syndrome or general fatigue, effort intolerance from lack of chronotropic support, and loss of AV synchrony.

Palpitations are also frequently reported by paced patients. These may be due to

- Intrinsic tachyarrhythmia
- Ventricular tracking of an atrial tachyarrhythmia (Fig. 9–55, 9–56, and 9–57)
- Excessive rate response from a sensor-driven pacemaker
- Search hysteresis

Before mode switching was available, ventricular tracking of atrial tachyrhyth-

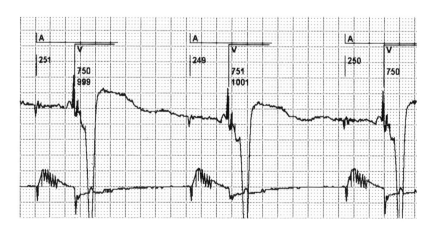

Fig. 9–54. Programmer-derived electrocardiographic tracing and diagnostic interpretation channel from a patient with fatigue and malaise after pacemaker implantation. The markers document markedly prolonged intra-atrial conduction. The ventricular pacing artifact was being delivered almost simultaneously with atrial depolarization, resulting in ineffective atrioventricular synchrony and clinical symptoms of pacemaker syndrome.

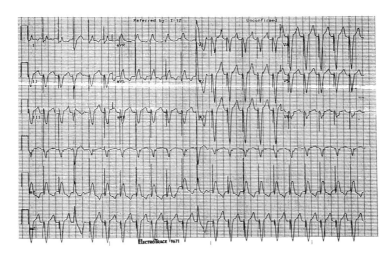

Fig. 9–55. Twelve-lead electrocardiogram from a patient with a DDD pacemaker demonstrating tracking of atrial flutter at a rate of approximately 137 bpm.

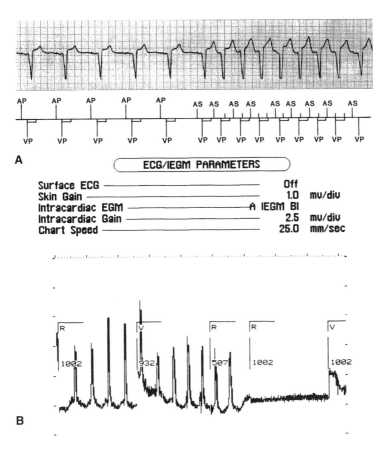

Fig. 9–56. *A,* Transtelephonic tracing and a schematic diagnostic channel consistent with atrioventricular sequential pacing followed by the onset of an atrial tachyarrhythmia with ventricular tracking. *B,* Atrial intracardiac electrogram (A IEGM) from the same patient captures the atrial tachyarrhythmia and its termination with return of a slower paced ventricular rhythm. AP, atrial pacing; AS, atrial sensing; BI, bipolar; ECG, electrocardiogram; EGM, electrogram; VP, ventricular pacing.

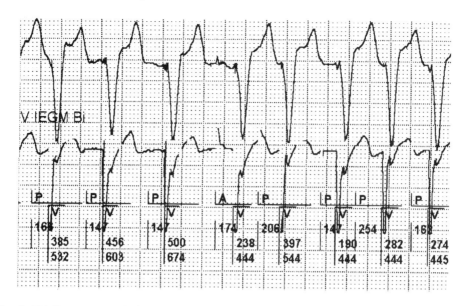

Fig. 9–57. Programmer-derived surface electrocardiogram, ventricular intracardiac electrogram (V IEGM), and markers demonstrating atrial fibrillation with ventricular tracking at a ventricular rate varying from 444 to 674 msec VV intervals. A, paced atrial event; P, sensed atrial event; V, paced ventricular event.

mias was a frequent source of palpitations. Without mode switching, treatment often required programming the pacemaker to a nontracking mode. Figures 9–55 and 9–56 demonstrate ventricular tracking of atrial tachyarrhythmias.

A rate-adaptive pacemaker that is programmed too aggressively and search hysteresis may also cause symptoms (see above). Some patients with pacing after prolonged periods of chronotropic incompetence may have poor tolerance of the new rate response. Although paced rates may be appropriate, patients may have a sensation of relative tachycardia and complain of palpitations. This may require reprogramming the pacemaker to a less aggressive rate response and allowing the patient to slowly adjust to faster rates. The rate response can then be reprogrammed as tolerated.

As discussed in Chapter 8, an inappropriately programmed rate-adaptive sensor may result in suboptimal cardiac output, which can be corrected by optimization of sensor settings.

Patients who have abrupt 2:1 AV block at the upper rate limit may have symptoms from the sudden change in ventricular rate. A sudden decrease in heart rate obviously affects cardiac output (cardiac output = heart rate × stroke volume). If this upper rate behavior is recognized as the cause of the patient's symptoms, reprogramming the pacemaker may alleviate the problem. Programming changes may include

- Shortening the total atrial refractory period to allow a higher achievable upper rate limit
- Shortening the postventricular atrial refractory period
- Programming rate-adaptive AV delay "on"
- Programming "on" or optimizing sensor-driven pacing, or both
- Programming "on" another feature, such as rate smoothing or fallback, to minimize sudden changes in cycle length

Primary cardiac abnormalities may also result in suboptimal cardiac output.

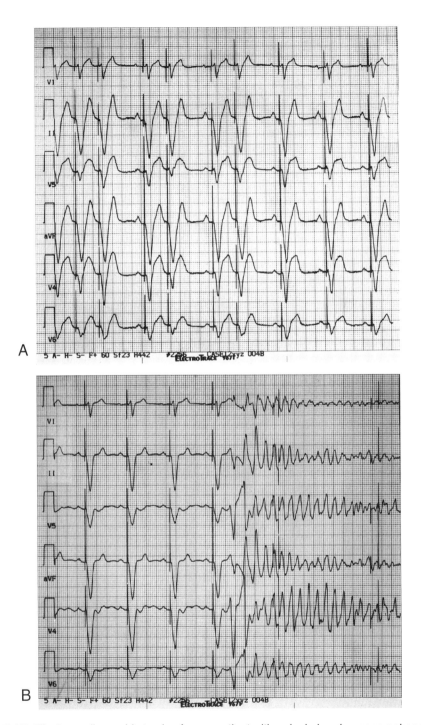

Fig. 9–58. Electrocardiographic tracing from a patient with a dual-chamber pacemaker. The patient had noted exertional fatigue after working very hard. The clinician suspected that the patient was having symptoms when the maximum tracking rate reached the upper rate limit and 2:1 upper rate behavior occurred, resulting in a sudden decrease in heart rate. *A,* With exercise testing, pacemaker behavior was normal and the patient was asymptomatic with 2:1 upper rate behavior. *B,* During cooldown, however, the patient had ventricular tachycardia that correlated with his typical exertional symptoms. (From Hayes DL: Pacemaker electrocardiography. *In* A Practice of Cardiac Pacing. Third edition. Edited by S Furman, DL Hayes, DR Holmes Jr. Mount Kisco, NY, Futura Publishing Company, 1993, pp 309–359. By permission of Mayo Foundation.)

Development of a primary cardiomyopathic process, left ventricular dysfunction due to ischemic disease, or tachyarrhythmias may be manifested by symptoms compatible with low cardiac output (Fig. 9–58).

Conclusion

The number and versatility of current pulse generators and lead systems available challenge the physician to understand all the various devices and their features when assessing a system for potential malfunction. A thorough understanding of pacemaker timing cycles and electrocardiography (Chapter 6), pacemaker radiography (Chapter 11), and programming (Chapter 7) is critical for successful troubleshooting. An understanding of the clinical situation, a systematic approach to troubleshooting, assessment of pacing system integrity, and judicious use of manufacturers' technical support teams can help distinguish between malfunction and apparent malfunction.

Implantable Defibrillator Troubleshooting

Implantable defibrillators have clearly been shown to reduce the risk of death from lethal tachyarrhythmias in high-risk individuals. As with pacemakers, ensuring continuous therapeutic efficacy requires periodic assessment of device function to detect battery depletion, mechanical system disruption, and suboptimal programming before any of these conditions becomes manifest. This routine device follow-up is covered in Chapter 13. At times, however, a patient comes to medical attention because of frequent (possibly inappropriate) device discharges or delayed, ineffective, or absent therapy in the face of a clearly documented ventricular tachyarrhythmia. In these circumstances, a systematic approach must be followed to determine the cause of the problem and offer an appropriate solution.

This chapter describes a stepwise approach to evaluation in patients with suspected device malfunction and reviews the diagnostic tools available and their interpretation. It then reviews the two most common problems seen: excessive device therapy and insufficient or inadequate therapy. Thus, the chapter is divided into three sections:

- Diagnostic tools and patient approach (patient history; telemetered device status, including battery voltage and charge time; pacing parameter assessment; real-time telemetry; system radiography; stored electrogram analysis; and surface electrocardiography)
- Differential diagnosis and management of frequent or recurrent ICD shocks
- Differential diagnosis and management of delayed, absent, or ineffective therapy for documented ventricular tachyarrhythmias

The evaluation of medical complications associated with device use—infection, pericarditis, pneumothorax, and so on—is covered in Chapter 5. The assessment of apparently inappropriate pacing function is covered in the preceding section.

Diagnostic Tools and Patient Approach

A systematic approach is essential for correctly identifying the cause of suspected defibrillator malfunction. Table 9–6 summarizes our approach. The interpretation of each of the diagnostic steps is discussed in this section; patient management is discussed in the subsequent sections. Advances in ICD technology have greatly

Table 9–6.
Systematic Approach to the Patient With Suspected Defibrillator Malfunction

Diagnostic Step	Comments and Suggestions
History	• Severe symptoms or frank syncope before shock strongly suggests ventricular arrhythmia. • Absence of symptoms is not specific; symptoms are absent or minimal in nearly all shocks caused by supraventricular tachycardia and most shocks caused by ventricular tachycardia. • Reaching, stretching, deep breathing at time of event may suggest lead fracture exacerbated by mechanical pull or myopotential oversensing associated with the maneuver. • Number of shocks or cluster: a large number of shocks (more than two) increase the likelihood that shocks are inappropriate (nonventricular arrhythmia or system malfunction). • Pulse generator location: abdominal devices have significantly increased risk of lead failure. • Audible tones emitted spontaneously by the device may suggest lead impedance abnormality, battery depletion, or other potential device problems
Telemeter device status	• Low battery voltage (end of life) may result in erratic behavior, delayed or ineffective therapies. • Prolonged charge time may delay therapy.
Pacing and shocking impedance (Fig. 9–61)	• Increased impedance suggests conductor fracture. • Decreased impedance suggests insulation defect. • Normal pacing impedance range is 200 to 1,000 Ω. • Because of normal changes with lead maturation, a change in pacing impedance <30% is often consistent with normal lead function. • Normal shocking lead impedance is 20 to 100 Ω for delivered shocks; values may be lower for low-energy automatic tests of shocking leads (in which case comparison with previous values is useful). Shocking lead impedance is a function of lead configuration.
Pacing threshold	• Increased pacing threshold can be caused by fibrosis at lead tip, microdislodgment, macrodislodgment, medications, or change in myocardial substrate (e.g., infarct including lead tip site). • Increased threshold can result in ineffective antitachycardia pacing, with subsequent shock.
Real-time telemetry (Fig. 9–66, 9–67, and 9–68)	• Manipulation, provocative maneuvers in various positions can bring out myopotential oversensing or fracture malfunction. • Monitoring of near-field and far-field electrograms, surface electrocardiogram, and marker channels during maneuvers can best detect lead malfunction.
Device radiography (Fig. 9–62 through 9–65)	• Can identify conductor defect; entire lead system must be visualized. • Macrodislodgment can be detected. • Subclavian crush—lead defect from compression between first rib and clavicle—can be found by careful examination of lead in vicinity of the first rib. • Poor pin connection in header may be seen. • Twiddler's syndrome—mechanical twisting of device and leads by patient—can disrupt lead integrity; seen as wound and twisted lead.

continues

Table 9–6. (*Continued*)
Systematic Approach to the Patient With Suspected Defibrillator Malfunction

Diagnostic Step	Comments and Suggestions
Stored electrogram analysis (Fig. 9–70 through 9–75 and Fig. 9–79)	• Can correctly identify ventricular and nonventricular arrhythmias, >90% of episodes. • Electrograms serve as continuous monitor for lead failure; if intermittent failure creates enough "noise," the episode is recorded.
Surface electro-cardiography, Holter, telemetry (Fig. 9–77 and 9–91)	• Therapy during normal sinus rhythm is diagnostic of device malfunction (but cannot distinguish lead fracture or noise from T-wave oversensing, etc.). • Can facilitate identification of arrhythmia leading to therapy if a device programmer is not available.

enhanced the ability to determine the cause of suspected system malfunction.[48]

Patient History and Physical Examination

The patient's history can provide important information about whether shocks are inappropriate (due to nonventricular arrhythmias or system malfunction) or appropriate (triggered by a ventricular tachyarrhythmia). Some defibrillators perform periodic self-diagnostic tests and generate an audible tone if an abnormality, such as low battery voltage or abnormal lead impedance is found; therefore, patients should be asked whether audible device tones were noted[49,50] (Fig. 9–59). Syncope preceding defibrillator discharge occurs in only 10% to 20% of patients[51] but is highly indicative of therapy for a ventricular tachyarrhythmia. Severe symptoms are present in the minority of episodes; when they occur before shocks, they strongly suggest appropriate therapy (Fig. 9–60). The converse is not true: absence of symptoms does not indicate absence of ventricular arrhythmias. In a study with electrocardiographic documentation of the rhythm leading to shock, more than 60% of ventricular tachycardia (VT) episodes and more than 90% of supraventricular tachycardia (SVT) episodes were associated with minimal or no antecedent symptoms.[52] For the asymptomatic patient who receives shocks, additional information is required to determine the appropriateness of therapy.

The temporal pattern of shock delivery may also offer information about whether shocks are appropriate. Clusters of shocks occurring within seconds or minutes in rapid succession are a strong indicator of inappropriate therapies. Intuitively, this makes sense; the success rate for two shocks for termination of VT or ventricular fibrillation (VF) exceeds 90% in a patient with an acceptable defibrillation threshold at implantation.[53] Additional shocks in a patient who is clearly free of fatal tachyarrhythmias suggest that the therapy most likely is inappropriately triggered by a rapidly conducting supraventricular rhythm not terminated by the first shock, by device malfunction (such as lead fracture noise), or by electromagnetic noise mimicking VT or VF and resulting in inappropriate detection. Indeed, inappropriate therapies have been associated with clusters of 4.0 ± 2.0 shocks per episode, compared with 1.6 ± 0.9 shocks per appropriate episode.[54,55] Knowledge of a patient's arrhythmia history is also useful. Persons with known atrial fibrillation or with previously documented SVT are at increased risk of having one of these arrhythmias as the cause of shocks.

Patient activity at the time of device

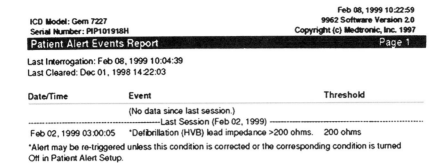

Patient Alert Events Report   Page 1

Last Interrogation: Feb 08, 1999 10:04:39
Last Cleared: Dec 01, 1998 14:22:03

Date/Time	Event	Threshold
	(No data since last session.)	
	------------------Last Session (Feb 02, 1999)------------------	
Feb 02, 1999 03:00:05	*Defibrillation (HVB) lead impedance >200 ohms.	200 ohms

*Alert may be re-triggered unless this condition is corrected or the corresponding condition is turned
Off in Patient Alert Setup.

Fig. 9–59. Printout of device interrogation after audible alert for lead failure. The patient's defibrillator (Medtronic 7227) emitted an audible warning tone because a measured defibrillation lead impedance was out of range (> 200 Ω). A chest radiograph confirmed the existence of a subclavian crush that required revision of the system.

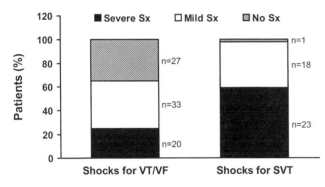

Fig. 9–60. Graph showing the frequency of symptoms (Sx) and their severity in patients with electrocardiographically documented supraventricular tachycardia (SVT) and ventricular tachycardia-ventricular fibrillation (VT/VF). Mild symptoms could include palpitations and mild presyncope. In contrast, severe symptoms consisted of marked presyncope and syncope and were strongly suggestive of VT/VF. (Modified from Rosenthal et al.[63] By permission of Kluwer Academic Publishers.)

discharge may also be helpful. Stretching or deep breathing may unmask a latent conductor defect, with "make-break" noise that can lead to inappropriate VF detection. Similarly, deep breathing or sitting up may lead to myopotential oversensing, with similar results. Physical activity such as walking up hill or jogging raises the possibility of sinus tachycardia crossing into the VT detection zone, but an exercise-induced arrhythmia or lead noise due to a fracture and mechanical motion must be excluded.

History and physical examination (along with radiography) can usually determine the location of the pulse generator and whether the patient has more than one device. As discussed in Chapter 13, there is a significantly increased risk of lead failure with the use of abdominal devices compared with pectoral devices.[56] Therefore, lead malfunction should be particularly considered in patients with frequent shocks and abdominal implantable defibrillators. Patients with separate pacemakers and defibrillators are at increased risk for device-device interactions, which could lead to overdetection or underdetection (discussed in greater detail in Chapter 13).[57]

Telemetered Data

Device telemetry reveals battery status and the most recent charge time. If the device battery reaches end of life, function may become unreliable. Additionally, a depleted battery or excessive capacitor charge time may lead to absent, delayed, or ineffective therapy. Battery and capacitor assessment are discussed in greater detail in Chapter 13. Telemetry also provides the programmed parameters, including programmed pacing rate, VT and VF detection zones, and detection enhancements, all of which are important to determine whether device function is appropriate for a given situation.

Pacing Parameters

Impedance. Abnormal pacing parameters may suggest lead conductor fracture, insulation breach, microdislodgment or macrodislodgment, ineffective antitachycardia pacing, or impaired sensing (Table 9–6). As in pacemakers, a significant elevation of the pacing impedance suggests a discontinuity in the lead or its connection to the pulse generator, and a low impedance suggests an insulation defect or short within the lead. Lead discontinuities in ICDs, unlike those in pacemakers, may not only lead to pacing failure (which may remain asymptomatic in a patient who is not pacemaker-dependent) but also result in ineffective termination of VT (if antitachycardia pacing is attempted) or in inappropriate shocks if "make-break" noise is detected by the pulse generator as VT/VF. Impedance values are available noninvasively by device telemetry. Normal pacing impedance may vary among lead types, but the usual range is from 200 to 1,000 Ω. After implantation, lead impedance may change, but a value 50% greater than the measurement at implantation suggests fracture. In a mature lead, impedance changes greater than 30% may suggest lead malfunction. With impedance values above 1,000 Ω, lead fracture is almost certain; with impedance values greater than 2,000 Ω, fracture is certain.[58] It is important to note that normal lead impedance values are a

function of the lead design. The development of "high pacing impedance" leads for defibrillators (as has already occurred in pacemakers) will result in different absolute values indicative of fracture.

Information on the trend of lead impedance can be immensely useful in diagnosing lead fracture. Figure 9–61 depicts stored episode data from a patient in whom multiple shocks without symptoms were associated with a sudden increase in lead impedance, confirming the diagnosis. Similarly, a decrease in impedance greater than 30% raises the possibility of an insulation defect that permits current to escape to the surrounding tissue (which can result in local muscle stimulation) or between conductors.[58] Importantly, some conductor and most insulation defects are not well visualized radiographically, so that abnormal impedance can correctly diagnose lead malfunction despite an apparently normal radiographic appearance.

In contrast to pacemakers, defibrillators have shocking elements incorporated into their leads. Abnormalities of shocking lead impedance are also useful in troubleshooting lead malfunctions.[59] In early-generation defibrillators, a test shock was required to assess shocking lead impedance. Normal shocking lead impedance ranges from 20 to 100 Ω for transvenous systems. Values outside this range suggest a conductor defect (high impedance) or insulation breach or short circuit (low impedance). Late-generation devices painlessly assess shocking lead impedance with a small test pulse, and some can be programmed to generate an audible tone if impedance measurements are abnormal.[49,50] In Medtronic defibrillators, the normal range for low-energy test pulses is lower than that for actual test shocks delivered through the system (normally, 11 to 20 Ω, depending on the lead system used), and it is therefore important to compare subsequent values with the implantation test pulse value and

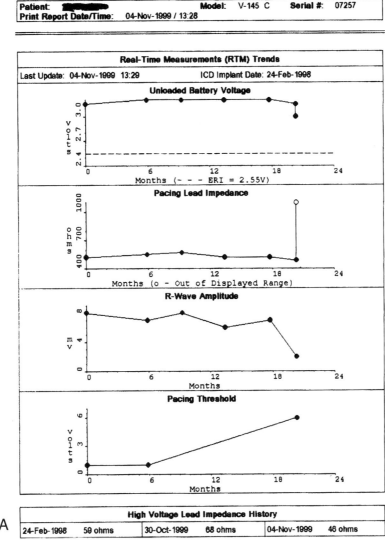

Fig. 9–61. Use of impedance values and electrograms to diagnose lead failure in a patient who presented with a cluster of implantable defibrillator (ICD) shocks. *A,* Trend plot showing (top to bottom) unloaded battery voltage, pacing lead impedance, R-wave amplitude, and pacing threshold. Note the abrupt increase in pacing lead impedance and drop in R-wave amplitude with the last measurement. *Continues.*

not with the impedance of any intervening shocks.

R Wave (P Wave) and Pacing Threshold.

The amplitude of the R wave during sinus rhythm should be at least 5 mV for assurance that the lower amplitude electrograms that occur during VF are appropriately sensed. A number of factors may result in electrogram diminution, including medications, myocardial infarction, failed shock, lead tip fibrosis, microdislodgment, and macrodislodgment. If the R-wave peak-to-peak voltage is less than 5 mV,

Real-Time Measurements (RTM) Trends Report   Ventritex, Inc.

Patient:		Model: V-145 C	Serial #: 07257
Print Report Date/Time:	04-Nov-1999 / 13:28		

Real-Time Measurement Data Display

Last Update: 04-Nov-1999 13:29   ICD Implant Date: 24-Feb-1998

Date / Time		Unloaded Battery Voltage (Volts)	R-Wave Amplitude (mV)	Pacing Lead Impedance (ohms)	Pacing Threshold (Volts)
04-Nov-1999	13:29	3.00	2	1950	N/A
04-Nov-1999	10:48	3.15		485	6.0 V
04-Nov-1999	10:48	3.15		485	N/A
17-Aug-1999	09:16	3.20	7	520	N/A
07-Apr-1999	09:36	3.20	6	520	N/A
02-Dec-1998	11:11	>3.2	8	570	N/A
21-Aug-1998	11:19	>3.2	7	550	1.0 V
24-Feb-1998	10:21	3.15	8	520	1.0 V

B

Stored EGM Report   Ventritex, Inc.

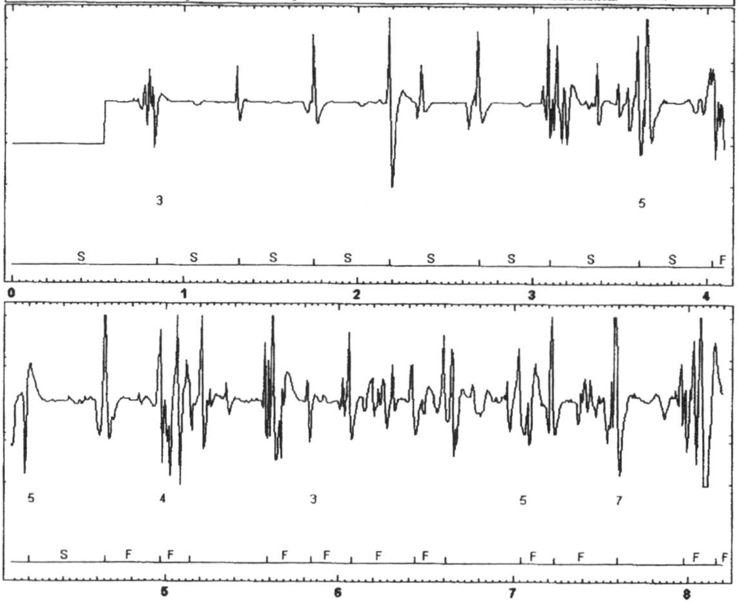

C

Fig. 9–61 *continued. B,* Printout of a table of values from the same patient showing the date and time and corresponding measurements (left to right) in battery voltage, R-wave amplitude, pacing lead impedance, and pacing threshold. The patient was seen in the clinic on Nov. 4, 1999, at 10:48, at which time device function was normal (note normal battery voltage, pacing impedance, and pacing threshold). That afternoon, the patient experienced a cluster of shocks without antecedent symptoms. Note the abrupt increase in pacing lead impedance and the drop in R-wave amplitude recorded at 13:29, consistent with conductor fracture. *C,* Review of stored electrograms of the episodes leading to shocks confirms nonphysiologic "make-break" noise consistent with lead fracture, which is oversensed, leading to inappropriate detection of ventricular fibrillation and shocks.

electrophysiologic testing to confirm adequate detection is warranted, particularly if arrhythmia detection has been delayed or absent.

The same factors that affect the R wave may also increase the pacing threshold. Increases in pacing threshold due to some drugs (particularly Vaughn-Williams class I agents, such as flecainide) may be rate-dependent. Therefore, the increases may not be detected during bradycardia pacing but may be manifested as ineffective antitachycardia pacing. In patients with infrequent pacing, an elevated pacing threshold may be acceptable so long as appropriate sensing function is confirmed, lead malfunction is excluded, and, if used, the ability to capture during antitachycardia pacing (for which outputs are independently programmable in many devices) is confirmed.

Radiography

In our experience,[60] radiographic manifestations of lead failure were present in 43% of patients found to have lead malfunction. Defibrillators should be examined radiographically when failure is suspected and after significant trauma. A number of abnormalities may be found on system radiographs. Macrodislodgment is diagnosed when the lead tip is in a clearly different location (often pulled back) than that on a previous film. Since the lead appearance may shift from radiograph to radiograph because of differences in systole and diastole or degree of inspiration, only gross changes can be diagnosed (Fig. 9–62). Subclavian crush occurs when a lead is compressed in the narrowly confined space between the first rib and the clavicle; this is a common site of fracture, and this region should be carefully examined on all device radiographs (Fig. 9–63). Radiography may also detect conductor defects, a loose pin connection in the header, or abandoned or incom-

pletely removed leads, which may give rise to contact noise (Fig. 9–64). Patients with twiddler's syndrome often unconsciously manipulate their systems, frequently rotating the pulse generator in the pocket. This can lead to twisted, dislodged, or fractured leads, and the resultant torsion and tension are radiographically visible (Fig. 9–65). When lead malfunction is suspected and system radiography is unrevealing, fluoroscopy may be considered. System radiography is covered in greater detail in Chapter 11, and briefly covered in Chapter 13.

Real-Time Telemetry

Late-generation ICDs can record electrograms from the near field (via the lead tip and a ring or distal coil) and the far field (between shocking elements).[48] Both types of electrograms should be evaluated in real time with the patient in several positions. During real-time recording, the effects of body position on the electrograms recorded by the device can be seen. Noise on the shocking elements may be the only manifestation of a lead failure affecting shocking electrodes without delivery of a shock (Fig. 9–66). Conversely, electrical signals on the near-field electrogram that do not correspond to far-field events may reflect a defect in the sensing portion of the lead rather than actual cardiac activity. Additionally, if a patient describes a stereotypical maneuver that reproduced the event (for example, reaching or coughing), the maneuver should be repeated while electrograms are telemetrically recorded. Electrical signals that do not correlate with surface electrocardiographic events suggest the possibility of myopotential oversensing or of "make-break" noise related to lead failure[61] (Fig. 9–67). Comparison of electrograms recorded in real time while the patient is known to be in normal sinus rhythm or atrial fibrillation with electrograms of

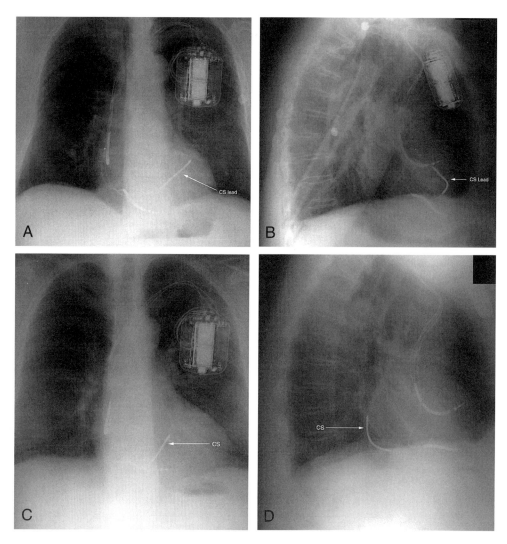

Fig. 9–62. Lead dislodgment. In *A* and *B,* the coronary sinus (CS) lead is dislodged into the right ventricle. In *C* and *D,* the lead has been repositioned into the CS. Note that dislodgment is very subtle in the posteroanterior view (*A*), which mimics the normal lead position (*C*). In the lateral view, however, the dislodged CS lead is clearly in an anterior right ventricular position (*B*) rather than its appropriate posterior CS position (*D*). Also present in *A* and *B* is a left pneumothorax.

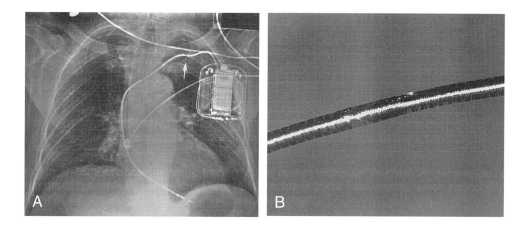

stored events is useful for differentiating SVT from VT. In contrast to stored ventricular arrhythmia episodes, the morphology of stored SVT episodes typically resembles that of the usual supraventricular rhythm[52,62] (Fig. 9–68).

Stored Episode Data

Current-generation defibrillators store electrograms of arrhythmias before and after therapy and a host of additional information—hundreds (sometimes thousands) of intervals preceding arrhythmia episodes, heart rate histograms, and event logs of atrial arrhythmias and nonsustained arrhythmia episodes. Stored information is immensely helpful in determining the cause of a shock and often leads to correct determination of the cause of suspected malfunction.[48,52] Accurate interpretation of a stored episode requires careful assessment of episodes in the ICD report and determination of the source of electrograms displayed. Two major considerations are important for appropriate electrogram interpretation: whether tracings are atrial or ventricular and whether they are near-field or far-field. In many devices, the electrogram source is labeled on the episode printouts (Fig. 9–69).

The first consideration is the chamber of origin of the recordings. Dual-chamber defibrillators often store both atrial and ventricular electrograms. When present, atrial electrograms may make rhythm diagnosis trivial. A sudden acceleration in ventricular rate with a persistently stable sinus rate in the atrium clearly indicates VT. The development of atrial fibrillation with an irregular and rapid ventricular response may also become self-evident.

Some devices generate plots of the atrial and ventricular rates, which can greatly facilitate event diagnosis (Fig. 9–70).

The second consideration is whether recordings are near-field or far-field (Fig. 9–71). Far-field electrograms are recorded between widely spaced electrodes (such as the right ventricular coil and the pulse generator can) and thus incorporate a large amount of electrical information, including QRS morphology. The far-field electrogram more closely resembles the surface electrocardiogram, and often demonstrates P waves when they are present (Fig. 9–71). Since far-field electrograms are recorded by the shocking electrodes, nonphysiologic signals (noise) on these leads may suggest malfunction of a shocking lead and warrant further testing, including shock delivery (Fig. 9–66). Recording the far-field electrogram, at times with the patient in various positions, can also be useful for comparison with stored electrograms to determine whether an event was supraventricular or ventricular in origin. In contrast, near-field electrograms are recorded between the lead tip and the adjacent ring or coil; they provide little morphologic information but are used for heart rate determination by the device. Since these represent the signal "seen" by the device, they can be particularly useful for diagnosing lead malfunction. Importantly, ventricular and supraventricular arrhythmias may appear very similar when examined with near-field electrograms (Fig. 9–72), and 5% to 10% of VT near-field electrograms mimic the electrogram recorded during normal sinus rhythm.[62]

Because the correlation between symptoms and the etiology of device therapies is incomplete, stored episode infor-

---

Fig. 9–63. Subclavian crush. *A,* Note the sharp bend on the lead at the site where it passes between the subclavian vein and the first rib (*arrow*). *B,* Lead extracted from a patient with subclavian crush. Note the disrupted insulation and the disarray of the filers (the circumferentially coiled conductor) at the site of the crush.

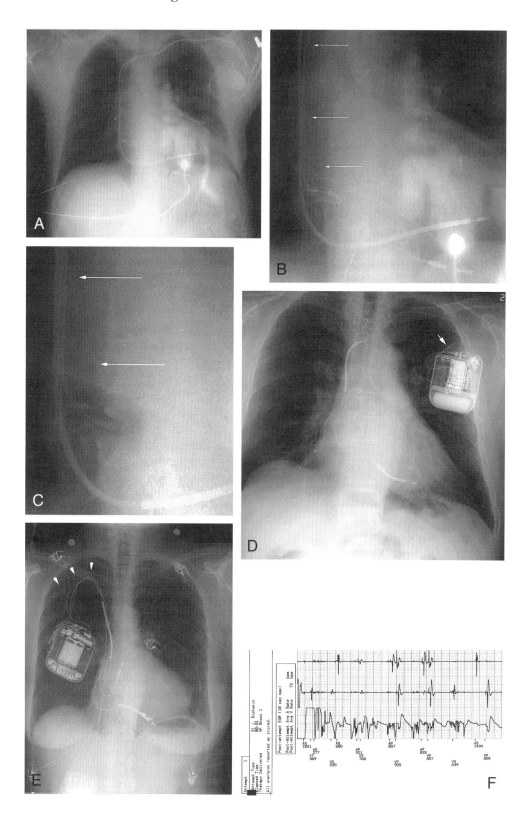

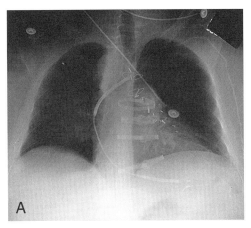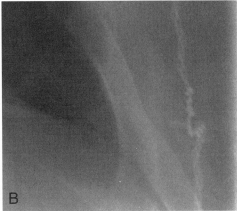

Fig. 9–65. *A*, Chest radiograph from a patient with twiddler's syndrome. *B*, Close-up view of lead body clearly illustrates the looped, twisted, tensed lead consequent to the patient's continuing rotation of the pulse generator in the pocket.

mation, analogous to the report from an omnipresent event recorder, is invaluable for troubleshooting.[48] Once the consideration of whether a tracing is atrial or ventricular and near-field (little morphologic information) or far-field (morphologic information) is determined, tracings can be analyzed with use of principles similar to those applied to traditional rhythm strip interpretation. This approach is summarized in Table 9–7. Generally, a ventricular rate greater than 240 bpm and exceeding

the atrial rate, a polymorphic morphology, or capture beats on ventricular far-field electrograms point to the diagnosis of VT.[55,63] A wider QRS morphology than that at baseline on far-field electrograms favors VT, although this can be seen at times during SVT with aberrancy. A markedly sudden onset excludes sinus tachycardia but does not differentiate VT from SVT or atrial fibrillation (Fig. 9–73). A gradual onset, with P waves preceding QRS complexes, is typical for sinus tachy-

Fig. 9–64. Causes of system malfunction detected by radiography. *A*, Remnant lead fragment from previous lead extraction results in intractable contact noise, ultimately requiring extraction of the newly implanted defibrillator. *B* and *C*, Enlarged views of the same radiograph demonstrating the remnant filament of conductor (*arrows*) responsible for the noise. The electrogram with noise is shown in Figure 9–92. *D*, Routine follow-up radiograph showing that the proximal defibrillation pin is not plugged into the defibrillator header (*arrow*). Review of the chart revealed that the proximal coil was intentionally excluded from the defibrillation circuit during implantation testing to achieve an acceptable defibrillation threshold. *E*, Radiograph from a patient with lead noise on the far-field electrogram recorded from the shocking leads. A stent (*arrowheads*) was placed in the subclavian vein because of venous thrombosis and stenosis after implantable cardioverter-defibrillator placement. The stent may have traumatized the defibrillator lead. *F*, Stored electrogram after a shock from the patient whose radiograph is shown in *E*. From top to bottom are shown the atrial electrogram, ventricular near-field electrogram (tip to distal coil), and far-field electrogram (distal coil to proximal coil and can). Note the bizarre postshock electrical noise prominent on the far-field electrogram. The predominance of the noise on this tracing suggests a defect involving the conductor of the proximal coil. An alternative explanation is contact between the stent and the proximal coil, but the radiograph excludes this possibility. (*A*, Courtesy of Dr. Michael Glikson, Heart Institute, Sheba Medical Center, Tel Hashomer, Israel.)

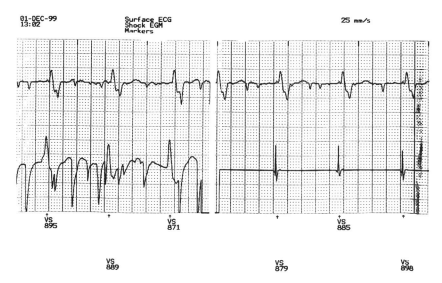

Fig. 9–66. Real-time telemetry during implantation of a pectoral system depicts noise on the shocking coil alone. The patient had a fractured abdominal lead that was abandoned and un-capped in the abdominal pocket. A shock through the new pectoral system failed to terminate ventricular fibrillation with a low impedance (17 Ω), and an external rescue shock was delivered. Subsequently, these electrograms were obtained through the pectoral system. On the *left* are shown (top to bottom) the real-time surface electrocardiogram (ECG), far-field shocking elec-trogram (recorded from the distal coil to the proximal coil and can), and markers. The abandoned uncapped lead probably is making contact with the proximal coil, resulting in contact noise seen on both the surface lead tracing and the shocking lead (far-field) electrogram. The markers show normal sensing of the QRS, suggesting that the sensing electrodes (tip and distal coil) are not involved. The contact between the proximal coil and the abandoned lead "shorted" the circuit, resulting in the failed defibrillation with a low impedance. On the *right*, from top to bottom, are the surface ECG, rate sensing (near-field) electrogram, and marker channels. The noise is still evident on the surface ECG, but the near-field electrogram tracing is clean, confirming absence of involvement of the distal coil and lead tip. After repositioning of the pectoral lead to avoid con-tact with the abandoned lead and capping of the abandoned lead, the noise was no longer pres-ent, and defibrillation was successful with a normal impedance of 36 Ω.

cardia. A tachycardia beginning with an atrial complex in which every QRS is pre-ceded by an atrial electrogram and the VV interval is determined by the preced-ing AA interval most likely is an atrial tachycardia. A very rapid irregular and fractionated atrial electrogram repre-sents atrial fibrillation. Termination by antitachycardia pacing favors VT and ex-cludes sinus tachycardia and atrial fibril-lation. However, antitachycardia pacing can terminate AV nodal reentrant tachy-cardia or SVTs utilizing an accessory pathway, although these arrhythmias are not commonly found de novo in patients with ICDs. In short, by systematic appli-cation of electrophysiologic principles, as summarized in Table 9–7, the correct di-agnosis for most episodes can be made (Fig. 9–74).

At times, very rapid or noncardiac noisy electrical activity is recorded. It suggests myopotential oversensing or lead fracture (Fig. 9–75). Differentiation of these mechanisms may be difficult, and information on lead impedance, pacing threshold, radiography, and real-time telemetry should be studied to make this distinction.[59,61] Reprogramming (decreas-ing sensitivity) may eliminate oversens-ing, whereas it is unlikely to eliminate problems related to lead fracture. If

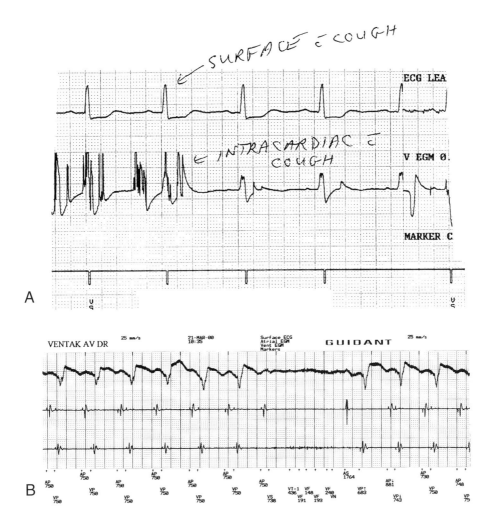

Fig. 9–67. Provocative maneuvers during real-time telemetry to diagnose system malfunction. *A,* Cough during real-time telemetry. From top to bottom are the surface electrocardiogram (ECG), far-field ventricular electrogram, and marker channel. During the cough, electrical noise is seen on the far-field electrogram (recorded between the coil and the device can) while the surface ECG displays continuing normal sinus rhythm, confirming that the electrical noise is noncardiac. The marker channel shows appropriate QRS sensing (one sensed event for each QRS), indicating that the fracture involves the shocking coil but spares the conductors to the tip or ring used for sensing. *B,* Oversensing of diaphragmatic myopotentials during deep inspiration. The patient has marked underlying sinus bradycardia and high-grade atrioventricular block. From top to bottom are shown the surface ECG, atrial electrogram, ventricular electrogram, and markers. With deep inspiration, diaphragmatic myopotentials are sensed as ventricular tachycardia (VT) and ventricular fibrillation (VF) events (beginning at marker VT-1 436). During VT/VF detection, pacing is suspended, resulting in a pause. This patient had received a shock during deep breathing exercises. Reprogramming from "nominal" to "least" sensitivity eliminated the problem. Assessment of adequate ventricular fibrillation detection should be performed when sensitivity is diminished.

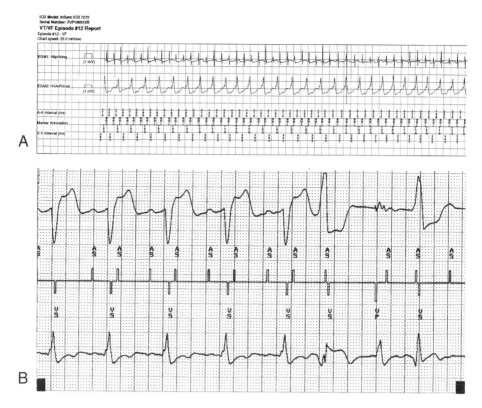

Fig. 9–68. Use of real-time telemetry to assess baseline electrogram morphology during sinus rhythm. *A,* Stored electrograms from an episode of wide-complex tachycardia. From top to bottom are the atrial electrograms, far-field (can to right ventricular [RV] coil) electrogram, and marker channels. Atrial electrograms show continuing atrial flutter, whereas ventricular electrograms show a regular wide-complex tachycardia, which could represent conducted atrial flutter or concomitant ventricular tachycardia. *B,* Real-time recordings during sinus rhythm showing (top to bottom) surface electrocardiogram marker channels, and far-field (can to RV coil) electrogram. Note the similarity between the far-field electrogram during sinus rhythm and the electrogram morphology during the episode in *A,* indicating that the tachycardia was rapidly conducted atrial flutter. Also incidentally noted in *B* is far-field R-wave oversensing (sensing of the QRS on the atrial channel), seen as an "AS" marker immediately following the "VS" marker. The PR Logic detection algorithm can take far-field R-wave oversensing into consideration if it is consistently present.

"noise" is seen on more than one lead (e.g., atrial and ventricular electrograms, simultaneously), electromagnetic interference should be considered.

Differential Diagnosis and Management in Patients With Frequent or Recurrent Shocks

A patient with an ICD may present with frequent or recurrent discharges. Appropriate diagnosis and treatment are crit-ical, since repetitive shocks can have a significant adverse effect on quality of life, and since recurrence can be prevented with proper management.[64] Broadly, multiple shocks may be due to one of four causes:

- Ventricular arrhythmias
- Supraventricular arrhythmias
- Device malfunction or dysfunction
- Electromagnetic interference

Differentiating the causes is important. Shocks due to VT or SVT may be

ICD Model: InSync ICD 7272
Serial Number: PJP100513R

VT/VF Episode #12 Report

Episode #12 - VF
Chart speed: 25.0 mm/sec

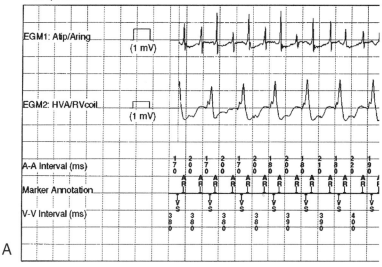

A

From top trace to bottom trace, traces are:
Atrial
Ventricular
Shock

Onset EGM (10 sec max)

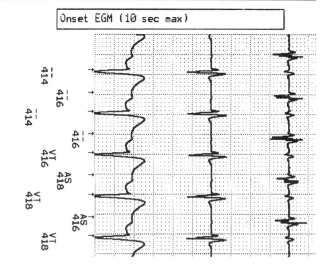

B

Fig. 9–69. Determining the source of an electrogram is essential for proper interpretation. Electrogram source is usually indicated on the episode printouts. *A,* Stored episode from a Medtronic 7272 biventricular defibrillator. The electrogram source is labeled on the left. EGM1 is recorded between the tip and ring of the atrial lead to provide a near-field atrial electrogram; EGM2 is recorded between the distal right ventricular coil and the proximal coil and can (HVA). Markers and intervals are shown at the bottom. *B,* Stored episode from a Guidant Ventak AV series defibrillator. The electrogram source is identified on the box at the far left. From top to bottom are the atrial near-field electrogram, ventricular (near-field, tip to distal coil) electrogram, and shock electrogram (far-field, recorded between the shocking elements).

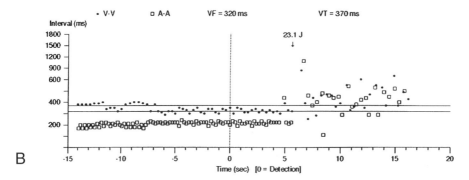

ICD Model: Gem DR 7271
Serial Number: PIM306843R

VT VF Episode #25 Report Page 1

ID#	Date/Time	Type	V. Cycle	Last Rx	Success	Duration
25	Oct 04 16:24:56	VT	470 ms	VT Rx 1	Yes	10 sec

A

ICD Model: InSync ICD 7272
Serial Number: PJP100513R

VT/VF Episode #12 Report Page 1

ID#	Date/Time	Type	V. Cycle	Last Rx	Success	Duration
12	Mar 15 19:58:56	VF	330 ms	VF Rx 1	Yes	13 sec

B

Fig. 9–70. Heart rate plots of stored episodes to facilitate arrhythmia diagnosis. *A,* Episode of ventricular tachycardia (VT). In this Medtronic 7272 dual-chamber defibrillator, the AA intervals are shown as hollow boxes and the VV intervals as solid circles. The interval (in milliseconds) is shown on the ordinate, and the time in seconds (with detection = time 0) is on the abscissa. A nonsustained VT episode is present between time −29 and −24, in which the ventricular cycle length shortens while the atrial cycle lengths remain long. Sinus rhythm returns and is present between −24 and −8 seconds, during which the atrial and ventricular intervals are identical and overlap on the plot. At −8 seconds, there is a sudden shortening in the ventricular cycle length with no change in the atrial cycle length (i.e., VT develops in the ventricles while sinus rhythm continues in the atria). Detection leads to delivery of antitachycardia pacing (a Ramp, which starts at time 0), with restoration of sinus rhythm at time 4 seconds. *B,* An episode of atrial flutter, leading to an inappropriate shock (same episode shown in Figure 9–68). Note that the atrial cycle length is 200 msec (equivalent to 300 bpm) while the ventricular cycle length hovers around 400 msec (150 bpm), which is also the cutoff rate for VT detection. When the ventricular rate is consistently faster than 150 bpm (cycle length shorter than 400), VT is inappropriately detected and a shock delivered (23.1 J at 6 seconds), which terminates the atrial flutter, slowing the heart rate. The cycle length variablility suggests considerable ectopy following the shock.

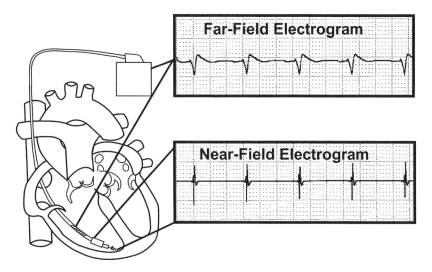

Fig. 9–71. Near-field and far-field electrograms. The near-field electrograms are recorded between the lead tip electrode and a proximal ring in true bipolar sensing, as shown here. In integrated lead systems, near-field electrograms are recorded between the tip and the distal defibrillation coil. Note the narrow, sharp electrogram recorded by the near-field electrodes; this signal is used for rate detection but has little morphologic information. In contrast, the far-field signals are recorded between the distal coil and the pulse generator can, integrating a large area of myocardium, so that P waves and morphologic information can be seen.

treated by medications for arrhythmia suppression or rate control, by device reprogramming for enhanced specificity or utilization of painless pacing therapies, or by catheter ablation to modify the arrhythmogenic substrate or to control the ventricular response in atrial arrhythmias. In contrast, device malfunction can be treated only by reprogramming (to prevent oversensing or correct algorithmic rhythm "misinterpretation") or by surgical correction (of a lead or other mechanical malfunction), and electromagnetic interference may require inactivation of the device (e.g., during electrocautery) or avoidance of environmental sources. Table 9–8 lists potential causes for frequent shocks in patients with minimal symptoms. These are discussed in greater detail below.

Emergency Management

When a patient receives one or two shocks, has no residual symptoms, and otherwise feels well, elective evaluation and interrogation are reasonable. In contrast, multiple or continually repeated shocks represent a medical emergency, as multiple shocks are painful and frightening and may also result in proarrhythmia when delivered inappropriately[64,65] (Fig. 9–76). Although some episodes of multiple ICD shocks, as noted above, may be due to intractable recurrent ventricular arrhythmias (VT storm), most episodes in which more than two shocks are delivered occur as a result of inappropriate therapy.[54]

Before definitive therapy, the patient actively receiving ICD shocks requires urgent management. If a programmer is not immediately available, the treatment steps include monitoring, medicating, and magnet application. Placing a patient on a hospital monitor immediately allows determination of whether therapies are delivered for VT, as a result of SVTs, or during sinus rhythm. Although the definitive cause of the shocks may not be ap-

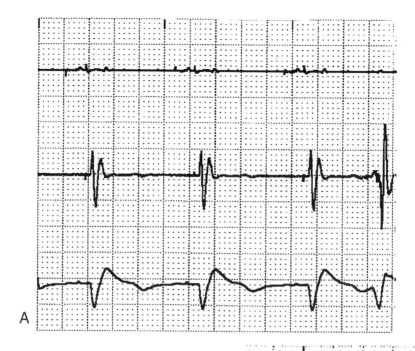

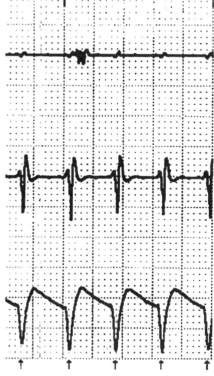

Fig. 9–72. Difficulty in distinguishing between supraventricular rhythm (or at times paced rhythm) and ventricular tachycardia (VT) seen only by near-field electrograms. Top to bottom are shown the atrial, rate (near-field), and shock (far-field) electrograms. *A,* Recording before arrhythmia onset. *B,* Tracing during VT; note that the ventricular rate (bottom two tracings) is greater than the atrial rate (top tracing). The amplitude and morphology of the near-field (middle) tracings are similar in *A* and *B,* with only minor differences in the electrogram onset, despite VT in *B*. In contrast, the morphologic differences are more evident on the far-field (bottom) tracing. The morphologic difference between supraventricular tachycardia and VT may be subtle when only near-field electrograms are available, and in contrast to this example, the differences are usually best seen in the terminal portion of the electrogram.

Table 9–7.
Analysis of Stored Electrogram to Discriminate Between Ventricular
and Supraventricular Tachycardias

	VT	ST	AF	SVT
Rate				
Ventricular >240 bpm	+++	−	−[1]	−[1]
Atrial < ventricular	+++	−	−	−
Atrial = ventricular	±[2]	++	−	+
Atrial > ventricular	±[3]	±[4]	++	±
RR intervals				
Stable	+	++	±	+
Sudden onset	++[5]	−	±	++
First in the ventricle	+++	−	−	−
Slowly crossing detection interval	±[6]	++	−	±[6]
Endocardial electrogram				
Polymorphic	+++	−	−[1]	−
Broad during tachycardia	++[7,8]	±	±	±
Different during tachycardia	+	±	±	±
Capture beat[7]	+++	−	−	−
Outcome of therapy				
Termination by cardioversion	+	−	±	±
Termination by ATP	+	−	−	±

AF, atrial fibrillation; ATP, antitachycardia pacing; ST, sinus tachycardia; SVT, supraventricular tachycardia; VT, ventricular tachycardia.

Classification in relation to class of tachycardia; +++, specific; ++, always but not specific; +, frequent; ±, might occur; −, does not occur.

[1]If an accessory pathway has been excluded.

[2]In 1:1 ventriculoatrial conduction

[3]If atrial arrhythmia occurs at the same time as VT, atrial rate can be greater than VT.

[4]If atrioventricular block is present.

[5]In some cases, VT is triggered by exercise showing only a small change of the tachycardia cycle length.

[6]When tachycardia begins below the programmed detection rate and later accelerates, ectopy occurring before onset may slow the "abruptness" of the crossing detection interval.

[7]Criterion should be used only with far-field electrogram.

[8]Rarely, a VT originating in the basal interventricular septum can be narrow.

Modified from Block M, Lamp B, Weber M, Breithardt G: Follow-up techniques in patients with implantable cardioverter/defibrillators. *In* Cardiac Arrhythmias, Pacing & Electrophysiology: The Expert View. Edited by PE Vardas. Dordrecht, The Netherlands, Kluwer Academic Publishers, 1998, pp 317–327. By permission of the publisher.

parent (shocks delivered during sinus rhythm may be due to dislodgment, lead fracture, or T-wave oversensing, for example), supraventricular or ventricular arrhythmias can be detected and treated pharmacologically (Fig. 9–77). Simultaneously, the patient can receive sedatives or anxiolytics. Once the patient is monitored and resources for arrhythmia therapy are at hand, magnet application over any ICD immediately inactivates the tachycardia sensing function, ending automatic therapies without affecting pacing function.

Some ICDs remain inactivated after magnet application, so that patients should continue to be monitored once a magnet is applied until the device is interrogated and its appropriate function assured.[66]

Specific Causes of and Management for Shocks

Ventricular Arrhythmias. Ventricular arrhythmias may cause recurrent ICD shocks—despite lack of symptoms—in

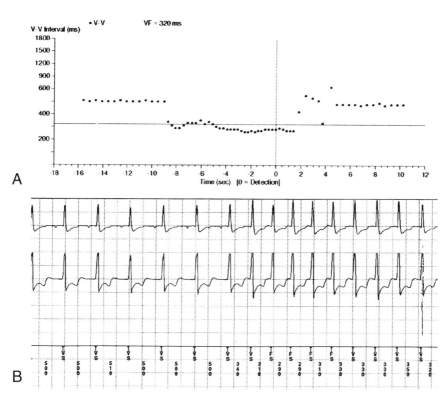

Fig. 9–73. Sudden onset (abrupt increase in heart rate) excludes sinus tachycardia but does not differentiate ventricular tachycardia from supraventricular tachycardia. *A,* Trend report from a patient with a single-chamber defibrillator shows a nonsustained tachycardia episode beginning abruptly at −9 seconds, excluding sinus tachycardia. *B,* Stored electrograms of the same episode show that after the onset of tachycardia, P waves are lost but the morphology is unchanged, consistent with atrial fibrillation.

Fig. 9–74. Use of stored episode data for diagnosis of arrhythmia. All tracings are from the same patient. From top to bottom are atrial, rate (near-field), and shock (far-field) electrograms. *A,* Episode of atrial tachycardia. Beginning with the fifth atrial complex (cycle length, 430), the atrial rate accelerates and is conducted rapidly to the ventricles. The changes in AA intervals precede the changes in VV intervals, as expected in atrial tachycardia (AA 430 leads to VV 430, AA 342 leads to VV 348, AA 330 leads to VV 336, and so on). Also, the far-field morphology is unchanged, consistent with supraventricular tachycardia. The atrial tachycardia is detected as ventricular fibrillation (VF), leading to a shock. *B,* After the shock, nine atrial tachycardia complexes are conducted with a wide QRS (most likely a result of the shock) and are followed by resumption of sinus rhythm. Despite the wide QRS complex, the fact that the AA intervals "drive" the VV intervals confirms a supraventricular rhythm. *C,* Subsequent development of ventricular tachycardia (VT). The tachycardia begins with a ventricular complex (with cycle length 285). The ventricular rate is greater than the atrial rate, and the morphology of both near-field and far-field electrograms is different from the sinus morphology (as seen in the first four ventricular complexes). *D,* After a successful shock (the first four complexes are sinus tachycardia with aberrant QRS, as seen in *B*), VT recurs. The tachycardia begins with a ventricular complex (VF 281), has a ventricular rate exceeding the atrial rate, and has a morphology that is different from the aberrantly conducted sinus tachycardia, all consistent with the diagnosis of VT. This example demonstrates how the initiation of VT during an aberrant supraventricular rhythm can be diagnosed.

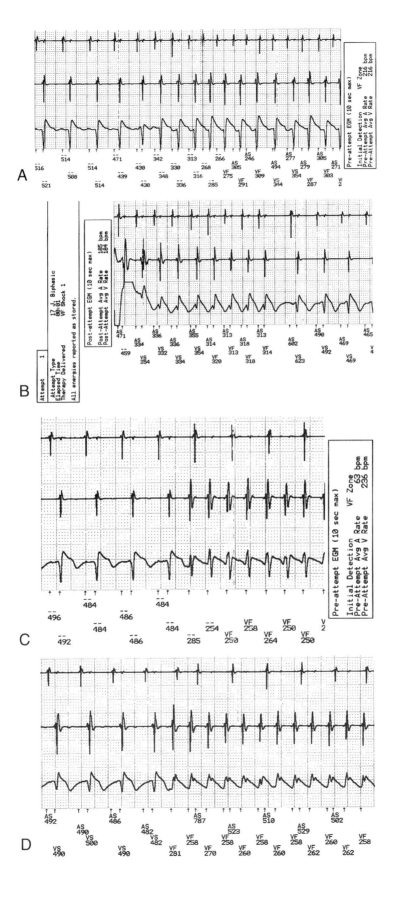

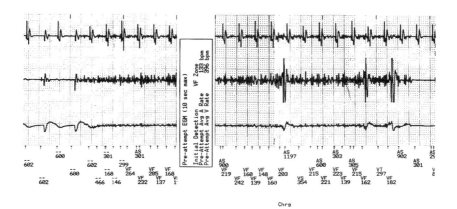

Fig. 9–75. Lead noise consistent with fracture or oversensing. From top to bottom are the atrial, rate (near-field), and shock (far-field) electrograms. Electrical noise inhibits pacing and is detected as ventricular fibrillation. The noise is much greater on the near-field electrogram than on the far-field electrogram. Note that a concomitant atrial tachyarrhythmia is present. Distinguishing between oversensing and fracture can be challenging at times. The distinction is made by assessment of pacing parameters (including pacing and shocking lead impedances), provocative maneuvers during real-time telemetry, and system radiography. This patient was ultimately found to have a lead fracture.

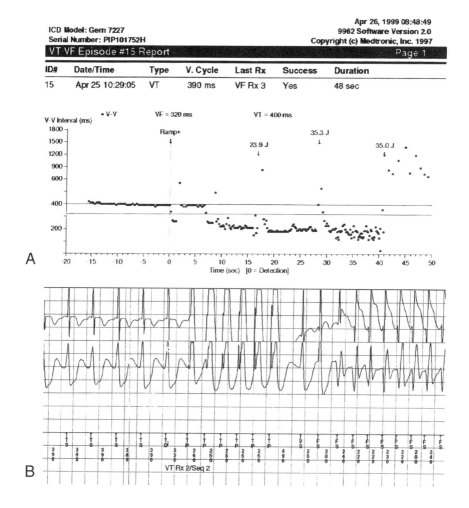

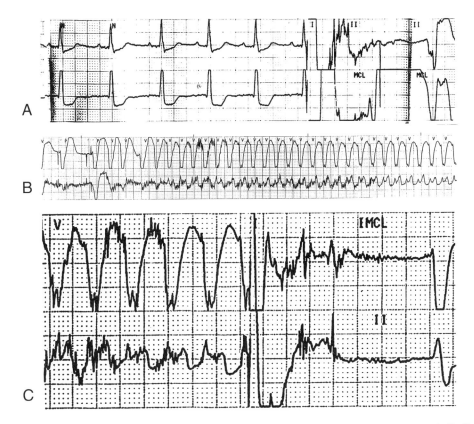

Fig. 9–77. Use of telemetry to rapidly determine whether implantable cardioverter-defibrillator shocks are appropriate as a guide for urgent management. *A,* Hospital monitor shows shock delivery during normal sinus rhythm. Although interrogation and further evaluation are necessary to diagnose the cause, in the interim a magnet can be placed over the device to prevent additional shocks, which could be proarrhythmic. This patient was found to have a dislodged lead. *B,* Hospital monitor reveals initiation of ventricular tachycardia (VT). *C,* VT is successfully terminated by a defibrillator shock. In this situation, urgent therapy is warranted to prevent recurrent VT.

Fig. 9–76. Implantable cardioverter-defibrillator proarrhythmia from inappropriate detection of sinus tachycardia. *A,* Interval plot shows gradually increasing heart rate, consistent with sinus tachycardia. At time 0, a Ramp+ is delivered with no success. At 7 seconds, a second sequence of Ramp+ is delivered, which induces a ventricular tachyarrhythmia. After unsuccessful 23.9-J and 35.3-J shocks, a 35.0-J shock at 39 seconds restores sinus rhythm. This device can use an electrogram width criterion to differentiate supraventricular tachycardia from ventricular tachycardia (VT). During this episode, the electrogram width criterion had been programmed to the passive mode, demonstrating that it would have correctly classified the arrhythmia as supraventricular had it been programmed "on." Preventing recurrent inappropriate detection in this patient was accomplished by turning this algorithm "on." Alternative approaches include administering medications (e.g., beta-blocking drugs) to blunt the sinus rate and increasing the programmed VT detection rate (if no slow VTs are present). *B,* Electrograms confirm that a tachycardia of supraventricular origin, in this case sinus tachycardia (the morphology of the first five complexes on the left matches sinus rhythm morphology), is accelerated to VT by antitachycardia pacing (indicated by markers "TP"). TS, tachycardia sense; TD, tachycardia detection; VS, ventricular sensed event; FS, fibrillation sense.

patients with hemodynamically tolerated VT, with very rapidly detected and treated VT, or with nonsustained VT triggering the shocks (Table 9–8). The diagnosis of ventricular tachyarrhythmias is suggested by severe symptoms and confirmed by diagnostic stored-event information, as described above. When the frequency of ventricular tachyarrhythmias dramatically increases, a screen for medical causes should be considered (Table 9–9), although a specific secondary cause is not often found.

If no clear or treatable cause for the recurrent arrhythmias is found, adjunctive medical therapy (i.e., in addition to the ICD) may be needed. The choice of agent is based on comorbid conditions and effectiveness (Table 9–10). Because of demonstrated tolerance and efficacy across a broad array of patients with significant heart disease,[67–70] amiodarone is often used. When this agent is given as adjunctive therapy in a patient with an ICD, lower dosages may be used than those applied as primary therapy. Nonetheless,

---

Table 9–8.
Causes of Frequent Implantable Cardioverter-Defibrillator Shocks in
Minimally Symptomatic Patients

Ventricular arrhythmias
  • Hemodynamically tolerated monomorphic sustained VT
  • Very rapidly detected and terminated VF or VT
  • Nonsustained VT with a committed device
Supraventricular arrhythmias
  • Sinus tachycardia
  • Atrial flutter
  • Atrial fibrillation
  • Other SVTs (e.g., AVNRT, AVRT)
Device malfunction or dysfunction
  • Algorithm "error" in rhythm interpretation
  • Oversensing of physiologic but non-QRS signals
      T-wave or P-wave oversensing
      Myopotential oversensing (e.g., diaphragm)
  • Device-device interaction (sensing of pacemaker stimuli)
  • Mechanical system malfunction
      Lead or adaptor fracture ("make-break potentials")
      Lead or adaptor insulation failure
      Loose generator or adaptor setscrew connections
      Lead dislodgment
Electromagnetic interference, e.g., electrocautery, welding

AVNRT, atrioventricular nodal reentrant tachycardia; AVRT, atrioventricular reentrant tachycardia; SVT, supraventricular tachycardia; VF, ventricular fibrillation; VT, ventricular tachycardia.

Table 9–9.
Potential Causes of Recurrent Ventricular Tachyarrhythmias

  • Progressive heart disease, ventricular dysfunction
  • Thyroid dysfunction (particularly in patients receiving amiodarone)
  • Electrolyte abnormalities (consider in patients who are taking diuretics or who have acute gastrointestinal illness)
  • Ischemia (favored by polymorphic ventricular tachycardia and ventricular fibrillation)
  • Noncompliance with medications or with diet
  • Over-the-counter medications, possible drug-drug interactions

Table 9–10.
Adjunctive Pharmacologic Therapy: Major Considerations

Vaughn-Williams class	Agents	Comments
IA	Procainamide, quinidine, disopyramide	• Can suppress atrial and ventricular arrhythmias • Enhance AVN conduction, so that rate-slowing agents must also be used when administered for atrial fibrillation • Disopyramide is a strong negative inotrope; useful in hypertrophic cardiomyopathy but should be avoided in depressed ventricular function • Quinidine can be used in renal failure, is tolerated in depressed ventricular function, and can usually be used in patients with lung disease • None are typically first-line agents • These agents slow VTs, which may increase ATP effectiveness but also necessitates device testing to ascertain appropriate programming of VT detection rate
IB	Lidocaine, mexiletine, tocainide	• Treat ventricular arrhythmias only • Mexiletine and tocainide not usual first-line agents for long-term oral administration • Lidocaine useful for short-term therapy of recurrent VT • These agents slow VTs, which may increase ATP effectiveness but also necessitates device testing to ascertain appropriate programming of VT detection rate
IC	Flecainide, propafenone	• Can suppress atrial and ventricular arrhythmias • Generally well tolerated in patients without structural heart disease • Avoid use in patients with ischemia or significant structural heart disease; both agents are negative inotropes • Flecainide better tolerated in COPD and reactive airway disease • These agents slow VTs, which may increase ATP effectiveness but also necessitates device testing to ascertain appropriate programming of VT detection rate
II	Beta-adrenergic blockers	• Slow AVN conduction • Also useful for sinus tachycardia; 1:1 supraventricular tachycardias • Hepatic (metoprolol) and renally excreted (atenolol) agents available

continues

Table 9–10. (*Continued*)
Adjunctive Pharmacologic Therapy: Major Considerations

Vaughn-Williams class	Agents	Comments
III	Sotalol, amiodarone, dofetilide	• Shown to reduce mortality after myocardial infarction in multiple large prospective, randomized studies (MIAMI, ISIS) • Shown to reduce mortality in patients with depressed ventricular function and heart failure (metoprolol, carvedilol) • May not be tolerated in COPD and reactive airway disease • Suppress atrial and ventricular arrhythmias • Slow AVN conduction • Sotalol is also anti-ischemic and antihypertensive but may not be tolerated in COPD because of β-blocking properties • Sotalol lowers the ventricular defibrillation threshold • Amiodarone may reduce mortality in coronary artery disease and dilated cardiomyopathy; often the agent of first choice in patients with structural heart disease • Amiodarone may cause lung toxicity, liver toxicity, thyroid dysfunction, and skin toxicity, requiring periodic biochemical screening • Amiodarone increases the defibrillation threshold; can be significant in patients with borderline thresholds • Early studies suggest that dofetilide is well tolerated after myocardial infarction and in patients with heart failure • All agents slow VTs, which may increase ATP effectiveness but also necessitates device testing to ascertain appropriate programming of VT detection rate
IV	Calcium channel antagonists	• Slow AVN conduction • Negative inotropic agents; should be use cautiously in depressed ventricular function • Hepatic excretion (diltiazem, verapamil) • Dihydropyridine agents (nifedipine, nicardipine, felodipine) do not slow AVN conduction and have no role in rhythm management

ATP, antitachycardia pacing; AVN, atrioventricular node; COPD, chronic obstructive pulmonary disease; ISIS, International Study of Infarct Survival; VT, ventricular tachycardia.

because of the side effects of amiodarone, newer class III agents, such as dofetilide,[71] also well tolerated in patients with ventricular dysfunction, may find a place in the management of these patients, although this application of these agents has not yet been evaluated. If administration of antiarrhythmic medications is initiated, noninvasive electrophysiologic study should be performed through the device to avoid drug-device interactions (discussed in greater detail in Chapter 13).

Catheter ablation, because of its arduousness and limited applicability for VT in patients with coronary artery disease, has been limited to patients with slow and stable VTs who are not helped by medical therapy and continue to receive frequent ICD shocks.[72] Advances in ablation technology may make this form of adjuvant therapy more tolerable and widely applicable, although this remains to be proven.[73–75] Medical, catheter, and surgical therapies for arrhythmias are covered in greater detail elsewhere.[76]

In patients with frequent shocks due to VT, the defibrillator must be optimally programmed to minimize painful therapy. Since antitachycardia pacing can terminate 57% to 95% of spontaneous VT episodes,[77,78] it should be used in patients with recurrent monomorphic VT. This is particularly true with "slower" VTs (heart rate under 200 bpm) because they more commonly respond to antitachycardia pacing. Subsequent testing of the antitachycardia pacing by device-based electrophysiologic study may be useful to assess efficacy for patients with frequent VT.[79,80] Programming of antitachycardia pacing is discussed in greater detail in Chapter 7.

Occasionally, patients may receive ICD shocks because of nonsustained VT. In older "committed" ICD units (e.g., Ventak 1550, 1555, 1600; PCD 7217) and in newer devices programmed to a committed mode, once initial detection criteria are met, the defibrillator charges and delivers a shock, irrespective of spontaneous arrhythmia termination during the charging period.[63] In "committed" devices, prolongation of detection criteria, adjunctive medical therapy to suppress episodes, or (rarely) upgrading to a newer device may be required. With newer devices, programming to a noncommitted mode may solve the problem. However, even with noncommitted devices, therapy may be delivered on rare occasions. Despite spontaneous arrhythmia termination after detection criteria are met, an ill-timed premature ventricular contraction may "fool" the device into inappropriate confirmation of continuing VT, with subsequent shock delivery[81] (Fig. 9–78). Algorithm "errors" may also lead to inappropriate shocks for nonsustained VT in pacemaker-dependent patients with noncommitted devices, discussed below.

Supraventricular Arrhythmias. Supraventricular arrhythmia is the most common cause of inappropriate device discharges, responsible for up to 80% of inappropriate shocks.[82,83] The diagnosis is suggested by exertion at the time of the event (sinus tachycardia), by a history of atrial arrhythmias, and by more than two shocks in a cluster, and it is confirmed by characteristic stored electrograms, as described above. Additionally, the far-field electrogram morphology remains unchanged (if there is no aberrancy), the rhythm may not respond to antitachycardia pacing (atrial fibrillation), and the heart rate may increase after shocks (especially for sinus tachycardia). Sinus tachycardia shows a characteristic gradually increasing heart rate, and P waves precede QRS complexes on far-field electrograms or an atrial channel. Atrial fibrillation is characterized by irregular ventricular intervals, and when an atrial lead is present, rapid, fractionated atrial electrograms are seen. However, if the

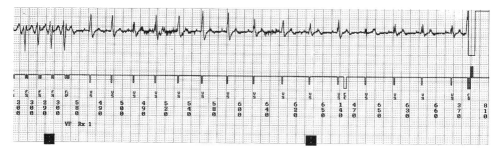

Fig. 9–78. Noncommitted therapy. Reconfirmation algorithm is "fooled" by a single ill-timed premature ventricular contraction (PVC). This single-chamber defibrillator (Medtronic 7223) requires four consecutive sinus cycle length complexes (defined as tachycardia detection interval plus 60 msec) to confirm arrhythmia termination. A run of nonsustained VT spontaneously terminates immediately after detection (at marker FD). After marker CE (charge end), the first interval is 470 msec. Because of an obligatory 300-msec blanking period and additional 100-msec refractory period after completion of the capacitor charge (at CE), the first interval is determined to be tachycardic by the device (although it is displayed as VS 470). Next, three sinus intervals (650, 630, and 660) are recorded. One additional cycle length longer than the tachycardia detection interval (TDI; 320 msec in this case) + 60 msec is required to abort therapy. A PVC occurs with a coupling interval of 370 msec (which is shorter than TDI + 60, or 320 + 60), so that a shock is delivered despite arrhythmia termination.

ventricular rate becomes regular and the ventricular morphology changes from baseline, the possibility of a double arrhythmia—development of VT during atrial fibrillation—is likely.

Inappropriate therapies due to SVTs must be eliminated because of discomfort to the patient (if shocks are delivered) and the risk of proarrhythmia, as shown in Figure 9–79. There are three approaches to preventing recurrent inappropriate therapies due to SVTs: (1) reprogramming the detection rate or adding detection enhancements to avoid delivery of ventricular therapy (and to appropriately deliver atrial therapy in devices in which it is available), (2) controlling the ventricular rate with medications or catheter therapy, and (3) controlling the supra-

ventricular rhythm with medications or catheter therapy. The ideal approach depends in part on how well the supraventricular arrhythmia is tolerated. Many patients with significant structural heart disease do not tolerate rapid atrial fibrillation, even without ICD shocks, so that specific therapy is required. In contrast, sinus tachycardia infrequently causes symptoms, and elimination of ICD therapies by detection enhancements may be preferable to medical or invasive interventions.

Detection enhancements use an abrupt change in heart rate to exclude sinus tachycardia (onset criterion), irregularity of heart rate to differentiate atrial fibrillation from VT (stability criterion), changes in electrogram width or morphology to differentiate supraventricular

Fig. 9–79. Implantable cardioverter-defibrillator proarrhythmia due to an inappropriately treated supraventricular tachycardia. From top to bottom are the atrial, near-field (rate) ventricular, and the far-field (shock) ventricular electrograms. *A,* Onset of supraventricular tachycardia. Arrhythmia begins with atrial acceleration (AS 502 and then AS 414), and AA interval changes precede VV interval changes. This is detected as ventricular tachycardia (VT), and a burst therapy is delivered. Changes in the near-field electrogram (middle tracing) amplitude are due to the autoadjusting gain used by this device (Guidant Ventak AV). *B,* The antitachycardia pacing burst induces polymorphic VT. *C,* The ventricular tachyarrhythmia is terminated by a high-energy shock.

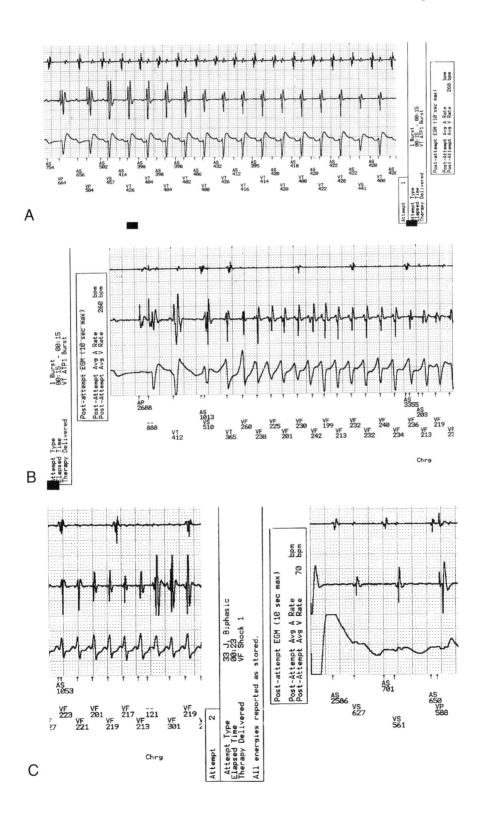

from ventricular rhythms (electrogram width and template criteria), or atrial rate and AV relationships (dual-chamber criteria) to prevent delivery of therapy for rhythms of supraventricular origin. With appropriate programming, detection enhancements can decrease detection of atrial arrhythmia by 95% to 99% while underdetecting only 0.5% of VTs.[84] Use of detection enhancement criteria is extensively covered in Chapter 7. Generally, patients with inappropriate therapies due to SVTs should have detection enhancement programmed "on."

Rate control medications are selected on the basis of the patient's concomitant heart disease. Digitalis preparations are well tolerated in left ventricular dysfunction and may ameliorate heart failure symptoms; however, since they often fail to effectively control the heart with exertion, they are frequently used in conjunction with other agents.[85] Beta-receptor antagonists, because they reduce mortality in patients with ventricular dysfunction and in patients with prior myocardial infarction,[86,87] should be used when these conditions are present.[85] Beta-blockers are also effective in the long QT syndrome (in which episode frequency and mortality are reduced) and in hypertrophic cardiomyopathy (in which the outflow gradient may be lowered). In patients without significant ventricular dysfunction who do not tolerate β-blocking agents very well, calcium channel antagonists are also effective for rate control. When medical therapy fails or is not tolerated, transcatheter AV nodal ablation may be performed.[88] Importantly, since AV block is created, a defibrillator capable of dual-chamber pacing with mode switching should be used in patients with episodic atrial arrhythmias, and a ventricular device with rate-responsive pacing used in patients with chronic atrial arrhythmias.

Rhythm control is preferable in patients who do not tolerate atrial fibrillation despite rate control and in patients with concomitant ventricular arrhythmias that also require therapy, in which case a single agent to treat both arrhythmias can be used. Atrial fibrillation is usually treated pharmacologically, and many of the same considerations in choosing a drug for ventricular arrhythmias apply (Table 9–10). In contrast to atrial fibrillation, atrial flutter and most 1:1 SVTs are effectively treated with catheter ablation.

Device Malfunction or Dysfunction. Algorithm "Error."—Rarely, therapies are inappropriately delivered because of errors in the device algorithm. When this occurs, analysis of stored electrograms, which show the cardiac activity at the time of the event, and of the marker channels, which reveal the defibrillator's "interpretation" of the events, enables this diagnosis to be made.[55] In Figure 9–80, for example, a patient with a GEM DR defibrillator has a long PR interval during sinus tachycardia that is faster than the VT detection rate. Because of the long PR interval during sinus tachycardia, the patient has a "short RP" tachycardia (i.e., the P wave is closer to the preceding QRS complex than to the QRS that follows it). Since a P wave shortly following a QRS complex is more commonly seen in VT with retrograde atrial activity than in sinus tachycardia, the algorithm inappropriately detects the rhythm as VT, and therapy is delivered. Newer versions of the algorithm permit the user to program the length of the RP interval to eliminate this inappropriate detection, which is more common in patients with a long PR interval. However, when PR interval reprogramming is not an option, alternative solutions, such as using medications to slow the sinus rate or increasing the VT detection rate (when possible), are necessary. Increasingly, defibrillators apply detection algorithms with software, so

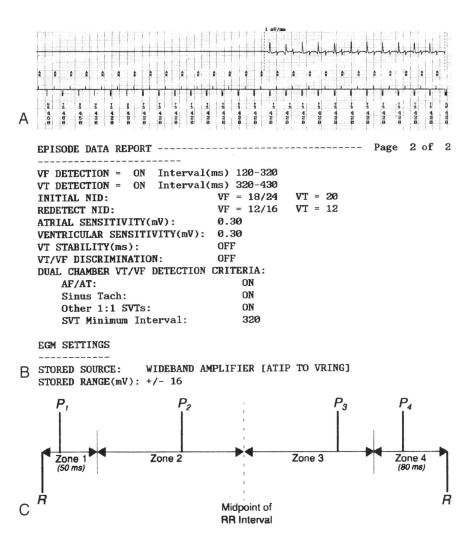

Fig. 9–80. Sinus tachycardia inappropriately detected as ventricular tachycardia (VT). The patient received a shock during exertion. *A,* Top to bottom are stored far-field electrogram, marker channel, and ventricular intervals (from the Medtronic 7250 implantable cardioverter-defibrillator). The ventricular rate is gradually increasing, and a P wave precedes each QRS. Because of a long PR interval, each P wave occurs immediately after the preceding QRS and is detected as an atrial refractory event (AR). When the cycle length is shorter than 430 msec (the tachycardia detection interval), VT is detected at TD (tachycardia detection) and a shock is subsequently delivered (not shown). *B,* Device settings. Note that the VT detection interval is 320–430 and that the "Sinus Tach" criterion is "on." This criterion is used to differentiate sinus tachycardia from VT. *C,* The "syntax" used by the PR Logic algorithm to assist in arrhythmia detection. Two R waves and the zones used to categorize atrial events are shown. Atrial events in Zone 1 are expected from junction rhythms, premature atrial contractions (PACs), premature ventricular contractions (PVCs), atrial fibrillation, and atrial flutter; in Zone 2 from retrograde conduction; in Zone 3 from sinus rhythm or sinus tachycardia; and in Zone 4 from junction rhythms, PACs, PVCs, and atrial fibrillation or flutter. In *B,* atrial events were in Zone 2, consistent with VT with retrograde atrial conduction, leading to VT detection. P_1, P wave in Zone 1, etc. (*C,* Modified from Medtronic 7250 manual.)

that conceivably algorithm errors would be correctable noninvasively by injection of new software into the defibrillator. This approach has already been used to correct one algorithm malfunction[89] (Fig. 9–81).

Another algorithm error is shown in Figure 9–82. In this patient, who has a Ventak AV II DR programmed to deliver non-committed shocks, four consecutive "sinus" intervals during charging signify termination of arrhythmia and abort the delivery of therapy. However, after the charge is completed, a sensed event must occur within 2 seconds or a shock is delivered. The rationale for the requirement of a sensed event is that failure to detect ventricular activity may represent fine ventricular fibrillation that is undersensed.[90] Although this rationale may make sense in single-chamber ICDs, now that dual-chamber devices are increasingly implanted in patients with AV block, a more likely explanation for the lack of a sensed event is asystole, since the defibrillator

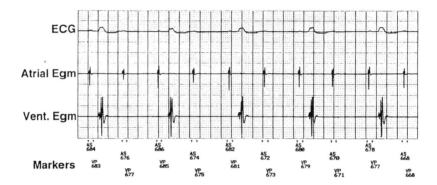

Fig. 9–81. Lack of ventricular output due to software error. Surface leads demonstrate absence of pacing artifact despite the suggestion of ventricular pacing by the interpretive markers. Non-invasive software injection corrects this malfunction permanently. ECG, electrocardiogram; Egm, electrogram. (From Coppess et al.[89] By permission of Futura Publishing Company.)

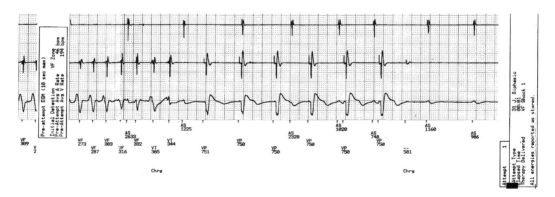

Fig. 9–82. Nonsustained ventricular tachycardia (VT) in a patient with atrioventricular (AV) block leading to transient asystole and inappropriate shock. Top to bottom are the atrial, ventricular near-field (rate), and ventricular far-field (shock) electrograms. An episode of fast VT is detected as ventricular fibrillation (VF) and then terminates during capacitor charge. During the remainder of the charge, the defibrillator provides appropriate ventricular pacing support (starting at VP 751). At the completion of the charge (the second "Chrg" marker), pacing is withheld as the device attempts to reconfirm the presence of VT or VF. Because of the AV block, asystole occurs while pacing is withheld. Since the algorithm inappropriately regards asystole as fine VF, a shock is delivered instead of a pacing pulse.

withholds pacing during the reconfirmation of VT or VF. Thus, a more appropriate device response would be delivery of a ventricular pacing pulse. In the absence of programmability for this confirmation behavior, alternative approaches must be used to prevent shock delivery for nonsustained VT in pacemaker-dependent patients. These include increasing the time to VT detection to prevent detection of shorter nonsustained episodes, adding

medications to suppress the nonsustained VT, and implanting a separate pacemaker.

Infrequently, several device problems may interact, leading to inappropriate shock. In Figure 9–83, for example, oversensing in a patient with a Ventak AV defibrillator leads to inappropriate VF detection. Since the patient also has AV block, even though the oversensing ceases when pacing is withheld during reconfirmation, asystole ensues. This is

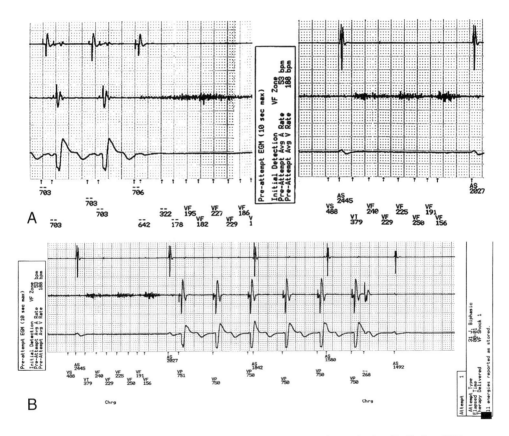

Fig. 9–83. Oversensing leading to inappropriate detection of ventricular fibrillation (VF), transient asystole, and shock delivery. The patient was performing deep breathing exercises when she felt dizzy and received a shock. These are stored episode data from the patient whose real-time telemetry findings are shown in Figure 9–67 *B*. From top to bottom are the atrial, ventricular near-field (rate), and the ventricular far-field (shock) electrograms. *A*, Diaphragmatic myopotential oversensing leads to inappropriate detection of VF. Pacing is withheld during ventricular tachycardia (VT)/VF detection, leading to asystole (note that QRS complexes are absent on the far-field electrogram [bottom tracing] but noise is present on the near-field electrogram [middle tracing]). *B*, Oversensing resolves and pacing resumes (at VP 751), presumably because the patient stopped the deep breathing exercises after the dizzy spell. During reconfirmation (at the second "Chrg" marker), pacing is withheld to determine whether VT or VF is still present. Since this patient has high-grade atrioventricular block, asystole recurs and is shocked by the algorithm, which inappropriately assumes that asystole represents fine VF.

followed by a shock, on the algorithm's presumption that asystole may represent undersensed fine VF.

The performance of an algorithm is closely tied to sensing and blanking characteristics of the defibrillator system. For example, in the Ventak AV defibrillators, an atrial blanking period is applied after a ventricular sensed event to avoid far-field R wave overdetection. In some situations, however, this blanking period can lead to detection errors, as shown in Figure 9–84. In this patient, atrial blanking after a sensed ventricular event results in "dropout" of atrial events, inappropriately leading the device to determine that the ventricular rate is greater than the atrial rate. Since the algorithm delivers therapy for any rhythm with a rate above the VT detection cutoff when the ventricular rate is greater than the atrial rate (when "V>A" is programmed "on"), shocks are delivered. Turning off the "V>A" feature permits application of onset and stability detection enhancements, which assess only changes in the ventricular rate irrespective of the atrial rate, and may eliminate the problem. A detailed understanding of the algorithm of each defibrillator is required to diagnose complex detection problems. As shown in these examples and in Figure 9–85, apparent device malfunction may in fact represent normal function for the defibrillator. The details of detection enhancement programming are covered in Chapter 7.

Determination of algorithm error requires a detailed understanding of device function. Given the complexity of modern-generation implantable defibrillators and the rapid rate of innovation, it is very useful in suspected instances of algorithm error to call technical support representatives of the manufacturer. In our experience, the support has generally been timely and the representatives knowledgeable about minutiae of device function. Additionally, some device behavior may be undocumented in the manual but known to the manufacturer's personnel.[90]

Oversensing.—Implantable defibrillators use dynamic gain or sensing to appropriately sense relatively large QRS complexes, to avoid detecting the subsequent midsized T wave (which would result in double counting of a single contraction), and at the same time to maintain adequate sensitivity to detect fibrillatory electrograms of small amplitude[78] (Fig. 9–86). Occasionally, defibrillators inappropriately detect the T waves, leading to an erroneous doubling of the heart rate and inappropriate therapies.[91,92] Any condition that increases the QT interval or results in a relatively small ventricular electrogram increases the likelihood of T-wave oversensing (Fig. 9–87). Additionally, since the effective sensitivity after a sensed R wave increases with each passing millisecond until the maximum sensitivity is reached[78] (Fig. 9–86), patients with slow heart rates, which allow more time after a QRS complex for the effective sensitivity to increase, are at increased risk for far-field oversensing. Since sensitivity (or gain) is rapidly maximized after a paced event, patients with pacing at slow rates are at greatest risk of far-field P-wave, T-wave, or myopotential oversensing (Fig. 9–88). Rarely, a very wide QRS may be double-counted (Fig. 9–89).

Oversensing, particularly of myopotentials, must be differentiated from lead fracture. When significant impedance or radiographic abnormalities are present, fracture is diagnosed. It is also helpful to review both near-field and far-field channels and to manipulate the pulse generator during real-time telemetry. Figure 9–90 illustrates apparent T-wave oversensing that with additional observation and review of near-field electrograms proved to be due to a lead defect, confirmed operatively. In our study of 379 patients with transvenous ICD systems and mean follow-up of 20 ± 16 months, 18% experienced lead failure at

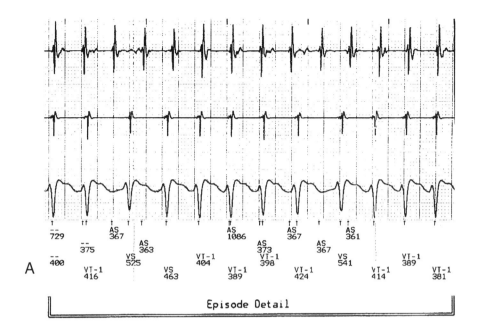

A

Episode Detail

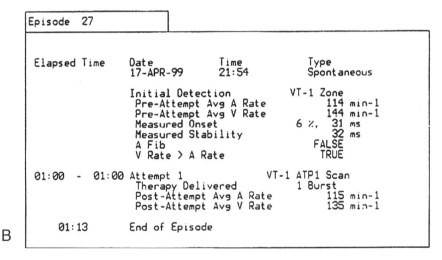

B

Fig. 9–84. Interaction between device sensing and algorithm performance. From top to bottom are the atrial, ventricular near-field (rate), and ventricular far-field (shock) electrograms and the markers. *A,* Atrial flutter with variable conduction is present. The ventricular rate is unstable, so that the stability algorithm alone would withhold therapy. However, because of dropout of the atrial complexes that occurs during the postventricular atrial blanking period, (e.g., after VS 463 and VT-1 404), the device inappropriately determines that the ventricular rate exceeds the atrial rate and delivers a shock. *B,* Episode information. Note that the episode has an unstable ventricular rate consistent with a conducted atrial arrhythmia (stability is 32 msec) and that the "V Rate > A Rate" is "TRUE." The preattempt average A rate shown is 114 bpm, whereas review of the atrial electrograms in *A* reveals that the rate is actually greater than 150 bpm. (Courtesy of Dr. Michael Glikson, Heart Institute, Sheba Medical Center, Tel Hashomer, Israel.)

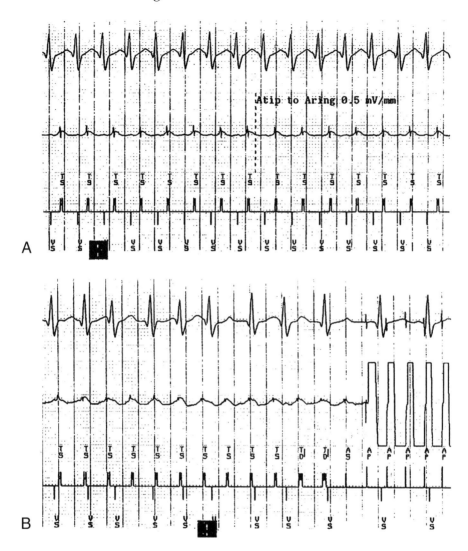

Fig. 9–85. Atrial tachycardia detection in an atrial and ventricular defibrillator (Medtronic 7250). Real-time telemetry is shown, with surface electrocardiogram, A-tip to A-ring atrial electrogram, and markers from top to bottom. Atrial markers are upgoing, and ventricular markers are down-going. *A,* Continuing atrial tachycardia is not detected. Despite the upgoing TS (tachycardia sense) markers indicative of an atrial rate in the atrial tachycardia zone, detection is not achieved, since the algorithm requires a P:R pattern with > 1:1 conduction to the ventricles. *B,* With the development of a > 1:1 P:R pattern, detection occurs (at TD, tachycardia detection) and atrial antitachycardia pacing is delivered. A detailed understanding of algorithm function is required to determine whether the device is functioning appropriately. (Courtesy of Dr. Michael Glikson, Heart Institute, Sheba Medical Center, Tal Hashomer, Israel.)

50 months.[60] Therefore, this defect should be looked for routinely. The approach to screening for lead failure is covered in detail in Chapter 13.

Device-Device Interactions.—Patients with a defibrillator and a separate pacing system are at risk for a number of device-device interactions. Some interactions, such as detection of both atrial and ventricular pacing spikes on the ventricular channel of the ICD, may result in inappropriate therapies. Since up to 50% of patients may

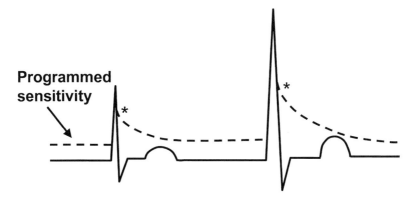

Fig. 9–86. Automatic adjusting sensitivity. At the (*), a QRS is sensed, and sensitivity is lowered to prevent T-wave oversensing. The sensitivity progressively increases over the cardiac cycle to permit sensing of small-amplitude fibrillation wavelets, should they occur. Some defibrillators dynamically adjust the gain while maintaining a fixed sensitivity, with a similar effect on sensing cardiac events over time.

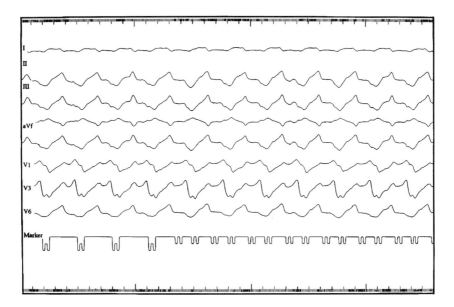

Fig. 9–87. Quinidine resulting in inappropriate classification of rhythm. The first four complexes on the left are appropriately sensed as ventricular tachycardia. In subsequent complexes, the broad QRS and prolonged repolarization on quinidine cause both the QRS and the T wave to be sensed. This double counting leads the device to sense ventricular fibrillation, which results in shock delivery instead of antitachycardia pacing (not shown). More commonly, antiarrhythmic drugs slow ventricular tachycardia below the heart rate cutoff, so that the arrhythmia is not detected at all.

have significant pacemaker-ICD interactions that can be avoided if properly identified, testing is warranted.[93] This subject is also covered in Chapter 13.

Mechanical System Malfunction.— Malfunction of the mechanical system includes lead failures, loose setscrews, and dislodgment. In our experience, lead dislodgment occurs earlier after implantation than lead failure due to other causes

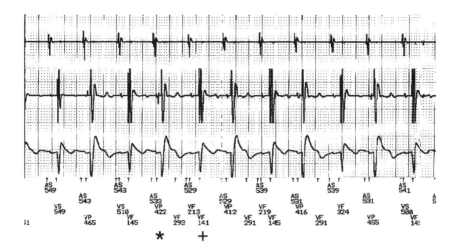

Fig. 9–88. Oversensing of P waves and T waves related to dynamic gain in a Ventak series implantable cardioverter-defibrillator. Note that oversensing occurs after ventricular pacing, since dynamic gain for sensing is increased rapidly following paced events. From top to bottom are the atrial, near-field ventricular (rate), and far-field ventricular (shock) electrograms. After a paced event (VP 422, asterisk), the T wave and P wave are both oversensed on the ventricular channel. Because of the short time between the pacing pulse and the T wave, these are detected as fibrillation-sensed events (VF 293 and VF 213). The next QRS complex is also sensed as a ventricular fibrillation event (VF 141) and is not paced. The absence of pacing (and its effect on dynamic sensing gain) leads to a normally sensed atrial event (AS 529), followed by a paced ventricular event after elapse of the atrioventricular interval (VP 412). This ventricular paced event, in turn, leads to repetition of the oversensing of the T wave at VF 291, the P wave at VF 219, and so on.

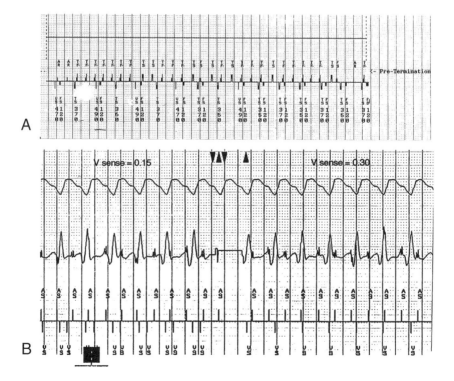

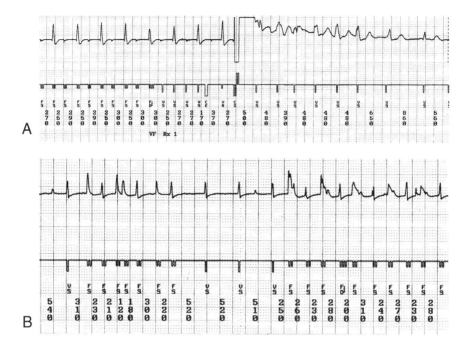

Fig. 9–90. Lead fracture masquerading as T-wave oversensing. *A,* Top to bottom are far-field electrograms, markers, and ventricular intervals from a stored episode (Medtronic 7223 single-chamber defibrillator). The far-field signal suggests T-wave oversensing, leading to inappropriate detection. Note that the shock is synchronized to a T wave—a potentially dangerous event. The apparent T-wave oversensing suggests that reprogramming the device to a less sensitive setting may eliminate the problem. *B,* The patient was admitted for monitoring, and the device was reprogrammed to record near-field electrograms. With the near-field recordings, electrical noise diagnostic of lead fracture is seen. This noise appears to coincide with the T wave, possibly resulting from a relationship between cardiac motion and electrical noise generated by the fracture. A fractured lead was confirmed at operation and a new lead placed.

Fig. 9–89. Oversensing of wide QRS complexes during ventricular tachycardia (VT), leading to detection of VT as ventricular fibrillation (VF). *A,* Stored episode data from a Medtronic 7250 atrial and ventricular defibrillator. From top to bottom are the stored electrograms (flat line; none stored for segment shown), marker channels (atrial markers are upgoing, ventricular downgoing), and ventricular intervals. Ventricular sensitivity is set high because of a relatively small R wave. The VF events (FS, fibrillation sense) are tightly coupled to the preceding sensed events, with a fixed interval of 120 msec. The blanking interval after a sensed ventricular interval is 120 msec, suggesting that these events are actually double counting of the same continuing wide QRS complex, which could be the result of an atrial arrhythmia with aberrancy or VT. *B,* Real-time electrograms recorded in the electrophysiology laboratory. During atrial fibrillation, no double sensing was noted (not shown). However, after VT induction (shown), double counting was detected. From top to bottom are the surface electrocardiogram, intracardiac electrogram, and markers. On the left, the ventricular sensitivity is 0.15 mV, and oversensing of the wide QRS occurs. After the up-down arrows at the top of the strip (indicating telemetry transmission), the ventricular sensitivity is reprogrammed to 0.30 mV, and oversensing is no longer present. (Courtesy of Dr. Michael Glikson, Heart Institute, Sheba Medical Center, Tel Hashomer, Israel.)

(2 ± 2 and 23 ± 15 months, respectively; $P < 0.0001$).[60] The diagnosis of lead dislodgment is nearly always apparent on radiographs, so that they should be routinely obtained after implantation and at 1-month follow-up. With routine x-ray screening, only 20% of patients with lead dislodgment present with inappropriate shocks. In contrast, more than 50% of patients with lead conductor fracture or insulation defect present with ICD shocks[60] (Fig. 9–75). Dislodgment may also be detected by hospital telemetry or stored episode data (Fig. 9–91). As noted above, screening for lead failure is covered in detail in Chapter 13.

Other forms of mechanical dysfunction occur rarely. When abandoned lead fragments contact active leads, contact noise may be generated that can be overdetected, leading to inappropriate therapies.[61,94] Figure 9–92 depicts an incompletely abandoned lead fragment contacting the active lead and thereby inhibiting pacing and overdetecting VF. In Figure 9-93, the distal screw of an Endotak 0125 lead was not fully deployed despite the fluoroscopic appearance of an extended screw. After the lead was connected to the defibrillator, recurrent contact-type noise appeared on the sensing circuit despite confirmation of a good lead connection in the header. Retraction and redeployment of the screw eliminated the problem, which presumably was due to contact noise between the distal screw and the lead itself.

Electromagnetic Interference. Electromagnetic interference can lead to electrical impulses on the ICD leads that can suppress pacing function or result in inappropriate detection of VF. This is reviewed in Chapter 12.

Phantom Shocks. Some patients report experiencing shocks, at times associated with flashes of light, myoclonic jerks, verbal outcries, and chest soreness, without actual discharge of the defibrillator, as confirmed by device interrogation.[95] This phenomenon usually occurs in the twilight preceding sleep, more commonly in patients with previous ICD discharges, and may represent anxiety or maladjustment to the defibrillator. Patients experiencing these symptoms should be reassured, and if symptoms persist, psychiatric evaluation should be considered.

Fig. 9–91. Patient with a single-chamber defibrillator (Medtronic 7227) and a dislodged lead. *A*, Hospital monitoring shows pacing of the *atrium*. Atrial pacing in a single-chamber ventricular defibrillator indicates that a lead tip is in an inappropriate location. The varying pacing intervals are due to the ventricular rate stabilization algorithm, which is "on." *B*, Trend report of an event. Note the rapidly alternating VV intervals (300 msec alternating with 150 msec) beginning at −4 seconds, giving the appearance of "railroad tracks." This alternating pattern is suggestive of far-field signal oversensing. The "railroad tracks" terminate at + 4 seconds, before the shock is delivered at 8 seconds (labeled 32.2 J), suggesting that a nonsustained ventricular tachycardia (VT) episode was shocked. *C*, Electrograms corresponding to the trend report shown in *B*. From top to bottom are far-field electrograms, near-field electrograms, and markers with VV intervals. The first complex is a sinus beat, followed by a run of nonsustained VT. The last two complexes are sinus beats. The lead is dislodged, with the tip in the atrium (hence the atrial capture with pacing in *A*) near the tricuspid annulus, so that atrial and ventricular activity is sensed. With the onset of VT, the short 150-msec intervals represent the ventriculoatrial interval, and the longer 310-msec cycle lengths represent the atrioventricular interval. Atrial oversensing leads to detection of ventricular fibrillation (VF) (at FD). *D*, Continuation of electrograms from *C*. The nonsustained VT has terminated. After capacitor charging is completed (CE for "charge end"), the defibrillator attempts to reconfirm whether VT or VF is still present. Since atrial oversensing results in two short intervals after CE (each of 170 msec), the device assumes that VF is still present and delivers a shock during sinus rhythm (CD for "charge delivered"). The lead was surgically repositioned without further problems.

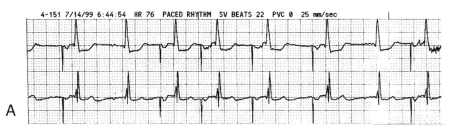

4-151 7/14/99 6:44:54 HR 76 PACED RHYTHM SV BEATS 22 PVC 0 25 mm/sec

A

Jul 14, 1999 07:49:12
9962 Software Version 2.0
Copyright (c) Medtronic, Inc. 1997

ICD Model: Gem 7227
Serial Number: PIP108098H

VT VF Episode #4 Report   Page 1

ID#	Date/Time	Type	V. Cycle	Last Rx	Success	Duration
4	Jul 14 09:14:33	VF	220 ms	VF Rx 1	Yes	3.2 min

• V-V   VF = 320 ms   VT = 400 ms

V-V Interval (ms)

32.2 J

Time (sec) [0 = Detection]

B

C

VF Rx 1 Defib

D

32.2 J

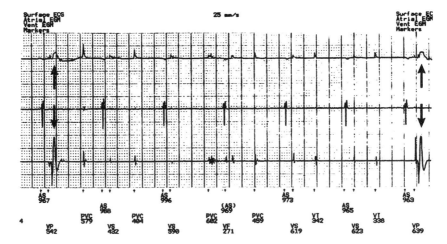

Fig. 9–92. Intractable electrical noise created by an incompletely extracted pacemaker lead that interfered with subsequent defibrillator implantation. Channels show (from top to bottom) the surface electrocardiogram, atrial electrogram, ventricular electrogram, and event markers. Only the complexes marked by arrows represent effective ventricular pacing; all other ventricular events (with markers indicating ventricular sensing [VS], premature ventricular contraction [PVC], ventricular fibrillation [VF], and ventricular tachycardia [VT]) are actually noise signals sensed by the ventricular channel and thus inhibiting pacing. The noise was strong enough to affect the surface electrocardiogram as well. Surface potentials most likely were evident, since the abandoned lead fragments were not capped, permitting transmission of the contact potentials close to the skin surface. Radiographs from this patient are shown in Figure 9–64 *A* through *C*. (From Friedman et al.[61] By permission of Futura Publishing Company.)

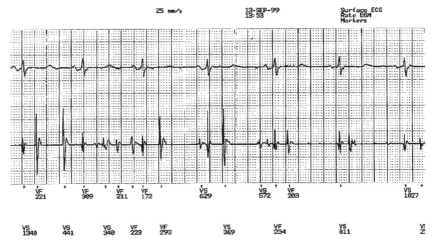

Fig. 9–93. Noise and overdetection at the time of implantation due to a distal screw that is not fully deployed on an Endotak 0125 lead. Details in the text.

Delayed, Absent, or Ineffective Therapy

Absent or lethally delayed ICD therapy is infrequent, as suggested by a series of observational studies demonstrating nearly uniform device effectiveness[96–98] and by prospective randomized trials showing reduced mortality compared with the best medical therapy in high-risk patients.[99,100] This is particularly true when an appropriate follow-up program is used, which often detects important malfunctions before they result in clinical events.[60] Nonetheless, therapy may be absent or delayed at times in patients with documented ventricular arrhythmias. This differential diagnosis is listed in Table 9–11. Patients with this problem should be carefully evaluated by the approach outlined earlier in this chapter. Often, this examination unearths the cause of the malfunction. Interrogation may show that the device is programmed "off," radiography or impedance values may reveal a lead fracture, the documented VT may be slower than the programmed detection cutoff, and so on. If a clear cause is not evident, electrophysiologic study should be done through the device to assess sensing, detection, and therapy delivery. The causes of absent or delayed therapy are further discussed below.

Inactivated Implantable Cardioverter-Defibrillator

An ICD may be inactivated by being programmed "off"—for example, preceding surgery to avoid overdetection of cautery—or, in some models, by prolonged contact with an external magnet. Close communication with other physicians and with the patient ensures that devices turned off intentionally for surgical interventions are reactivated before the patient is dismissed from a monitored hospital bed. Guidant defibrillators offer a "Change Tachy Mode with Magnet" feature that enables the mode of the device to be changed by holding a mag-

---

Table 9–11.
Causes of Absence or Delay in Effective Implantable Cardioverter-Defibrillator (ICD) Therapy With Documented Ventricular Tachycardia (VT) or Ventricular Fibrillation (VF)

Inactivated ICD
- Programmed off
- Sustained (possibly inadvertent) contact with an external magnet

Undersensing of ventricular electrogram
- Diminished amplitude of sensed ventricular electrogram (e.g., lead-tissue interface fibrosis)
- Postshock electrogram diminution
- Electrogram amplitude fluctuation in ICD with slow automatic gain control
- Lead malfunction or displacement
- Generator malfunction
- Device-device interaction (VF not detected because of pacing artifacts)

Underdetection
- VT below detection cutoff rate
- VT therapy withheld because of programmed specificity criteria
  Onset
  Stability
  Electrogram width or template matching
  Dual-chamber criteria
  Algorithm "error" in rhythm interpretation
- Detection in inappropriate zone (e.g., antitachycardia pacing for VF)

Mechanical failure preventing delivery of therapy
- Lead fracture or failure
- Poor lead connection in header

Algorithm failure preventing delivery of therapy

Ineffective delivered therapy
- Pacing threshold increase (medications, metabolic)
- Defibrillation threshold increase (medications or mechanical)

net over it for at least 30 seconds.[66,101] Initially, tones synchronous with R waves are heard (while the device is in the monitor plus therapy mode), and they become continuous when the device is off. Since environmental magnets (e.g., in stereo speakers, motors) have in rare instances inactivated devices, with life-threatening consequences, we routinely program this feature "off." This prevents environmental magnets from permanently reprogramming the ICD. Additionally, patients are advised to call their physician if tones are heard emanating from their ICD.

Undersensing and Underdetection of Ventricular Arrhythmias

Undersensing occurs when the electrical signals used by the defibrillator are absent or inadequate to permit appropriate detection. The cause can be diminished amplitude of sensed R wave, lead malfunction, or device-device interactions (Table 9–11). In contrast, underdetection occurs when despite appropriate sensing, arrhythmia is not detected (because the rate is too slow or specificity algorithms inappropriately determine that the rhythm is not ventricular) (Table 9–11).

The factors that can lead to R-wave diminution in pacemakers can do the same in defibrillators: local inflammation and fibrosis, myocardial infarction at the lead tip site, and medication effect. Additionally, electrograms in defibrillators may be further diminished after shocks from the effect of the high-voltage gradient on the nearby myocardium[102] (Fig. 9–94). Although postshock electrogram diminution with failed redetection was a problem in some older ICDs used with integrated leads and a distal coil near the lead tip (Ventritex Cadence ICD on an Endotak-C 60 series lead), the issue is no longer significant in modern systems.[102–106] Nonetheless, redetection may be impaired in patients with marginal R-wave amplitudes (< 5 mV). In general, if an R wave is small and there is any question of system malfunction, redetection after a failed shock should be assessed at electrophysiologic study. If impaired sensing impedes detection, a separate sensing lead should be implanted or the present lead should be repositioned. It is important when the R-wave amplitude is assessed to be certain that the near-field (rate sensing or pace-sense) electrogram is measured; this is the signal used by the device for detection. The far-field and near-field amplitudes may be very differ-

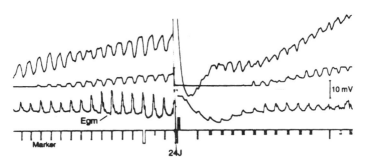

Fig. 9–94. Postshock electrogram diminution. After a failed 24-J shock, the endocardial electrogram (Egm) amplitude is diminished. The scale refers to the endocardial electrogram recording. In addition to the endocardial electrogram, diagnostic markers (bottom) from the defibrillation implant support device and two surface electrocardiographic leads are shown. Ventricular fibrillation was initiated by a low-energy shock delivered during ventricular repolarization. (From Brady et al.[102] By permission of Excerpta Medica.)

ent, but the near-field detection electrogram is critical.

Undersensing may also occur because of lead failure or insulation breakdown in both epicardial and transvenous systems.[63] Thus, system radiography, analysis of stored episodes, real-time telemetry with provocative maneuvers, and assessment of pacing threshold and impedance and high-voltage impedance (in devices that offer this feature) may all be fruitful, as discussed in Chapter 13. Similarly, since defibrillators decrease the sensitivity (or gain) immediately after a detected QRS to avoid T-wave oversensing, the large pacing spikes in patients with a separate pacing system may mimic QRS complexes and result in significant undersensing of continuing VF (also discussed in Chapter 13). Electrophysiologic testing to assess for device-device interactions is required in the patient with two separate systems and untreated ventricular tachyarrhythmias.[57]

Underdetection may occur because ventricular arrhythmias are below the VT cutoff rate, particularly if medications that may slow the VT rate are added. Real-time telemetry during an episode of stable VT may confirm this diagnosis. Often, the VT must be terminated (pharmacologically or by external cardioversion) before the device can be interrogated. However, careful measurement of the heart rate during VT can determine whether it is slower than the detection cutoff rate, confirming the cause of absent therapy.

Therapy for VT may also be withheld by detection enhancements designed to improve specificity. Detection of irregular VT, for example, may be impaired by the use of the stability criterion, which uses RR irregularity to differentiate atrial fibrillation-flutter from VT. Swerdlow et al.,[84] who defined underdetection as a delay of 5 seconds or longer, found underdetection in 0.4% of VT episodes during long-term follow-up of patients with PCDs (Pacemaker Cardioverter Defibrillator, Medtronic) using onset and stability criteria. In a study of patients with Ventak PRx I, PRx II, and PRx III defibrillators, Schaumann et al.[107] found that 2% of VTs were initially untreated because of variability greater than the programmed stability; however, all patients had a programmed sustained-rate-duration algorithm programmed "on" for 30 seconds, so that therapy was delivered at the end of 30 seconds despite the unstable RR intervals. Interestingly, patients treated with antiarrhythmic drugs, particularly class IC agents, may be at increased risk for underdetection of VT with use of the stability criterion. Le Franc et al.[108] found an important delay in VT detection in 12.5% of patients receiving class IC agents compared with 0% for nontreated patients or patients receiving sotalol.

Undersensing may lead to detection of a tachyarrhythmia in an inappropriate zone. In Figure 9–95, VF was induced with sensitivity programmed to "least" in a patient with a Guidant MINI ICD. Because of undersensing of the fibrillation electrograms, the arrhythmia was detected in the VT zone, and antitachycardia pacing—ineffective during VF—was delivered. Reprogramming to "nominal" sensitivity eliminated the problem.

Mechanical, Pulse Generator, or Algorithm "Failure" Preventing Delivery of Therapy

Isolated failure of shocking leads may prevent delivery of effective therapy despite appropriate detection. This phenomenon occurs predominantly in epicardial systems, in which the leads for sensing and for shocking are mechanically distinct.[61,109] Infrequently, mechanical connections (e.g., an improperly inserted lead pin) can result in nondelivery of a shock. Figure 9–96 is from an episode of induced VF in which one of the lead

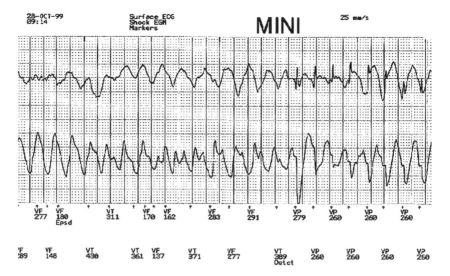

Fig. 9–95. Undersensing resulting in ventricular fibrillation detected as ventricular tachycardia (at VT 389 Detct). This leads to antitachycardia pacing delivery (starting with VP 279), which is ineffective for ventricular fibrillation. The problem was corrected by reprogramming sensitivity from "least" to "nominal."

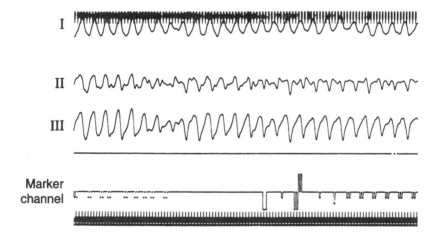

Fig. 9–96. Diagnosis of lack of shock delivery using a marker channel. Surface leads I, II, and III and the marker channel are displayed. Ventricular fibrillation (VF) was induced (not shown), and no defibrillation shock was delivered to the patient from the pacemaker-cardioverter-defibrillator system. Analysis of the marker channel shows appropriate detection of VF (short double markers). Loss of marker channel telemetry then occurs, which is normal during capacitor charging. The wide long marker denotes the end of capacitor charging followed by a refractory sensed event (short single marker). Attempted shock delivery by the pulse generator is denoted by the long double-down/double-up marker, but no shock artifact is seen on the surface leads, and VF continues with appropriate redetection after the refractory and normal sense markers. Thus, the marker channel revealed quickly that detection and attempted delivery of therapy was not the problem. Re-examination of the pulse generator header showed that in the two-lead system used, one lead had been inadvertently placed in the pulse 1 port and the plug placed in the pulse 2 port. Single shocks are delivered between the common and pulse 2. This problem was easily corrected by switching the leads in the header. This case further emphasizes the importance of performing a final VF induction before closing the pulse generator pocket. (From Friedman and Stanton.[78] By permission of Futura Publishing Company.)

pins is not properly seated in the header. VF is detected, and a shock is delivered by the pulse generator (as shown on the marker channels), without delivery of effective energy, as is evident on the surface electrocardiogram, which remains free of shock artifacts. Re-seating the pin in the header eliminated the problem.

Quite rarely, algorithm errors prevent delivery of therapy after an arrhythmia is appropriately detected. Figure 9–97 depicts VT in a patient with a 7217 PCD in which detection was appropriate, antitachycardia pacing (ATP) was programmed "on," and yet therapy was withheld. This result occurred because the VT cycle length was less than the programmed allowable minimum ATP cycle length. The rationale for a minimum ATP cycle length is the avoidance of proarrhythmia by preventing excessively fast pacing rates. In this case, however, the device did not deliver ATP (or any ther-

apy) and would not unless the tachycardia had spontaneously changed cycle length. The algorithm has since been modified, so that in current-generation devices, a shock is delivered if ATP is withheld because of the programmed minimum length of the pacing cycle. VT with an irregular cycle length may lead to delayed detection in the absence of specificity enhancements if the long cycle lengths are not in the detection window (Fig. 9–98).

Ineffective Delivered Therapy

ATP may be ineffective because the paced impulses cannot reach critical arrhythmogenic substrates as a result of medication effects on pacing thresholds, emergence of new arrhythmia circuits, or a change in the substrate. If repeated sequences of ATP fail to terminate VT, the

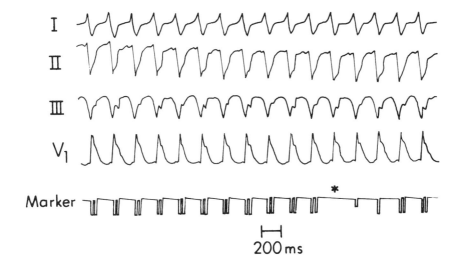

Fig. 9–97. Apparent lack of ventricular tachycardia (VT) therapy delivery actually due to inability of the pacemaker-cardioverter-defibrillator to deliver antitachycardia pacing therapy when the calculated coupling interval of the first pulse is less than the minimum programmed pacing interval. Surface leads I, II, III, and VI and the marker channel are displayed. The asterisk denotes the absent marker pulse when QRS occurred during the blanking period following attempted antitachycardia pacing. Double marker pulses are VT sensed events. The short single marker pulse is a sensed event during a refractory period, and the longer single marker pulse is a normal (non-VT) sensed event. See text for details. (From Friedman and Stanton.[78] By permission of Futura Publishing Company.)

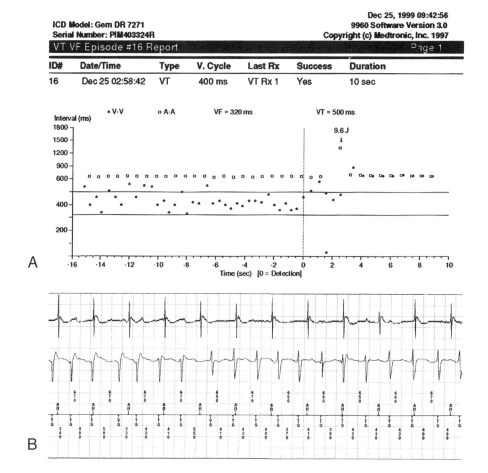

Fig. 9–98. Delayed detection of ventricular tachycardia (VT) due to an irregular VT with intervals falling outside the detection zone. *A,* Trend report from a Medtronic 7271 dual-chamber defibrillator. The atrial cycle length (approximately 660 msec, *open boxes*) is stable, whereas VT with unusually variable VV intervals continues. At times −15, −12, −11, and −7, intervals longer than 500 msec occur. These are outside the tachycardia zone and reset the VT counter, delaying detection. After detection, a shock is delivered (9.6 J at + 3 seconds), restoring sinus rhythm. Note the overlap of the VV and AA intervals after the shock. *B,* Electrograms from the episode shown in *A.* From top to bottom are the atrial electrogram, ventricular electrogram, and atrial (upgoing) and ventricular (downgoing) markers. The ventricular rate is faster than the atrial rate, consistent with VT. However, note the long intervals (e.g., VS 550) and the shifting ventricular morphology. In the Medtronic algorithm, a single long interval outside the VT zone resets the VT counter to zero. This often prevents detection of atrial fibrillation, but when VT is irregular, it may delay its detection.

device should be reprogrammed, and if new sequences of ATP are assigned, electrophysiologic study should be performed to assess ATP efficacy.[61]

Of greatest concern is the occurrence of ineffective defibrillation shocks, as these arrhythmias are immediately life-threatening. Shocks may fail from battery depletion, component failure, epicardial patch crumpling, transvenous lead dislodgment, or a pneumothorax, which adversely affects energy delivery across the myocardium[110,111] (Table 9–12 and Fig. 9–99, 9–100, and 9–101). Device interro-

Table 9–12.
Causes of Failed Defibrillation Shocks

Device-related
  • Battery depletion
  • Component failure
  • Crumpling of epicardial patch
  • Dislodgment of transvenous lead
Medical or biologic
  • Evolution of defibrillation threshold over time (especially if threshold at implantation exceeded 15 J)
  • Pneumothorax
  • Myocardial infarction
  • Drug proarrhythmia or alteration of defibrillation threshold
  • Electrolyte abnormalities

gation and chest radiographs diagnose these conditions. Defibrillation thresholds may also spontaneously vary over time; our experience has been that patients with initial defibrillation thresholds above 15 J are at increased risk for subsequent ineffective defibrillation, warranting routine assessment of defibrillation efficacy.[80,112] Conversely, in patients with implantation defibrillation

thresholds under 15 J, failure to defibrillate is exceedingly rare with current-generation devices (with maximum output $\geq$ 30 J) without a concomitant risk factor.[112] Importantly, medications may alter the defibrillation threshold. In particular, long-term oral administration of amiodarone increases the defibrillation threshold, so that we routinely reassess the threshold after initiation of this therapy.[31] In patients with borderline defibrillation thresholds, administration of amiodarone may need to be discontinued or additional defibrillation elements added to the system to improve safety margins.

In a patient who has had ineffective shocks, acute conditions that can impair therapy by modifying the substrate must be excluded. These conditions include myocardial infarction, active ischemia, drug proarrhythmia, and electrolyte abnormalities. Once they have been excluded, full evaluation of the device as described above is required. If no clear cause remains, electrophysiologic testing to determine the defibrillation threshold is helpful for guiding the need

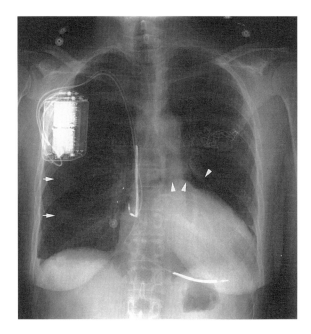

Fig. 9–99. Pneumothorax, as seen in this chest radiograph (*arrows*), can result in ineffective defibrillation. Also present is a pneumopericardium (*arrowheads*).

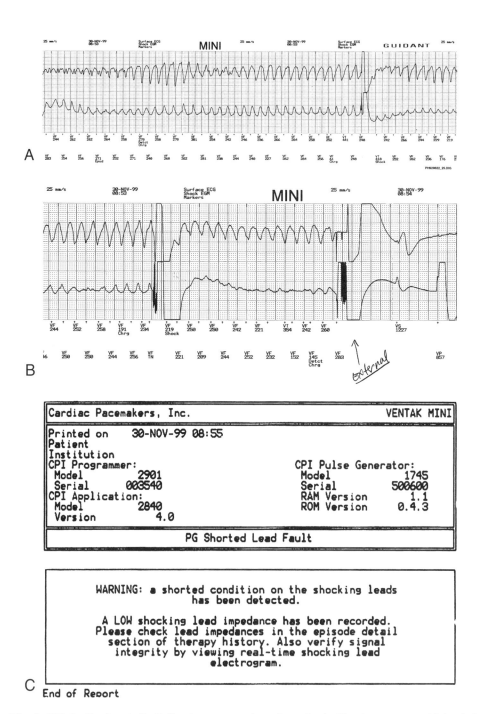

Fig. 9–100. Ineffective defibrillation in an asymptomatic patient with a transvenous biphasic implantable cardioverter-defibrillator (Guidant MINI) and an abdominal lead system. *A*, An induced episode of ventricular fibrillation is not terminated by the device shock. *B*, Continuation of same episode in *A*. A second device shock at maximal output also fails, and external rescue is required. *C*, Interrogation after the event reveals that a shorted lead was responsible for the failed shocks. *Continues.*

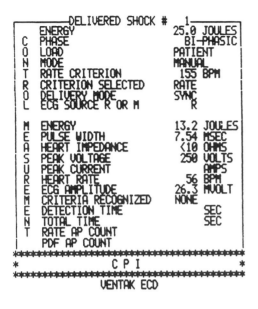

```
         DELIVERED SHOCK #    1
         ENERGY              25.0 JOULES
    C    PHASE                BI-PHASIC
    O    LOAD                 PATIENT
    N    MODE                 MANUAL
    T    RATE CRITERION        155 BPM
    R    CRITERION SELECTED   RATE
    O    DELIVERY MODE        SYNC
    L    ECG SOURCE R OR M      R

    M    ENERGY              13.2 JOULES
    E    PULSE WIDTH          7.54 MSEC
    A    HEART IMPEDANCE       <10 OHMS
    S    PEAK VOLTAGE          250 VOLTS
    U    PEAK CURRENT              AMPS
    R    HEART RATE             56 BPM
    E    ECG AMPLITUDE        26.3 MVOLT
    M    CRITERIA RECOGNIZED  NONE
    E    DETECTION TIME            SEC
    N    TOTAL TIME               SEC
    T    RATE AP COUNT
         PDF AP COUNT

  *************************************
  *               C P I               *
  *************************************
                 VENTAK ECD

PATIENT

PHYSICIAN

DATE

D  NOTES
```

Fig. 9–100 *continued. D,* Lead testing after the abdominal pocket is opened. A shock is delivered during sinus rhythm through the suspect lead by use of an external defibrillation testing system. The impedance of less than 10 Ω confirms a lead short circuit. The patient received a new pectoral system. This is the same patient whose tracings through the new system are shown in Figure 9–66. Because of the increased risk of lead failure with abdominal pulse generators, we recommend routine arrhythmia inductions in patients with these systems (discussed in detail in Chapter 13).

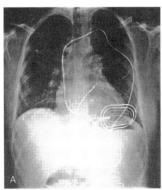

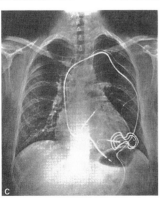

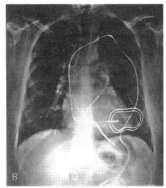

Fig. 9–101. Serial chest radiographs showing progressive crinkling of the subcutaneous patch at 8 days (*A*), 24 days (*B*), and 16 months (*C*) after implantation. The defibrillation thresholds were 18, 18, and 15 J, respectively. Although this patient's defibrillation threshold did not change with progressive patch crinkling, assessment of defibrillation efficacy is nevertheless recommended when this occurrence is noted. (From Friedman and Stanton.[78] By permission of Futura Publishing Company.)

for medication changes or addition of defibrillation electrodes to the system to lower the threshold. In patients with older, monophasic systems, upgrading to a biphasic system results in significant enhancement of defibrillation efficacy and should be considered.

Conclusion

Advances in ICD technology, including the use of multilumen leads and pectoral placement of the device, have greatly enhanced defibrillator reliability. Additionally, when troubleshooting is required, sophisticated event and data storage, coupled with real-time telemetry and automated assessment of pacing thresholds and impedance values, provides information leading to rapid diagnosis. The addition of self-diagnostic tests and audible warning tones holds promise for earlier detection of potential problems. Despite these significant enhancements, the growing complexity of defibrillators, lead systems, and algorithms mandates a systematic approach to troubleshooting and a detailed understanding of device function so that system malfunction can be diagnosed and effectively corrected.

References

1. Love CJ, Hayes DL: Evaluation of pacemaker malfunction. *In* Clinical Cardiac Pacing. Edited by KA Ellenbogen, GN Kay, BL Wilkoff. Philadelphia, WB Saunders Company, 1995, pp 656–683
2. Levine PA: Differential diagnosis, evaluation, and management of pacing system malfunction. *In* Cardiac Pacing. Edited by KA Ellenbogen. Boston, Blackwell Scientific Publications, 1992, pp 309–382
3. Parsonnet V, Neglia D, Bernstein AD: The frequency of pacemaker-system problems, etiologies, and corrective interventions (abstract). Pacing Clin Electrophysiol 15:510, 1992
4. Sweesy MW, Forney CC, Hayes DL, Batey RL, Forney RC: Evaluation of an in-line bipolar polyurethane ventricular pacing lead. Pacing Clin Electrophysiol 15:1982–1985, 1992
5. Moller JE, Moller M, Arnsbo P, Simonsen EH: Insulation defects in the Siemens 1010T and 1050T bipolar leads: occurrence and control measures for prevention of acute complications. Eur J Cardiac Pacing Electrophysiol 7:15–19, 1997
6. Stokes K, Staffenson D, Lessar J, Sahni A: A possible new complication of subclavian stick: conductor fracture (abstract). Pacing Clin Electrophysiol 10:748, 1987
7. Fyke FE III: Simultaneous insulation deterioration associated with side-by-side subclavian placement of two polyurethane leads. Pacing Clin Electrophysiol 11:1571–1574, 1988
8. Lloyd MA, Hayes DL, Holmes DR Jr, Stanson AW, Espinosa RE, Osborn MJ, McGoon MD: Extraction of the Telectronics Accufix 330–801 atrial lead: the Mayo Clinic experience. Mayo Clin Proc 71:230–234, 1996
9. Rankin JM, Davis MJ: Protrusion of retention wire from Encor-Dec passive fixation atrial pacing lead (letter). Lancet 346:1169–1170, 1995
10. Clarke M, Liu B, Schuller H, Binner L, Kennergren C, Guerola M, Weinmann P, Ohm OJ: Automatic adjustment of pacemaker stimulation output correlated with continuously monitored capture thresholds: a multicenter study. European Microny Study Group. Pacing Clin Electrophysiol 21:1567–1575, 1998
11. O'Hara GE, Kristensson B-E, Lundstrom R Jr, Kempen K, Soucy B, Lynn MS, on behalf of the worldwide Kappa 700 Investigators: First clinical experience with a new pacemaker with ventricular Capture Management™ feature (abstract). Pacing Clin Electrophysiol 21:892, 1998
12. Lee MT, Baker R: Circadian rate variation in rate-adaptive pacing systems. Pacing Clin Electrophysiol 13:1797–1801, 1990
13. van Mechelen R, Ruiter J, de Boer H, Hagemeijer F: Pacemaker electrocardiography of rate smoothing during DDD pacing. Pacing Clin Electrophysiol 8:684–690, 1985
14. Benditt DG, Sutton R, Gammage MD, Markowitz T, Gorski J, Nygaard GA, Fetter J: Clinical experience with Thera DR rate-drop response pacing algorithm in carotid sinus syndrome and vasovagal syncope. The International Rate-Drop Investigators Group. Pacing Clin Electrophysiol 20:832–839, 1997

15. Levine PA, Sanders R, Markowitz HT: Pacemaker diagnostics: measured data, event marker, electrogram, and event counter telemetry. *In* Clinical Cardiac Pacing. Edited by KA Ellenbogen, GN Kay, BL Wilkoff. Philadelphia, WB Saunders Company, 1995, pp 639–655

16. Levine PA: The complementary role of electrogram, event marker and measured data telemetry in the assessment of pacing system function. J Electrophysiol 1:404–416, 1987

17. Kruse I, Markowitz T, Ryden L: Timing markers showing pacemaker behavior to aid in the follow-up of a physiological pacemaker. Pacing Clin Electrophysiol 6:801–805, 1983

18. Irwin ME, Gulamhusein SS, Senaratne MP, St. Clair WR: Outcomes of an ambulatory cardiac pacing program: indications, risks, benefits, and outcomes. Pacing Clin Electrophysiol 17:2027–2031, 1994

19. Kenny RA, Krahn AD: Implantable loop recorder: evaluation of unexplained syncope. Heart 81:431–433, 1999

20. Irnich W: Pacemaker-related patient mortality (editorial). Pacing Clin Electrophysiol 22:1279–1283, 1999

21. Ector H, Rickards AF, Kappenberger L, Vardas P, Oto A, Santini M, Sutton R: The registry of the European working group on cardiac pacing (abstract). Eur Heart J 20 Abstract Suppl:469, 1999

22. Hauser R, Hayes D, Parsonnet V, Furman S, Epstein A, Hayes J, Saksena S, Almquist A, Gross J, Kallinen L: Feasibility and initial results of an internet-based North American pacemaker and ICD pulse generator and lead registry (abstract). Pacing Clin Electrophysiol 23:597, 2000

23. Puglisi A, Ricci R, Azzolini P, Peraldo Neja C, Fioranelli M, Speciale G, Angrisani G: Ventricular cross stimulation in a dual chamber pacing system: phenomenon analysis. Pacing Clin Electrophysiol 13:993–1001, 1990

24. Levine PA, Rihanek BD, Sanders R, Sholder J: Cross-stimulation: the unexpected stimulation of the unpaced chamber. Pacing Clin Electrophysiol 8:600–606, 1985

25. Altamura G, Bianconi L, Lo Bianco F, Toscano S, Ammirati F, Pandozi C, Castro A, Cardinale M, Mennuni M, Santini M: Transthoracic DC shock may represent a serious hazard in pacemaker dependent patients. Pacing Clin Electrophysiol 18:194–198, 1995

26. Beanlands DS, Akyurekli Y, Keon WJ: Prednisone in the management of exit block,

27. Risby O, Meibom J, Nyboe I, Schüller H: The influence of prednisolon on pacemaker threshold (abstract). Pacing Clin Electrophysiol 4:A-68, 1981

28. Hellestrand KJ, Burnett PJ, Milne JR, Bexton RS, Nathan AW, Camm AJ: Effect of the antiarrhythmic agent flecainide acetate on acute and chronic pacing thresholds. Pacing Clin Electrophysiol 6:892–899, 1983

29. Bianconi L, Boccadamo R, Toscano S, Serdoz R, Carpino A, Iesi AP, Altamura G: Effects of oral propafenone therapy on chronic myocardial pacing threshold. Pacing Clin Electrophysiol 15:148–154, 1992

30. Dohrmann ML, Goldschlager N: Metabolic and pharmacologic effects on myocardial stimulation threshold in patients with cardiac pacemakers. *In* Modern Cardiac Pacing. Edited by SS Barold. Mount Kisco, NY, Futura Publishing Company, 1985, pp 161–170

31. Carnes CA, Mehdirad AA, Nelson SD: Drug and defibrillator interactions. Pharmacotherapy 18:516–525, 1998

32. Nielsen AP, Griffin JC, Herre JM, Luck JC, Mann DE, Cashion RW, Spencer WH, Schuenemeyer TD, Magro S, Wyndham CR: Effect of amiodarone on acute and chronic pacing thresholds (abstract). Pacing Clin Electrophysiol 7:462, 1984

33. Schlesinger Z, Rosenberg T, Stryjer D, Gilboa Y: Exit block in myxedema, treated effectively by thyroid hormone therapy. Pacing Clin Electrophysiol 3:737–739, 1980

34. Lee D, Greenspan K, Edmands RE, Fisch C: The effect of electrolyte alteration on stimulus requirement of cardiac pacemakers (abstract). Circulation 38 Suppl:VI-124, 1968

35. O'Reilly MV, Murnaghan DP, Williams MB: Transvenous pacemaker failure induced by hyperkalemia. JAMA 228:336–337, 1974

36. Sowton E, Barr I: Physiological changes in threshold. Ann N Y Acad Sci 167:679–685, 1969

37. Hughes JC Jr, Tyers GF, Torman HA: Effects of acid-base imbalance on myocardial pacing thresholds. J Thorac Cardiovasc Surg 69:743–746, 1975

38. Preston TA, Judge RD: Alteration of pacemaker threshold by drug and physiological factors. Ann N Y Acad Sci 167:686–692, 1969

39. Levine PA: Clinical manifestations of lead insulation defects. J Electrophysiol 1:144–155, 1987

40. Batey FL, Calabria DA, Shewmaker S, Sweesy MW: Crosstalk and blanking periods in a dual-chamber (DDD) pacemaker: a case report. Clin Prog Electrophysiol Pacing 3:1314–1318, 1985

41. Jain P, Kaul U, Wasir HS: Myopotential inhibition of unipolar demand pacemakers: utility of provocative manoeuvres in assessment and management. Int J Cardiol 34:33–39, 1992

42. Gabry MD, Behrens M, Andrews C, Wanliss M, Klementowicz PT, Furman S: Comparison of myopotential interference in unipolar-bipolar programmable DDD pacemakers. Pacing Clin Electrophysiol 10:1322–1330, 1987

43. Gross JN, Platt S, Ritacco R, Andrews C, Furman S: The clinical relevance of electromyopotential oversensing in current unipolar devices. Pacing Clin Electrophysiol 15:2023–2027, 1992

44. Toivonen L, Valjus J, Hongisto M, Metso R: The influence of elevated 50 Hz electric and magnetic fields on implanted cardiac pacemakers: the role of the lead configuration and programming of the sensitivity. Pacing Clin Electrophysiol 14:2114–2122, 1991

45. Peters RW, Kushner M, Knapp K: Giant pacemaker spikes. An electrocardiographic artifact. Chest 87:256–257, 1985

46. Souliman SK, Christie J: Pacemaker failure induced by radiotherapy. Pacing Clin Electrophysiol 17:270–273, 1994

47. Teskey RJ, Whelan I, Akyurekli Y, Eapen L, Green MS: Therapeutic irradiation over a permanent cardiac pacemaker. Pacing Clin Electrophysiol 14:143–145, 1991

48. Auricchio A, Hartung W, Geller C, Klein H: Clinical relevance of stored electrograms for implantable cardioverter-defibrillator (ICD) troubleshooting and understanding of mechanisms for ventricular tachyarrhythmias. Am J Cardiol 78:33–41, 1996

49. O'Hara GE, Rashtian MY, Lemke B, Philippon F, Gilbert M, Brown AB, Cuijpers A, Koehler J, Soucy B, and the 7271 Gem DR Worldwide Investigators: Patient alert: clinical experience with a new patient monitoring system in a dual chamber defibrillator (abstract). Pacing Clin Electrophysiol 22:709, 1999

50. Philippon F, Johnson BW, Waldecker B, O'Hara GE, Gilbert M, Brown AB, Ayeni F, Soucy B: Painless lead impedance in a dual chamber defibrillator (abstract). Pacing Clin Electrophysiol 22:825, 1999

51. Kou WH, Calkins H, Lewis RR, Bolling SF, Kirsch MM, Langberg JJ, de Buitleir M, Sousa J, el-Atassi R, Morady F: Incidence of loss of consciousness during automatic implantable cardioverter-defibrillator shocks. Ann Intern Med 115:942–945, 1991

52. Hook BG, Callans DJ, Kleiman RB, Flores BT, Marchlinski FE: Implantable cardioverter-defibrillator therapy in the absence of significant symptoms. Rhythm diagnosis and management aided by stored electrogram analysis. Circulation 87:1897–1906, 1993

53. Degroot PJ, Church TR, Mehra R, Martinson MS, Schaber DE: Derivation of a defibrillator implant criterion based on probability of successful defibrillation. Pacing Clin Electrophysiol 20:1924–1935, 1997

54. Fogoros RN, Elson JE, Bonnet CA: Actuarial incidence and pattern of occurrence of shocks following implantation of the automatic implantable cardioverter defibrillator. Pacing Clin Electrophysiol 12:1465–1473, 1989

55. Nisam S, Fogoros RN: Troubleshooting of patients with implantable cardioverter-defibrillators. In Interventional Electrophysiology. Edited by I Singor. Baltimore, Williams & Wilkins, 1997, pp 793–824

56. Luria DM, Chugh SS, Lexvold NY, Hammill SC, Shen WK, Friedman PA: High rate of long-term endovascular lead failure with abdominally placed implantable defibrillators (abstract). Circulation 100 (Suppl I):I-568, 1999

57. Glikson M, Trusty JM, Grice SK, Hayes DL, Hammill SC, Stanton MS: A stepwise testing protocol for modern implantable cardioverter-defibrillator systems to prevent pacemaker-implantable cardioverter-defibrillator interactions. Am J Cardiol 83:360–366, 1999

58. Furman S, Hayes DL, Holmes DR Jr: A Practice of Cardiac Pacing. Third edition. Mount Kisco, NY, Futura Publishing Company, 1993

59. Haddad L, Padula LE, Moreau M, Schoenfeld MH: Troubleshooting implantable cardioverter defibrillator system malfunctions: the role of impedance measurements. Pacing Clin Electrophysiol 17:1456–1461, 1994

60. Luria D, Rasmussen MJ, Hammill SC, Friedman PA: Frequency and mode of detection of nonthoracotomy implantable defibrillator lead failure (abstract). Pacing Clin Electrophysiol 22:705, 1999

61. Friedman PA, Glikson M, Stanton MS: Defibrillator challenges for the new millen-

nium: the marriage of device and patient—making and maintaining a good match. J Cardiovasc Electrophysiol 11:697–709, 2000

62. Marchlinski FE, Callans DJ, Gottlieb CD, Schwartzman D, Preminger M: Benefits and lessons learned from stored electrogram information in implantable defibrillators. J Cardiovasc Electrophysiol 6:832–851, 1995

63. Rosenthal ME, Alderfer JT, Marchlinski FE: Troubleshooting suspected ICD malfunction. *In* Implantable Cardioverter Defibrillator Therapy: The Engineering-Clinical Interface. Edited by MW Kroll, MH Lehmann. Norwell, MA, Kluwer Academic Publishers, 1996, pp 435–476

64. Grimm W, Flores BF, Marchlinski FE: Electrocardiographically documented unnecessary, spontaneous shocks in 241 patients with implantable cardioverter defibrillators. Pacing Clin Electrophysiol 15:1667–1673, 1992

65. Dunbar SB, Warner CD, Purcell JA: Internal cardioverter defibrillator device discharge: experiences of patients and family members. Heart Lung 22:494–501, 1993

66. Miller JM, Hsia HH: Management of the patient with frequent discharges from implantable cardioverter defibrillator devices. J Cardiovasc Electrophysiol 7:278–285, 1996

67. Julian DG, Camm AJ, Frangin G, Janse MJ, Munoz A, Schwartz PJ, Simon P: Randomised trial of effect of amiodarone on mortality in patients with left-ventricular dysfunction after recent myocardial infarction: EMIAT. European Myocardial Infarct Amiodarone Trial Investigators. Lancet 349:667–674, 1997

68. Cairns JA, Connolly SJ, Roberts R, Gent M: Randomised trial of outcome after myocardial infarction in patients with frequent or repetitive ventricular premature depolarisations: CAMIAT. Canadian Amiodarone Myocardial Infarction Arrhythmia Trial Investigators. Lancet 349:675–682, 1997

69. Doval HC, Nul DR, Grancelli HO, Perrone SV, Bortman GR, Curiel R: Randomised trial of low-dose amiodarone in severe congestive heart failure. Grupo de Estudio de la Sobrevida en la Insuficiencia Cardiaca en Argentina (GESICA). Lancet 344:493–498, 1994

70. Massie BM, Fisher SG, Radford M, Deedwania PC, Singh BN, Fletcher RD, Singh SN: Effect of amiodarone on clinical status and left ventricular function in patients with congestive heart failure. CHF-STAT Investigators. Circulation 93:2128–2134, 1996

71. Torp-Pedersen C, Moller M, Bloch-Thomsen PE, Kober L, Sandoe E, Egstrup K, Agner E, Carlsen J, Videbaek J, Marchant B, Camm AJ: Dofetilide in patients with congestive heart failure and left ventricular dysfunction. Danish Investigations of Arrhythmia and Mortality on Dofetilide Study Group. N Engl J Med 341:857–865, 1999

72. Stevenson WG, Friedman PL, Kocovic D, Sager PT, Saxon LA, Pavri B: Radiofrequency catheter ablation of ventricular tachycardia after myocardial infarction. Circulation 98:308–314, 1998

73. Friedman PA, Packer DL, Hammill SC: Catheter ablation of mitral isthmus ventricular tachycardia using electroanatomically guided linear lesions. J Cardiovasc Electrophysiol 11:466–471, 2000

74. Friedman P, Beinborn D, Schultz J, Hammill S: Ablation of noninducible idiopathic left ventricular tachycardia using a non-contact map acquired from a premature complex with tachycardia morphology. Pacing Clin Electrophysiol (in press)

75. Marchlinski FE, Callans DJ, Gottlieb CD, Zado E: Linear ablation lesions for control of unmappable ventricular tachycardia in patients with ischemic and nonischemic cardiomyopathy. Circulation 101:1288–1296, 2000

76. Zipes DP, Jalife J: Cardiac Electrophysiology: From Cell to Bedside. Third edition. Philadelphia, WB Saunders Company, 2000

77. Schaumann A, von zur Muhlen F, Herse B, Gonska BD, Kreuzer H: Empirical versus tested antitachycardia pacing in implantable cardioverter defibrillators: a prospective study including 200 patients. Circulation 97:66–74, 1998

78. Friedman PA, Stanton MS: The pacer-cardioverter-defibrillator: function and clinical experience. J Cardiovasc Electrophysiol 6:48–68, 1995

79. Glikson M, Stanton MS, Friedman PA, Benderly M, Trusty JM, Hammill SC: Is routine programmed ventricular stimulation necessary with pectoral ICDs? (Abstract.) Arch Mal Coeur Vaiss 91 (Suppl 3):349, 1998

80. Glikson M, Luria D, Friedman PA, Trusty JM, Benderly M, Hammill SC, Stanton MS: Are routine arrhythmia inductions necessary in patients with pectoral implantable cardioverter defibrillators? J Cardiovasc Electrophysiol 11:127–135, 2000

81. Goldberger JJ, Horvath G, Challapalli R, Kadish AH: Inappropriate implantable cardioverter-defibrillator therapy due to the detection of premature ventricular complexes. Pacing Clin Electrophysiol 22:825–828, 1999

82. Neuzner J, Pitschner HF, Schlepper M: Programmable VT detection enhancements in implantable cardioverter defibrillator therapy. Pacing Clin Electrophysiol 18:539–547, 1995

83. Grimm W, Flores BF, Marchlinski FE: Symptoms and electrocardiographically documented rhythm preceding spontaneous shocks in patients with implantable cardioverter-defibrillator. Am J Cardiol 71:1415–1418, 1993

84. Swerdlow CD, Chen PS, Kass RM, Allard JR, Peter CT: Discrimination of ventricular tachycardia from sinus tachycardia and atrial fibrillation in a tiered-therapy cardioverter-defibrillator. J Am Coll Cardiol 23:1342–1355, 1994

85. Friedman PA: Atrial fibrillation: diagnosis, management and stroke prevention. In Mayo Clinic Cardiology Review. Second edition. Edited by JG Murphy. Philadelphia, Lippincott, Williams & Wilkins, 2000, pp 633–645

86. Di Lenarda A, Sabbadini G, Salvatore L, Sinagra G, Mestroni L, Pinamonti B, Gregori D, Ciani F, Muzzi A, Klugmann S, Camerini F: Long-term effects of carvedilol in idiopathic dilated cardiomyopathy with persistent left ventricular dysfunction despite chronic metoprolol. The Heart-Muscle Disease Study Group. J Am Coll Cardiol 33:1926–1934, 1999

87. First International Study of Infarct Survival Collaborative Group: Randomised trial of intravenous atenolol among 16 027 cases of suspected acute myocardial infarction: ISIS-1. Lancet 2:57–66, 1986

88. Brignole M, Menozzi C, Gianfranchi L, Musso G, Mureddu R, Bottoni N, Lolli G: Assessment of atrioventricular junction ablation and VVIR pacemaker versus pharmacological treatment in patients with heart failure and chronic atrial fibrillation: a randomized, controlled study. Circulation 98:953–960, 1998

89. Coppess MA, Miller JM, Zipes DP, Groh WJ: Software error resulting in malfunction of an implantable cardioverter defibrillator. J Cardiovasc Electrophysiol 10:871–873, 1999

90. Mann DE, Kelly PA, Reiter MJ: Inappropriate shock therapy for nonsustained ventricular tachycardia in a dual chamber pacemaker defibrillator. Pacing Clin Electrophysiol 21:2005–2006, 1998

91. Frazier DW, Stanton MS: Pseudo-oversensing of the T wave by an implantable cardioverter defibrillator: a nonclinical problem. Pacing Clin Electrophysiol 17:1311–1315, 1994

92. Perry GY, Kosar EM: Problems in managing patients with long QT syndrome and implantable cardioverter defibrillators: a report of two cases. Pacing Clin Electrophysiol 19:863–867, 1996

93. Glikson M, Trusty JM, Grice SK, Hayes DL, Hammill SC, Stanton MS: Importance of pacemaker noise reversion as a potential mechanism of pacemaker-ICD interactions. Pacing Clin Electrophysiol 21:1111–1121, 1998

94. Lickfett L, Wolpert C, Jung W, Spehl S, Pizzulli L, Esmailzadeh B, Luderitz B: Inappropriate implantable defibrillator discharge caused by a retained pacemaker lead fragment. J Interv Card Electrophysiol 3:163–167, 1999

95. Kowey PR, Marinchak RA, Rials SJ: Things that go bang in the night (letter). N Engl J Med 327:1884, 1992

96. Saksena S, Prakash A, Madan N, Giorgberidze I, Munsif AN, Mathew P, Kaushik R, Krol RB: New generations of implantable pacemaker defibrillators for ventricular and atrial tachyarrhythmias. Arch Mal Coeur Vaiss 89 Spec No 1: 149–154, 1996

97. Zipes DP, Roberts D: Results of the international study of the implantable pacemaker cardioverter-defibrillator. A comparison of epicardial and endocardial lead systems. The Pacemaker-Cardioverter-Defibrillator Investigators. Circulation 92:59–65, 1995

98. Bardy GH, Yee R, Jung W: Multicenter experience with a pectoral unipolar implantable cardioverter-defibrillator. Active Can Investigators. J Am Coll Cardiol 28:400–410, 1996

99. Moss AJ, Hall WJ, Cannom DS, Daubert JP, Higgins SL, Klein H, Levine JH, Saksena S, Waldo AL, Wilber D, Brown MW, Heo M: Improved survival with an implanted defibrillator in patients with coronary disease at high risk for ventricular arrhythmia. Multicenter Automatic Defibrillator Implantation Trial Investigators. N Engl J Med 335:1933–1940, 1996

100. The Antiarrhythmics Versus Implantable Defibrillators (AVID) Investigators: A comparison of antiarrhythmic-drug therapy with implantable defibrillators in patients resuscitated from near-fatal ven-

tricular arrhythmias. N Engl J Med 337:1576–1583, 1997

101. Pinski SL, Trohman RG: Implantable cardioverter-defibrillators: implications for the nonelectrophysiologist. Ann Intern Med 122:770–777, 1995

102. Brady PA, Friedman PA, Stanton MS: Effect of failed defibrillation shocks on electrogram amplitude in a nonintegrated transvenous defibrillation lead system. Am J Cardiol 76:580–584, 1995

103. Jung W, Manz M, Moosdorf R, Luderitz B: Failure of an implantable cardioverter-defibrillator to redetect ventricular fibrillation in patients with a nonthoracotomy lead system. Circulation 86:1217–1222, 1992

104. Cooklin M, Tummala RV, Peters RW, Shorofsky SR, Gold MR: Comparison of bipolar and integrated sensing for redetection of ventricular fibrillation. Am Heart J 138:133–136, 1999

105. Isbruch FM, Block M, Bocker D, Dees H, Hammel D, Borggrefe M, Scheld HH, Breithardt G: Improved sensing signals after endocardial defibrillation with a redesigned integrated sense pace defibrillation lead. Pacing Clin Electrophysiol 19:1211–1218, 1996

106. Goldberger JJ, Horvath G, Donovan D, Johnson D, Challapalli R, Kadish AH: Detection of ventricular fibrillation by transvenous defibrillating leads: integrated versus dedicated bipolar sensing. J Cardiovasc Electrophysiol 9:677–688, 1998

107. Schaumann A, von zur Muhlen F, Gonska BD, Kreuzer H: Enhanced detection criteria in implantable cardioverter-defibrillators to avoid inappropriate therapy. Am J Cardiol 78:42–50, 1996

108. Le Franc P, Kus T, Vinet A, Rocque P, Molin F, Costi P: Underdetection of ventricular tachycardia using a 40 ms stability criterion: effect of antiarrhythmic therapy. Pacing Clin Electrophysiol 20: 2882–2892, 1997

109. Brady PA, Friedman PA, Trusty JM, Grice S, Hammill SC, Stanton MS: High failure rate for an epicardial implantable cardioverter-defibrillator lead: implications for long-term follow-up of patients with an implantable cardioverter-defibrillator. J Am Coll Cardiol 31:616–622, 1998

110. Luria D, Stanton MS, Eldar M, Glikson M: Pneumothorax: an unusual cause of ICD defibrillation failure. Pacing Clin Electrophysiol 21:474–475, 1998

111. Friedman PA, Stanton MS: Thoracotomy elevates the defibrillation threshold and modifies the defibrillation dose-response curve. J Cardiovasc Electrophysiol 8:68–73, 1997

112. Luria D, Glikson M, Hammill S, Friedman P: Stability of long-term defibrillation thresholds in patients with nonthoracotomy implantable defibrillators. Cardiac Arrhythmias 1999. Proceedings of the 6th International Workshop on Cardiac Arrhythmias, Springer, 1999

10

Complications

David L. Hayes, M.D.

Pacemaker complications can be classified in many ways. One approach is to consider complications by clinical presentation.[1]

- Implantation-related complications
- Recurrence of preimplantation symptoms
- New symptoms that correlate temporally with pacemaker implantation
- Asymptomatic electrocardiographic abnormalities (see Chapters 6 and 9)

Implantation-Related Complications

As noted in Table 10–1, multiple potential complications are related to implantation. During preimplantation description of the procedure with the patient, potential complications should be discussed. Our practice is to routinely include the complications that are statistically the most common and those that potentially carry the greatest threat to the patient. Specifically, lead dislodgment, pneumothorax, infection, and cardiac perforation with tamponade are discussed.

Lead Placement

Complications of lead placement result from catheterization of the heart and from placement of a permanent lead itself.

Lead Dislodgment

Historically, the most common complication of transvenous pacing has been lead dislodgment. Improved fixation mechanisms have significantly reduced the frequency of this complication for both atrial and ventricular pacing leads. It is difficult to state precisely what rate of lead dislodgment is acceptable, but secondary intervention rates for all reasons should be below 2% for ventricular leads and probably below 3% for atrial leads. In the Pacemaker Selection in the Elderly (PASE) trial, lead dislodgment was the most common complication, occurring in 9 of the 407 patients, or 2.2%.[2]

Dislodgment has been classified by some as "macrodislodgment" and "microdislodgment." Macrodislodgment is radiographically evident, and microdislodgment is not (Fig. 10–1). Adequate lead position is assessed by posteroanterior and lateral chest radiographs (see Chapter 11). Lead placement by chest radiography

Table 10–1.
Classification of Pacemaker Complications by Clinical Presentation

Implantation-related complications	Recurrence of preimplantation symptoms	New symptoms secondary to PMP	Asymptomatic ECG abnormalities
• Pneumothorax due to subclavian puncture • Other complications of subclavian puncture • Hematoma formation • Lead perforation • Lead dislodgment • Painful pocket • Lead placement in the systemic circulation • Twiddler's syndrome	• Lead fracture • Lead insulation defect • Loose lead-connector block interface • Oversensing	• Extracardiac stimulation • Pacemaker syndrome • Pacemaker-mediated tachycardia • Infection • Pain	• Failure to capture • Failure to sense • Oversensing (failure to output) • Change in paced rate

ECG, electrocardiographic; PMP, pacemaker placement.

may appear excellent in the patient with a microdislodgment. Slightly higher dislodgment rates may be acceptable in pediatric patients, whose activity is more difficult to control, and in patients with unusual ana-tomy, such as congenital cardiac anomalies.

Atrial lead dislodgment has traditionally been higher. With current lead technology, the rate of atrial lead dislodgment should be less than 3% (Fig. 10–2). The dis-lodgment rates of active and passive fixation atrial leads are reported to be similar, and dislodgment is clearly related more to implanter experience than to the fixation mechanism.

Pneumothorax

Complications of venous entry, in-herent in any approach to venous struc-

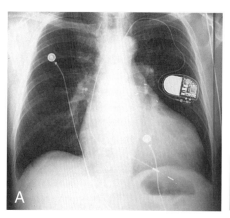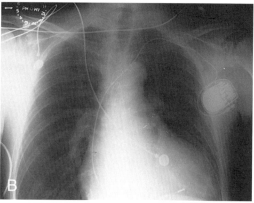

Fig. 10–1. Posteroanterior radiographs on the day after implantation (*A*) and 2 days later (*B*), when there was evidence of malfunction. *A,* The lead is directed inferiorly toward the right ventricular apex. *B,* The lead is now directed superiorly, indicating that the lead has definitely moved (macrodislodgment). (From Hayes DL: Pacemaker radiography. *In* A Practice of Cardiac Pacing. Third edition. Edited by S Furman, DL Hayes, DR Holmes Jr. Mount Kisco, NY, Futura Publishing Company, 1993, pp 361–400. By permission of Mayo Foundation.)

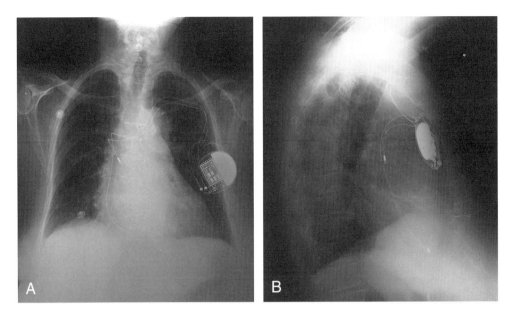

Fig. 10–2. Posteroanterior (*A*) and lateral (*B*) radiographs on the morning after implantation of a dual-chamber pacemaker. The active-fixation atrial lead has clearly dislodged and is now positioned in the superior vena cava.

tures, include damage to associated arterial or neural structures, extensive bleeding, air embolism, and thrombosis. In the subclavian approach, the potential for pneumothorax also exists; it can be minimized by knowledge of the patient's anatomy, attention to details, and contrast venography (Fig. 10–3). In the PASE trial, pneumothorax occurred in 1.97% of patients.[2] Analysis of unpublished data from our institution found the overall risk of pneumothorax from subclavian puncture to be approximately 1.5%. Although statistical proof is not possible, our data also show that contrast venography appears to lower the incidence of pneumothorax.

If the subclavian artery is also lacerated, hemopneumothorax may occur (Fig. 10–4). Anatomy must be considered before subclavian puncture is undertaken. In a patient with unusual anatomy of the chest wall or clavicle, the subclavian vein can be displaced and the usual landmarks used for subclavian puncture can be altered. Peripheral injection of contrast media and fluoroscopic guidance of the sub-

clavian puncture may help to minimize complications[3] (Fig. 10–5).

If pneumothorax occurs, manifestation may be during the pacemaker procedure or as late as 48 hours after implantation. Indications of pneumothorax are aspiration of air during subclavian puncture when the exploring needle is either introduced or removed, unexplained hypotension, chest pain, and respiratory distress.

After subclavian puncture, a chest radiograph should be obtained and inspected specifically for pneumothorax. A pneumothorax estimated to involve less than 10% of the pleural space can probably be observed without chest tube placement. A chest tube should be considered if more than 10% of the lung is involved, the patient has continued respiratory distress, or hemopneumothorax is present.

Other potential complications of subclavian venous entry are air embolism, arteriovenous fistula, thoracic duct injury, and brachial plexus injury. Although all are uncommon, it is essential that the

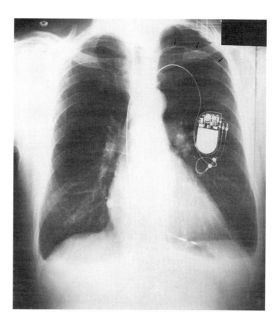

Fig. 10–3. Posteroanterior radiograph taken within a few hours after implantation in a patient complaining of mild dyspnea and left-sided chest discomfort. The patient has an apical pneumothorax as a complication of subclavian puncture.

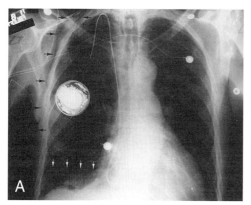
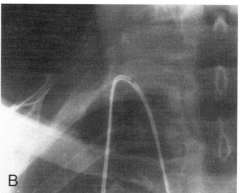

Fig. 10–4. Posteroanterior radiograph (*A*) from a patient with a hemothorax (fluid level noted by *white arrows*) and subcutaneous emphysema (*black arrows*) as complications of subclavian puncture. (Size of the pacemaker indicates older radiograph.) There is also an abandoned lead that has been transected and left in place. Close observation reveals a fracture of the abandoned lead, which is more evident in the close-up view (*B*). (From Hayes DL: Pacemaker complications. *In* A Practice of Cardiac Pacing. Edited by S Furman, DL Hayes, DR Holmes Jr. Mount Kisco, NY, Futura Publishing Company, 1986, pp 253–271. By permission of the publisher.)

implanter using the subclavian puncture technique be familiar with the potential problems.

Lead Perforation

Myocardial perforation is caused by improper force on the lead. It may be a particular problem in elderly patients because of a thin-walled right ventricle. Perforation of the coronary sinus also has been described, and awareness of this potential complication will become increasingly more important as the coronary veins are more commonly used for permanent lead placement.

In the PASE trial, perforations oc-

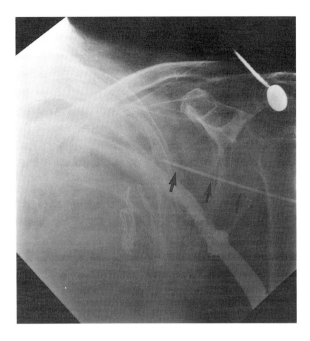

Fig. 10–5. Fluoroscopic image obtained during dye injection. This image can be used to facilitate subclavian puncture, thus minimizing the risk of pneumothorax. *Arrows* denote needle.

curred in 4 of the 407 randomized patients, 0.98%.[2] Myocardial perforation during lead placement is an uncommon but potentially serious complication. The true frequency of lead perforation is difficult to determine.

Perforation can potentially remain asymptomatic or be detected by an increasing stimulation threshold. In other patients, the signs may include right bundle branch block paced rhythm if the lead has been placed in the right ventricle (depending on lead position, the right bundle branch block pattern is possible when the lead is within the right ventricular cavity), intercostal muscle or diaphragmatic contraction, friction rub after implantation (Fig. 10–6), pericarditis, pericardial effusion, and cardiac tamponade. Hemodynamic deterioration may occur at the time of perforation, but a "slow" pericardial leak may also arise, and symptoms may not appear for 24 to 48 hours. With atrial perforation, tamponade may be more frequent.

If the patient has mild symptoms or signs compatible with lead perforation, such as pericardial pain and friction rub, but a persistent perforation cannot be identified, observation is reasonable. If the symptoms or signs resolve within 24 to 48 hours, lead repositioning probably is not necessary. If an echocardiogram reveals a small pericardial effusion but no definite perforation, serial echocardiograms should be obtained to be certain that the effusion is not hemodynamically significant or enlarging.

Management of lead perforation depends, in part, on the clinical sequelae. Perforation associated with hemodynamic compromise must be dealt with as an emergency. If clinical and echocardiographic findings are consistent with tamponade, echocardiographically guided pericardiocentesis should be performed. Usually, placing an indwelling pigtail catheter is reasonable to avoid recurrent hemodynamic compromise and to accurately measure drainage. If neither significant additional drainage nor reaccumulation by echocardiographic imaging occurs, the catheter can be removed in 48 to 72 hours and the patient managed by observation and reimaging. If no reaccumulation occurs, the leads may not have to be

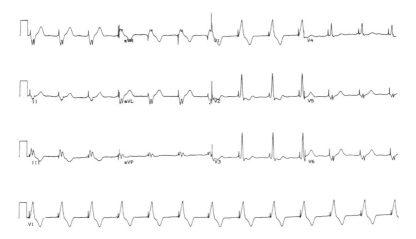

Fig. 10–6. Twelve-lead electrocardiogram obtained immediately after VVI pacemaker implantation. The paced ventricular complex has a right bundle branch block configuration compatible with left ventricular lead placement.

repositioned so long as thresholds remain stable. Any significant rise in threshold necessitates lead withdrawal and repositioning. Anytime a lead suspected of perforation is withdrawn, there is the potential for pericardial bleeding.

Arrhythmias

A frequent complication during lead implantation is development of supraventricular or ventricular arrhythmias related to lead manipulation. These effects are usually transient, ending promptly when the lead position is changed. Rarely, they may be sustained. Atrial manipulation may rarely result in sustained atrial tachycardia, fibrillation, or flutter, which complicates placement of a permanent atrial system. Atrial tachycardia may revert to normal sinus rhythm with gentle manipulation of the electrode against the atrial wall or by overdrive pacing. Management of atrial flutter or fibrillation is more difficult and may require antiarrhythmic agents or cardioversion to restore normal sinus rhythm. Brief ventricular arrhythmias are

more common, particularly during ventricular lead manipulation. They are usually easily controlled. However, patients with a history of spontaneous sustained ventricular tachycardia may experience these during lead manipulation. Occurrence is obviously more likely during implantation of an implantable cardioverter-defibrillator (ICD). For this reason, all pacemaker and ICD recipients are monitored, and life-support equipment and a defibrillator are immediately available.

Ventricular extrasystoles may occur in the early postimplantation period as a result of irritation at the electrode-myocardium interface. These premature beats, termed "tip extrasystoles," are usually of the same morphology as the paced ventricular beat (Fig. 10–7). They usually subside within 24 hours after implantation and rarely, if ever, require treatment.

In addition to tachycardia, bradyarrhythmias may occur. In patients with intermittent atrioventricular (AV) block and left bundle branch block, catheter trauma to the right bundle may result in an AV block. More commonly, bradycardia results from overdrive suppression of an escape ventricular focus dur-

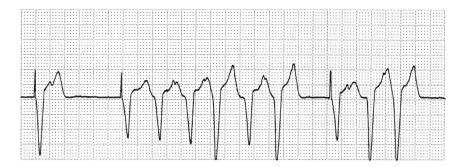

Fig. 10–7. Electrocardiographic tracing obtained within hours after VVI pacemaker implantation. The pacemaker is programmed to a lower rate of 50 bpm. There are frequent ventricular extrasystoles morphologically similar to the paced beats, and at least one of the premature beats is undersensed.

ing threshold testing. In a patient at high risk for development of asystole or complete heart block during the procedure, a temporary pacemaker may be placed before implantation at the discretion of the implanter. Alternatively, external-pacing pads can be placed during the procedure should temporary pacing be needed, and this method may obviate adjunctive transvenous temporary pacing.

Pulse Generator Pocket

Because local ecchymoses are common after pacemaker implantation, an ecchymosis, regardless of size, that is not expanding is treated by observation only. It occurs particularly in patients receiving anticoagulants or antiplatelet agents. Aspirin and other inhibitors of platelet aggregation, such as ticlopidine, may be significant, and often unrecognized, offenders. Careful local hemostasis is essential. In patients requiring oral anticoagulants, we insist that the prothrombin time be nearly normal before implantation. (An international normalized ratio of 1.5 to 1.7 is usually considered acceptable.)

There are reports of successful pacemaker implantation in fully anticoagulated patients with the adjunctive use of topical thrombin applied to the pocket before closure.[4] We have not adopted this technique. For any patient, however, previously anticoagulated or not, who seems to have excessive "oozing" within the pocket, we have found that topical application of thrombin is highly effective in stopping the bleeding.

Discrete hematoma formation at the site must be dealt with on the basis of its secondary consequences (Fig. 10–8 and 10–9). If bleeding continues, pain cannot be managed with mild analgesics, or the integrity of the incision is threatened, evacuating the hematoma should be considered. Aspiration of the hematoma should not be attempted, because it is often ineffective, and regardless of the care taken to maintain sterile technique, aspiration increases the risk of introducing an infection.

Administration of anticoagulants can be resumed within 48 to 72 hours after implantation if there is no evidence of significant hematoma formation. Should a significant hematoma occur, conservative treatment is preferred if possible. Needle aspiration or placement of a drain should be avoided to minimize the risk of infection. If evacuation of the hematoma is required to manage local pain or stop progression because of a threat to the integrity of the incision, the procedure should be thoroughly sterile.

Late complications, including erosion

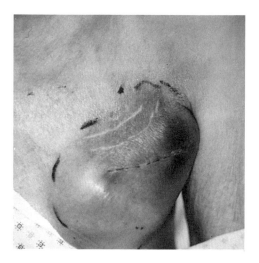

Fig. 10–8. Large hematoma of the pacemaker pocket. The boundaries of the hematoma are marked to determine whether the hematoma is continuing to expand.

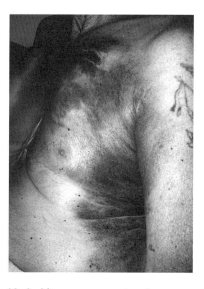

Fig. 10–9. After coronary artery bypass grafting and subsequent pacemaker implantation, evidence of a hematoma appeared at the pacemaker site. There is also extensive ecchymosis (present after the bypass grafting) along the lateral aspect of the chest.

and migration, are often the result of suboptimal initial surgery (Fig. 10–10). These can be minimized by careful technique at the time of initial pacemaker implantation and by the formation of an adequate pocket. Also, a painful pocket, as previously discussed, may result from inadequate positioning of the pacemaker below the subcutaneous tissues, and the pulse generator may have to be repositioned.

Pain

Patients should be told to expect some local discomfort at the pacemaker implantation site. This gradually subsides and can usually be managed with mild analgesics, such as acetaminophen. For several reasons, a patient could experience a painful pacemaker site, commonly called a "painful pocket," and the complaint should be taken seriously. The differential diagnosis includes

- Infection
- Pacemaker implanted too superficially
- Pacemaker implanted too laterally
- Pacemaker allergy

An indolent infection may be signaled by a painful pocket long before any other signs of infection. This diagnosis may be difficult. Needle aspiration of a pacemaker site that is not obviously infected is not advised for fear of introducing infection. However, if a painful pocket is explored for any reason, specimens for culture should be obtained at that time.

The pacemaker pocket should be formed in the prepectoralis fascia, that is, deep to adipose tissue in the subcutaneous space. If it is placed anterior to the adipose layer, that is, within subcutaneous tissues, significant pain may result. This is one of the most common causes of a painful pocket and justifies revision of the pacemaker pocket.

If the pacemaker is positioned too laterally, impingement on the axillary space may cause discomfort (Fig. 10–11). Although there are published series on axillary pocket placement, significant experience is required to position the pacemaker in such a way that there is no discomfort.

Allergic reaction to the pacemaker

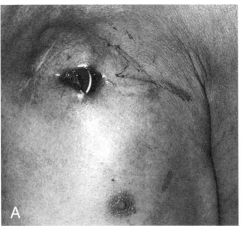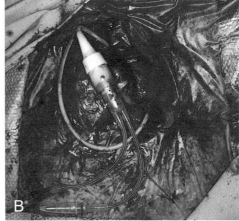

Fig. 10–10. *A,* Erosion of a pacemaker. *B,* At explantation, it was found that a large adaptor had been used to allow an older lead to be connected to a newer lead. The large adaptor was placed without further enlargement of the pocket, resulting in a pocket that was too small and subsequent erosion.

can or other components of the pacing system is a rare but reported complication. Pain at the pocket site may occur if the allergic reaction is to the pacemaker can or other component located within the pocket site. Proof of such an allergy requires sophisticated allergy testing, and correction of the problem may require changing certain components of the hardware. Some of the instances of "allergy" are, in reality, low-grade infections, which

should be treated as infections rather than allergies. No diagnosis of allergy should be made until infection has been ruled out.

Inadvertent Left Ventricular Lead Placement

Inadvertent placement of the transvenous lead in the left ventricular cavity is not uncommon.[5] This occurrence is

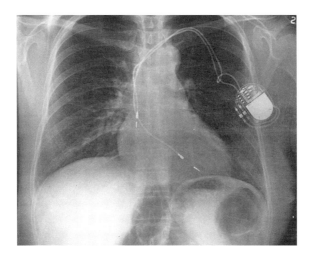

Fig. 10–11. Posteroanterior radiograph from a patient with chronic pain and arm limitation after pacemaker implantation. An attempt had been made to place the pacemaker in an axillary position for cosmetic reasons.

most likely when a lead is passed across an atrial or ventricular septal defect that is not known to exist (Fig. 10–12). It can also occur by inadvertent puncture and cannulation of the subclavian artery. A systemic position of the lead can be suspected by an unusually high "takeoff" of the ventricular lead, that is, it begins to pass to the left side of the heart at a point higher than the lowermost portion of the atrial J. If lateral fluoroscopy or lateral chest radiography is done, the left ventricular position is fairly obvious because the lead is directed posteriorly.

The concern with left ventricular lead placement is the potential for thromboemboli. Small thromboemboli arising from the pacing leads on the right side of the heart are probably not uncommon but are rarely of clinical significance. Conversely, a small thromboembolus in the system circulation could be catastrophic. Therefore, a lead in the system circulation is of clinical concern. If such a position is realized within the first few days after implantation, the lead should be withdrawn and repositioned if the patient does not have a right-to-left shunt across the defect that allowed the lead to cross. With a shunt, epimyocardial lead placement must be considered. If left ven-

tricular lead positioning is not recognized in the first few days, it is not likely to be realized for some time. If months have passed, the approach must be individualized for the patient. If the lead is to be left in the system circulation, the patient should receive anticoagulation with warfarin and be told of the potential risk of embolic phenomena. Lead extraction can be considered, although controversy exists. Because of the potential for embolization of small clots during extraction, some physicians opt for removal of the leads only during an open chest approach. Those who are expert in extraction procedures believe that the risk of emboli is small and proceed with standard extraction techniques. All options should be discussed with the patient.

Thrombosis

Thromboembolic complications after permanent pacemaker implantation are rare.[6] If thrombosis involves the superior vena cava, axillary vein, or area around the pacemaker lead in the right atrium or right ventricle, several problems can develop (Fig. 10–13). These include occlusion of the superior vena cava

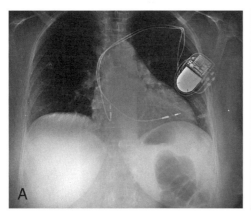 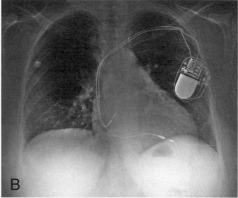

Fig. 10–12. *A,* Posteroanterior chest radiograph obtained the day after pacemaker implantation. The lead has a "high takeoff" as it begins to cross to the left from the atrial position. This lead had been passed across an unknown patent foramen ovale and positioned in the left ventricle. *B,* Posteroanterior chest radiograph obtained the day after the lead had been withdrawn and repositioned in the right ventricular apex.

and superior vena cava syndrome; thrombosis of the superior vena cava, right atrium, or right ventricle, with hemodynamic compromise or pulmonary embolism; and symptomatic thrombosis of the subclavian vein with an edematous painful upper extremity.

Partial or silent thrombosis is common and is usually clinically insignifi-cant except at the time of pacing system revision; an alternative venous route may be required. Venoplasty has been used when partial thrombosis limits venous access and a new lead must be placed[7] (Fig. 10–14).

If the patient presents with symptomatic venous thrombosis, several thera-peutic approaches can be considered.

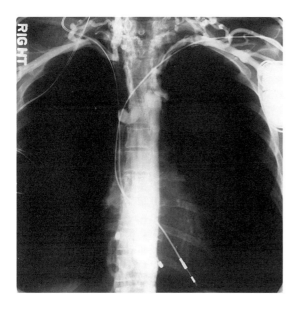

Fig. 10–13. Venogram from a patient with an abandoned pacing lead on the left and a functional but failing pace-maker lead through the left subclavian vein. Extensive thrombosis is present in the subclavian vein with bilateral innom-inate vein occlusion.

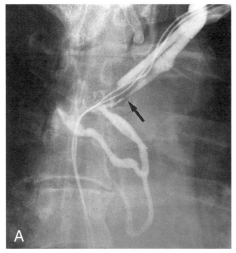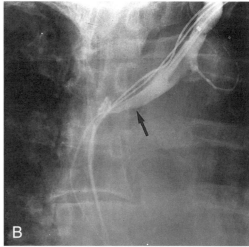

Fig. 10–14. *A,* Initial venogram reveals high-grade stenosis of the left innominate vein and large bridging collateral venous channels around the area of stenosis (*arrow*). *B,* Venogram after venoplasty shows large opening in area of previously noted stenosis (*arrow*). Dilation was suf-ficient to allow passage of the pacemaker lead. (From Spittell et al.[7] By permission of Futura Publishing Company.)

The most common presentation is a mildly edematous arm and complaints of "aching" or a "heavy" sensation in the arm. Conservative treatment with bed rest, arm elevation, and intravenous heparin often results in relief of symptoms. There are reports of thrombolytic therapy for symptomatic thrombosis after device implantation. Although this method may work well, the patient should be advised that there is some risk of bleeding within the pocket if the procedure had been recently performed. Whether long-term anticoagulation is of benefit in patients with subclavian thrombosis is controversial. Although the information available is anecdotal only or consists of single case reports, we favor the use of warfarin for approximately 3 months after immediate heparin therapy. In the patient with more extensive thrombosis, such as superior vena cava syndrome, other interventions may be required.

Loose Connector Block Connection

Intermittent or complete failure of output can occur because of a loose connection at the pacing lead-connector block interface. This failure usually occurs because the lead was inadequately secured at the time of pacemaker implantation. It may also occur because of a poor fit between the lead and the pacemaker even though they are allegedly compatible. Specifically, a side-lock connector has been demonstrated to be insecure in connecting with one model of VS-1 connector. When there is a loose connection, manipulating the pacemaker may reproduce the problem. The poor connection may be evident radiographically (Fig. 10–15).

Lead Damage

Lead damage during pacemaker implantation may be more common than is recognized. Pacing leads are easily cut by scissors or scalpel, and repair is difficult. Polyurethane leads can be easily damaged by placement of a ligature directly around the lead itself. To secure the lead, the protector sleeve provided on most polyurethane leads or a "butterfly" sleeve that can be secured around the lead and then to the underlying support structures should be used (Fig. 10–16).

It is also possible to damage the lead with the stylet during implantation, that is, the stylet may be forced at an angle through the conductor and the surrounding insulating material. If this is recognized during the procedure, the lead should be removed and discarded.

Skin Adherence

Adherence of the pulse generator to the skin strongly suggests an infection, and salvage of the site may not be possible. Impending erosion (skin thinned to the point of transparency) should be dealt with as an emergency. Once the skin is broken, infection is virtually certain; while it is still closed, the pacemaker is protected. If revision is accomplished before the pacemaker has fully eroded and become contaminated, the original pacemaker can be reimplanted if infection is not present. In this situation, the original site can be successfully revised and reused. Culture specimens should be obtained in all such circumstances.

Erosion

Although erosion of the pulse generator through the skin usually occurs long after implantation, it is most often related to the implantation technique (Fig. 10–10). Erosion is an uncommon complication that may occur in four situations.

- The patient has an indolent infection.
- The pacemaker pocket formed at the time of surgery is too small for the implanted pulse generator.

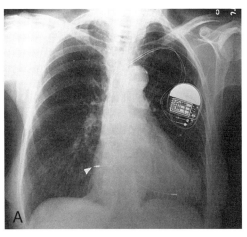
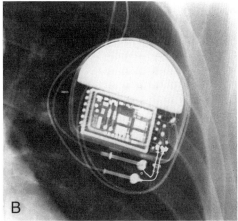

Fig. 10–15. Posteroanterior (*A*) and close-up (*B*) radiographic views from a patient with intermittent failure to pace. Comparison of the upper and lower pins reveals that the lower of the two unipolar leads is not completely advanced. This difference is more evident on the close-up view. By convention, the lower of the two leads in the connector block is the ventricular lead, so that this patient must have had intermittent or permanent ventricular failure to output. Incidentally, the atrial lead is positioned laterally and the J curve is suboptimal (*arrowhead*). (From Hayes DL: Pacemaker radiography. *In* A Practice of Cardiac Pacing. Third edition. Edited by S Furman, DL Hayes, DR Holmes Jr. Mount Kisco, NY, Futura Publishing Company, 1993, pp 361–400. By permission of Mayo Foundation.)

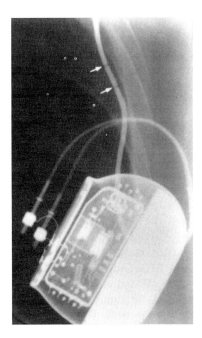

Fig. 10–16. Close-up view from a posteroanterior radiograph shows a pacemaker and the proximal portion of a lead. At two sites (*arrows*), the insulation is compressed by ligatures placed around a securing sleeve. (From Hayes.[1] By permission of Mayo Foundation.)

• The pulse generator is implanted too superficially, especially in children and small-framed adults, in whom lack of adipose tissue results in "tightness" of the pacemaker despite adequate pocket size.

• The generator is implanted too far laterally in the anterior axillary fold.

Infection is the most common cause of erosion, and the other causes are uncommon by comparison. When pacemaker erosion occurs, the only choice is surgical revision of the pacemaker site. If erosion is associated with infection, the entire system (both pulse generator and lead) must be removed and a completely new pacing system implanted at a clean site. It may be possible to revise the pacemaker site, enlarge the pocket, and fashion a satisfactory skin flap. Revision can be undertaken only if there is no infection. Infection may be present even without purulent material; therefore, cultures should be done and results proven negative before pocket revision.

Infection

The incidence of infection after pacemaker implantation should certainly be less than 2% and in most series has been less than 1%. Careful attention to surgical details and sterile procedures is of paramount importance in avoiding pacemaker site infection. The prophylactic use of antibiotics before implantation and in the immediate postoperative period remains controversial. Most studies do not show any significant difference in the rate of infection between patients who have had prophylactic administration of antibiotics and those who have not. Irrigation of the pacemaker pocket with an antibiotic solution at the time of pacemaker implantation may help to prevent infection.

Pacemaker infection must be recognized and be treated properly. It may appear as

- Local inflammation and abscess formation in the area of the pulse generator pocket
- Erosion of part of the pacing system through the skin with secondary infection
- Fever associated with positive blood cultures with or without a focus of infection elsewhere

The most common clinical presentation is infection around the generator; septicemia is an uncommon mode of presentation. Early infections usually are caused by *Staphylococcus aureus,* are aggressive, and are often associated with fever and systemic symptoms. Late infections commonly are caused by *Staphylococcus epidermidis* and are more indolent, usually without fever or systemic manifestations. Treatment for both organisms requires removal of the entire infected pacing system, pulse generator, and leads. Other organisms may be involved in either early or late infections.

There is some controversy about how to proceed once the infected system has been removed. A one-stage surgical approach involves implantation of a new pacing system at a distant clean site after explantation of the infected pacing system. Others favor removal of the infected system, temporary pacing, if required, and antibiotic management in the interim, with implantation of a new system at a later date.

Multiple techniques can be used for lead extraction.[8] Leads should be extracted only by someone well-trained in the technique and in the potential complications of extraction.

Retained Lead Fragments

Whether abandoned, nonfunctioning, and noninfected leads should be extracted is controversial. Abandoned leads must be removed if they are part of an infected system. If the pacing system is infected, it is essential that the entire lead be removed. In other situations, extraction may be desirable, for example, tricuspid regurgitation caused by multiple leads, symptomatic thrombosis, impediment to placement of a new pacing lead, interaction between pacing and ICD leads, and leads in pediatric patients, who require multiple lead changes and in whom abandonment would result in excessive hardware. If none of these conditions exists, it is possible to abandon leads in place without compromise to the patient[9] (Fig. 10–17).

At the time of lead extraction, a portion of the lead, specifically, portions of the "tines," may be left in an endocardial position. A distal electrode also may not be removed and be left somewhere within the vascular tree (Fig. 10–18). A clinical problem usually does not result.

Twiddler's Syndrome

Purposeful or absent-minded "twiddling"—manipulation of the pulse generator by the patient—has been named "twiddler's syndrome." Manipulation may cause axial rotation of the pacemaker, twisting of the lead, and eventual fracture or dislodgment of the lead. The pulse generator usually is not damaged. The syndrome commonly occurs when the pacemaker sits loosely in the pacemaker pocket (Fig. 10–19), either because the pocket was too large or because the pacemaker migrated.

If the problem has occurred because of pacemaker migration or a poorly

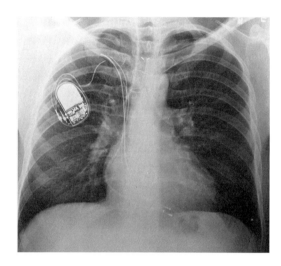

Fig. 10–17. Posteroanterior chest radiograph shows three ventricular leads in place. All three leads are fractured. Two of the leads were transected at the time they were replaced. At the time of this radiograph, the patient presented with fracture of the third lead. No clinical problems could be attributed to the excessive abandoned hardware. (From Hayes DL: Pacemaker radiography. *In* A Practice of Cardiac Pacing. Third edition. Edited by S Furman, DL Hayes, DR Holmes Jr. Mount Kisco, NY, Futura Publishing Company, 1993, pp 361–400. By permission of Mayo Foundation.)

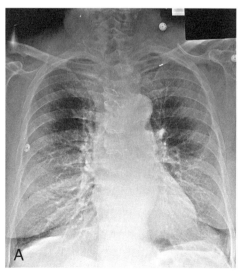
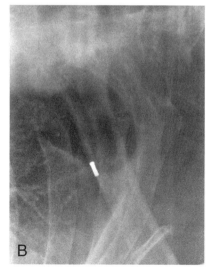

Fig. 10–18. Posteroanterior chest radiograph (*A*) and close-up view (*B*) of a retained lead fragment, the distal electrode, after partial lead extraction. The fragment is wedged in an infraclavicular portion of the subclavian vein. The retained fragment has not produced long-term complications.

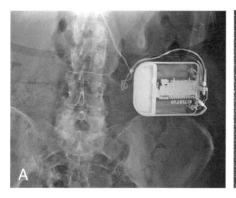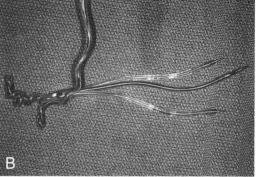

Fig. 10–19. Anterior abdominal radiograph (*A*) of a tightly twisted lead close to the implantable cardioverter-defibrillator and photograph (*B*) of the explanted lead. Although there was no definite evidence that the patient had "twiddled" the lead, the radiographic and direct appearances of the lead are compatible with this syndrome.

fashioned pacemaker pocket, the pocket should be revised. Avoiding the creation of an excessively large pocket, fixing the pulse generator by an anchoring suture, or anchoring the lead to the prepectoral fascia by a sleeve may prevent this problem. Others advocate placing the pacemaker in a snugly fitting Dacron pouch to reduce migration and torsion of the pacing system by promoting tissue ingrowth and stabilization of the pacemaker.

Recurrence of Preimplantation Symptoms

Loss of Circuit Integrity

Any abnormality that can permanently or intermittently interrupt the integrity of the pacing circuit can allow recurrent bradycardia and therefore recurrence of symptoms. Likewise, interruption of the circuit in an ICD can result in recurrent bradyarrhythmia or tachyarrhythmia. This can occur with fracture of the lead conductor coil, breach of lead insulation, or loose connection where the lead pin joins the connector block. Failure of the pacemaker circuitry, which would also allow recurrent bradycardia, is extraordinarily rare unless the

pacemaker is exposed to some external source. For example, exposure to a strong electrical source, such as defibrillation, can result in circuit failure. A component failure is, at times, a diagnosis of exclusion, and the specific problem may not be clear until the device has been removed, returned to the manufacturer, and subjected to destructive analysis. In a patient with suspected pacemaker failure (Fig. 10–20), destructive analysis of the device revealed a fracture of the atrial feed-through wire. (Feed-through wires, small wires that can be seen on close inspection of the header of the device, extend from the header to within the pacemaker can.)

Exposing a pacemaker or an ICD to therapeutic radiation may also result in unpredictable component failure and a "runaway" or "sudden no output" response. A pacemaker in or very near the field of therapeutic radiation should be moved to avoid damage to the circuitry and to prevent compromise of the field as defined by the radiation oncologist. This situation is most common in a female patient with a malignant tumor of the breast on the same side as the pacemaker or ICD. The simplest and least invasive approach is to explant the device, form a new pocket on the contralateral side, and tunnel the leads subcutaneously to the other side. If

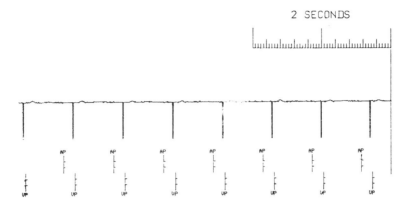

Fig. 10–20. Surface electrocardiogram and diagnostic interpretation markers from an older pacemaker, one of the first to have telemetric capabilities. The surface tracing demonstrates ventricular pacing only, but the marker channel shows atrioventricular sequential pacing. When no reason was found to explain failure to output on the atrial channel, the pacemaker was explanted. Destructive analysis of the device demonstrated a "make-or-break" fracture of the atrial feed-through wire. The pacemaker was indeed expending an atrial output, but fracture of this small wire prevented its conduction via the lead. AP, atrial pacing; VP, ventricular pacing.

the leads are not long enough to reach, "lead extenders" can be connected to span the additional distance (Fig. 10–21).

Lead Fracture and Insulation Defect

Lead malfunction due to fracture or insulation defect is most commonly seen in the late postimplantation period. Lead fracture, common in the early years of cardiac pacing, has become less common as conductor technology has evolved (Fig. 10–22). Lead fractures most often occur adjacent to the pulse generator or near the site of venous access, that is, at a stress point, although fracture has also been reported of more distal portions of the pacing lead. Although uncommon, direct trauma may result in damage to the pacing lead. When lead fracture does occur, it is usually necessary to replace the lead. If the fracture is in a bipolar lead and the pacemaker is polarity programmable, it may be possible to restore pacing by reprogramming to the unipolar configuration. This is a short-term solution and should not be a substitute for replacing the lead (Fig. 10–23).

Polyurethane and silicone are used as insulating materials for most permanent pacing leads. In the early 1980s, concern arose about the long-term performance of the polyurethane lead because of the early failure of several specific polyurethane leads. In these leads, difficulties in manufacturing were identified that apparently were limited to those leads and not indicative of overall polyurethane experience. Insulation defects in polyurethane leads have also been described at stress points; with crush injury, specifically at the costoclavicular space after placement by the subclavian puncture technique (Fig. 10–24); and at the site of ligatures, even with a suture sleeve. In bipolar coaxial leads, the insulation defect often occurs internally, in the layer of insulation between coils, rather than externally, on the outer surface.

Exit Block

Exit block has been defined in several ways. The most commonly accepted clinical definition is high pacing thresholds, often progressive, that cannot be

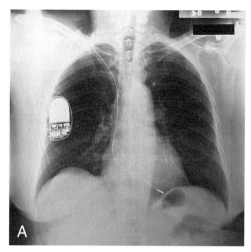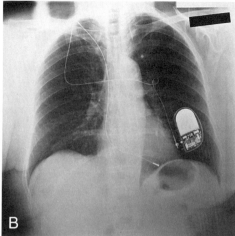

Fig. 10–21. Posteroanterior chest radiographs of a VVIR pacing system. *A,* The pacemaker is located in the right prepectoral position. *B,* The pacemaker is now located on the left, and the previous wire has been tunneled subcutaneously across the chest. This relocation removed the pacemaker from the field for therapeutic radiation.

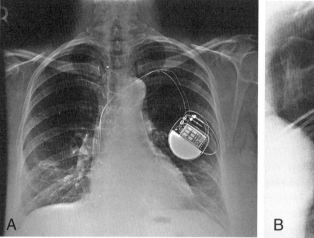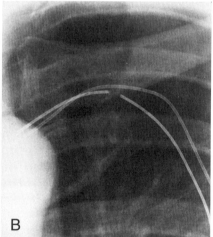

Fig. 10–22. Posteroanterior chest radiograph (*A*) and close-up view (*B*) of a fractured atrial lead. What appears to be complete fracture of the conductor coil was accompanied by failure to pace in the atrium. Atrial sensing, however, remained intact. The most likely explanation is that intact insulation and a fluid column between the fractured ends of the conductor coil allowed maintenance of sensing function.

explained by radiographic dislodgment or perforation. (If normal thresholds are achieved and maintained after repositioning of the lead, the term "exit block" does not apply.) In true exit block, stimulation thresholds are often excellent at the time of implantation but instead of the usual early rise at 3 to 6 weeks with a subsequent decrease and plateau, the threshold remains high. Exit block is uncommon and appears to represent an abnormality at the myocardial tissue-electrode interface. The cause is controversial. Some believe that the problem is with the lead de-

Bipolar

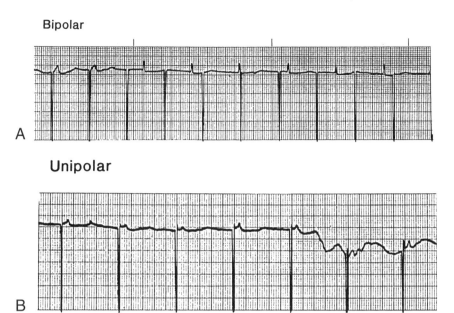

A

Unipolar

B

Fig. 10–23. *A,* Transtelephonically obtained tracing from a patient with a VVI pacemaker in a bipolar pacing and sensing configuration. This magnet tracing reveals capture for the first two beats followed by failure to capture thereafter. *B,* Nonmagnet tracing from the same patient after programming to the unipolar pacing and sensing configuration. There is now consistent ventricular capture.

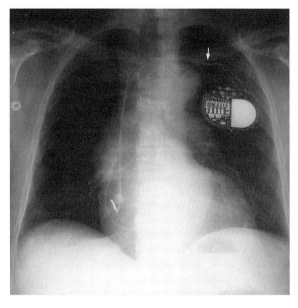

Fig. 10–24. Posteroanterior chest radiograph in a patient with kinking or crushing of the lead as it passes under the clavicle. The patient presented with evidence of lead-insulation failure. Close inspection of the distal tip of the lead identified three poles, and inspection of the connector block of the pulse generator also identified a third port. The third "pole" was required for a special rate-adaptive sensor. (From Hayes.[1] By permission of Mayo Foundation.)

sign, and others believe that it is intrinsic to the patient's myocardium, resulting in excessive reaction to the electrode. Steroid-eluting leads are often effective in preventing exit block.

Failure to Capture and Oversensing

Either failure to capture or significant oversensing could result in bradycardia and recurrent symptoms. The differential diagnosis for both of these abnormalities is relatively extensive. Troubleshooting to determine the cause of failure to capture and oversensing is discussed in Chapter 9.

New Symptoms Secondary to Pacemaker Placement

Extracardiac Stimulation

Extracardiac stimulation usually involves the diaphragm or pectoral muscle. Diaphragmatic stimulation may be due to direct stimulation of the diaphragm (usually stimulation of the left hemidiaphragm) or stimulation of the phrenic nerve (usually stimulation of the right hemidiaphragm). The potential for diaphragmatic stimulation should be tested at the time of implantation. If any stimulation is noted with 10 V, the pacing lead should be repositioned. Because this testing is usually accomplished with the patient in a supine position, it does not eliminate the possibility of diaphragmatic stimulation when the patient is upright. Diaphragmatic stimulation occurring during the early postimplantation period may be due to either microdislodgment or macrodislodgment of the pacing lead. (Although perforation of the myocardium by the pacing lead may result in extracardiac stimulation, perforation occurs uncommonly.) Stimulation may be diminished or alleviated by de-

creasing the voltage output or the pulse width. (An adequate pacing margin of safety must be maintained after the output settings are decreased.) Local muscle stimulation occurs much more commonly with unipolar than with bipolar pacemakers and is usually noted in the early postimplantation period.

Pectoral muscle stimulation may also be due to an insulation defect of the pacing lead, current leakage from the connector or sealing plugs, erosion of the pacemaker's protective coating, or rapid high-amplitude atrial output in a unipolar dual-chamber pacemaker. If the problem is due to an insulation defect on either a unipolar pacemaker or the pacemaker lead, decreasing the voltage output or the pulse width (or both) may minimize the stimulation, but the defective portion of the system may have to be replaced. (If an activity-sensing rate-adaptive pacemaker is in place, muscle stimulation may result in sensor activation and inappropriately rapid pacing rates for a given level of activity.) Pectoral muscle stimulation is less common with bipolar than with unipolar pacemakers. If pectoral muscle stimulation occurs in a polarity-programmable pacemaker that is programmed to be unipolar, reprogramming to the bipolar configuration may alleviate the problem.

If pectoral muscle stimulation occurs in the late postimplantation period in a patient with a unipolar pacing system, erosion of the pacemaker's protective coating should be suspected (Fig. 10–25). Unipolar pulse generators are insulated on one side, generally that opposite to the side engraved with the pulse generator identification. The insulated side should be placed toward muscle and the noninsulated side toward the subcutaneous tissue. The integrity of the insulation material can be compromised by damage during handling or, it seems, deterioration with time.

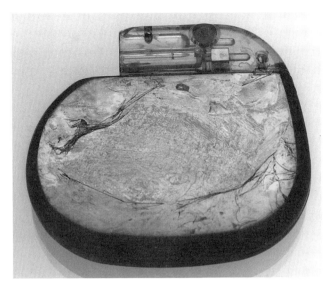

Fig. 10–25. Deterioration of the insulating cover of a unipolar pacing device. Pectoral muscle stimulation developed when the insulating material was no longer intact. (From Hayes DL: Pacemaker complications. *In* A Practice of Cardiac Pacing. Second revised and enlarged edition. Edited by S Furman, DL Hayes, DR Holmes Jr. Mount Kisco, NY, Futura Publishing Company, 1989, pp 485–507. By permission of Mayo Foundation.)

Endless-Loop, or Pacemaker-Mediated, Tachycardia

Endless-loop tachycardia is a well-recognized pacemaker-related rhythm disturbance.[10,11] In any pacemaker capable of P-synchronous pacing, endless-loop tachycardia, also called "pacemaker reentrant tachycardia" or "pacemaker-mediated tachycardia," may result. If AV synchrony is dissociated by any event, most commonly a premature ventricular contraction, retrograde ventriculoatrial conduction may result in a retrograde P wave. If the retrograde P wave is sensed by the atrial sensing circuit of the pacemaker, the AV interval is initiated, resulting in a paced ventricular complex at a cycle length approximately equal to the maximum tracking rate. The paced ventricular event may again result in retrograde ventriculoatrial conduction, perpetuating this rapid reentrant circuit (Fig. 10–26). Endless-loop tachycardia can be prevented by a postventricular atrial refractory period that is long enough to prevent sensing of the retrograde P wave. Most pacemakers also have specific algorithms that attempt to recognize and abort endless-loop tachycardia.

Pacemaker Syndrome

Adverse hemodynamics associated with a normally functioning pacing system that cause overt symptoms or limit the patient's ability to achieve optimal functional status are referred to as "pacemaker syndrome." Pacemaker syndrome was initially recognized with ventricular (VVI) pacing but may occur with any pacing mode if there is AV dissociation. The incidence of pacemaker syndrome is difficult to determine and depends on how the syndrome is defined. If the definition is confined to clinical limitations during any pacing mode that results in AV dissociation, the incidence is proba-

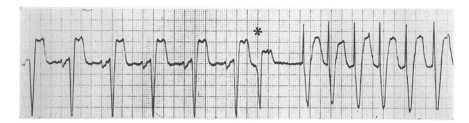

Fig. 10–26. Resting electrocardiographic tracing of pacemaker-mediated, or endless-loop, tachycardia from a patient with a pacemaker programmed to the VDD mode. A premature ventricular contraction (*) occurs and dissociates atrioventricular synchrony. The pacemaker escapes with ventricular pacing, retrograde ventriculoatrial conduction occurs, the retrograde P wave is sensed, initiating the atrioventricular interval, and ventricular pacing occurs at the programmed maximum tracking rate of 125 bpm; this cycle persists.

bly 7% to 10% in patients with VVI pacing.[12] In a study of patients with DDD pacemakers who were randomized to the DDD or VVI pacing mode, some degree of pacemaker syndrome was thought to be present in 83%.[13] The most common symptoms reported were shortness of breath, dizziness, fatigue, pulsations in the neck or abdomen, cough, and apprehension. In addition to these symptoms, a decrease in blood pressure with ventricular pacing but not with normal sinus rhythm or dual-chamber pacing suggests hemodynamic compromise (Fig. 10–27).

Battery Depletion

Battery depletion is expected, because the power supply of a pulse generator is consumable, and should not be considered a complication in most patients. If the pulse generator displays end-of-life characteristics much earlier than expected, other potential problems should be explored. Early battery depletion may be due to inappropriate programming at unnecessarily high output or to excess current drain caused by a loss of lead integrity. The manufacturer should also be

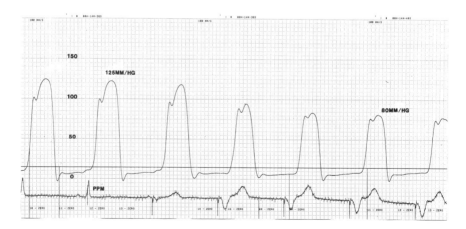

Fig. 10–27. Arterial pressure tracing with simultaneous surface electrocardiogram from a patient who underwent coronary angiography for chest pain. Initially, the systolic pressure is approximately 125 mm Hg and corresponds to intrinsic QRS complexes. The second QRS complex is a pseudofusion beat and the third a fusion complex. As paced ventricular depolarizations occur, the systolic pressure decreases to approximately 80 mm Hg. This hemodynamic compromise with loss of atrioventricular synchrony is compatible with pacemaker syndrome.

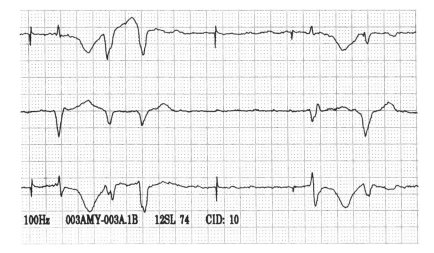

Fig. 10–28. Electrocardiographic tracing from a patient with a 10-year-old pacemaker and intermittent failure to capture. The pacemaker was nearing total battery depletion and was generating insufficient voltage to maintain capture at all times.

consulted for data on performance of the pulse generator, that is, pulse generator longevity predicted or observed in other patients.

If battery depletion is very advanced, it may not be possible to program the pacemaker. At other times, attempting to program a pacemaker at an advanced stage of battery depletion may result in sudden complete loss of output (Fig. 10–28).

Lead Extraction

Extraction of pacing and ICD leads is included here but could as easily have been in the chapter on device implantation. Pacemaker lead extraction has been performed, by necessity, for many years but in rather limited numbers. This procedure has received increased attention in recent years because of advances in extraction techniques[14,15] and recall of the Accufix atrial J lead (Telectronics Pacing Systems, Inc., Englewood, CO). The procedure is not without significant potential risks, including death, and should not be undertaken lightly or without a

thorough understanding of the technique and possible difficulties. Several aspects of lead extraction have yet to be clearly defined. Specifically, what are the absolute indications for lead extraction, including the Accufix lead, should there be training requirements for performing lead extractions, and is there a preferred technique for lead extraction?

Indications for Lead Extraction

Although some controversy exists about indications for lead extractions, absolute indications can be categorized as class 1, conditions for which there is general agreement that leads should be removed. In class 2 are conditions for which leads are often removed but for which opinion differs somewhat on whether the benefit outweighs the risk of removal. Class 3 comprises conditions for which there is general agreement that removal of leads is unnecessary. The following classification is taken from the North American Society of Pacing and Electrophysiology (NASPE) Policy Statement on Recommendations for Extraction of

Chronically Implanted Transvenous Pacing and Defibrillator Leads.[8]

Class 1

- Sepsis (including endocarditis) as a result of documented infection of any intravascular part of the pacing system or as a result of a pacemaker pocket infection when the intravascular portion of the lead system cannot be aseptically separated from the pocket.
- Life-threatening arrhythmias secondary to a retained lead fragment.
- A retained lead, lead fragment, or extraction hardware that poses an immediate or imminent physical threat to the patient, for example, Accufix atrial J.
- Clinically significant thromboembolic events caused by a retained lead or lead fragment.
- Obliteration or occlusion of all usable veins, with the need to implant a new transvenous pacing system.
- A lead that interferes with the operation of another implanted device (e.g., pacemaker or ICD).

Class 2

- Localized pocket infection, erosion, or chronic draining sinus that does not involve the transvenous portion of the lead system, if the lead can be cut through a clean incision that is totally separate from the infected area.*
- An occult infection for which no source can be found and for which the pacing system is suspected.

- Chronic pain at the pocket or lead insertion site that causes significant discomfort for the patient, that cannot be managed by medical or surgical technique without lead removal, and for which there is no acceptable alternative means of relief.
- A lead that, due to its design or its failure, may pose a threat to the patient that is not immediate or imminent if left in place.
- A lead that interferes with the treatment of a malignant lesion.
- A traumatic injury to the entry site of the lead that cannot be reconstructed without interference from the lead.
- Leads preventing access to the venous circulation for newly required implantable devices.
- Nonfunctional leads in a young patient.

Class 3

- Any situation in which the risk posed by removal of the lead is significantly higher than the benefit of removing the lead.
- A single lead in a vessel that has become nonfunctional in an older patient.
- A normally functioning lead that has a reliable performance history at the time of pulse generator replacement.

If the lead can potentially harm the patient, extraction should be considered. Infection and mechanical complications of retained leads have been the obvious lead complications with the potential to harm the patient. The more recent recall of the Telectronics Accufix atrial J lead is in this category.[16] Of the multiple lead advisories issued in the past decade, most have been for leads with unacceptably high failure rates due to insulation problems. Although these failed leads

---

*The lead can be cut and the clean incision closed. Then, the infected area can be opened, the clean distal portion of the lead pulled into the infected area, and that portion removed. This allows total separation of the retained lead fragment from the infected area.

may have required abandonment and implantation of a new lead, extraction of the defective lead was usually not necessary. The recall of the Accufix atrial J lead differs significantly because simply abandoning the lead and placing a new atrial lead does not protect the patient.[16] The Accufix lead incorporates a small wire to retain the J shape of the atrial lead. The wire has been shown to have the potential to fracture. If the wire breaks and extrudes through the insulation, it can lacerate the aorta or perforate the atrial myocardium, injuries leading to fatal bleeding or cardiac tamponade. With deaths and other near-catastrophic events documented as a result of this mechanism, a lead recall was issued. The recall and the reason it was issued resulted in the extraction of many Accufix leads.

Subsequently, there have been multiple anecdotal reports of deaths due to the extraction attempt. How, then, does one decide when to extract this lead? This has been the subject of significant controversy, and no consensus has been reached. The decision to extract or not to extract must be made individually. Fluoroscopic techniques have been shown to be reliable in detecting fracture of a retention wire.[16] Patients with fluoroscopically normal leads can be managed by serial fluoroscopic examinations and counseling. If the wire is fractured but has not extruded through the lead insulation, serial fluoroscopy also appears appropriate. If the wire is fractured and extruded, the potential risks and benefits of lead extraction should be discussed thoroughly with the patient and a clinical decision made. Before any extraction is attempted, whether it is the Accufix or any other lead, the procedure, including all potential complications, must be explained in detail to the patient.

The indications for lead extraction listed above are meant to be used as a guideline. Each patient's situation must be individualized, and the procedure and potential complications should be discussed in detail with the patient. The NASPE policy statement lists the following clinical factors that should be taken into consideration:

- Patient's age
- Patient's sex (published complication rates are higher in females)
- Patient's overall health, both physical and mental
- Calcification involving the lead or leads
- Vegetations in the heart
- Number of leads in the intravascular space
- Length of time the lead or leads have been in place
- Fragility, condition, and physical characteristics of the lead
- Experience of the physician
- Patient's preference, that is, extraction or not

Facility Requirements for Lead Extraction

Lead extraction should generally not be considered if the necessary equipment is not available, the patient is not a candidate for emergency thoracotomy should a complication require surgery, or there is known anomalous placement of the lead or leads through structures other than the normal venous and right-sided cardiac chambers (for example, the leads are in an arterial position, left-sided cardiac chambers, pericardial space).

Who should perform extraction once the decision has been made to extract a lead? The extraction registry data[17] clearly show that with less experienced operators, the chance of a successful outcome is lower, the incidence of complications is higher, and the procedure time is longer. What qualifications are necessary for performance of lead extraction? Although guidelines are established for pacemaker implantation,[17] they are vague in referring to appropriate training for lead extraction.

They state that it is preferable to have exposure to lead extraction techniques, and if a trainee cannot learn such techniques during the training period and wants to perform the procedure at a later date, that experience should be sought with someone expert in extraction.

Ideally, lead extraction procedures require specialized training in a center that frequently performs extraction. As noted above, stringent guidelines for training requirements for pacemaker implantation are in place but similar guidelines for lead extraction are less precise. More rigorous guidelines for training requirements in lead extraction are needed. The current NASPE policy statement[8] recommends that physicians being trained in lead extraction perform a minimum of 20 lead extractions as the primary operator under the direct supervision of a qualified training physician. The supervising physician, that is, the one doing the training, should have performed more than 100 lead extractions with an efficacy safety record consistent with published data.

Complications of Lead Extraction

On the basis of data from the Cook Lead Extraction Registry, we tell patients that the risk of potentially life-threatening complications is 2.1% and the risk of death is 0.6%.[18] These numbers are based on extraction data gathered before the advent of laser-assisted extraction. Potential complications as outlined in the NASPE policy statement are as follows:

Major

- Death
- Cardiac avulsion or tear requiring thoracotomy, pericardiocentesis, chest tube, or surgical repair
- Vascular tear requiring thoracotomy, pericardiocentesis, chest tube, or surgical repair

- Hemothorax or severe bleeding from any source requiring transfusion
- Pneumothorax requiring chest tube drainage
- Pulmonary embolism requiring thrombectomy or surgical intervention
- Respiratory arrest
- Septic shock
- Cerebrovascular accident

Minor

- Pericardial effusion not requiring pericardiocentesis or surgical intervention
- Hemodynamically significant air embolism
- Pulmonary embolism not requiring intervention
- Vascular repair near the implantation site or venous entry site
- Arrhythmia requiring cardioversion

Facility requirements have also been outlined by the NASPE document.[8] These include

- An accredited cardiac surgery program on site
- An accredited cardiac catheterization program
- At least one physician who is properly trained and proficient in the technique of transvenous lead extraction
- Cardiothoracic surgeon on site and capable of initiating an emergency procedure within 5 minutes
- Anesthesiologist with working anesthesia equipment
- A full set of basic instruments for lead extraction
- High-quality fluoroscopy
- Transthoracic ultrasound and transesophageal ultrasound capability immediately available
- Physiologic data acquisition equipment for arterial pressure monitoring and oxygen saturation monitoring

- Pericardiocentesis tray in the procedure room
- Thoracotomy tray in the procedure room
- Temporary pacing and defibrillation-cardioversion equipment in the procedure room
- Fluids, pressors, and other emergency medication available in the procedure room

Extraction Techniques

Of the several approaches to lead extraction that have been described, is there a preferred approach? Multiple techniques can be used, including simple traction, locking stylet and telescoping sheaths with countertraction, an inferior approach with various catheter techniques to snare the lead,[19] laser-assisted extraction,[20] and open surgical techniques. Individual operators have definite biases about technique, for example, superior approach with locking stylet with or without telescoping sheaths, femoral approach

with snare technique, or Dotter retriever technique.[19–21] So long as the operator has a thorough understanding of the equipment and options at his or her disposal, the approach should be defined by comfort level and expertise.

Before any attempt at extraction, the lead must be freed from underlying tissue in the pocket, and any sleeve around the lead securing it to underlying tissue must be released. A stylet should be placed in the lead before any traction is applied. Traction should be gentle. Fluoroscopic observation may indicate the extent of fibrosis holding the lead to the underlying vascular structures. Figure 10–29 shows how fibrous tissue surrounds the lead. Fibrosis may occur in specific areas or along the entire course of the lead.

As traction is applied (Fig. 10–30), the electrocardiogram should be monitored for ectopy, and the patient's blood pressure should also be observed for any hypotension. Even if gentle traction is not initially successful, continued steady traction for several minutes may be successful.

If traction fails, our next approach is to transect the lead just beyond the con-

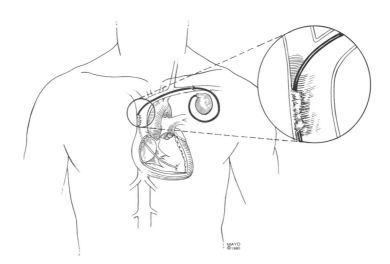

Fig. 10–29. Drawing of a chronically implanted pacing lead. The enlarged inset depicts fibrosis that occurs around the lead where it abuts the superior vena cava. Fibrosis may be minimal or extend throughout the entire course of the lead. (From Spittell and Hayes.[6] By permission of Mayo Foundation.)

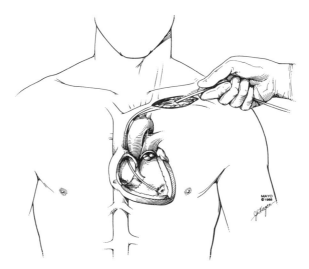

Fig. 10–30. After the lead has been freed from the underlying tissue, a stylet is placed in the lead and gentle traction is applied while the electrocardiogram and blood pressure are monitored. (By permission of Mayo Foundation.)

nector pin and nonisodiametric portion of the lead, trying to leave as much as possible with which to work. A locking stylet is placed (Fig. 10–31). There are now several varieties of locking stylets. Ideally, the locking stylet can be locked and unlocked if necessary. Traction can again be attempted with the locking stylet in place. If this is not successful, ei-

ther countertraction techniques or laser extraction can be attempted. We tend to proceed straight to laser extraction. Quite appropriately, however, others experienced in lead extraction prefer to place a countertraction sheath and attempt to pass this along the lead without laser. If successful, this is a more economical approach to extraction.

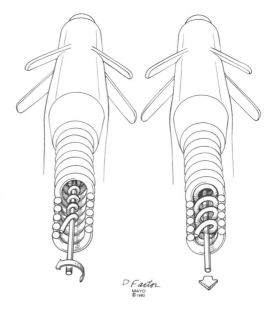

Fig. 10–31. The locking stylet functions by some mechanism that results in the stylet being caught or entwined in the inner electrode coil. In the original Cook locking stylet, after the lead was sized and the appropriately sized locking stylet chosen, the stylet was advanced as far as possible, ideally the length of the lead, and counterclockwise turning of the stylet "locked" it into place (*left panel*). Traction could then be applied (*right panel*). (From Furman S: Troubleshooting. *In* A Practice of Cardiac Pacing. Third edition. Edited by S Furman, DL Hayes, DR Holmes Jr. Mount Kisco, NY, Futura Publishing Company, 1993, pp 685–723. By permission of Mayo Foundation.)

Results with the laser extraction technique have been excellent, and we believe that in experienced hands it can significantly decrease the time required for lead extraction. Laser extraction is not without potential morbidity and mortality and requires adequate training and a careful approach, the same as any other extraction technique.[20] Laser-assisted lead extraction has been the subject of a multicenter study, the Pacing Lead Extraction with the Excimer Laser System (PLEXES) trial. Randomization of patients to laser-assisted extraction technique or to standard extraction techniques demonstrated efficacy of laser-assisted lead extraction.[20] Lead extraction can also be accomplished in an inferior approach, that is, through the femoral vein. A variety of traction and snare techniques can be applied after vascular access is achieved. After placement of a relatively large sheath—16 French, or so-called workstation—a Dotter retriever, pigtail catheters, various sizes of snares, or other devices can be used to grasp and retract the lead. Figures 10–32, 10–33, and 10–34 demonstrate a technique that uses a pigtail catheter and a Dotter retriever.[19]

Whoever is performing percutaneous lead extraction, cardiologist or surgeon, should not overlook the possibility of surgical removal of the leads.[21] Although most leads can be extracted by a percutaneous technique, some cannot, and thoracotomy or some other limited surgical approach may be the best option for the patient.[22]

The next challenge in lead extraction is the increasing requirement for experience in extraction of defibrillation leads.

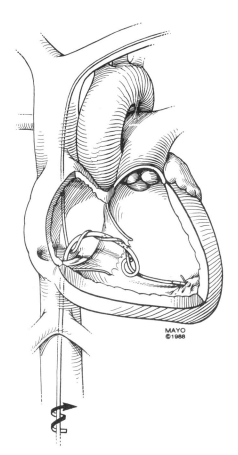

Fig. 10–32. An inferior extraction technique involves placing a pigtail catheter through the femoral vein and advancing it into the right side of the heart. The old lead is "snagged" by the pigtail catheter and the catheter turned clockwise to effectively entwine the pigtail catheter and the permanent pacing lead. (From Furman S: Troubleshooting. *In* A Practice of Cardiac Pacing. Second revised and enlarged edition. Edited by S Furman, DL Hayes, DR Holmes Jr. Mount Kisco, NY, Futura Publishing Company, 1989, pp 611–650. By permission of Mayo Foundation.)

Fig. 10–33. *A,* With the pigtail catheter and the permanent pacing lead firmly entwined, traction is applied on the pigtail catheter in an attempt to free the lead tip from the endocardial surface. *B,* If traction is successful in freeing the tip of the lead, the lead is pulled into the inferior vena cava. The pigtail catheter is rotated in a counterclockwise direction to free it, and it is then removed through the femoral vein. *C,* The pigtail catheter is replaced with a Dotter retriever. (Alternatively, other snares could be used.) The wire basket is extended and under fluoroscopy positioned so that the pacing lead is firmly caught in the Dotter retriever. Traction is then applied to the Dotter retriever in an attempt to extract the whole lead through the femoral vein. The most proximal portion of the pacing system (the lead connector) should be transected prior to extraction. (From Furman S: Troubleshooting. *In* A Practice of Cardiac Pacing. Second revised and enlarged edition. Edited by S Furman, DL Hayes, DR Holmes Jr. Mount Kisco, NY, Futura Publishing Company, 1989, pp 611–650. By permission of Mayo Foundation.)

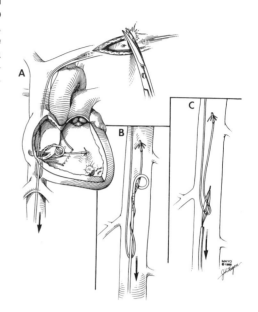

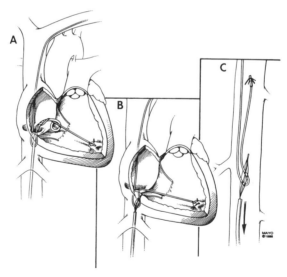

Fig. 10–34. *A,* With the pigtail catheter firmly entwined with the permanent pacing lead, traction is applied, but the lead tip cannot be dislodged from the endocardial surface. Traction is applied on the pigtail catheter and the still attached lead in an effort to position a small loop of the pacing catheter within the inferior vena cava. The pigtail catheter is then rotated in a counterclockwise direction in an effort to separate the catheter from the pacing lead. The pigtail catheter is then removed. *B,* The Dotter retriever is passed into the inferior vena cava. With the Dotter retriever extended, an attempt is made to snare the loop of the pacing lead in the Dotter retriever. Once this is accomplished, the basket portion of the Dotter retriever is retracted, firmly securing a portion of the pacing lead in the retriever. Traction is then applied on the Dotter retriever to free the tip of the pacing lead from the endocardial surface. *C,* If the tip of the pacing lead is successfully dislodged from the endocardial surface, the lead is extracted through the femoral vein. (From Furman S: Troubleshooting. *In* A Practice of Cardiac Pacing. Second revised and enlarged edition. Edited by S Furman, DL Hayes, DR Holmes Jr. Mount Kisco, NY, Futura Publishing Company, 1989, pp 611–650. By permission of Mayo Foundation.)

Endocardial leads that are currently part of ICD systems are, in general, larger in caliber and longer than standard pacing leads. These differences can add difficulty to the extraction procedure.

Extraction techniques will undoubtedly continue to evolve and improve. For now and the foreseeable future, this procedure must be approached with great respect by personnel committed to developing expertise.

References

1. Hayes DL: Pacemaker complications. *In* A Practice of Cardiac Pacing. Third edition. Edited by S Furman, DL Hayes, DR Holmes Jr. Mount Kisco, NY, Futura Publishing Company, 1993, pp 537–569

2. Link MS, Estes NA III, Griffin JJ, Wang PJ, Maloney JD, Kirchhoffer JB, Mitchell GF, Orav J, Goldman L, Lamas GA: Complications of dual chamber pacemaker implantation in the elderly. Pacemaker Selection in the Elderly (PASE) Investigators. J Interv Card Electrophysiol 2:175–179, 1998

3. Higano ST, Hayes DL, Spittell PC: Facilitation of the subclavian-introducer technique with contrast venography. Pacing Clin Electrophysiol 13:681–684, 1990

4. Irwin M, Harris L, Cameron D, Glynn MFX, Mycyk T, Kennedy C, Goldman B: Topical cryoprecipitate in the anticoagulated patient undergoing pacing system implantation (abstract). Pacing Clin Electrophysiol 12:642, 1989

5. Ghani M, Thakur RK, Boughner D, Morillo CA, Yee R, Klein GJ: Malposition of transvenous pacing lead in the left ventricle. Pacing Clin Electrophysiol 16:1800–1807, 1993

6. Spittell PC, Hayes DL: Venous complications after insertion of a transvenous pacemaker. Mayo Clin Proc 67:258–265, 1992

7. Spittell PC, Vlietstra RE, Hayes DL, Higano ST: Venous obstruction due to permanent transvenous pacemaker electrodes: treatment with percutaneous transluminal balloon venoplasty. Pacing Clin Electrophysiol 13:271–274, 1990

8. North American Society of Pacing and Electrophysiology Lead Extraction Conference Faculty: Recommendations for extraction of chronically implanted transvenous pacing and defibrillator leads: indications, facilities, training. Pacing Clin Electrophysiol 23:544–551, 2000

9. Furman S, Behrens M, Andrews C, Klementowicz P: Retained pacemaker leads. J Thorac Cardiovasc Surg 94:770–772, 1987

10. Furman S, Fisher JD: Endless loop tachycardia in an AV universal [DDD] pacemaker. Pacing Clin Electrophysiol 5:486–489, 1982

11. Hayes DL: Endless-loop tachycardia: the problem has been solved? *In* New Perspectives in Cardiac Pacing. Edited by SS Barold, J Mugica. Mount Kisco, NY, Futura Publishing Company, 1988, pp 375–386

12. Furman S: Pacemaker syndrome (editorial). Pacing Clin Electrophysiol 17:1–5, 1994

13. Heldman D, Mulvihill D, Nguyen H, Messenger JC, Rylaarsdam A, Evans K, Castellanet MJ: True incidence of pacemaker syndrome. Pacing Clin Electrophysiol 13:1742–1750, 1990

14. Byrd CL, Schwartz SJ, Hedin NB, Goode LB, Fearnot NE, Smith HJ: Intravascular lead extraction using locking stylets and sheaths. Pacing Clin Electrophysiol 13:1871–1875, 1990

15. Byrd CL, Schwartz SJ, Hedin N: Intravascular techniques for extraction of permanent pacemaker leads. J Thorac Cardiovasc Surg 101:989–997, 1991

16. Lloyd MA, Hayes DL, Holmes DR Jr: Atrial "J" pacing lead retention wire fracture: radiographic assessment, incidence of fracture, and clinical management. Pacing Clin Electrophysiol 18:958–964, 1995

17. Hayes DL, Naccarelli GV, Furman S, Parsonnet V: Report of the NASPE Policy Conference training requirements for permanent pacemaker selection, implantation, and follow-up. North American Society of Pacing and Electrophysiology. Pacing Clin Electrophysiol 17:6–12, 1994

18. Smith HJ, Fearnot NE, Byrd CL, Wilkoff BL, Love CJ, Sellers TD: Five-years experience with intravascular lead extraction. U.S. Lead Extraction Database. Pacing Clin Electrophysiol 17:2016–2020, 1994

19. Espinosa RE, Hayes DL, Vlietstra RE, Osborn MJ, McGoon MD: The Dotter retriever and pigtail catheter: efficacy in extraction of chronic transvenous pacemaker leads. Pacing Clin Electrophysiol 16:2337–2342, 1993

20. Wilkoff BL, Byrd CL, Love CJ, Hayes DL, Sellers TD, Schaerf R, Parsonnet V, Epstein LM, Sorrentino RA, Reiser C: Pacemaker lead extraction with the laser

sheath: results of the Pacing Lead Extraction with the Excimer Sheath (PLEXES) trial. J Am Coll Cardiol 33:1671–1676, 1999

21. Colavita PG, Zimmern SH, Gallagher JJ, Fedor JM, Austin WK, Smith HJ: Intravascular extraction of chronic pacemaker leads: efficacy and follow-up. Pacing Clin Electrophysiol 16:2333–2336, 1993

22. Frame R, Brodman RF, Furman S, Andrews CA, Gross JN: Surgical removal of infected transvenous pacemaker leads. Pacing Clin Electrophysiol 16:2343–2348, 1993

11

Pacemaker and ICD Radiography

Margaret A. Lloyd, M.D.,
David L. Hayes, M.D.

The chest radiograph remains an important tool in the preoperative and postoperative evaluation of a pacing or defibrillation system. Additionally, the chest radiograph is essential during assessment of the integrity of a pacing or implantable cardioverter-defibrillator (ICD) system. Both a posteroanterior (PA) view and a lateral view should be obtained. A systematic approach should be used, with various anatomical and device components evaluated in an orderly fashion.[1-3]

Preoperatively, clips, wires, prosthetic valves, and other hardware can provide clues to previous cardiac or thoracic surgery, which may be important in the planning of the operative procedure. After implantation of the pacing or ICD system, both PA and lateral radiographs should be obtained to confirm correct position of the lead or leads and to note potential surgical complications, such as pneumothorax, pleural effusion, and pericardial effusion (Fig. 11–1). A chest radiograph should be obtained as part of any device troubleshooting; assessment includes lead position, lead continuity, and connection of the lead with the connector block (Table 11–1).

It is not uncommon for a patient to have a pacing system, an ICD, and a variety of functional and abandoned leads, both epicardial and transvenous (Fig. 11–2). The type and position of the generator or generators and the type, position, and integrity of all leads should be determined. For some patients, additional abdominal radiographs are required to visualize abdominally implanted devices. Comparison with any previous radiographs is frequently useful.

One systematic approach is to address the radiograph's components in the following order:

1. Bony structures
2. Aorta
3. Cardiac shadow
4. Trachea
5. Diaphragm
6. Lung fields
7. Other (including the pacing and ICD systems)

Pulse Generators

The initial evaluation includes the location of the pacemaker or the ICD,

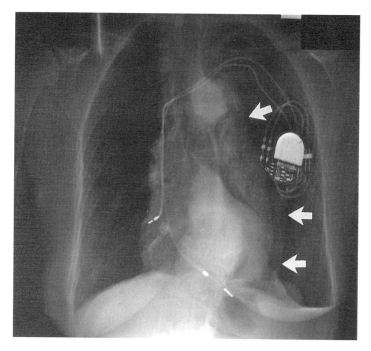

Fig. 11–1. Posteroanterior chest radiograph taken the day after pacemaker implantation. *Arrows* denote a pneumothorax.

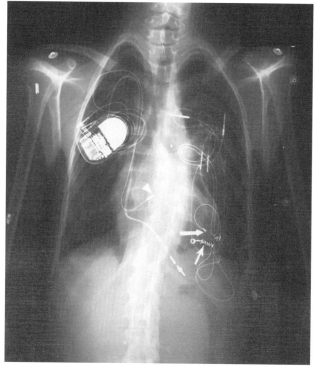

Fig. 11–2. Posteroanterior chest radiograph from a patient with multiple leads. *Arrowhead,* transvenous atrial lead; *largest arrow,* abandoned stab-in ventricular epicardial lead; *midsized arrow,* abandoned screw-in ventricular epicardial lead; *smallest arrow,* transvenous ventricular lead. (From Hayes DL: Pacemaker radiography. *In* A Practice of Cardiac Pacing. Third edition. Edited by S Furman, DL Hayes, DR Holmes Jr. Mount Kisco, NY, Futura Publishing Company, 1993, pp 361–400. By permission of Mayo Foundation.)

Table 11–1.
Systematic Approach to Radiographic Assessment of Pacemakers and
Implantable Cardioverter-Defibrillators

Systematic approach	Clinical considerations
Determine the pulse generator site.	Is there any suggestion of a significant shift from intended position? A displaced generator could be associated with lead dislodgment or twiddler's syndrome.
Determine the pulse generator manufacturer, polarity, and model, if possible.	Radiographic identifiers allow determination of the manufacturer, information that is helpful if the patient comes without the identification card. The polarity of the pulse generator should be determined and compared with the polarity of the leads.
Inspect the connector block.	Is the connector pin (or pins) completely through the connector block? Loose connection could explain intermittent or complete failure to output or intermittent failure to capture.
Consider the venous route used.	This step is especially important if a pacemaker system revision is being considered. Can the same venous route be accessed, and how many leads are already placed in a single vein?
Determine lead polarity.	Does lead polarity match pulse generator polarity, or has some type of adaptor been used to allow combination of the system hardware?
Determine lead position.	Determine where the lead was postioned. For the ventricular lead, is it in the apex, outflow tract, septal position, or coronary sinus? For the atrial lead, is it in the atrial appendage, lateral wall, septal position, or coronary sinus?
Does the lead position appear radiographically acceptable?	Inadequate lead position may explain failure to capture or to sense. Compare current and previous radiographs, if possible. Is ventricular lead redundancy, or "slack," adequate? Is the atrial J adequate?
Inspect the entire length of the lead for integrity, looking for fracture, compression, crimping, and so forth.	Intermittent or complete failure to capture or sense or to output could be secondary to fracture of the lead conductor coil or loss of integrity of the insulation. Attempt to follow each lead along its course, assessing the conductor coil. In addition, inspect for any crimping of the lead as it passes under the clavicle.
Is there any other chest x-ray abnormality that is potentially related?	For a recent implantation, be certain there is no pneumothorax or hemopneumothorax. For the patient with an implantable cardioverter-defribrillator who has a change in defibrillation thresholds, whether acute or chronic, remember that a pneumothorax can alter these thresholds.
If no abnormality is appreciated radiographically but there is a clinical abnormality, reassess the chest radiograph in a problem-oriented fashion.	As an example, for intermittent failure to output, the differential diagnosis includes a problem with the connector pin, such as a loose set screw, or conductor coil fracture. Go back once again and inspect these elements of the pacing system.

or both. Most current implantations are prepectoral, and the pulse generator is located in the upper chest, inferior to the clavicle and medial to the axilla. At one time, many implantations in children and many implantations of ICDs were made subpectorally or in a subrectus position in the abdominal wall; radiographic evaluation requires an anteroposterior radiograph of the abdomen as well as PA and lateral chest radiographs. Other potential implantation sites are the retromammary and subpectoralis positions for a better cosmetic result. However, given the very small pacemakers available today, such surgical approaches are rarely necessary.[4] Subpectoral placement of an ICD is occasionally necessary in the small adult or pediatric patient. True axillary position has also been used in an effort to obtain a better cosmetic result (Fig. 11–3).

The pulse generator manufacturer and model can usually be identified from the chest radiograph. Specific models may have a unique shape, size, and internal circuitry pattern; at one time, these features were sufficient to identify a manufacturer and model. All current devices have a radiopaque code identifying the manufacturer and model of the device, and all companies publish charts and tables detailing radiographic identification of their devices (Fig. 11–4). After identification of the manufacturer, the technical support division of that manufacturer can identify the device and may be able to provide additional information obtained at the time of implantation and kept on file with the pulse generator registration (e.g., leads used, configurations, thresholds). If a patient has both pacing and ICD systems implanted, the pulse generators and leads may come from different manufacturers, and careful inspection of both are important.

The relationship of redundant, coiled leads to the generator in the pocket should be noted. Usually, redundant leads are coiled under the generator, but they may work their way superficially over time. It

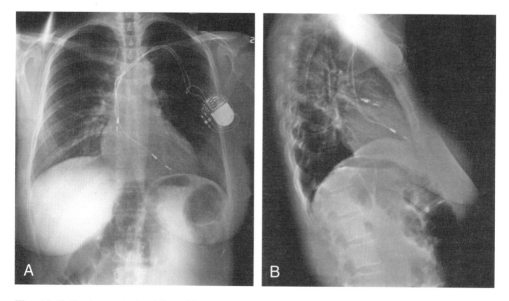

Fig. 11–3. Posteroanterior (A) and lateral (B) radiographs from a patient with chronic pain and arm limitation after pacemaker implantation. An attempt had been made to place the pacemaker in an axillary position for cosmetic reasons.

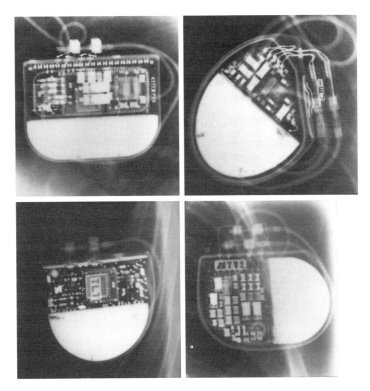

Fig. 11–4. Examples of radiographic identification of the pacemaker by radiographic codes embedded within the device. *Upper left,* A CPI generator is identified by the notation "CPI0925," the actual model number of the generator. *Upper right,* An Intermedics, Inc., pacemaker is identified by "IEJ." *Lower left,* A Telectronics device is identified by "TLT." *Lower right,* A Medtronic generator is identified by the company logo and "TV2," which designates the specific model. (From Hayes DL: Pacemaker radiography. *In* A Practice of Cardiac Pacing. Third edition. Edited by S Furman, DL Hayes, DR Holmes Jr. Mount Kisco, NY, Futura Publishing Company, 1993, pp 361–400. By permission of Mayo Foundation.)

may be difficult to determine which lead is connected to the pulse generator and which lead is abandoned. With careful inspection, differentiation should be possible, but it is also necessary to determine the polarity of the pacing pulse generators. This can be ascertained by the number and type of connector pins (unipolar, coaxial bipolar, bifurcated bipolar) (Fig. 11–5 and 11–6). Most current devices have independently programmable polarity, so that bipolar leads do not necessarily imply bipolar function.

Migration of a pulse generator is uncommon with the smaller devices used today. However, comparison of previous and current radiographs for pulse genera-

tor position is useful. The clinical concern about pulse generator migration is that tension may be placed on the lead, possibly causing dislodgment or fracture. It is not possible to determine from a radiograph whether the patient is a "twiddler," but without significant migration of a device, a twisted appearance of the lead suggests twiddler's syndrome[5] (Fig. 11–7).

The generator connector block should also be inspected. The lead connector pin should be advanced beyond the set screw or screws in the connector block, and the screws should be in direct contact with the pin. One cause of intermittent pacing failure is a loose connection between the set screws and the connector pin (Fig. 11–8).

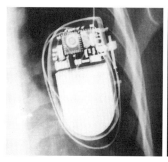
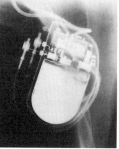
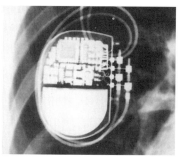

Fig. 11–5. Examples of three different pulse generator polarity configurations. *Left,* A single connector pin identifies this as a unipolar device. *Middle,* The two connector pins could indicate a unipolar dual-chamber pacemaker or an older single-chamber pacemaker that accepts a bifurcated bipolar lead. *Right,* Two leads with two pins, each representing a bipolar in-line lead; therefore, the device is a dual-chamber bipolar generator. (From Hayes DL: Pacemaker radiography. *In* A Practice of Cardiac Pacing. Edited by S Furman, DL Hayes, DR Holmes Jr. Mount Kisco, NY, Futura Publishing Company, 1986, pp 333–378. By permission of the publisher.)

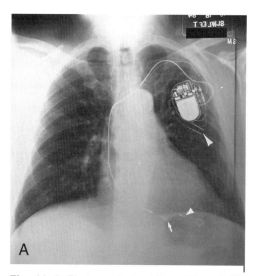
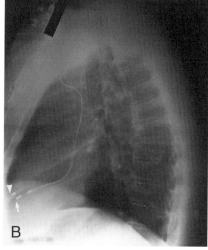
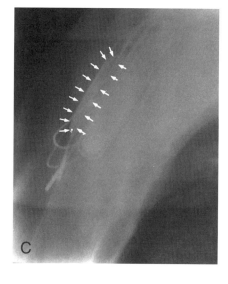

Fig. 11–6. Posteroanterior (*A*) and lateral (*B*) chest radiographs showing two leads in the ventricle, a single-chamber bifurcated lead and an abandoned ventricular lead. The abandoned ends of the lead can be seen to the side of the pulse generator (*large arrowhead*). One of the leads is bipolar (*arrow*), and one is unipolar (*small arrowhead*). The bipolar lead is abandoned, and the unipolar lead is connected to a bifurcated single-chamber pacemaker. *C,* On a close-up view of the lateral projection, an object highlighted by *arrows* is shown parallel to the pacemaker. To allow use of a unipolar lead with the bipolar generator, an indifferent electrode has been placed in the positive connector and the unipolar pin in the negative connector of the pacemaker. (From Hayes DL: Pacemaker radiography. *In* A Practice of Cardiac Pacing. Edited by S Furman, DL Hayes, DR Holmes Jr. Mount Kisco, NY, Futura Publishing Company, 1986, pp 333–378. By permission of the publisher.)

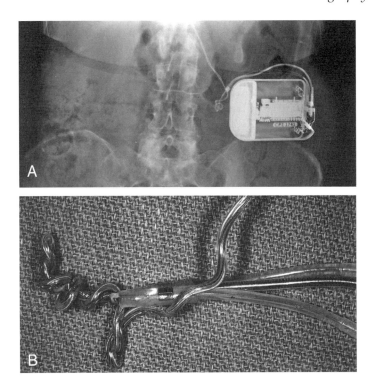

Fig. 11–7. *A,* Abdominal radiograph in a patient with a malfunctioning implantable cardioverter-defibrillator. Inspection of the lead showed tight twisting, which resulted in device malfunction. Twiddler's syndrome was suspected. *B,* The explanted "twisted" lead.

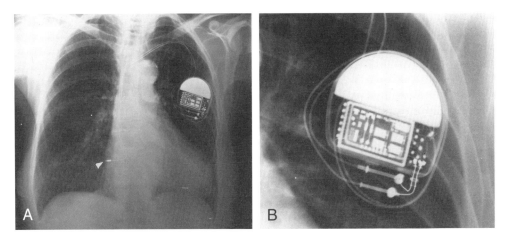

Fig. 11–8. Posteroanterior (*A*) and close-up (*B*) radiographic views from a patient with intermittent failure to pace. The lower of the two unipolar leads is not completely advanced (compare upper and lower pins). This is more evident on the close-up view. By convention, the lower of the two leads in the connector block is the ventricular lead, so that this patient must have presented with intermittent or permanent ventricular failure to output. Incidentally noted (*arrowhead*), the atrial lead has inadequate redundancy (inadequate J). The ventricular lead also lacks adequate redundancy. (From Hayes DL: Pacemaker radiography. *In* A Practice of Cardiac Pacing. Third edition. Edited by S Furman, DL Hayes, DR Holmes Jr. Mount Kisco, NY, Futura Publishing Company, 1993, pp 361–400. By permission of Mayo Foundation.)

Leads

Many, if not most, pacing system malfunctions are due to lead malfunction. For this reason, lead assessment is a critical component of the radiographic assessment of a pacing or ICD system. Standard radiographic techniques may not clearly demonstrate lead components, and higher radiographic penetration or coning of the radiographic field may be required. Unfortunately, lead-insulating materials are not visualized radiographically, and insulation breech is a frequent cause of lead failure. The number, type, location, and radiographic integrity of all leads should be determined after studying the PA and lateral radiographs. Unlike pulse generators, leads do not have characteristic radiopaque markers to aid in identification; however, much information on the type and functional status of various leads can be obtained by radiographic appearance.

Pacemaker Leads

The vast majority of contemporary pacing leads are placed transvenously, although patients may still have epicardial (myocardial) pacing wires placed after certain types of cardiac surgical repair or because of congenital cardiac anomalies. Intravascular insertion of transvenous leads is usually through either the right or the left subclavian, axillary, or cephalic vein, although the internal or external jugular vein may be used. Clues to the insertion site may be obtained from the chest radiograph by a change in the directional contour of the lead (Fig. 11–9). A more medial insertion site suggests a subclavian approach; a more lateral site suggests a cephalic or axillary approach. Jugular vein insertion sites are usually easily identified by the lead coursing over or under the clavicle (Fig. 11–10).

The radiopaque conductor coil

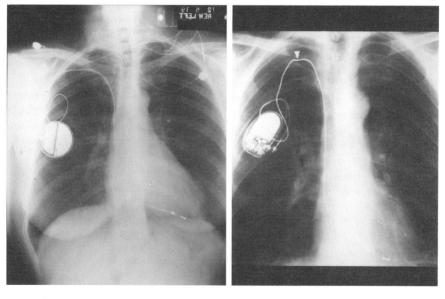

Fig. 11–9. Side-by-side comparison of subclavian and cephalic approaches to lead implantation. See text. (*Arrowhead* notes crimping of the lead as it passes under the clavicle.) (From Hayes DL: Pacemaker radiography. *In* A Practice of Cardiac Pacing. Edited by S Furman, DL Hayes, DR Holmes Jr. Mount Kisco, NY, Futura Publishing Company, 1986, pp 333–378. By permission of the publisher.)

should be inspected in its entirety. There should be no discontinuity of the coil; any kinking or sharp angulation may represent lead fracture. Special attention should be paid to the area between the first rib and the clavicle, as this is a frequent site of lead fracture (subclavian crush syndrome)[6] (Fig. 11–11).

A pseudofracture is shown in Figure 11–12.[7,8] This intact lead shows discontinuity at the point of bifurcation (white arrow). This is not a fracture but rather the normal x-ray appearance of this lead, which simply reflects the two conductors of a bipolar lead coming together.[6] The term "pseudofracture" has also been inappropriately applied to a different circumstance: the indentations caused by ligatures compressing the insulating material of a lead[9] (Fig.11–13).

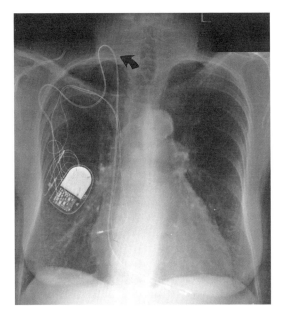

Fig. 11–10. Posteroanterior chest radiograph shows two leads placed in the subclavian vein on the right. The *arrow* denotes a third lead inserted through the right jugular vein.

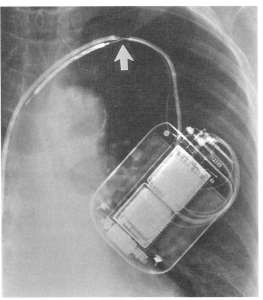

Fig. 11–11. Posteroanterior chest radiograph reveals subclavian crush of the high-voltage defibrillation electrode. The *arrow* marks the point of wire fracture. (From Lloyd MA, Hayes DL: Pacemaker and implantable cardioverter-defibrillator radiography. *In* Clinical Cardiac Pacing and Defibrillation. Second edition. Edited by KA Ellenbogen, GN Kay, BL Wilkoff. Philadelphia, WB Saunders Company, 2000, pp 710–723. By permission of the publisher.)

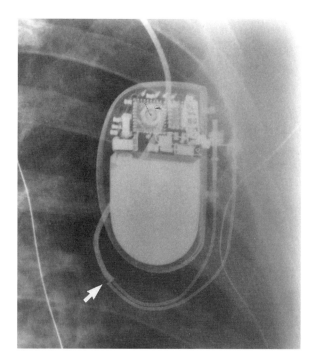

Fig. 11–12. Close-up from a posteroanterior chest radiograph demonstrating a pseudofracture (*arrow*). This radiographic appearance occurs at the point where the two conductor coils come together. (From Hayes DL: Pacemaker radiography. *In* A Practice of Cardiac Pacing. Edited by S Furman, DL Hayes, DR Holmes Jr. Mount Kisco, NY, Futura Publishing Company, 1986, pp 333–378. By permission of the publisher.)

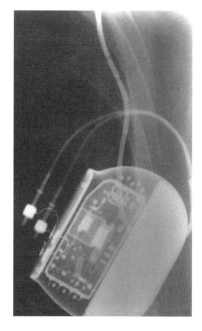

Fig. 11–13. Close-up from a chest radiograph shows an indentation of the insulation material. This is caused by excessive tightening of the ligature around the sleeve. (From Hayes DL: Pacemaker radiography. *In* A Practice of Cardiac Pacing. Second revised and enlarged edition. Edited by S Furman, DL Hayes, DR Holmes Jr. Mount Kisco, NY, Futura Publishing Company, 1989, pp 323–368. By permission of Mayo Foundation.)

Intracardiac Position

For appreciation of abnormal lead position, a detailed description of the normal radiographic appearance is necessary.

Leads should have a modest amount of redundancy and not be too shallow. Undue tension on leads may result in poor pacing thresholds or frank dislodgment from the endocardial surface (Fig. 11–14). In Figure 11–15, placement of both leads is too shallow. The atrial lead is most likely in the right atrial appendage. The atrial lead is not optimally positioned and is best appreciated on the lateral view. The angle of the J is significantly greater than 90°. The ventricular lead is also much too shallow, and this can be appreciated in both views.

Generous lead redundancy is preferred in pediatric patients in an attempt to accommodate subsequent growth and minimize the number of lead revisions during a lifetime of pacing therapy[10] (Fig. 11–16).

The type of lead fixation can often be determined by the chest radiograph (Fig. 11–17). Active fixation leads have a radiopaque screw, which is usually visible radiographically. Passive fixation leads have a variety of tines and fins that cannot be visualized. Unipolar leads have a single electrode (cathode) at the tip, whereas bipolar leads have two electrodes separated by an interelectrode space. Extracardiac location of the lead tip usually signifies cardiac perforation with extracardiac migration of the lead; this circumstance may require other imaging modalities or clinical troubleshooting techniques to verify extracardiac lead position.

Transvenous Atrial Leads

Most atrial leads have a J shape and are placed in the atrial appendage unless it has been surgically amputated. Regardless of whether a preformed J or a straight lead is implanted in the atrium, if implantation is in the right atrial appendage, the J portion of the lead is slightly medial on the PA projection and anterior on the lateral projection. Optimally, the limits of

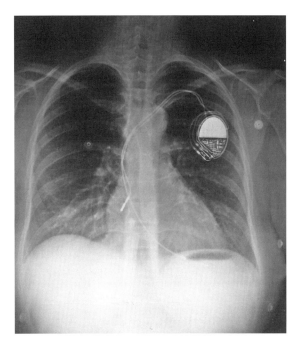

Fig. 11–14. Both the atrial and the ventricular leads shown on this posteroanterior chest radiograph lack adequate redundancy. The patient presented with loss of atrial capture and symptoms of pacemaker syndrome.

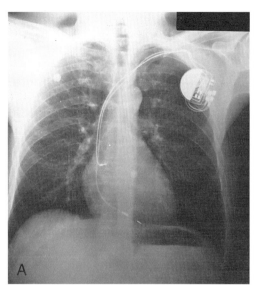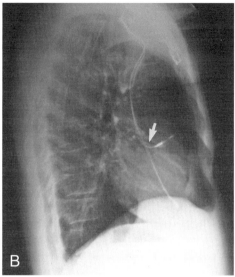

Fig. 11–15. Posteroanterior (*A*) and lateral (*B*) chest radiographs of a dual-chamber pacing system. Both the atrial and the ventricular leads have inadequate redundancy, which may result in poor pacing thresholds or lead dislodgment. (*Arrow* notes the wide angle of the J lead resulting from inadequate redundancy.) (From Hayes DL: Pacemaker radiography. *In* A Practice of Cardiac Pacing. Third edition. Edited by S Furman, DL Hayes, DR Holmes Jr. Mount Kisco, NY, Futura Publishing Company, 1993, pp 361–400. By permission of Mayo Foundation.)

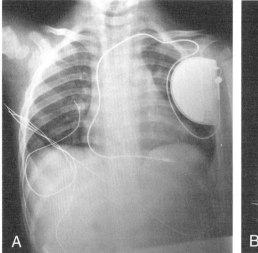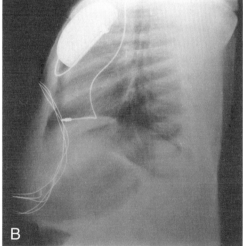

Fig. 11–16. Posteroanterior (*A*) and lateral (*B*) chest radiographs from a pediatric patient with a newly implanted pacemaker. Excessive redundancy has been left on the ventricular lead to allow for future growth.

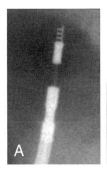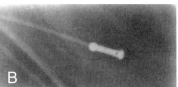

Fig. 11–17. Close-up radiographic appearance of lead tips. *A,* Active fixation bipolar lead. Note the screw mechanism. *B,* Unipolar passive fixation lead. (From Lloyd MA, Hayes DL: Pacemaker and implantable cardioverter-defibrillator radiography. *In* Clinical Cardiac Pacing and Defibrillation. Second edition. Edited by KA Ellenbogen, GN Kay, BL Wilkoff. Philadelphia, WB Saunders Company, 2000, pp 710–723. By permission of the publisher.)

the J should be no greater than approximately 80° apart. Redundancy proximal to the J within the atrium or superior vena cava should not be seen. A large posterior curve suggests placement in the coronary sinus or placement across a patent foramen ovale or atrial septal defect into the left atrium. If the appendage has been surgically truncated, the lead may be placed septally (Fig. 11–17 *A*) or on any portion of the free wall (Fig. 11–17 *B*), wherever mechanical stability and satisfactory thresholds can be obtained. Unlike the appendage, the remainder of the

atrium is not trabeculated, and active fixation leads are usually required to obtain mechanical stability.

Investigational pacing for the prevention of atrial fibrillation may utilize dual-site atrial leads; in this case, one lead is usually placed in the right atrium and the second (usually active fixation) on the posterior septum[11,12] (Fig. 11–18).

Special note should be made of the appearance of the atrial lead if it is one of the Telectronics Pacing Systems leads currently under advisory[13,14] (Fig.11–19). Both the Accufix active fixation atrial

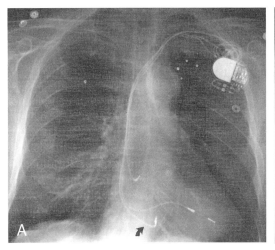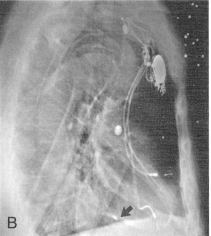

Fig. 11–18. Posteroanterior (*A*) and lateral (*B*) radiographs of dual-site atrial pacing system. The *arrow* denotes the second atrial lead placed on the posterior septum.

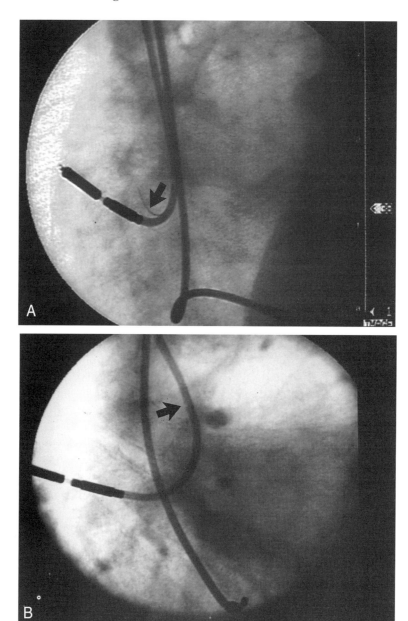

Fig. 11–19. Digital fluoroscopic images of Telectronics (Englewood, CO) atrial leads. *A,* Accufix 330–801 active fixation atrial lead. The *arrow* denotes fractured and protruding retention wire. *B,* The wire fracture of this Accufix lead is not visible, but the breach in the insulation (*arrow*) in the area of the retention wire indicates fracture. *C,* The angulation in the interelectrode area (*arrow*) of an Encor passive fixation lead indicates fracture of the retention wire. *D,* The wire in an Encor lead is fractured and protrudes through the insulation in the interelectrode space (*arrow*). Note the sharp angulation of the lead. *E,* The retention wire in this Encor lead is not visible. The lead is severed in the interelectrode space (*arrow*), indicating de facto fracture of the retention wire. (From Lloyd MA, Hayes DL: Pacemaker and implantable cardioverter-defibrillator radiography. *In* Clinical Cardiac Pacing and Defibrillation. Second edition. Edited by KA Ellenbogen, GN Kay, BL Wilkoff. Philadelphia, WB Saunders Company, 2000, pp 710–723. By permission of the publisher.) *Continues.*

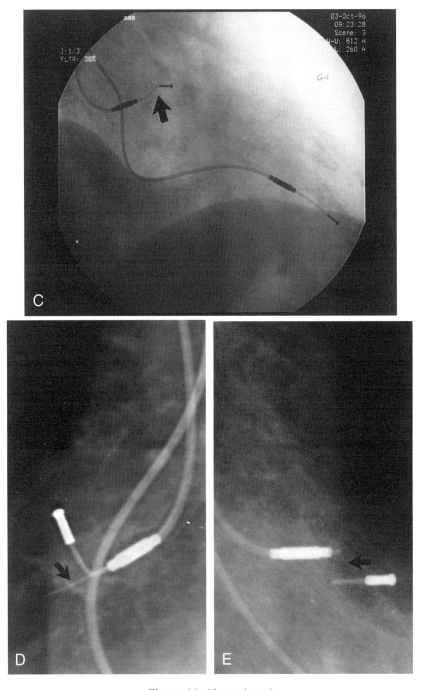

Figure 11–19 *continued.*

lead and the Encor passive fixation atrial lead have retention wires in the distal portion of the lead to maintain the J shape; the retention wire is within the insulation in the Accufix lead and within the coil in the Encor lead. The retention wire may fracture and protrude through the insulation, possibly resulting in cardiac or vascular laceration, or may migrate into extracardiac locations.

The shape of the distal portion of the Accufix lead should be inspected, because some studies have suggested that a wide-open J shape may predispose to fracture. The retention wire itself may be difficult to visualize radiographically, even with significant protrusion or migration of the wire. Multiple views, high penetration, and coned-in views may aid visualization. Digital fluoroscopy has proven to be a more reliable technique for assessing the status of the retention wire.

Fracture of the Encor lead is difficult to detect even by digital fluoroscopy because of the position of the wire within the coil. Fracture and protrusion of the retention wire in these leads commonly occur in the interelectrode space, and this area should be scrutinized for linear angulation or frank fracture and protrusion of the retention wire.

Transvenous Ventricular Leads

Transvenous ventricular leads are traditionally placed in the right ventric-ular apex. Radiographically, the lead should have a gentle contour, with the tip of the lead pointing downward in the PA view and located between the left border of the vertebral column and the cardiac apex. The position of the heart, vertical or relatively more horizontal, largely determines the position of the lead in relation to the cardiac apex and varies among patients. The lateral view is necessary to distinguish an apical position in which the lead tip is anterior and caudally directed, is directed posteriorly in the right ventricle, or is on the posterior surface of the heart, that is, within the coronary sinus. The ventricular lead should have a gentle curve along the lateral wall of the right atrium and cross the tricuspid valve to the ventricular apex (Fig. 11–20). Occasionally, it may be preferable to place the lead on the right ventricular septum or in the outflow tract (Fig. 11–21). These alternative positions are commonly used when adequate thresholds cannot be obtained at the apex or when a separate pace-sense lead is used in combination with an ICD

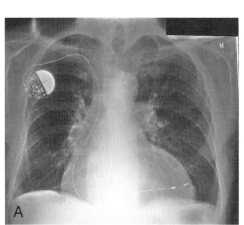
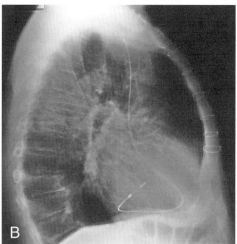

Fig. 11–20. *A,* In a posteroanterior chest radiograph of a VVI pacing system, the ventricular lead appears to be in the right ventricle. *B,* In a lateral chest radiograph from the same patient, the ventricular lead clearly traverses the coronary sinus, and the tip is in a coronary vein. (From Lloyd MA, Hayes DL: Pacemaker and implantable cardioverter-defibrillator radiography. *In* Clinical Cardiac Pacing and Defibrillation. Second edition. Edited by KA Ellenbogen, GN Kay, BL Wilkoff. Philadelphia, WB Saunders Company, 2000, pp 710–723. By permission of the publisher.)

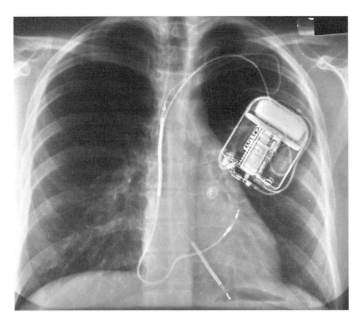

Fig. 11–21. In a posteroanterior chest radiograph of an implantable cardioverter-defibrillator system, a high-voltage lead is in the right ventricle and a separate pace-sense lead is high in the right ventricular outflow tract. Sensing thresholds were inadequate elsewhere in the right ventricle.

lead. Ventricular leads are secured by previously mentioned fixation techniques.

Undesirable positions for the ventricular lead are in the left ventricular cavity, that is, through perforation of the ventricular septum, the lead having inadvertently crossed a patent foramen ovale, atrial septal defect, or ventricular septal defect during transvenous placement, and in the pericardial space as a result of perforation (Fig. 11–22). If it is recognized at once that a lead has inadvertently been placed in the left atrium or left ventricle, the lead should be withdrawn and repositioned in the right side of the heart.

Lead dislodgment is a common cause of failure to pace or sense. Dislodgment may be obvious, that is, macrodislodgment. Such dislodgment can be anywhere other than the original position, that is, the pulmonary artery, coronary sinus, ventricular cavity, or superior or inferior vena cava. Dislodgment may not be identifiable radiographically. This has been labeled "microdislodgment," but without x-ray documentation, there is no evidence that it exists. The diagnosis, therefore, is presumptive. A "macrodislodged" atrial lead is shown in Figure 11–23. The atrial lead is difficult to appreciate on the PA view, but on the lateral view, dislodgment is obvious.

In Figure 11–24, a large loop is seen in the ventricular lead. The patient's thresholds were excellent, and no problems had been encountered. Even though the positioning is suboptimal, if function is normal, no intervention is necessary. By comparison, the lateral chest radiograph in Figure 11–25 was taken the day after pacemaker implantation. The large loop in the ventricular lead was not appreciated at the time of implantation. Pacing thresholds were found to be elevated, and the lead was repositioned.

It is often helpful to compare chest radiographs to confirm lead dislodgment. In Figure 11–26, PA chest radiographs from two consecutive days demonstrate a change in ventricular lead position.

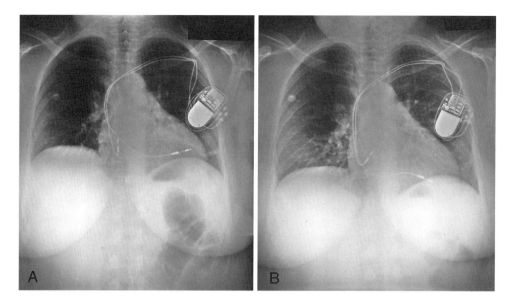

Fig. 11–22. *A,* Posteroanterior chest radiograph obtained the day after pacemaker implantation demonstrates an unusual course of the ventricular lead. The lead has a "high take-off" as it begins to cross to the left from the atrial position. This lead had been passed across an unknown patent foramen ovale and positioned in the left ventricle. *B,* Posteroanterior chest radiograph obtained the following day after the lead had been withdrawn and repositioned in the right ventricular apex.

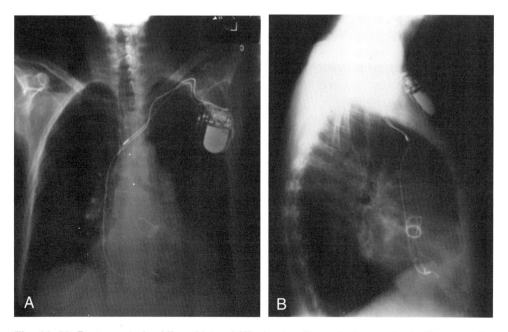

Fig. 11–23. Posteroanterior (*A*) and lateral (*B*) chest radiographs in a patient with gross dislodgment of the atrial lead, best appreciated on the lateral view.

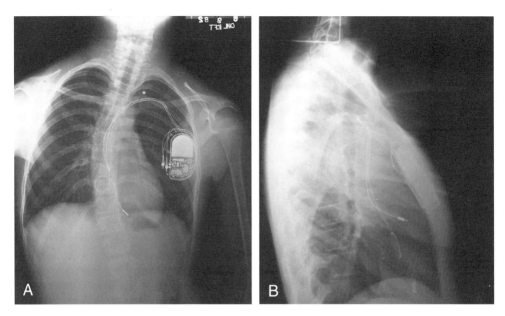

Fig. 11-24. Posteroanterior (*A*) and lateral (*B*) chest radiographs from a patient with a large loop in the ventricular lead. If this anomaly is noted soon after implantation, repositioning should be considered. If it is found later and the lead is functioning normally, no action is necessary. (From Hayes DL: Pacemaker radiography. *In* A Practice of Cardiac Pacing. Edited by S Furman, DL Hayes, DR Holmes Jr. Mount Kisco, NY, Futura Publishing Company, 1986, pp 333–378. By permission of the publisher.)

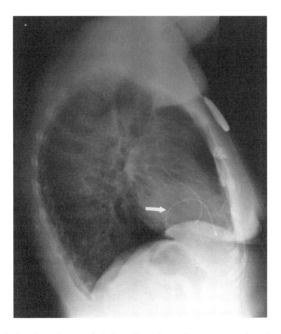

Fig. 11–25. Lateral chest radiograph taken the day after pacemaker implantation. There is a large loop (*arrow*) in the ventricular lead, and the pacing thresholds were found to be increased. The patient underwent repositioning of the ventricular lead.

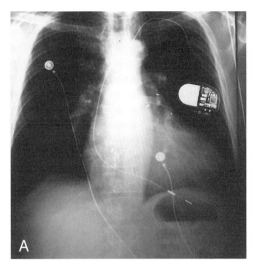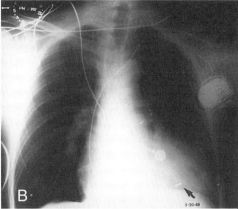

Fig. 11–26. *A,* Posteroanterior chest radiograph the day after pacemaker implantation. The ventricular lead appears to be adequately positioned, with the lead tip in the right ventricular apex. *B,* Portable posteroanterior chest radiograph obtained the next day. Despite the significant difference in the patient's position (rotated to the left), there is a definite change in ventricular lead position. The lead tip (*arrow*) is now pointing superiorly, not toward the apex. (From Hayes DL: Pacemaker radiography. *In* A Practice of Cardiac Pacing. Third edition. Edited by S Furman, DL Hayes, DR Holmes Jr. Mount Kisco, NY, Futura Publishing Company, 1993, pp 361–400. By permission of Mayo Foundation.)

Single-lead VDD or DDD systems can be identified by an additional floating bipolar sensing electrode in the right atrial area (Fig. 11–27).

Epicardial Leads

Currently, epicardial pacing leads are used in patients with specific congenital cardiac abnormalities, some pediatric patients, and patients with right atrioventricular valve prostheses (Fig. 11–28). The leads are then tunneled to the pulse generator or ICD, in either the pectoral or the abdominal area. Radiographic evaluation may require both chest and abdominal views to inspect the entire system. Historically, epicardial leads have had a higher incidence of lead failure, and a transvenous approach is generally preferred if possible[15,16] (Fig. 11–29).

Implantable Cardioverter-Defibrillator Leads

ICD systems have advanced rapidly over the past decade. Initially, epicardial patches were the only option for such systems; however, the introduction and refinement of transvenous systems have vastly simplified the operative procedure. As a result of these technical advances, expanding indications for ICD therapy, and data confirming the efficacy of these devices, the number of implants has increased tremendously.[3]

Epicardial Leads

Although currently used infrequently, epicardial defibrillation patches remain functional in many patients (Fig. 11–30). Such systems usually have easily

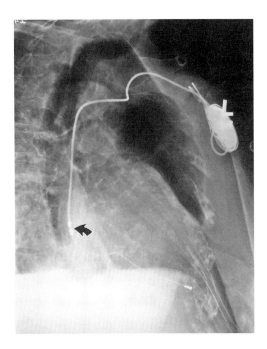

Fig. 11–27. Oblique chest radiograph of a VDD pacing system. The *arrow* denotes the floating bipolar atrial sensing lead; the ventricular lead functions in the unipolar mode. (From Lloyd MA, Hayes DL: Pacemaker and implantable cardioverter-defibrillator radiography. *In* Clinical Cardiac Pacing and Defibrillation. Second edition. Edited by KA Ellenbogen, GN Kay, BL Wilkoff. Philadelphia, WB Saunders Company, 2000, pp 710–723. By permission of the publisher.)

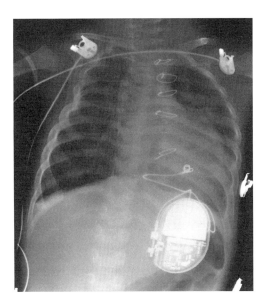

Fig. 11–28. Anteroposterior radiograph of chest and abdomen. This infant has a screw-in ventricular epicardial lead attached to a generator positioned in the abdomen.

recognizable, externally located patches over the heart as well as epicardial or transvenous pacing leads for sensing and pacing. Depending on the manufacturer, the defibrillation coils may or may not be easily visualized. One manufacturer's epicardial patches have a radiopaque marker around the periphery of the patch; it is not active, and a fracture of the marker does not affect the integrity of the patch. The coils of these patches are radiolucent and not visible on the radiograph. A frequent site of fracture in all epicardial patches is the patch-lead junction, and this area should be carefully inspected.

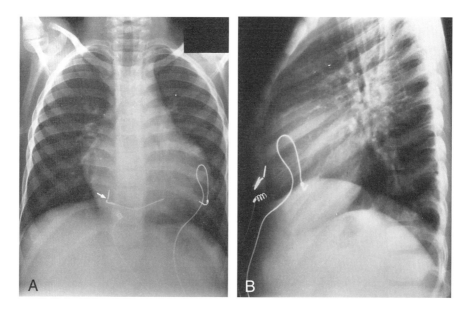

Fig. 11–29. Posteroanterior (*A*) and lateral (*B*) chest radiographs from a patient with three epicardial pacing leads. There are two "stab-in" leads, one of which is fractured (*arrow*), and one screw-in ventricular epicardial lead. (From Hayes DL: Pacemaker radiography. *In* A Practice of Cardiac Pacing. Edited by S Furman, DL Hayes, DR Holmes Jr. Mount Kisco, NY, Futura Publishing Company, 1986, pp 333–378. By permission of the publisher.)

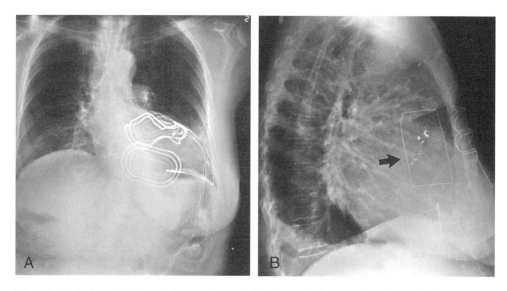

Fig. 11–30. Epicardial defibrillator patches. *A,* Posteroanterior chest radiograph. The generator is implanted in the abdomen. Note the screw-in pace-sense leads under the superior patch. *B,* Lateral chest radiograph from another patient. A barely visible radiographic marker around the perimeter of the patch (*arrow*) is not electrically active; fractures in this marker have no bearing on the integrity of the system. The generator is implanted in the abdomen.

Transvenous Leads

Most current systems utilize a single transvenous lead placed in the right ventricular apex and connected to a generator located in the pectoral area. The lead may be actively or passively fixed and, like pacing leads, should have a gentle redundancy. Leads may have a single high-voltage coil in the right ventricle or may have an additional coil in the superior vena cava area (Fig. 11–31). An additional subclavian lead, subcutaneous patch, or array may be used to obtain satisfactory defibrillation thresholds (Fig. 11–32). Because of their larger diameter, transvenous ICD leads may be more susceptible to sub-clavian crush syndrome; the area where the clavicle and first rib join should be carefully inspected. As with pacing leads, the insertion into the connector block and the connection with the set screws should be noted. All leads and patches should be inspected for obvious fracture and for unusual bending or kinking. Subcutaneous patches and arrays are usually placed inferior and posterior to the axilla; lateral or customized oblique views may be required to obtain satisfactory visualization.

The design of defibrillation leads and the radiographic "edge effect" create characteristic sites of pseudofracture with which the physician should be familiar (Fig. 11–33).

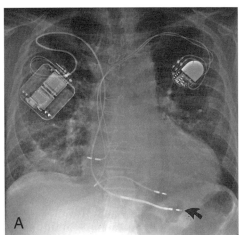

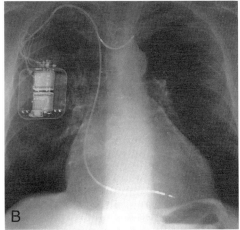

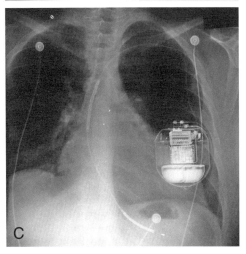

Fig. 11–31. Posteroanterior chest radiographs showing transvenous defibrillation leads. *A,* A dual-chamber pacing system is on the left and an implantable cardioverter-defibrillator (ICD) on the right. The *arrow* notes the defibrillator lead in the right ventricle. *B,* The ICD is implanted on the right, and the ventricular lead has a single high-voltage coil in the right ventricle. A separate defibrillator lead has been placed across the superior vena cava into the left subclavian vein. *C,* The single defibrillator lead has two high-voltage coils, proximally in the region of the superior vena cava and distally in the right ventricle. *Continues.*

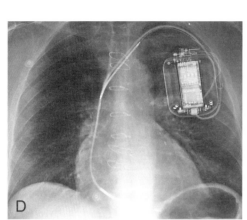 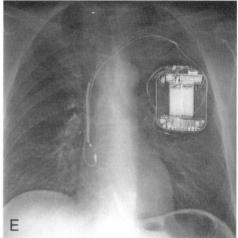

Figure 11–31 *continued. D,* There is a defibrillator lead in the right ventricle; a separate proximal defibrillator lead has been placed in the superior vena cava. *E,* A dual-chamber pacing and ICD system has a pacing lead in the right atrium and a defibrillator lead in the right ventricle. (From Lloyd MA, Hayes DL: Pacemaker and implantable cardioverter-defibrillator radiography. *In* Clinical Cardiac Pacing and Defibrillation. Second edition. Edited by KA Ellenbogen, GN Kay, BL Wilkoff. Philadelphia, WB Saunders Company, 2000, pp 710–723. By permission of the publisher.)

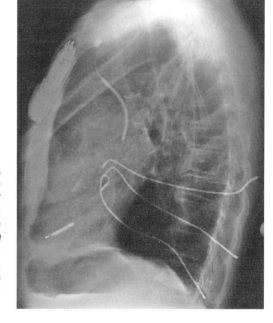

Fig. 11–32. Lateral chest radiograph of a subcutaneous array. Note the large increase in the area of the shocking vector created by the array. (From Lloyd MA, Hayes DL: Pacemaker and implantable cardioverter-defibrillator radiography. *In* Clinical Cardiac Pacing and Defibrillation. Second edition. Edited by KA Ellenbogen, GN Kay, BL Wilkoff. Philadelphia, WB Saunders Company, 2000, pp 710–723. By permission of the publisher.)

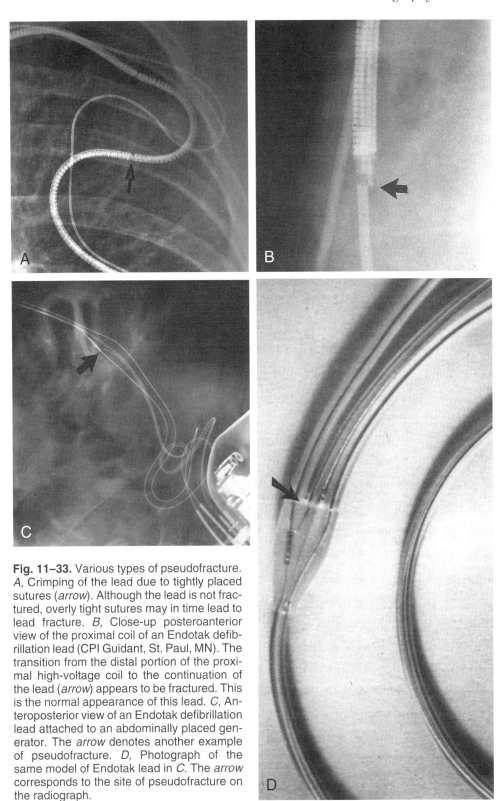

Fig. 11–33. Various types of pseudofracture. *A,* Crimping of the lead due to tightly placed sutures (*arrow*). Although the lead is not fractured, overly tight sutures may in time lead to lead fracture. *B,* Close-up posteroanterior view of the proximal coil of an Endotak defibrillation lead (CPI Guidant, St. Paul, MN). The transition from the distal portion of the proximal high-voltage coil to the continuation of the lead (*arrow*) appears to be fractured. This is the normal appearance of this lead. *C,* Anteroposterior view of an Endotak defibrillation lead attached to an abdominally placed generator. The *arrow* denotes another example of pseudofracture. *D,* Photograph of the same model of Endotak lead in *C*. The *arrow* corresponds to the site of pseudofracture on the radiograph.

Radiographic Appearance of New Device Applications

Coronary sinus lead placement was used many years ago but lost favor because of the high rate of lead dislodgment. However, expanding interest in pacing for the treatment of congestive heart failure and pacing for the prevention of atrial fibrillation has led to a resurgence of interest in coronary sinus pacing and leads designed to improve stability.

Recent years have seen the development of dual-site atrial pacing in an attempt to prevent atrial fibrillation.[11,12]

Two leads are placed in the right atrium, usually in the appendage and on the posterior septum near the coronary sinus ostium (Fig. 11–18). Alternatively, the second atrial lead or a single atrial lead is placed within the coronary sinus (Fig.11–34). Atrial defibrillators are also being developed; current devices have an atrial pace-sense lead as well as a coronary sinus defibrillation lead (Fig. 11–35). At this time, these devices are under investigation and must have backup ventricular defibrillation capability; therefore, a standard ventricular ICD lead is placed. Freestanding atrial defibrillators are under consideration but not yet available.

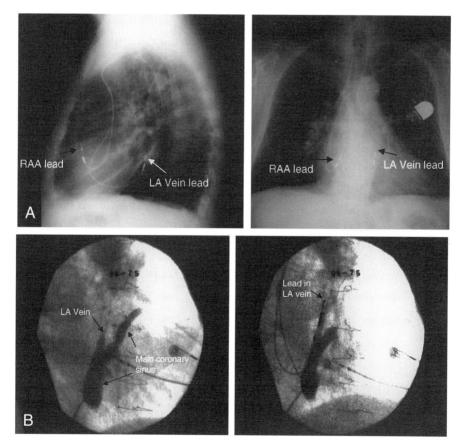

Fig. 11–34. *A,* Lateral and posteroanterior chest radiographs from a patient with a dual-chamber pacemaker. The atrial lead is positioned in the left atrial (LA) vein for left atrial pacing. RAA, right atrial appendage. *B,* Coronary sinus venogram and final LA vein lead position. The images were obtained in the right anterior oblique view. (Courtesy of Dr. Anthony Tang, Ottawa Heart Institute, Ottawa, Ontario, Canada.)

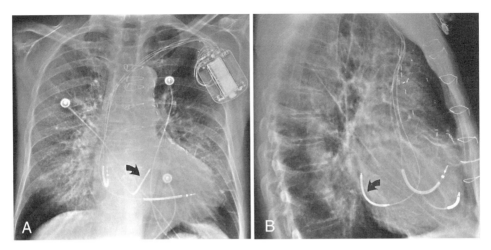

Fig. 11–35. Posteroanterior (*A*) and lateral (*B*) chest radiographs of a combination atrial and ventricular implantable cardioverter-defibrillator. Note defibrillation leads in both the right atrium and the right ventricle. An additional coronary sinus lead (*arrow*) is present for atrial defibrillation.

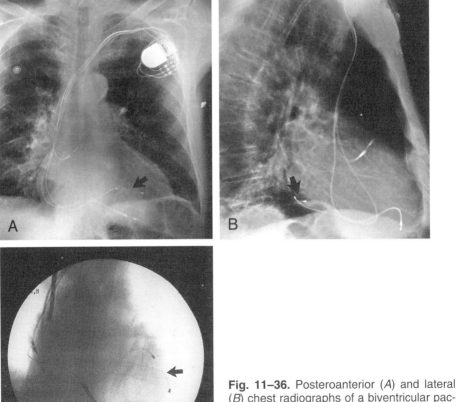

Fig. 11–36. Posteroanterior (*A*) and lateral (*B*) chest radiographs of a biventricular pacing system. The *arrow* denotes the lead in a lateral cardiac vein. *C*, Fluoroscopic view of biventricular pacing and implantable cardioverter-defibrillation system. The *arrow* denotes the left ventricular lead.

Biventricular pacing as a treatment for congestive heart failure is also investigational. In addition to a right ventricular lead, a pace-sense lead is placed into the coronary sinus and then into a cardiac vein for left ventricular pacing. The placement of the left ventricular lead varies on the basis of variations in coronary sinus anatomy (Fig. 11–36 and 11–37). A right atrial pacing lead is also placed if indicated.

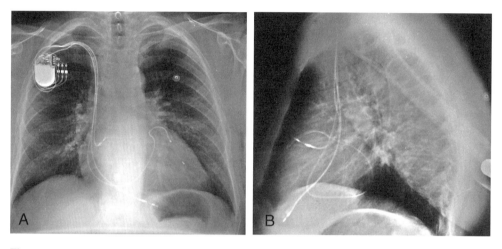

Fig. 11–37. Posteroanterior (*A*) and lateral (*B*) chest radiographs from a patient with right atrial, right ventricular, and coronary sinus leads. The coronary sinus lead is positioned in the anterior interventricular cardiac vein.

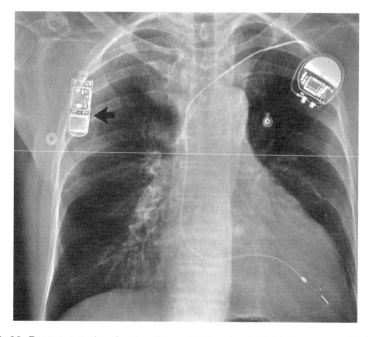

Fig. 11–38. Posteroanterior chest radiograph of an implantable loop recorder (*arrow*).

Implantable loop recorders are now available. The device appears as a small object, usually in the pectoral region (Fig. 11–38).

Miscellaneous Considerations

Occasionally, the subclavian vein may be difficult to locate, or the patency of the cephalic, axillary, or subclavian vein may be in question. Contrast material injected into a peripheral intravenous line in the ipsilateral upper extremity is outlined as it flows into the central circulation, determining patency and guiding access (Fig. 11–39). There is also evidence that routine use of the contrast-guided subclavian approach minimizes the incidence of pneumothorax.[17]

Management of the patient with a prosthetic tricuspid valve who requires permanent pacing must receive special consideration. We believe that a single ventricular pacing lead can be safely placed across a bioprosthetic valve. Placement of the ventricular lead with echocardiographic and fluoroscopic guidance has been suggested in an effort to minimize trauma to the bioprosthetic valve. The goal of echocardiographic guidance is preferential placement of the lead in a commissure of the bioprosthetic valve. Our experience with this approach is limited, but we have found that it is difficult, even with echocardiographic guidance, to be certain the lead is within a commissure.

A standard ventricular transvenous pacing lead cannot be placed across a prosthetic tricuspid valve. Several approaches have been used in this circumstance. If the need for permanent pacing is anticipated at the time of tricuspid valve replacement, some have advocated placing the transvenous lead outside the sewing ring of the tricuspid valve. The concern with this approach is the difficulties encountered if the lead needed to be extracted at some future date or if the lead failed and another lead was necessary. Alternatively, transmural placement of a ventricular pacing lead can be considered. In this approach, a cardiac surgeon places an active fixation lead through the free wall of the right ventricle, and the lead is actively fixated to the endocardial surface. A purse-string suture is placed around the lead where it passes through the right ventricular wall. Our limited but long-term success with this technique has been excellent[18] (Fig. 11–40).

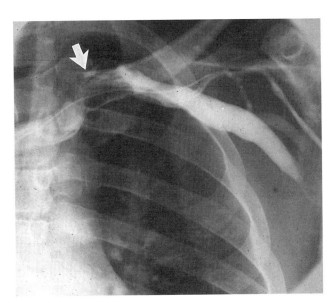

Fig. 11–39. Fluoroscopic view of the infraclavicular region after contrast material injected through a peripheral intravenous site has outlined the venous system. The *arrow* identifies an area of subclavian stenosis that would make access and placement of a lead difficult. (From Lloyd MA, Hayes DL: Pacemaker and implantable cardioverter-defibrillator radiography. *In* Clinical Cardiac Pacing and Defibrillation. Second edition. Edited by KA Ellenbogen, GN Kay, BL Wilkoff. Philadelphia, WB Saunders Company, 2000, pp 710–723. By permission of the publisher.)

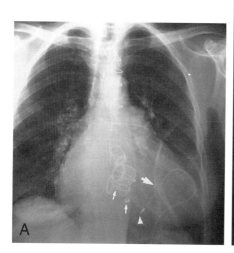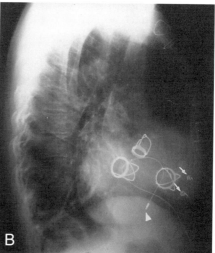

Fig. 11–40. Posteroanterior (*A*) and lateral (*B*) chest radiographs from a patient with prosthetic mitral and tricuspid valves. A ventricular lead passes through the free wall of the right ventricle (*arrowhead*) and is fixated on the endocardial surface. The two *small arrows* note abandoned screw-in epicardial leads and the *large arrow* on the posteroanterior projection notes a remnant of an epicardial "stab-in" lead. (From Hayes DL: Pacemaker radiography. *In* A Practice of Cardiac Pacing. Third edition. Edited by S Furman, DL Hayes, DR Holmes Jr. Mount Kisco, NY, Futura Publishing Company, 1993, pp 361–400. By permission of Mayo Foundation.)

Another option for patients who have had tricuspid valve replacement or surgery in whom it is desirable to avoid placing a lead across the tricuspid valve and for patients in whom ventricular access is limited because of congenital anomalies is to pace the ventricle via the coronary sinus. With newer, more reliable coronary sinus leads, this option should be viable.

The most common cardiovascular anomaly encountered by the implanting physician is persistent left superior vena cava. The leads are placed through the left vena cava, into the coronary sinus, and then into the right atrium.[19] The ventricular lead usually needs to be looped to direct it across the tricuspid valve into the right ventricle (Fig. 11–41). The diagnosis can be

Fig. 11–41. Posteroanterior chest radiograph showing persistent left superior vena cava. The atrial and ventricular leads both follow the course of the left superior vena cava into the coronary sinus. The atrial lead is then actively fixated to the lateral right atrial wall, and the ventricular lead loops in the right atrium before crossing the tricuspid valve into the right ventricle. (From Lloyd MA, Hayes DL: Pacemaker and implantable cardioverter-defibrillator radiography. *In* Clinical Cardiac Pacing and Defibrillation. Second edition. Edited by KA Ellenbogen, GN Kay, BL Wilkoff. Philadelphia, WB Saunders Company, 2000, pp 710–723. By permission of the publisher.)

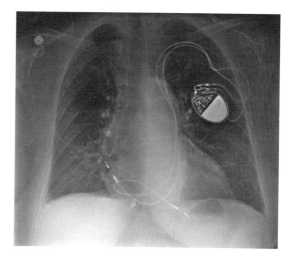

suspected by finding an enlarged coronary sinus at echocardiography or by injecting contrast material into an ipsilateral intravenous line in the left upper extremity.

Congenital cardiovascular anomalies may require novel implantation techniques and may result in unusual lead placement. Knowledge of the native and corrected anatomy is essential for planning a procedure and for interpreting the chest radiograph; consultation with the congenital cardiologist or cardiovascular surgeon may be helpful (Fig. 11–42, 11–43, and 11–44).

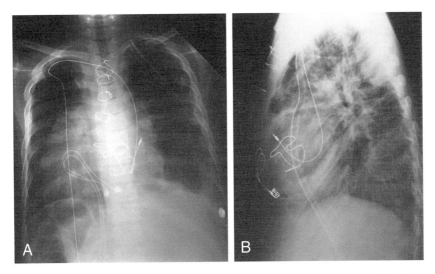

Fig. 11–42. Posteroanterior (*A*) and lateral (*B*) chest radiographs from a child after a Fontan procedure and implantation of a dual-chamber pacemaker. The ventricular lead has been placed in an epicardial position because the ventricle could not be accessed transvenously, and the atrial lead is transvenously positioned.

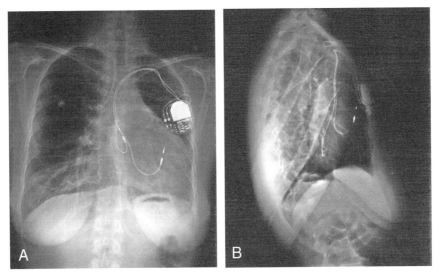

Fig. 11–43. Posteroanterior (*A*) and lateral (*B*) chest radiographs from a patient who has had a Senning procedure. The ventricular lead is placed through a baffle in the nonsystemic but morphologic left ventricle. The atrial lead is fixated in active atrial tissue.

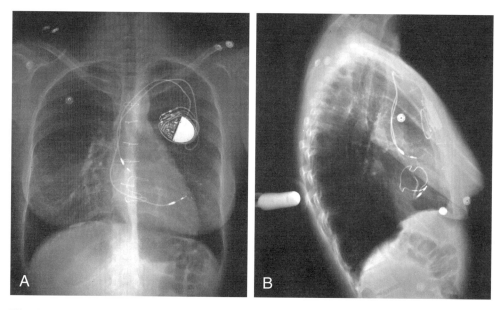

Fig. 11–44. Posteroanterior (*A*) and lateral (*B*) chest radiographs from a patient who has had a Mustard procedure. The ventricular lead is placed through a baffle into the nonsystemic but morphologic left ventricle. The atrial lead is fixated in active atrial tissue.

Conclusion

The chest radiograph provides important information about pacing and ICD systems. As systems become more complex and specialized and as indications for these devices expand, the importance of recognizing the normal and abnormal appearance of these systems is essential. A systematic evaluation of the anatomy and system components is necessary preoperatively, postoperatively, and during troubleshooting.

References

1. Hayes DL: Pacemaker radiography. *In* A Practice of Cardiac Pacing. Edited by S Furman, DL Hayes, DR Holmes Jr. Mount Kisco, NY, Futura Publishing Company, 1986, p 361
2. Steiner RM, Tegtmeyer CJ, Morse D, Moses ML, Goodman LR, Nanda N, Ravin CE, Parsonnet V, Flicker S: The radiology of cardiac pacemakers. Radiographics 6: 373–399, 1986
3. Epstein AE, Kay GN, Plumb VJ, Shepard RB, Kirklin JK: Combined automatic implantable cardioverter-defibrillator and pacemaker systems: implantation techniques and follow-up. J Am Coll Cardiol 13:121–131, 1989
4. Stanton MS, Hayes DL, Munger TM, Trusty JM, Espinosa RE, Shen WK, Osborn MJ, Packer DL, Hammill SC: Consistent subcutaneous prepectoral implantation of a new implantable cardioverter defibrillator. Mayo Clin Proc 69:309–314, 1994
5. Roberts JS, Wenger NK: Pacemaker twiddler's syndrome. Am J Cardiol 63:1013–1016, 1989
6. Fyke FE III: Simultaneous insulation deterioration associated with side-by-side subclavian placement of two polyurethane leads. Pacing Clin Electrophysiol 11:1571–1574, 1988
7. Dunlap TE, Popat KD, Sorkin RP: Radiographic pseudofracture of the Medtronic bipolar polyurethane pacing lead. Am Heart J 106:167–168, 1983
8. Hecht S, Berdoff R, Van Tosh A, Goldberg E: Radiographic pseudofracture of bipolar pacemaker wire. Chest 88:302–304, 1985
9. Witte AA: Pseudo-fracture of pacemaker lead due to securing suture: a case report. Pacing Clin Electrophysiol 4:716–718, 1981

10. Gheissari A, Hordof AJ, Spotnitz HM: Transvenous pacemakers in children: relation of lead length to anticipated growth. Ann Thorac Surg 52:118–121, 1991

11. Daubert C, Gras D, Leclercq C, Baïsset JM, Pavin D, Mabo P: Biatrial synchronous pacing: a new approach for prevention of drug refractory atrial flutter (abstract). Circulation 92 Suppl:I-532, 1995

12. Delfaut P, Saksena S, Prakash A, Krol RB: Long-term outcome of patients with drug-refractory atrial flutter and fibrillation after single- and dual-site right atrial pacing for arrhythmia prevention. J Am Coll Cardiol 32:1900–1908, 1998

13. Lloyd MA, Hayes DL, Holmes DR Jr: Atrial "J" pacing lead retention wire fracture: radiographic assessment, incidence of fracture, and clinical management. Pacing Clin Electrophysiol 18:958–964, 1995

14. Gross JN, Hildner F, Brinker J, Kawanishi D, Kay GN, Reeves RC, for the Independent Physician Advisory Committee and Multicenter Study Group: Multi-center passive fixation lead study: fluoroscopic screening and clinical event update (abstract). Pacing Clin Electrophysiol 20:1064, 1997

15. Helguera ME, Maloney JD, Woscoboinik JR, Trohman RG, McCarthy PM, Morant VA, Wilkoff BL, Castle LW, Pinski SL: Long-term performance of epimyocardial pacing leads in adults: comparison with endocardial leads. Pacing Clin Electrophysiol 16:412–417, 1993

16. Hayes DL, Holmes DR Jr, Maloney JD, Neubauer SA, Ritter DG, Danielson GK: Permanent endocardial pacing in pediatric patients. J Thorac Cardiovasc Surg 85:618–624, 1983

17. Higano ST, Hayes DL, Spittell PC: Facilitation of the subclavian-introducer technique with contrast venography. Pacing Clin Electrophysiol 13:681–684, 1990

18. Hayes DL, Vlietstra RE, Puga FJ, Shub C: A novel approach to atrial endocardial pacing. Pacing Clin Electrophysiol 12:125–130, 1989

19. Zerbe F, Bornakowski J, Sarnowski W: Pacemaker electrode implantation in patients with persistent left superior vena cava. Br Heart J 67:65–66, 1992

12

Electromagnetic Interference and Implantable Devices

David L. Hayes, M.D.

Some of the most common questions patients ask have to do with potential sources of interference. Often, their concerns are misdirected because of myth or sensationalism by the press. It is important to know not only what sources of interference are of potential concern but also how external interference actually affects pacemakers and implantable cardioverter-defibrillators (ICDs).

Pacemakers and ICDs are subject to interference from many sources. Most sources of electromagnetic interference (EMI) are nonbiologic, but in addition, biologic sources of interference, such as myopotentials and extremes of temperature or irradiation, may cause pacemakers to malfunction. In general, modern pacemakers are effectively shielded against EMI, and the increasing use of bipolar leads has reduced the problem even further. There has always been some concern about EMI that patients may encounter in the nonhospital environment, but because of improvements in pacemaker protection, that is, shielding and design changes, EMI is now of less concern. The principal sources of interference that affect pacemakers are in the hospital.

The portions of the electromagnetic spectrum that may affect pacemakers are *radio waves*, with frequencies between 0 and 10^9 Hz, including alternating current electricity supplies (50 or 60 Hz) and electrocautery, and *microwaves*, with frequencies between 10^9 and 10^{11} Hz, including ultrahigh-frequency radio waves, radar, and microwave ovens (2.45 to 10^9 Hz)[1] (Fig. 12–1). Higher frequency portions of the spectrum, including infrared, visible light, ultraviolet, x-rays, and gamma rays, do not interfere with pacemakers because their wavelength is much shorter than the pacemaker or lead dimensions. However, therapeutic radiation can damage pacemaker circuitry directly.

EMI enters a pacemaker by conduction if the patient is in direct contact with the source or by radiation if the patient is in an electromagnetic field with the pacemaker lead acting as an antenna. Pacemakers have been protected from interference by shielding of the pacemaker circuitry, filtering of the incoming signal, and reduction of the distance between the electrodes to minimize the "antenna." The contemporary pacemaker is protected from most sources of interference because the circuitry is shielded inside a stainless steel or titanium case. In addition, body tissues provide some protection by reflection or absorption of external radiation.

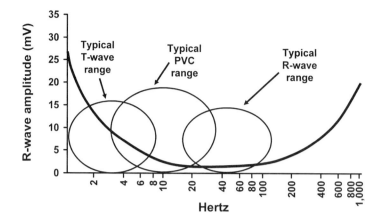

Fig. 12–1. Electromagnetic frequency spectrum of intracardiac events. PVC, premature ventricular contraction.

Bipolar leads sense less conducted and radiated interference because the distance between anode and cathode is smaller than that for unipolar leads. Bipolar sensing has, in large part, eliminated myopotential inhibition and cross-talk as pacemaker problems. In addition, studies have shown that with bipolar sensing, there is considerably less sensing of external electrical fields[2,3] and less effect from electrocautery during surgery.[4]

Sensed interference is filtered by narrow band-pass filters to exclude noncardiac signals. However, signals in the 5- to 100-Hz range are not filtered because they overlap the cardiac signal range. These signals can result in abnormal pacemaker behavior if they are interpreted as cardiac.

The possible responses to external interference include

- Inappropriate inhibition of pacemaker output (Fig. 12–2)
- Inappropriate triggering of pacemaker output (Fig. 12–3)
- Asynchronous pacing (Fig. 12–4)
- Reprogramming, usually to a backup mode (Fig. 12–5)
- Inappropriate initiation of "other" features, such as mode switching or rate drop response (Fig. 12–6)
- Damage to the pacemaker circuitry (Fig. 12–7)

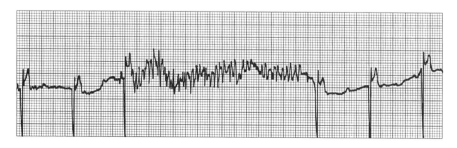

Fig. 12–2. Electrocardiographic recording from a patient with a pacemaker programmed to the VVI mode. Isometric maneuvers result in myopotentials and pacemaker inhibition.

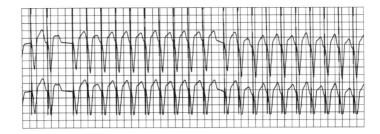

Fig. 12–3. Electrocardiographic recording taken at rest from a patient with a pacemaker programmed to the DDDR mode. During exposure to equipment emitting a radiofrequency signal close to that of the pacemaker, the external signal was sensed on the atrial sensing circuit of the pacemaker, resulting in tracking and a paced ventricular rate at the programmed upper rate limit.

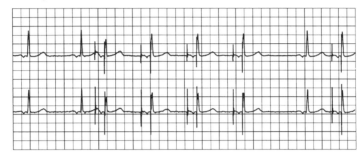

Fig. 12–4. Electrocardiographic recording taken at rest from a patient with a pacemaker programmed to the DDDR mode. During exposure to equipment emitting a radiofrequency signal close to that of the pacemaker, the external signal resulted in asynchronous (DOO) pacing.

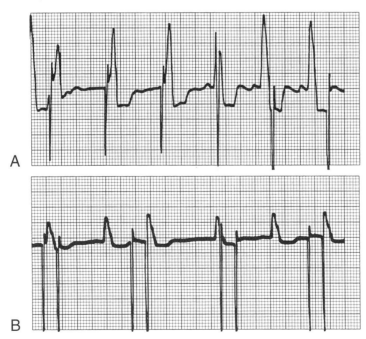

Fig. 12–5. Electromagnetic reprogramming. *A,* Transtelephonic electrocardiographic tracing from a patient with a pacemaker programmed to the DDD pacing mode. The transmission reveals VOO pacing instead of the expected DOO response. *B,* Electrocardiographic tracing obtained after reprogramming in the pacemaker clinic to the DDD mode; there is appropriate DOO pacing. A history obtained from the patient revealed that she had undergone magnetic resonance imaging of the head. This procedure had reprogrammed the pacemaker to the backup mode, that is, VVI at a rate of 65 bpm.

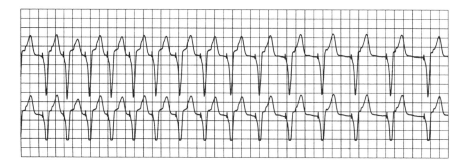

Fig. 12–6. Electrocardiographic tracing from a patient with a dual-chamber pacemaker. The electrocardiogram is obtained during exposure to a source of electromagnetic interference. The interference is sensed on the atrial sensing channel, and the pacemaker responds by rapid ventricular tracking. Criteria are met for mode switching, and the rate begins to fall back to the programmed lower rate.

```
294-03 SN 064860                    06 JAN 99 11:17
              RELAY      TELEMETRY DATA
     PACING RATE                      60 MIN-1
     PACING INTERVAL                1000 MS
     CELL VOLTAGE                    2.65 VOLTS
     CELL IMPEDANCE                  3.75 KOHMS
     CELL CURRENT                    19.0 UA
                   ATRIAL( B1)   VENTRICULAR( B1)
     SENSITIVITY       0.5          2.0 MV
     LEAD IMPEDANCE    HIGH         465 OHMS
     PULSE AMPLITUDE   2.68         3.95 VOLTS
     PULSE WIDTH       0.40         0.60 MS
     OUTPUT CURRENT    LOW          7.8 MA
     ENERGY DELIVERED  LOW          16.1 UJ
     CHARGE DELIVERED  LOW          4.68 UC
```

Fig. 12–7. Programmer printout after elective cardioversion in a patient with a DDD pacemaker. The telemetered data from the atrial lead are incomplete, with lead impedance noted to be "high" and output current, energy delivered, and charge delivered "low." In addition, there was failure to pace in the atrium. The device was explanted; direct measurements on the atrial lead were all within acceptable range. A new pacemaker was attached and functioned normally. Destructive analysis of the explanted device showed damage to the atrial pacing circuit.

Pacemaker Responses to Noise

Asynchronous Pacing

To protect the patient from inappropriate inhibition of pacemaker output, contemporary pacemakers have the capability of reverting to asynchronous pacing if exposed to sufficient interference. This change is usually activated by signals detected during a noise-sampling period (NSP) within the pacemaker timing cycle (Fig. 12–8). The NSP occurs immediately after the ventricular refractory period (VRP), which follows a ventricular sensed or paced event. The VRP is an "absolute" refractory period, during which the ventricular sensing channel does not detect any signals and in particular does not sense the afterpotential of the ventricular pacing artifact or the evoked QRS and T waves. The VRP usually lasts between 200 and 400 msec, and events occurring during this period have no effect on pacemaker timing. The NSP, or resettable refractory period, lasts between 60 and 200 msec. If an event is

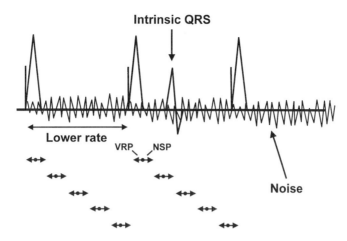

Fig. 12–8. Response of a VVI pacemaker to noise. There is no sensing during the ventricular refractory period (VRP). Noise detected in the noise-sampling period (NSP) immediately after the VRP causes restarting of the VRP. In the next NSP, noise is again detected, and the VRP is again restarted. This process continues until the lower rate interval (LRI) times out, and a ventricular pacing pulse is delivered. Because the sensing channel is refractory throughout the LRI, the intrinsic cardiac beat (R) is not sensed, and pacing is asynchronous. (Modified from Hayes and Strathmore.[1] By permission of WB Saunders Company.)

sensed during this period, it is interpreted as noise, and either the VRP or the NSP is restarted. In addition, in a dual-chamber mode, the postventricular atrial refractory period and the upper rate interval, but not the lower rate interval, are restarted. If a further noise event is detected in the NSP, the VRP or NSP again is restarted and the pacemaker does not recognize cardiac signals. Repetitive noise events eventually cause the lower rate interval to time out, and a pacing pulse is delivered. Continuous noise thus results in asynchronous pacing at the lower rate limit.

In some pacemakers, rather than timing out the lower rate interval, repetitive detection of noise in the NSP causes temporary switching to a specific "noise reversion mode," which is usually an asynchronous mode (VOO or DOO). In some pacemakers with programmable polarity, the pacing output is unipolar in the noise reversion mode, even if the device is programmed to bipolar pacing.

Whether noise causes inhibition or asynchronous pacing depends on the du-

ration and field strength of the signal. As the field strength increases, there is a greater tendency to inhibition, because the noise may be sensed intermittently and may not be sensed in the NSP but in the alert period between the NSP and the next pacing pulse. At higher field strengths, the noise is sensed continuously, including in the NSP, and asynchronous pacing occurs. Pacemaker models vary considerably in their susceptibility to noise.

Mode Resetting

EMI can reprogram the pacing mode, as opposed to the transient changes already described. This is usually the "backup mode" or "reset mode" and is often the same as the pacemaker elective replacement indicator or "battery depletion" mode (Fig. 12–5). Confusion can arise when the "backup mode" and the default settings at battery depletion are the same. Recognition of these parameters indicates that either the pacemaker has been af-

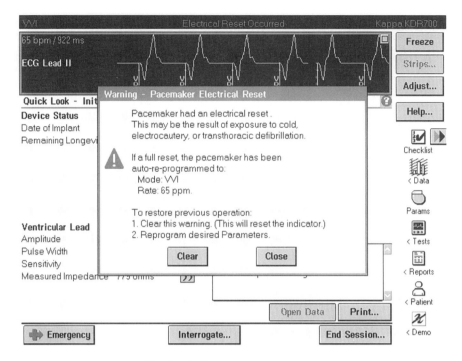

Fig. 12–9. Power on reset screen.

fected by interference or has truly reached battery depletion. In both cases, careful attention to the programmer telemetry, when available, is helpful. If the telemetered cell impedance remains low or the battery voltage is normal, the pacemaker battery is not exhausted and interference is the problem. In addition, if the pacemaker is reprogrammed to the original pacing mode with maximum output and an increased rate, it quickly reverts to the settings that indicate battery depletion if the pacemaker battery is truly near depletion.

The backup or reset mode is usually VVI, and if the pulse generator has programmable polarity, the backup polarity is unipolar. This factor may be significant in patients with ICDs. Some pacemakers may reset to VOO mode if subjected to interference, potentially resulting in competition with the intrinsic rhythm.

Exposure to low temperatures before implantation also may result in mode resetting. The cold temperatures cause an increase in the internal battery resistance, and the subsequent decrease in the battery voltage causes the end-of-life indicator or reset mode to be activated.[5] Because this effect occurs frequently during shipment in cold climates, all pacemakers should be routinely interrogated before implantation and reprogrammed if necessary (Fig. 12–9).

Environmental Electromagnetic Interference

Electric and magnetic signals are emitted by certain industrial, hospital-medical, and domestic sources. Each of these environments is discussed individually.

Hospital Environment

The hospital is the most common environment with sources of potential EMI that can cause significant interference with implantable devices (Table 12–1).

Electrocautery

Electrocautery continues to be one of the most common potential sources of EMI for patients with implanted devices. Electrocautery involves the use of radiofrequency current to cut or coagulate tissues. It is usually applied unipolarly between the cauterizing instrument (the cathode) and the indifferent plate (the anode) attached at a distance to the patient's skin. Bipolar cautery uses a bipolar instrument for coagulation. The frequency is usually between 300 and 500 kHz (at frequencies of less than 200 kHz, muscle and nerve stimulation may occur).[1] Cutting diathermy uses a modulated signal, so that bursts of energy are applied, whereas coagulation diathermy uses an unmodulated signal to heat the tissue. Coagulation diathermy is used in radiofrequency ablation of cardiac tissue for the treatment of arrhythmias.

The current generated by electrocautery is related to the distance and orientation of the cautery electrodes relative to the pacemaker and lead. High current is generated if the cautery cathode is close to the pacemaker, and particularly high currents are generated in the pacemaker if it lies between the two cautery electrodes.

Electrocautery can result in multiple clinical responses from a permanent pacemaker (Table 12–2). The electrocautery signal may induce currents in the pacing lead and cause local heating at the electrode, leading to myocardial damage with a subsequent increase in pacing or sensing threshold or in both. Threshold alteration is usually transient.

To prevent inappropriate inhibition of the pacemaker, a magnet is often applied to the chest over the pacemaker during cautery to convert it to the asynchronous mode. Although this maneuver may be successful, it may open some pacemakers to reprogramming by the electrocautery signal and is therefore controversial.

Pacemakers with rate-responsive functions may exhibit inappropriate responses during surgery due to vibration sensed from other intraoperative equipment or vibrations created by the surgical procedure. The electrocautery signal may overwhelm the impedance measuring circuit of a minute ventilation rate-responsive pacemaker and cause pacing at the upper rate limit.

Most reported complications of electrocautery are with unipolar pacemakers, and a prospective study of patients with pacemakers undergoing surgery suggested that bipolar devices are less susceptible to the effects of electrocautery.[4]

Patients with pacemakers who are to undergo surgery in which electrocautery may be used should be assessed preoperatively. Table 12–3 provides all the information necessary, but a few key points bear repeating. Preoperatively, it

---

Table 12–1.
Sources of Electromagnetic Interference in the Hospital

- Electrocautery
- Cardioversion-defibrillation
- Magnetic resonance imaging
- Lithotripsy
- Radiofrequency ablation
- Electroshock therapy
- Electroconvulsive therapy
- Diathermy

Table 12–2.
Potential Effects of Electrocautery

- Reprogramming
- Permanent damage to the pulse generator
- Pacemaker inhibition
- Reversion to a fallback or noise reversion mode, or electrical reset
- Myocardial thermal damage

Table 12–3.
Perioperative Management of Pacemakers

Preoperatively
- Identify pacemaker and determine "reset" mode
- Check pacemaker program, telemetry, thresholds, battery status
- Deactivate rate response or Vario
- Record pacemaker information

Intraoperatively
- Position electrocautery-indifferent plate away from pacemaker so that pacemaker is not between electrocautery electrodes
- Monitor pulse or oximeter (electrocardiogram is obscured by artifact)
- Have programmer readily available
- Use bipolar cautery when possible
- Do not use cautery near pacemaker
- Use cautery in short bursts
- Reprogram if necessary if reset mode is hemodynamically unstable
- Rarely consider use of VVT mode if necessary

Postoperatively
- Check pacemaker program, telemetry, thresholds
- Reprogram if necessary

is most important to determine the programmed settings and whether the patient is pacemaker-dependent.

In the operating room, it is most important that the indifferent plate of the electrocautery be placed at a distance from the pacemaker, usually on the thigh, and that good contact be ensured. The effect of electrocautery may be difficult to assess, because it causes interference on the electrocardiographic (ECG) monitor. Another method of assessing cardiac rhythm should be used: palpation of the pulse, pulse oximetry, or arterial blood pressure monitoring.

Cautery should be used with caution in the vicinity of the pacemaker and its leads. The cathode should be kept as far from the pulse generator as possible, the lowest possible amplitude should be used, and the surgeon should deliver only brief bursts.

During electrocautery, pacemaker function and cardiac rhythm should be carefully assessed. The most likely response is transient inhibition or asynchronous pacing during electrocautery, which should not cause a significant hemodynamic problem. If persistent pacemaker inhibition occurs, a magnet can be applied to the pacemaker during electrocautery.

Postoperatively, it is critical that the pacemaker be interrogated, and if it is in the reset mode, it should be reprogrammed to the original settings. Ideally, thresholds should be reassessed and compared with preoperative values. If problems are encountered during interrogation of the pacemaker or reprogramming to the original settings, the manufacturer should be consulted to determine whether a malfunction has occurred.

Defibrillation

External transthoracic defibrillation produces a large amount of electrical energy delivered in the vicinity of a pacemaker and has the potential to damage both the pulse generator and the cardiac tissue in contact with the lead. The pacemaker is protected from damage by high defibrillation energies through special circuitry incorporating a Zener diode that electronically regulates the voltage entering the pacemaker circuit and that should prevent high currents from being conducted by the lead to the myocardium. However, the extremely high energies can overwhelm this protection and cause damage to the pacemaker or the heart. Internal defibrillation via epicardial or subcutaneous patches or intracardiac defibrillation electrodes delivers smaller amounts of energy but may also interfere with pacemaker function. Bipolar pacemakers are less susceptible than unipolar pacemakers to interference from defibrillation.

As with electrocautery, defibrillation may result in reprogramming to the backup or reset mode, a transient increase in pacing or sensing threshold, or damage to pacemaker circuitry.

The degree of damage seems to be related to the distance of the defibrillation paddles from the pulse generator. The paddles should be placed as far as possible from the generator; when possible, an anterior-posterior configuration is preferred (Fig. 12–10). However, in the anterior-anterior configuration, the paddles should be 10 cm away from the pacemaker if possible. After defibrillation, the pacemaker should be interrogated and the programmed settings compared with those before defibrillation and cardioversion. A transient rise in threshold should be managed by increasing the energy output if necessary (Fig. 12–11). Rarely, prolonged, severe threshold increases occur that necessitate lead replacement. Recommendations for management of patients undergoing cardioversion and defibrillation are summarized in Table 12–4.

Catheter Ablation

Catheter ablation of intracardiac structures to control arrhythmias was first performed with direct current shock. This technique had a higher tendency to affect pacemakers than did external defibrillation, and patients frequently experienced problems, including reprogramming to the backup or reset mode, pacemaker circuit failure, and transient increases in pacing and sensing thresholds. Direct current catheter ablation should be avoided in patients with permanent pacemakers if alternative therapy is available.

Nearly all ablations are now done by radiofrequency current, which is the same as coagulation electrocautery, that is, unmodulated radiofrequency current at a frequency of 400 to 500 kHz. Effects similar to those of surgical electrocautery have been reported, including inappropriate inhibition, asynchronous pacing, and resetting to backup mode.[6,7]

The ablation catheter is usually some distance from the pacing lead, and radiofrequency ablation has been accomplished safely near implanted pacemakers and does not appear to result in any significant myocardial damage at the site of the pacemaker electrode. Some operators actually prefer to place the permanent pacemaker before atrioventricular nodal ablation. Performing the procedure in this sequence obviates temporary pacemaker placement.

Before radiofrequency ablation is performed, however, it is essential to interrogate the pacemaker, record its programmed settings, and measure thresh-

Apex-Anterior   **Apex-Posterior**

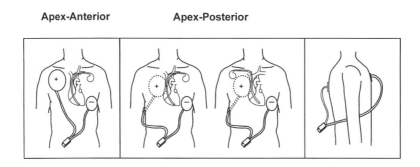

Fig. 12–10. For elective cardioversion, the paddles should ideally be kept at least 4 to 6 inches away from the pulse generator. In our practice, we use anterior-posterior paddle placement, but anterior-anterior paddle placement can also be used.

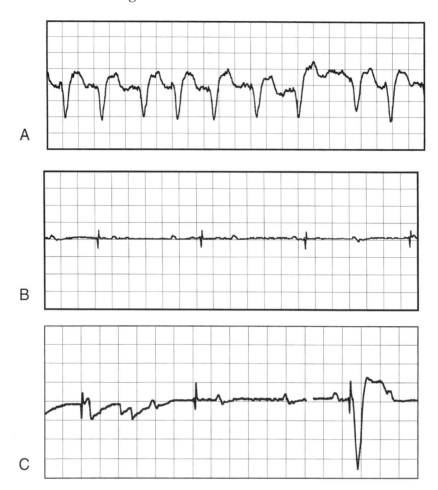

Fig. 12–11. External transthoracic defibrillation. *A,* Electrocardiographic recording from a patient with a DDD pacemaker. The underlying rhythm is atrial fibrillation, and the ventricular pacing channel is irregularly tracking the atrial fibrillation, with a resulting rate of approximately 100 bpm. *B,* Electrocardiographic recording immediately after elective cardioversion demonstrates ventricular asystole with ventricular pacing artifacts and failure to capture. *C,* A subsequent tracing demonstrates intermittent ventricular capture. (*C,* From Hayes DL, Wang PJ (editors): Cardiac Pacemakers and Implantable Defibrillators: A Multi-Volume Workbook. Vol 4. ICDs and Pacemakers. Armonk, NY, Futura Publishing Company, 2000, p 37. By permission of the publisher.)

olds. Activity sensing should be switched off. A programmer should be available during the procedure. After the procedure, the pacemaker should be checked and reprogrammed if necessary.

Magnetic Resonance Imaging

In magnetic resonance imaging (MRI), a large magnetic field is generated by an electromagnet modulated by a ra-diofrequency electrical signal. When a pacemaker is near an MRI scanner with the electromagnet "on," the reed switch closes, and asynchronous pacing occurs. Although there may be competition with the underlying cardiac rhythm, asynchronous pacing does not commonly cause a clinical problem.

Measuring the effect of the MRI scanner on pacemakers is difficult because the radiofrequency pulses cause ECG artifacts. However, several studies of pace-

Table 12–4.
Cardioversion-Defibrillation in the Patient
With a Pacemaker or Implantable
Cardioverter-Defibrillator

- Ideally, place paddles in the anterior-posterior position
- Try to keep paddles at least 4 inches from the pulse generator
- Have the appropriate programmer available
- Interrogate the device after the procedure

makers in dogs have demonstrated the potential effects. In some pacemakers, no effect other than asynchronous pacing occurred.[8] In other pacemakers, cardiac pacing at the same frequency or a multiple of the frequency of the radiofrequency current occurred; for example, if the MRI device was operating at 200 msec, pacing rates at 300 bpm were observed in some dogs.[8,9] The radiofrequency signal is detected by the leads acting as an antenna and is then amplified by the pacemaker circuitry to produce sufficient energy to pace the heart.

Reported problems of pacemakers in MRI scanners are magnet-activated asynchronous pacing, inhibition by the radiofrequency signal, rapid pacing induced by the radiofrequency signal,[8–12] discomfort at the pacemaker pocket, reprogramming (Fig. 12–5), and death in an unmonitored patient.[10] Transient reed switch malfunction has also been seen.[9] There are no published reports of pacemaker circuitry damage by MRI.

Temporary pacemakers are also subject to interference from MRI. In the most commonly used temporary pacing modes, VVI and DDD, the radiofrequency signal is sufficient to inhibit the pacemaker output.

Extracorporeal Shock Wave Lithotripsy

Extracorporeal shock wave lithotripsy (ESWL) is a noninvasive treatment for

nephrolithiasis and cholelithiasis that delivers multiple, focused hydraulic shocks, generated by an underwater spark gap, to a patient lying in a water bath. The shock is focused on the stones by an ellipsoidal metal reflector. Because the shock wave can produce ventricular extrasystoles, it is synchronized to the R wave.

ESWL is safe to use with implanted pacemakers, provided that the shock is given synchronously with the ECG and that dual-chamber pacemakers have safety pacing enabled. In the pacemaker-dependent patient, it is recommended that a dual-chamber pacemaker be programmed to the VVI, VOO, or DOO pacing mode to avoid ventricular inhibition.[13] Programming of a DDD pulse generator to the VVI, VOO, or DOO mode also avoids rare instances of irregularities of pacing rate, supraventricular arrhythmias that can be tracked or induced, and triggering of the ventricular output by electromechanical interference.

ESWL has not been reported to cause any damage to the pacemaker, except that if an activity-sensing pacemaker is placed at the focal point of the ESWL, the piezoelectric crystal could be shattered.[14] Patients with rate-adaptive pacemakers that have piezoelectric crystal activity can probably undergo lithotripsy safely if the device is implanted in the thorax, but lithotripsy should be avoided in these patients if the device is located in the abdomen.

Transcutaneous Electrical Nerve Stimulation

Transcutaneous electrical nerve stimulation (TENS) is a widely used method for the relief of acute and chronic pain from musculoskeletal and neurologic problems. A TENS unit consists of several electrodes placed on the skin and connected to a pulse generator that applies pulses of between 1 and 200 V and 0 to 60 mA at a frequency of 20 to 110 Hz. The output and frequency of the unit can be adjusted by the patient to provide maximum relief of pain.

The repetition frequency of the TENS output is similar to the normal range of heart rates, so it would be expected that TENS pulses might cause pacemaker inhibition. Although a study of 51 patients with pacemakers showed no inhibition during TENS stimulation,[15] cases have been reported of asymptomatic inhibition of pacemaker output by TENS.[16,17] Interference is most likely to occur in significantly older pacemakers and pacemakers in the unipolar sensing configuration.

TENS can probably be used safely in most patients with bipolar pacemakers. However, it is reasonable to take special precautions in the pacemaker-dependent patient and monitor the response during initial TENS application. If TENS results in interference in patients with unipolar pacemakers, the testing can be repeated after reprogramming the sensitivity to a less sensitive value.

Dental Equipment

Dental ultrasound scalers may cause inhibition or asynchronous pacing in older pacemakers, but a recent study showed no effect on pacing function.[18] Repetitive activation of other dental equipment may cause inhibition.[19] Dental drilling can cause enough vibration to increase the pacing rate of an activity-sensing pacemaker.

Therapeutic Radiation

The dose of radiation used in diagnostic x-ray procedures, including coronary angiography, barium enemas, and cerebral angiography, for example, does not appear to affect pulse generator function either immediately or cumulatively. Therapeutic radiation can cause failure in contemporary pacemakers that incorporate complementary metal oxide semiconductor and integrated circuit technology.[20–22] ICDs have also been shown to fail when exposed to radiation.[20]

The amount of therapeutic radiation that causes a device to fail is unpredictable and may involve changes in sensitivity, amplitude, or pulse width; loss of telemetry; failure of output; or runaway rates. If dysfunction occurs, pacemaker replacement is required. Although some changes may resolve in hours to days, the long-term reliability of the pacemaker is suspect, and it should be replaced. It should be emphasized that radiation therapy to any part of the body away from the site of the pulse generator should not cause a problem with the generator, but it should be shielded to avoid scatter.

Centers that perform therapeutic radiation should have a protocol for patients with pacemakers.[23] Before radiation begins, the pacemaker should be identified and evaluated. The most common clinical situation is development of malignant disease of the breast on the ipsilateral side in a patient with a permanent pacemaker. The pacemaker must be moved out of the field of radiation, because shielding the pacemaker would result in suboptimal radiation therapy. The pacemaker can be explanted and a new system implanted on the contralateral side. Alternatively, it is often possible to explant the pacemaker, tunnel the existing long-term pacing lead through the subcutaneous tissues to the contralateral side, and form a new pacemaker pocket on the contralateral side. The pacemaker is reattached to the now-tunneled lead and reimplanted.

Electroconvulsive Therapy

Electroconvulsive therapy appears safe with respect to pacemaker function, as only a minimal amount of electricity reaches the heart because of the high impedance of body tissues. ECG monitoring during the procedure and interrogation of the pacemaker after the procedure are advisable. In unipolar pacemakers, seizure activity may generate sufficient myopotentials to result in inhibition or ventricular tracking.

The equipment used may also generate an electrical field capable of causing 60-cycle interference (Fig. 12–12).

Diathermy

Short-wave diathermy consists of therapeutic application of current directly to the skin. Diathermy can be a source of interference, and because of its high frequency, it should be avoided near the implantation site. It has the potential to inhibit the pulse generator or damage the pulse generator circuitry by excessive heating.

Impedance Plethysmography

Some patient monitoring systems can cause interference with minute ventilation sensing pacemakers. Specifically, interference can occur with a monitor in which impedance plethysmography is used to document the patient's respiratory rate and detect ECG lead disconnection. Because the minute ventilation sensor also functions by detecting a change in intrathoracic impedance, the monitor may result in inappropriate sensor-driven pacing.

When connected to such a monitor, the pacemaker sensor measures the summated impedance signals coming from the monitor, falsely interprets the information as an increase in transthoracic impedance, and increases the heart rate accordingly. As soon as the patient is disconnected from the monitor, the heart rate returns to the programmed lower pacing rate. Figure 12–13 shows an example of such monitor-driven interference.

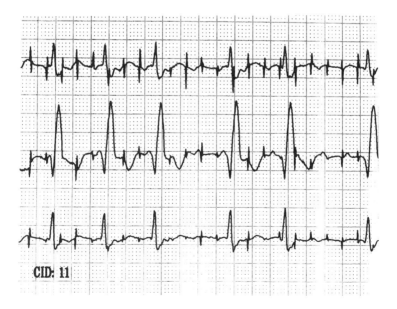

Fig. 12–12. Electrocardiographic tracing obtained after electroconvulsive therapy from a patient with a DDD pacemaker. The patient was hemodynamically stable at the time of electrocardiography. The artifacts were generated by the electroconvulsive therapy equipment, not by the pacemaker. When the power source for the equipment was turned off, the artifacts were no longer present.

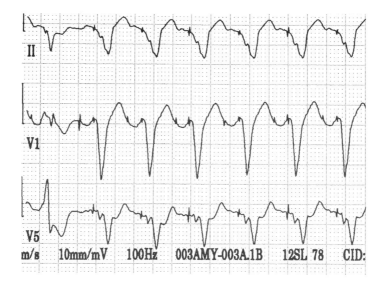

Fig. 12–13. Electrocardiographic tracing obtained postoperatively from a patient with a minute ventilation rate-adaptive DDDR pacemaker. The tracing reveals atrioventricular sequential sensor-driven pacing at a rate of approximately 120 bpm. The rate was driven by the respiratory monitor, which uses impedance plethysmography. When the monitor was disconnected, the paced rate returned to the programmed lower rate. (From Hayes DL, Wang PJ [editors]): Cardiac Pacemakers and Implantable Defibrillators: A Multi-Volume Workbook. Vol 4. ICDs and Pacemakers. Armonk, NY, Futura Publishing Company, 2000, p 32. By permission of the publisher.)

The Food and Drug Administration has issued an advisory about this phenomenon to manufacturers of monitoring equipment.[24] It is important that physicians working with such patients in the operating suite and intensive care unit be familiar with this circumstance.

Industrial Environment

Conventional wisdom has been to advise patients to avoid "arc welding" and close contact with combustion engines. This advice needs to be reexamined as pacemakers become more resistant to external interference. However, as previously discussed, pacemakers of unipolar sensing configuration remain more susceptible to EMI than pacemakers in a bipolar sensing configuration. For patients whose livelihood involves equipment with potential for EMI, a pacemaker with committed bipolar sensing configuration should be implanted.

Industrial environments with significant potential for clinically significant EMI with implantable devices include industrial-strength welding, that is, welding equipment exceeding 500 A, use of degaussing equipment, and induction ovens. If a patient works in one of these environments or potentially some other even more obscure environment that suggests significant potential for EMI, the work environment should be carefully evaluated. If the patient is pacemaker-dependent, consideration should be given to assessment of the work environment by an engineer from the pacemaker manufacturer. Some manufacturers are willing to send an engineer to the patient's work environment to conduct such testing. If the patient is not pacemaker-dependent, assessment may be achieved by ambulatory monitoring during exposure to the environment or by use of patient-triggered event records stored within the pacemaker (Fig. 12–14).

From a practical standpoint, most patients who claim to do "arc welding"

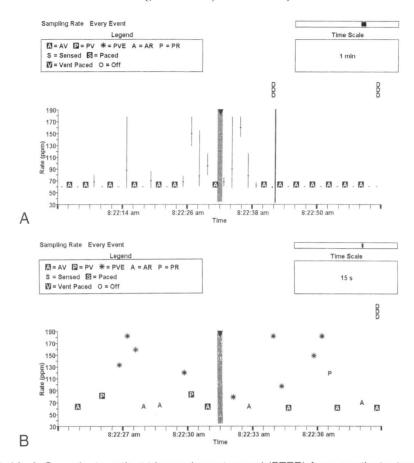

Fig. 12–14. *A,* One-minute patient-triggered event record (PTER) from a patient returning to the work environment after a pacemaker implantation. The work environment contained potential sources of electromagnetic interference (EMI). The PTER was obtained when the patient was in the vicinity of an EMI source. (The dark, thick central line is a reference point for the center of the recording. The lighter vertical lines indicate a rate variation at that point. The line with the designation "DDD" indicates the point of magnet application, and the pacemaker identifies the programmed mode at that time.) *B,* A "zoomed" 15-second portion of the preceding PTER. The pacemaker indicates frequent premature ventricular events (PVEs). This designation occurred only when the patient was near the EMI source, and it was suspected that these were not true PVEs but instead represented noise sensed on the ventricular sensing channel that led to inhibition. This explanation was confirmed by subsequent ambulatory monitoring. AR, paced atrial event to intrinsic ventricular event; AV, paced atrial event to paced ventricular event; PR, intrinsic atrial event to intrinsic ventricular event; PV, intrinsic atrial event to paced ventricular event.

use low-amperage equipment for hobby welding. If the patient uses welding equipment in the 100 to 150 A range, significant EMI is unlikely to occur.[25] However, before giving the patient permission to return to this activity, the pacemaker clinician must consider the type of hardware implanted and the dependency status.

Testing methods have been designed to allow exposure of the patient with a pacemaker or ICD to progressively stronger fields of EMI. Although this testing is not practical for the individual patient, the study cited[25] determined levels of interference at several programmed sensitivities (Table 12–5). This informa-

Table 12–5.
Electromagnetic Interference Levels in Work Environments
Capable of Pacemaker Interference

Sensitivity setting, mV	Atrial*		Ventricular*	
	Unipolar	Bipolar	Unipolar	Bipolar
0.5	4,509	17,984	1,720	14,240
0.75	5,744	20,000	NA	NA
1.0	7,679	20,000	4,705	18,100
1.5	10,143	20,000	NA	NA
2.0	11,790	20,000	7,454	19,630
3.0	15,034	20,000	10,003	20,000

NA, not available.
*Values in milligauss units

tion could be applied to an individual patient if readings of EMI strengths in the work environment could be obtained.

Nonindustrial and Home Environments

Many potential sources of EMI in the nonindustrial and home environments are capable of one-beat inhibition of the pacemaker (Table 12–6). However, it would be unusual for any of these sources to cause EMI of clinical significance. It would also be unlikely that any of the devices in Table 12–6 could cause sustained EMI resulting in clinically significant interference with an ICD. However, anecdotal reports exist.[26–28]

Although few sources can cause clinically significant EMI resulting in pacemaker malfunction, the potential for interference from cellular phones and electronic article surveillance equipment has been of intense interest because of possible public health issues. Before these are discussed in detail, several other potential sources, some of historical importance only, merit discussion.

One of the most common questions still asked by pacemaker recipients today is whether they can use a microwave oven. In many areas, signs are still in place warning the patient with a pace-

maker not to use a microwave oven. The original warnings were posted because ineffective microwave shielding and less effective shielding of early pacemakers created the potential for pacemaker interference. Microwave ovens are no longer considered a significant source of interference, partly because they have effective shielding and interlocking circuitry that prevents them from being switched on while the door is open; moreover, significant advances have been made in shielding the pacemaker circuitry.

Metal detectors are frequently mentioned as a potential problem, and warning signs are often seen at airport security stations. However, a study of patients wearing ambulatory ECG monitors while passing through metal detector gates with pacemakers at the most sensitive programmable option showed no effect on pacing.[29] Asynchronous pacing might occur for one or two beats without ill effect to the patient. The major reason to warn patients about metal detectors is that the pacemaker may "set off" the detector.

Electronic Article Surveillance Equipment

The antitheft device (electronic article surveillance equipment) in many depart-

Table 12–6.
Potential Sources of Electromagnetic Interference

Source	Pacemaker damage	Total inhibition	One-beat inhibition	Asynchronous pacing (noise)	Increased rate
Acupuncture	N	Y	Y	Y	N
Airport detector	N	N	Y	N	N
Antitheft equipment	?	?	Y	Y	?
Arc welder	N	Y	Y	Y	N
Cardioversion	Y	N	N	Y	Y
Cautery, coagulation	Y	Y	Y	Y	Y*,†
Cellular phone	N	Y	Y	Y	Y
CB radio	N	N	Y	N	N
CT scanner	N	N	N	N	N
Defibrillation	Y	N	N	Y	Y
Diathermy	Y	Y	Y	Y	Y
Drill, electric	N	N	Y‡	N	N
ECT, EST	N	Y	Y	Y	Y†
Electric blanket	N	N	Y‡	N	N
Electric shaver	N	N	Y‡	N	N
Electric switch	N	N	Y‡	N	N
Electrolysis	N	N	Y	Y	N
Electrotome	N	N	Y‡	N	N
Ham radio	N	N	Y	N	N
Heating pad	N	N	N	Y	N
Lithotripsy	Y†	Y‡	Y‡	Y‡	Y§
Metal detector	N	N	Y‡	N	N
Microwave	N	N	N	N	N
MRI	?	N	Y	Y	Y
PET scanner	?	N	N	N	N
Power line	N	N	N	Y	N
Radar	N	N	Y‡	N	N
Radiation, Dx	N	N	N	N	Y
Radiation, Rx	Y	N	N	N	Y
RF ablation	Y	Y	N	N	Y
TENS	N	Y	N	Y	Y
TV remote	N	N	N	N	N
Ultrasound, Dx	N	N	N	N	N

CB, citizens band; CT, computed tomography; Dx, diagnostic; ECT, electroconvulsive therapy; EST, electroshock therapy; MRI, magnetic resonance imaging; N, no; PET, positron emission tomography; RF, radiofrequency; Rx, therapeutic; TENS, transcutaneous electrical nerve stimulation; TV, television; Y, yes.

*Impedance-based pulse generators.

†Piezoelectric crystal-based pulse generators.

‡Remote potential for interference.

§DDD mode only.

ment stores consists of a tag or marker that is sensed by an electromagnetic field as the person walks through or by a "gate." Most systems consist of a "deactivator" that a cashier can use to remove or deactivate the tag after purchase of an item. This allows the customer to purchase an item and leave the store without activating an alarm. These electronic antitheft devices consist of multiple technologic systems that generate electromagnetic fields in various ranges, including the radiofrequency range of 2 to 10 mHz, magnetic material in the 50- to 100-kHz range, pulsed systems at various frequencies, and electromagnetic fields in the microwave range. In the Study of Pacemakers and Implantable Cardioverter-Defibrillator Triggering by Electronic Article Surveillance Devices (SPICED TEAS), 33 patients in whom 18 pacemakers and 17 ICDs had been implanted were exposed to six different electronic article surveillance (EAS) detectors.[30] Of the six, three were radiofrequency devices, one was magnetoacoustic, and two were magnetic. No reprogramming of or damage to pulse generators was noted. Sixteen of the pacemakers demonstrated noise reversion or inhibition when they were exposed to a magnetoacoustic system at a range shorter than 18 inches. Reprogramming the sensitivity of the pacemaker could not abolish this effect. In addition, one epicardial unipolar pacemaker exhibited inhibition or noise reversion in each magnetic device. No EMI effects on any of the ICDs were demonstrated. No EMI was detected in any patients during exposure to the radiofrequency system.

ICDs were assessed by exposure of 170 patients to three surveillance systems.[31] During extreme exposure, defined as 2 minutes of exposure within 6 inches of the surveillance system, interactions between the ICD and the EAS device were seen in only 19 patients. In 12 patients, the interaction was classified as minor. In the other seven patients, the interaction was clinically relevant, and in three of them, inappropriate ICD shocks probably would have occurred had the exposure continued. The authors concluded that it is safe for a patient with an ICD to walk through an EAS system but that lingering could result in an inappropriate ICD discharge.

In a case report, a patient with an ICD received inappropriate shocks because of oversensing of the pulsed electromagnetic signal.[32] The ensuing controversy resulted in a mailing from the Food and Drug Administration warning clinicians of potential interactions between EAS systems and implanted devices.[33] Although larger studies are needed to provide clinicians and patients with definitive guidelines, it is reasonable to advise patients to pass rapidly through any obvious EAS equipment and avoid leaning on or standing near the EAS equipment; that is, "Don't linger, don't lean."

Cellular Phones

A great deal of literature exists on cellular phones and the potential of pacemaker or ICD interference.[34–37] At least one case report detailed injury that occurred when a pacemaker-dependent patient used a digital cellular phone.[36]

In a multicenter study,[37] 980 patients were tested with as many as six phones for a total of 5,533 phone exposures. A highly variable incidence of interference was observed. The overall incidence of interference, 20%, was high, but to quote this single percentage out of context would be misleading clinically. Interference at the "normal" use ear position was very low, and none was clinically significant, supporting the safety of "normal" use. The incidences of interference and, specifically, clinically significant interference were also highly variable by combination of phone type, pacemaker manufacturer, and pacemaker model. When one phone (not commercially available) was eliminated from the analysis, the incidences of interference and clinically significant interference dropped significantly to 13.1% and 2.8%, respectively (Fig. 12–15).

Although symptoms were present during 7.2% of the phone exposures, most were due to palpitations. The incidence of interference was highly variable by pacemaker manufacturer. Even for a given manufacturer, the incidence varied by pacemaker model, reflecting the effect of design on susceptibility to interference.

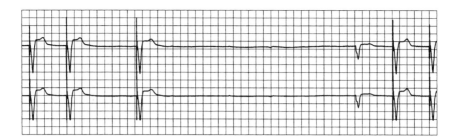

Fig. 12–15. Electrocardiographic tracing obtained during exposure to a cellular telephone from a patient with a VVIR pacemaker. The tracing reveals profound pacemaker inhibition. The patient became nearly syncopal, at which point the phone was removed. The phone used for testing is not commercially available.

The highest incidence of interference occurred when the phone was directly over the pacemaker. Although this position is possible if the activated phone were carried in a pocket directly over the pacemaker, it is certainly not a "normal" phone use position and could be consciously avoided. As stated earlier, minimal interference occurred at the ear position. Most adverse effects are eliminated if the phone is kept 8 to 10 cm from the implanted device.

Even though specific changes in pacemaker design, such as feed-through filters, have significantly reduced rates of interference, new phone technologies could result in the potential for pacemaker interference, thus requiring further testing.

Fewer data exist on ICD interference from cellular phones. Recent publications involving either a relatively small number of patients with ICDs or exposure to a limited variety of cellular phone technologies did not demonstrate any significant interference.[38,39]

Clinical Advice

Nearly all patients can be reassured that EMI will not affect their pacemakers during the course of daily life. Patients in specialized industrial environments should be assessed individually. Improvements in pacemaker and ICD resistance to EMI should continue to minimize clinical concerns. However, the potential for EMI should never be taken lightly, and appropriate screening and monitoring should be done to avoid adverse clinical outcomes. In addition, despite improvements in pacemaker resistance to EMI, emerging technologic advances result in new challenges for the patient with an implanted arrhythmia-control device. Newer technologies must be assessed for potential interference to the pacemaker or ICD.

References

1. Hayes DL, Strathmore NF: Electromagnetic interference with implantable devices. *In* Clinical Cardiac Pacing and Defibrillation. Second edition. Edited by KA Ellenbogen, GN Kay, BL Wilkoff. Philadelphia, WB Saunders Company, 2000, pp 939–952
2. Toivonen L, Valjus J, Hongisto M, Metso R: The influence of elevated 50 Hz electric and magnetic fields on implanted cardiac pacemakers: the role of the lead configuration and programming of the sensitivity. Pacing Clin Electrophysiol 14:2114–2122, 1991
3. Astridge PS, Kaye GC, Whitworth S, Kelly P, Camm AJ, Perrins EJ: The response of implanted dual chamber pacemakers to 50 Hz extraneous electrical interference. Pacing Clin Electrophysiol 16:1966–1974, 1993

4. Hayes DL, Trusty J, Christiansen J, Osborn MJ, Vlietstra RE: A prospective study of electrocautery's effect on pacemaker function (abstract). Pacing Clin Electrophysiol 10:686, 1987

5. Barold SS, Falkoff MD, Ong LS, Heinle RA, Willis JE: Resetting of DDD pulse generators due to cold exposure. Pacing Clin Electrophysiol 11:736–743, 1988

6. Pfeiffer D, Tebbenjohanns J, Schumacher B, Jung W, Luderitz B: Pacemaker function during radiofrequency ablation. Pacing Clin Electrophysiol 18:1037–1044, 1995

7. Ellenbogen KA, Wood MA, Stambler BS: Acute effects of radiofrequency ablation of atrial arrhythmias on implanted permanent pacing systems. Pacing Clin Electrophysiol 19:1287–1295, 1996

8. Holmes DR Jr, Hayes DL, Gray JE, Merideth J: The effects of magnetic resonance imaging on implantable pulse generators. Pacing Clin Electrophysiol 9:360–370, 1986

9. Hayes DL, Holmes DR Jr, Gray JE: Effect of 1.5 tesla nuclear magnetic resonance imaging scanner on implanted permanent pacemakers. J Am Coll Cardiol 10:782–786, 1987

10. Gimbel JR, Lorig RJ, Wilkoff BL: Safe magnetic resonance imaging of pacemaker patients (abstract). J Am Coll Cardiol 25:11A, 1995

11. Achenbach S, Moshage W, Diem B, Bieberle T, Schibgilla V, Bachmann K: Effects of magnetic resonance imaging on cardiac pacemakers and electrodes. Am Heart J 134:467–473, 1997

12. Lauck G, von Smekal A, Wolke S, Seelos KC, Jung W, Manz M, Luderitz B: Effects of nuclear magnetic resonance imaging on cardiac pacemakers. Pacing Clin Electrophysiol 18:1549–1555, 1995

13. Langberg J, Abber J, Thuroff JW, Griffin JC: The effects of extracorporeal shock wave lithotripsy on pacemaker function. Pacing Clin Electrophysiol 10:1142–1146, 1987

14. Cooper D, Wilkoff B, Masterson M, Castle L, Belco K, Simmons T, Morant V, Streem S, Maloney J: Effects of extracorporeal shock wave lithotripsy on cardiac pacemakers and its safety in patients with implanted cardiac pacemakers. Pacing Clin Electrophysiol 11:1607–1616, 1988

15. Rasmussen MJ, Hayes DL, Vlietstra RE, Thorsteinsson G: Can transcutaneous electrical nerve stimulation be safely used in patients with permanent cardiac pacemakers? Mayo Clin Proc 63:443–445, 1988

16. O'Flaherty D, Wardill M, Adams AP: Inadvertent suppression of a fixed rate ventricular pacemaker using a peripheral nerve stimulator. Anaesthesia 48:687–689, 1993

17. Chen D, Philip M, Philip PA, Monga TN: Cardiac pacemaker inhibition by transcutaneous electrical nerve stimulation. Arch Phys Med Rehabil 71:27–30, 1990

18. Agarwal A, Hewson J, Redding VJ: Ultrasound dental scalers and demand pacing (abstract). Pacing Clin Electrophysiol 11:853, 1988

19. Rahn R, Zegelman M: The influence of dental treatment on the Activitrax (abstract). Pacing Clin Electrophysiol 11:852, 1988

20. Rodriguez F, Filimonov A, Henning A, Coughlin C, Greenberg M: Radiation-induced effects in multiprogrammable pacemakers and implantable defibrillators. Pacing Clin Electrophysiol 14:2143–2153, 1991

21. Last A: Radiotherapy in patients with cardiac pacemakers. Br J Radiol 71:4–10, 1998

22. Souliman SK, Christie J: Pacemaker failure induced by radiotherapy. Pacing Clin Electrophysiol 17:270–273, 1994

23. Marbach JR, Sontag MR, Van Dyk J, Wolbarst AB: Management of radiation oncology patients with implanted cardiac pacemakers: report of AAPM Task Group No. 34. Med Phys 21:85–90, 1994

24. Burlington DB: Interaction between minute ventilation rate-adaptive pacemakers and cardiac monitoring and diagnostic equipment (10-14-98). Safety alerts, public health advisories, and notices from Center for Devices and Radiological Health, Federal Drug Administration. Retrieved January 13, 2000, from the World Wide Web: http://www.fda.gov/cdrh/safety.html

25. Marco D, Eisinger G, Hayes DL: Testing of work environments for electromagnetic interference. Pacing Clin Electrophysiol 15:2016–2022, 1992

26. Seifert T, Block M, Borggrefe M, Breithardt G: Erroneous discharge of an implantable cardioverter defibrillator caused by an electric razor. Pacing Clin Electrophysiol 18:1592–1594, 1995

27. Man KC, Davidson T, Langberg JJ, Morady F, Kalbfleisch SJ: Interference from a hand held radiofrequency remote control causing discharge of an implantable defibrillator. Pacing Clin Electrophysiol 16:1756–1758, 1993

28. Schmitt C, Brachmann J, Waldecker B, Navarrete L, Beyer T, Pfeifer A, Kubler W:

Implantable cardioverter defibrillator: possible hazards of electromagnetic interference. Pacing Clin Electrophysiol 14: 982–984, 1991

29. Copperman Y, Zarfati D, Laniado S: The effect of metal detector gates on implanted permanent pacemakers. Pacing Clin Electrophysiol 11:1386–1387, 1988

30. McIvor ME, Reddinger J, Floden E, Sheppard RC: Study of Pacemaker and Implantable Cardioverter Defibrillator Triggering by Electronic Article Surveillance Devices (SPICED TEAS). Pacing Clin Electrophysiol 21:1847–1861, 1998

31. Groh WJ, Boschee SA, Engelstein ED, Miles WM, Burton ME, Foster PR, Crevey BJ, Zipes DP: Interactions between electronic article surveillance systems and implantable cardioverter-defibrillators. Circulation 100:387–392, 1999

32. Santucci PA, Haw J, Trohman RG, Pinski SL: Interference with an implantable defibrillator by an electronic antitheft-surveillance device. N Engl J Med 339:1371–1374, 1998

33. Burlington DB: Important information on anti-theft and metal detector systems and pacemakers, ICDs, and spinal cord stimulators (9-28-98). Safety alerts, public health advisories, and notices from Center for Devices and Radiological Health, Federal Drug Administration. Retrieved October 5, 1999, from the World Wide Web: http://www.fda.gov/cdrh/safety.html

34. Hayes DL, Carrillo RG, Findlay GK, Embrey M: State of the science: pacemaker and defibrillator interference from wireless communication devices. Pacing Clin Electrophysiol 19:1419–1430, 1996

35. Irnich W, Batz L, Muller R, Tobisch R: Electromagnetic interference of pacemakers by mobile phones. Pacing Clin Electrophysiol 19:1431–1446, 1996

36. Yesil M, Bayata S, Postaci N, Aydin C: Pacemaker inhibition and asystole in a pacemaker dependent patient. Pacing Clin Electrophysiol 18:1963, 1995

37. Hayes DL, Wang PJ, Reynolds DW, Estes M III, Griffith JL, Steffens RA, Carlo GL, Findlay GK, Johnson CM: Interference with cardiac pacemakers by cellular telephones. N Engl J Med 336:1473–1479, 1997

38. Sanmartin M, Fernandez Lozano I, Marquez J, Antorrena I, Bautista A, Silva L, Ortigosa J, de Artaza M: The absence of interference between GSM mobile telephones and implantable defibrillators: an in-vivo study. Groupe Systemes Mobiles [Spanish]. Rev Esp Cardiol 50:715–719, 1997

39. Fetter JG, Ivans V, Benditt DG, Collins J: Digital cellular telephone interaction with implantable cardioverter-defibrillators. J Am Coll Cardiol 31:623–628, 1998

13

Follow-up

David L. Hayes, M.D.,
Paul A. Friedman, M.D.

The complexity of pacemaker and implantable cardioverter-defibrillator (ICD) follow-up has paralleled the increasing sophistication of the devices. Follow-up therefore requires a dedicated staff with a thorough understanding of managing implantable devices.

Follow-up of permanent pacemakers can be accomplished in more than one way: periodic visits to a pacemaker clinic, less frequent clinic visits in combination with transtelephonic monitoring (TTM), and TTM only. ICDs require in-clinic visits at this time, although TTM assessment of ICDs is technologically possible and will undoubtedly be possible in the near future.

In the United States, TTM in combination with periodic clinic visits is the most common follow-up method for larger centers. Some physicians who have a limited number of devices requiring follow-up prefer to see the patient periodically and avoid the need for TTM. In a very large follow-up center, follow-up by clinic visits only would quickly monopolize a large portion of the clinical resources.

TTM can be performed by the implanting center or by a commercial monitoring firm. Follow-up solely by TTM is suboptimal, because some patients undergoing pacemaker implantation may not be seen again until battery depletion indicators appear. Periodic clinic visits allow thorough evaluation and, if necessary, alteration of output settings, rate-adaptive settings, and so forth. Few patients would obtain maximum efficiency of their pacemaker if it remained at nominal or initially programmed values for the life of the pulse generator.

Requirements for a Device Follow-up Clinic

Space

Because of the specialized equipment necessary for pacemaker and ICD assessment and follow-up, dedicated space is desirable. There must be adequate space for

- Patient assessment, programming, and storage of all necessary programmers (Fig. 13–1).
- Electrocardiographic monitoring.
- Teaching tools, for example, written educational information, videotapes,

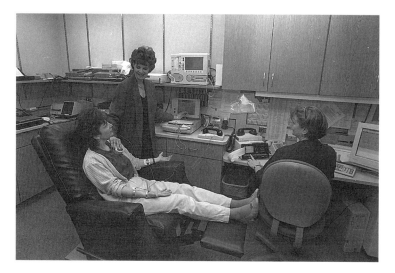

Fig. 13–1. Outpatient area for device programming. The chair reclines to a semisupine position. The programmers surround the area for easy access to any one of them.

videocassette recorder and screen, heart models (Fig. 13–2).

• Transtelephonic receiving station or stations. (The number of stations required is proportional to the overall volume of calls received.) (Fig. 13–3.)

• Record storage. (Even though most storage may be accomplished by computerized databases, in many centers some room is required for "paper storage.") (Fig. 13–4.)

• Resuscitative equipment.

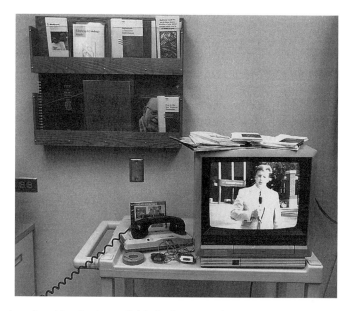

Fig. 13–2. Various teaching tools available in the outpatient area: videocassette recorder and videotapes (what the patient should expect at the time of implantation; transtelephonic monitoring), teaching brochures, heart model, etc.

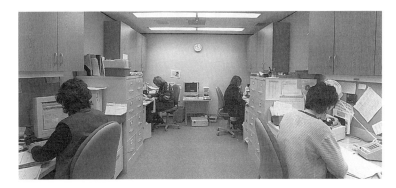

Fig. 13–3. Work area for nurses performing transtelephonic monitoring. The work area provides ready access to files, computer terminal, and receiving station.

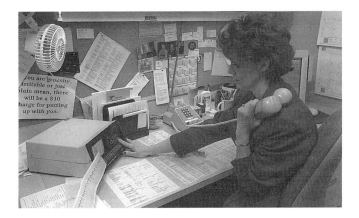

Fig. 13–4. Nurses' work area in pacemaker clinic.

Personnel

Personnel requirements in the pacemaker clinic include

- Allied professionals with expertise in pacemaker and ICD programming and follow-up. (Among them may be registered nurses, specially trained technicians, certified technologists [in some countries], physician assistants, and nurse practitioners.)
- Secretarial support.

Equipment

Equipment requirements include

- Electrocardiographic (ECG) monitoring. (This could be accomplished by the programmers. However, because some older programmers do not have this capability and independent monitoring is helpful in some situations, ECG monitoring should be available.)
- Programmers for all pacemakers and ICDs followed.
- Reclining chair or examining table for patient evaluation.
- Resuscitative equipment, including external cardioversion-defibrillation and external (transcutaneous) pacing.
- Transtelephonic receiving station or stations.
- Storage of technical manuals for all devices being followed. (Although most information can be obtained by calling the technical service department for the specific manufacturer, it

is best to have written reference material available in the pacemaker clinic. Some technical information is also available through manufacturers' web sites, and this source of technical information will undoubtedly become more important.)

Pacemaker Follow-up

Transtelephonic Monitoring

TTM has been part of pacemaker follow-up since approximately 1970.[1,2] For many years, this follow-up method was used only in the United States. Although still limited outside the United States, TTM is being used more widely.

Proponents of TTM believe that it is an effective method to monitor pacemaker battery status and to demonstrate normal or abnormal function. Admittedly, transtelephonic assessment of atrial events is much more difficult than assessment of ventricular events. In large part the reason is simply the small amplitude of the atrial signal, either paced depolarization or intrinsic depolarization. The pacemaker artifact may overwhelm the atrial event, whereas the usually larger ventricular event is not commonly overshadowed by the ventricular pacing artifact.

Obtaining TTM tracings of good quality is also an issue. Patients with pacemakers are often elderly, and without excellent initial teaching and possibly coaching during the TTM calls, they may have difficulty handling the transtelephonic equipment. We request that a family member or friend be present during the initial teaching session. It is often reassuring to the patients to know that someone else has the information necessary to complete the transmission should they forget a portion of the instructions. Transmission difficulties may be compounded if the patient has a significant hearing deficit. Incorrect use of the transtelephonic transmitter and im-

proper magnet placement may impair the quality of the transmission.

Some types of telephones may be suboptimal for TTM. For example, with cordless phones, the quality of transmission at times is decreased and there is a greater chance of being disconnected. Speaker phones and phones with altered volume controls may also present problems. Any source of electromagnetic interference close to the site of the patient's transtelephonic transmission may induce significant artifacts.

The frequency of TTM differs among centers. The Health Care Financing Administration (HCFA) has established guidelines for pacemaker follow-up and reimbursement for follow-up.[3] Reimbursement generally is not allowed for more frequent follow-up than that specified by the HCFA guidelines. The current guidelines are as follows:

Category I (These apply to most contemporary pacemakers)
Single-chamber pacemakers:

- 1st month—every 2 weeks
- 2nd through 36th month—every 8 weeks
- 37th month to failure—every 4 weeks

Dual-chamber pacemakers:

- 1st month—every 2 weeks
- 2nd through 6th month—every 4 weeks
- 7th through 36th month—every 8 weeks
- 37th month to failure—every 4 weeks

Category II (These apply only to pacemaker systems [pacemaker and leads] for which sufficient long-term clinical information exists to assure that they meet the standards* of the Inter-Society Commis-

---

*The ICHD standards are (1) 90% cumulative survival at 5 years after implantation and (2) an end-of-life decay of less than a 50% decrease in output voltage and less than a 20% deviation in magnet rate, or a decrease of 5 bpm or fewer, over 3 months or longer.

sion for Heart Disease Resources [ICHD] for longevity and end-of-life decay) Single-chamber pacemakers:

- 1st month—every 2 weeks
- 2nd through 48th month—every 12 weeks
- 49th through 72nd month—every 8 weeks
- Thereafter—every 4 weeks

Dual-chamber pacemakers:

- 1st month—every 2 weeks
- 2nd through 30th month—every 12 weeks
- 31st through 48th month—every 8 weeks
- Thereafter—every 4 weeks

Mayo Clinic Guidelines (Same guidelines apply to single- and dual-chamber pacemakers)

- 1st month—every week
- 2nd month until first signs of battery depletion—every 3 months
- Onset of battery depletion to elective replacement indication—every 4 weeks

The less frequent follow-up schedule used at our institution results in significant cost savings for providers, such as Medicare, over the life of the pulse generator.[4] We have also demonstrated that the less frequent schedule does not compromise follow-up.[5]

Equipment

To perform TTM, the patient must have access to the necessary TTM equipment. Typical transmitting equipment is shown in Figure 13–5. Transmission requires contact with the patient's skin, that is, electrodes on the wrists or the chest. After calling the pacemaker clinic or commercial follow-up center, the patient places the telephone over the transmitting equipment.

In the pacemaker clinic, a receiving center is used to obtain the ECG tracings the patient transmits. As shown in Figure 13–6, the typical receiving center is coupled with a telephone in the pacemaker clinic during the actual transmission.

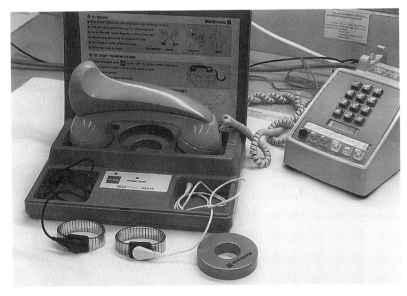

Fig. 13–5. Equipment used by the patient for transtelephonic monitoring. In addition to the telephone, the patient requires a transmitter and electrodes. Various types of electrodes can be used.

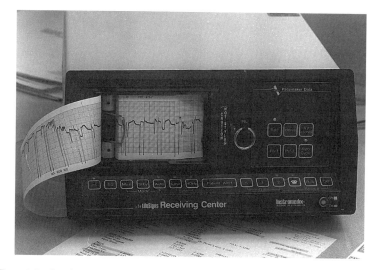

Fig. 13–6. Transtelephonic receiving center. During electrocardiographic transmission, the patient is instructed to transmit for approximately 30 seconds. However, if the transmission needs to be interrupted for any reason, an alarm can be sent from the receiving center. If the patient hears the alarm, he or she is instructed to stop the transmission attempt and pick up the phone.

Transtelephonic Monitoring Sequence

A significant amount of information can be obtained transtelephonically. The order in which the information is collected may vary. The following sequence is used by our clinic.

- Brief discussion with the patient to determine general well-being and elucidate any problems the patient believes may be related to the pacemaker
- Nonmagnet "free-running" tracing (duration, 30 seconds)[3]
- Magnet tracing (duration, 30 seconds)[3]
- Patient informed of pacemaker status; next TTM transmission or clinic visit scheduled
- TTM data stored

If the nonmagnet tracing displays intrinsic rhythm, the underlying rhythm should be noted and compared with previous transmissions. If there is intermittent pacing or pacing in only one chamber of a dual-chamber device, sensing can be assessed.

The magnet tracing should be used to assess

- Capture (for dual-chamber devices, capture should be determined for both chambers)
- Magnet rate
- Pulse width (for dual-chamber devices, pulse width should be determined for both chambers)

Magnet response varies not only from manufacturer to manufacturer but also among models from one manufacturer (Fig. 13–7). Specific magnet response for many different devices is difficult to commit to memory. Therefore, it is helpful to have the specific magnet response recorded on the patient's records (Fig. 13–8).

The health care professional taking the transmission should be familiar with the elective replacement indicators for the specific pacemaker. Measurements from the patient's previous transmission should be available for comparison.

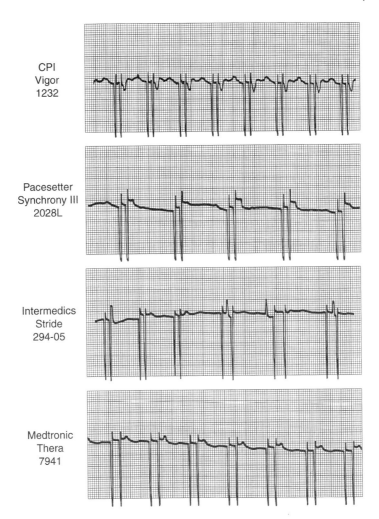

Fig. 13–7. Composite of magnet responses from four different dual-chamber pacemakers. Magnet response, *top* to *bottom:* CPI device to 100 bpm with an abbreviated atrioventricular interval (AVI). Pacesetter device to programmed lower rate with an abbreviated AVI. Intermedics pacemaker to rate of 100 bpm for 3 beats and an abbreviated AVI and then reversion to programmed AVI and programmed lower rate limit. Medtronic pacemaker to rate of 85 bpm.

Pacemaker Information:					
Implant Date: 08/11/1999	Model: 7088		Program Mode	DDDR	P. Amp. A 2.00
Manufacturer: Medtronic	ERI: VVI at 65		Program Rate:	60.00	P. Amp. V 2.50
Device Status: Current	Backup Mode: Rate 65 either pro mode or		Max Sensor Rate:	120.00	
Monthly Check: Pulse width increa			Max Track:	120.00	

ECG | Followup | Measured Values | **Threshold Values** | Complications | Providers | Encounter Note

Lead Threshold Values:

Type	Pulse Width	Voltage	Energy	Impedance	Current	Sensing
Atrial	0.15	1.00	0.40	467.00		1.00
Ventricular	0.09	1.00	0.20	687.00		11.20

Fig. 13–8. A computer screen that is part of the follow-up section of our computerized database. The screen provides generator identification, limited programming information, and magnet rate at elective replacement indicator (ERI).

Other specific information can be obtained from specific pacemakers. The proprietary Threshold Margin Test (TMT) provides some information on pacing threshold at the onset of magnet application[6] (Fig. 13–9). The first three pacemaker artifacts occur at a rate of 100 bpm. As part of the TMT, the pulse duration of the third pacemaker stimulus is 75% of the programmed pulse duration. Failure to capture with the reduced pulse duration provides some information about threshold and pacing margin of safety.

Vario is another proprietary method that provides threshold information.[7] With this feature, magnet application results in 16 asynchronous beats at the magnet rate of 100 bpm followed by 16 asynchronous beats at 125 bpm. During the 16 beats at 125 bpm, the voltage output is reduced by 1/15 progressively until zero output is reached (Fig. 13–10). Removal of the magnet returns full output at the next stimulus. The Vario mode can be activated for the test procedure only or programmed "on" permanently.

Telemetered data cannot be obtained transtelephonically at this time. However, technology to make this possible is currently undergoing investigation. In the relatively near future, it will be possible to obtain programmed parameters and stored and measured data transtelephonically for pacemakers and defibrillators.

Pacemaker Clinic Follow-up Visit

The detail required during the pacemaker clinic visit depends on the follow-up technique or techniques used.[8] Our practice is to see the patient in the pacemaker clinic at approximately 3 months

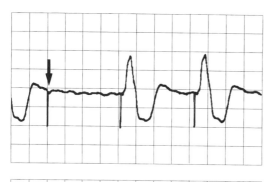

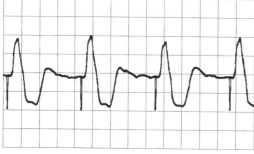

Fig. 13–9. Electrocardiographic tracings from a patient with a VVI Medtronic pacemaker programmed to a rate of 70 bpm and 5.0 V. The pacemaker is capable of a Threshold Margin Test (TMT) during magnet application. In the *upper panel*, the pulse duration is 0.5 msec. There is failure to capture with the first pacing artifact seen (*arrow*). This pacing artifact is the third of three asynchronous pulses at 100 bpm that occur with magnet application. As part of the Threshold Margin Test, the pulse duration of this pacemaker stimulus is 75% of the programmed pulse duration of 0.5 msec. A suprathreshold stimulus is at 0.5 msec, but at 75% of this output duration (equivalent to a pulse duration of 0.375 msec), failure to capture occurs. In the *lower panel*, the programmed pulse duration is 0.7 msec. The first pacing artifact is again the third of three asynchronous pulses and is therefore at 75% of the programmed duration, or 0.525 msec, and capture is maintained. (Modified from Hayes DL: Programmability. *In* A Practice of Cardiac Pacing. Edited by S Furman, DL Hayes, DR Holmes Jr. Mount Kisco, NY, Futura Publishing Company, 1986, pp 219–251. By permission of the publisher.)

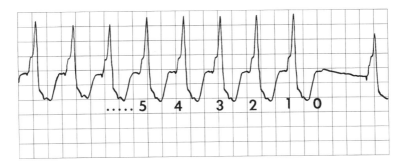

Fig. 13–10. Final portion of a Vario test of a pacemaker programmed to 5.0 V. Capture is maintained at 0.3 V, indicated here by "1," and appropriately there is no capture when output is 0 V (0). Following this, a paced ventricular event occurs at the programmed lower rate of 60 bpm. (From Hayes DL: Programmability. *In* A Practice of Cardiac Pacing. Third edition. Edited by S Furman, DL Hayes, DR Holmes Jr. Mount Kisco, NY, Futura Publishing Company, 1993, pp 635–663. By permission of Mayo Foundation.)

after implantation, at yearly intervals, and at any time a problem is noted by TTM or the patient has a concern that may be pacemaker-related. At the time of each pacemaker clinic visit, the following steps are completed.

- Retrieval of previous data and follow-up records
- Discussion and interview with the patient
- Interrogation of the pacemaker
- Assessment of stored data
- Programming sequence
- Assessment of rate-adaptive parameters
- Radiographic assessment
- Data storage

Retrieval of Previous Data and Records

At the onset of the pacemaker clinic visit, records should be available. These should include information from the patient's previous clinic visits and most recent transtelephonic transmissions.

Discussion and Interview

The patient should be interviewed in an attempt to elucidate any clinical problems that could potentially be related to pacemaker-related problems (Table 13–1). It is important to have some knowledge of the most commonly noted pacemaker problems.[9] These are discussed in detail in Chapter 9.

At our institution, the pacemaker clinic does not serve as the primary health care or cardiac care provider, and the extent of the physical examination is related to suspected problems. For example, if no clinical problem is suspected, the examination is limited to inspection of the pacemaker site. If the patient has hemodynamic symptoms suggestive of pacemaker syndrome, physical examination includes assessment of jugular veins and postural blood pressure measurements with and without pacing (Table 13–1).

At other centers, the pacemaker clinic may serve as the primary health care provider and may therefore provide a complete physical examination at periodic visits.

Assessment of Stored Data

In some pacemakers, initial interrogation results in a printout of stored data. In other pacemakers, these data must be specifically requested. It may be necessary to obtain stored data before programming, because a permanent change in programming may "clear" stored data.

Contemporary pacemakers may have

Table 13–1.
Common Symptoms and Possible Pacemaker-Related Causes

Symptoms	Considerations
Palpitations	• Rapid paced ventricular rates • Tracking of sinus tachycardia or supraventricular arrhythmia • Pacemaker-mediated tachycardia • Atrial failure to capture with retrograde conduction and tracking of the premature atrial contraction • Intrinsic (non-pacemaker-related) tachyarrhythmia or extrasystoles
Weakness, fatigue, malaise	• Pacemaker syndrome • Failure to capture • Inappropriately programmed rate-adaptive parameters • Disease process unrelated to the permanent pacemaker
Dyspnea	• Pacemaker syndrome • Underlying cardiac or pulmonary disease
Hiccups	• Phrenic nerve stimulation
Muscle stimulation	• Loss of generator coating in unipolar system • Loss of insulation integrity of the pacing lead
Presyncope, syncope	• Pacemaker syndrome • Failure to capture • Oversensing with inhibition • Vasodepression
Cough	• Pacemaker syndrome
Chest pain	• Pacemaker syndrome

Modified from Goldschlager et al.[8] By permission of WB Saunders Company.

the capability of storing a great deal of data. The data may provide invaluable assistance in achieving optimal programming and in diagnosing intermittent symptoms.[10] Categories of stored information include

- Event counters (Fig. 13–11)
- Rate histograms (Fig. 13–12)
- Electrograms (Fig. 13–13)
- Measured values (Fig. 13–14)
- Special diagnostic features (Fig. 13–15)

Programming Sequence

A specific sequence should be adopted and followed for programming. This sequence is discussed in detail in Chapter 7. It is not important that this specific sequence be followed, but it is crucial that all steps be completed in some orderly manner to avoid deletion of any necessary steps.

Rate-Adaptive Parameter Programming

As discussed in Chapter 8, the patient's rate requirements may change over time. For example, in the chronotropically incompetent patient in whom rate response is restored, the newly found rate response may allow the patient to begin an exercise program and improve conditioning. With subsequent improvement in conditioning, a change in rate-adaptive parameters may be desired, such as higher paced rates and a faster increment in heart rate.

Conversely, if symptomatic coronary artery disease were to develop in a patient with a rate-adaptive pacemaker, it may be desirable to make the rate-adaptive parameters less sensitive to avoid rate-related angina while the coronary artery disease is being evaluated and treated.

We routinely assess exercise infor-

```
┌─────────────────────────────────────────────────────────────────────────┐
│ Cardiac Pacemakers, Inc.                                        VIGOR     │
├─────────────────────────────────────────────────────────────────────────┤
│                            19-FEB-99        11:50                          │
│ Institution:                                                              │
│                                          Programmer:       007167         │
│ 1232 Generator:     Serial   203080      2880 Software:         4.1       │
└─────────────────────────────────────────────────────────────────────────┘
```

	Totals	Zone 1 <= 70	Zone 2 70- 85	Zone 3 85-100	Zone 4 100-130	Zone 5 130-200
ATRIUM						
Paced	17.7M	13.0M	3.5M	1.1M	153.5K	299
	86%	63%	17%	5%	1%	0%
Sensed	2.9M	2.5M	381.1K	17.8K	1.3K	163
	14%	12%	2%	0%	0%	0%
VENTRICLE						
Paced	20.6M	15.5M	3.9M	1.1M	153.8K	302
	100%	75%	19%	5%	1%	0%
Sensed	13.5K	1.8K	5.0K	3.8K	2.7K	219
	0%	0%	0%	0%	0%	0%

A-Tachy Response	0
PVCs	6.2K

Time Since Last Setup
   7.2 months

Fig. 13–11. Telemetered data classifying cardiac events as paced or sensed for both atrial and ventricular channels.

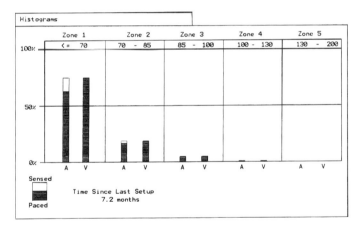

Fig. 13–12. Telemetered data displaying rate histograms, that is, distribution of heart rates since the counters were previously cleared.

mally at each clinic visit. The patient is also questioned about activity level. This is especially important the first time rate-adaptive parameters are initiated. However, since activity levels change—increase with better conditioning and improvement in well-being or decrease because of associated medical problems—it is wise to inquire about any change in activity before assessing and possibly changing rate-adaptive parameters.

After a standard programming sequence and assessment of rate histograms, informal exercise is performed. If the patient's subjective response to pacing and the rate histograms imply optimal rate response, no alteration in programming is made before exercise assessment. If the rate histogram suggests suboptimal rate response (Fig. 13–16), the rate-adaptive parameters are reprogrammed before informal exercise.

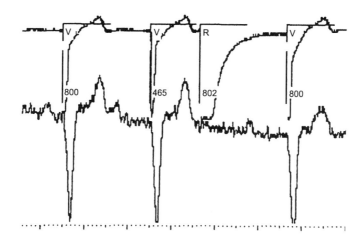

Fig. 13–13. Telemetered intracardiac ventricular electrogram (*top*) and simultaneous surface electrocardiographic tracing (*bottom*). In this example, the electrogram confirms intracardiac detection of some event, classified as "R" for an intrinsic QRS complex. The marked fluctuation of the electrogram and lack of a simultaneous event on the surface tracing suggest a "make-or-break" fracture. V, paced ventricular event.

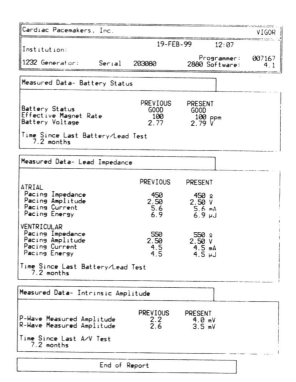

Fig. 13–14. Telemetered measurements of battery voltage, battery impedance, and lead impedance.

Informal exercise is completed in the following manner. The patient has previously been connected to the transtelephonic receiver by wrist electrodes to allow single-lead ECG monitoring during programming. The cable is disconnected from the receiver, bracelets are left in place, and the patient is asked to hold the end of the cable. The patient is then asked to walk the clinic halls at a pace that feels "casual" for a minimum of 2 minutes. At the end of the walk, the cable is imme-

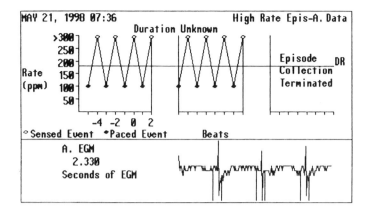

Fig. 13–15. Telemetered data of an atrial tachycardia episode. This is one of many special diagnostic features stored and telemetrically retrievable by various devices. This example details a specific episode of atrial tachycardia.

diately plugged in, and with the receiving mode at "standby," the ECG can be obtained at once and peak heart rate recorded. If telemetry is available, it is the preferred method of monitoring the patient during exercise. We use telemetry if rate-adaptive programming is performed in the inpatient setting. Alternatively, the rate histogram can be assessed for the focused period of informal exercise.

For the patient who exercises vigorously, formal exercise may be important. If formal (treadmill) exercise is performed and the rate-adaptive pacemaker being optimized has an activity sensor, the patient should avoid holding on to the treadmill. Holding the treadmill railing may blunt the sensor response and lead to inappropriate programming (see Chapter 8).

```
Cardiac Pacemakers, Inc.                                      VIGCR

                              19-FEB-99        11:50
Institution:
                                         Programmer:      007167
1232 Generator:     Serial   203080      2880 Software:       4.1
```

	Totals	Zone 1 <= 70	Zone 2 70- 85	Zone 3 85-100	Zone 4 100-130	Zone 5 130-200
ATRIUM						
Paced	17.7M	13.0M	3.5M	1.1M	153.5K	299
	86%	63%	17%	5%	1%	0%
Sensed	2.9M	2.5M	381.1K	17.8K	1.3K	163
	14%	12%	2%	0%	0%	0%
VENTRICLE						
Paced	20.6M	15.5M	3.9M	1.1M	153.8K	302
	100%	75%	19%	5%	1%	0%
Sensed	13.5K	1.8K	5.0K	3.8K	2.7K	219
	0%	0%	0%	0%	0%	0%

```
A-Tachy Response         0
PVCs                     6.2K

Time Since Last Setup
   7.2 months
```

Fig. 13–16. Rate data from a patient with sensor-driven pacing. The information collected demonstrates that 80% of the paced atrial activity was less than or equal to 85 bpm. Depending on the patient's activity level, this may be consistent with suboptimal rate response and suggests possible need for reprogramming the sensor to more aggressive settings.

Radiographic Assessment

Radiographic assessment of the pacemaker or ICD may provide critical information. This is discussed in detail in Chapter 9, and additional comments on radiography of ICDs are made later in this chapter. We do not routinely obtain a chest radiograph for every pacemaker clinic visit. For the patient with a pacemaker, one is obtained yearly or before any invasive procedure, such as replacement of the pulse generator.

Data Storage

It is critical that the programmed data and battery and lead measurements be stored in some manner for future reference. Depending on the size of the follow-up clinic and available facilities, possibilities include paper storage and computerized database.

Printouts of measured data and initial and final programmed parameters can be posted in a permanent record to allow comparison with subsequent pacemaker evaluations. This method may work well for centers with smaller volumes of patients. For large numbers of patients, paper storage becomes cumbersome. Computer storage of data is more efficient. The data can be entered into various data screens (Fig. 13–17 through 13–20), or with some programs, it may be possible to download data directly from the pacemaker programmer to the database.

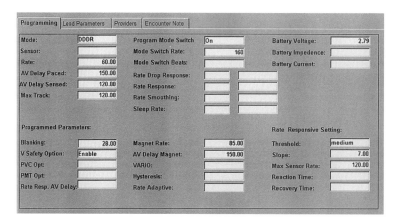

Fig. 13–17. Computerized data storage providing programming information that can be referred to during transtelephonic monitoring or a clinic visit.

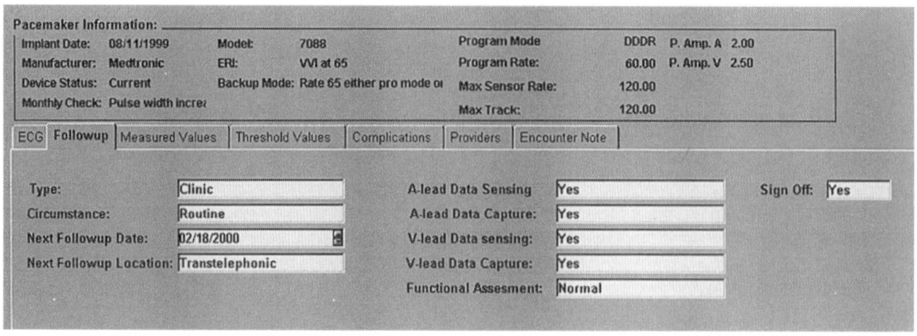

Fig. 13–18. Computer entry site for details of a specific follow-up visit. Menus provide various designations, such as type of follow-up visit, routine or emergency, and verification of normal sensing and pacing.

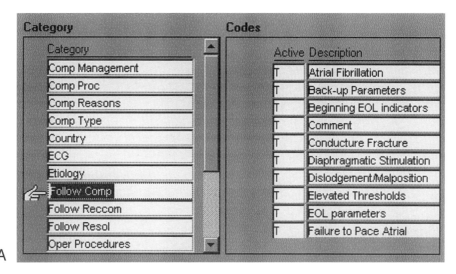

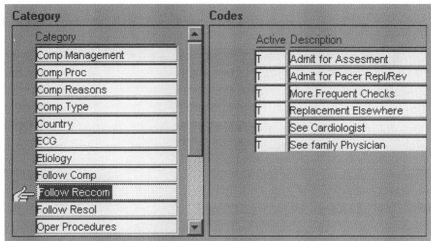

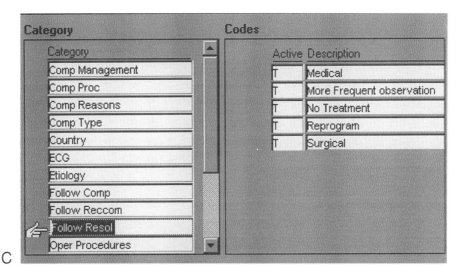

Fig. 13–19. Menus of categories related to pacemaker complications and follow-up. *A,* Menu of follow-up complications. *B,* Menu of follow-up recommendations. *C,* Menu of follow-up resolutions.

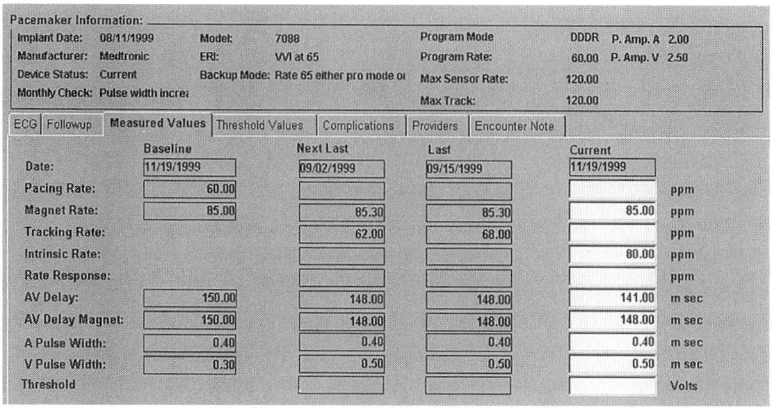

Fig. 13–20. Follow-up entry of current measured values and comparison with the two previous measurements and with baseline values.

If patient data are computerized, several additional functions may be available for data management, including

- Keeping track of follow-up schedules
- Automatic reminders of patients delinquent in follow-up
- Ability to query for outcome data or to assess performance of specific leads or pulse generators
- Billing functions

Implantable Cardioverter-Defibrillator Follow-up

Follow-up of patients with implantable defibrillators is in many respects similar to that of patients with pacemakers. Indeed, with the progressive integration of pacemaker and defibrillator technology, assessing the "pacemaker" function of the defibrillator has become a standard part of ICD evaluation. However, the evaluation also has specific ICD components, discussed below.

In general, follow-up of patients with ICDs has two components: assessment of patient status and assurance of normal device function, with screening for potential complications. Since most patients with defibrillators have significant structural heart disease, cardiovascular medical evaluation is important. Assessing the defibrillator function can be further divided into assessing pulse generator function, assessing lead integrity, ensuring appropriate patient-specific therapy (defibrillation threshold, therapy for ventricular tachycardia, and review of stored episodes) (Table 13–2). This comprehensive approach can be done expeditiously in a dedicated pacemaker-ICD clinic, ensures proper device function, and can unmask device-related complications before they become clinically manifest.

Assessment of Patient Clinical Status

Of the 460 patients receiving biphasic waveform implantable defibrillators at the Mayo Clinic through July 1998, only 3% had primary electrical disease (Fig. 13–21); the others had structural heart disease of one form or another. Most patients had coronary artery disease (64%) or dilated cardiomyopathy (23%); previous myocardial infarction was present in 41% of the patients, and 29% had previous coronary artery bypass grafting.[11] Since pharmacologic therapy can significantly reduce mortality in patients with structural heart disease, a defibrillator clinic check provides an opportunity for review

Table 13–2.
Routine Follow-up Evaluation of
Implantable Cardioverter-Defibrillators

Cardiovascular-medical condition of the patient
- Changes in status (myocardial infarction, new congestive heart failure, syncope, change in medications, etc.)
- Screening for use of appropriate mortality-reducing medications for cardiovascular disease or depressed ventricular function (or both)

Defibrillator function
- Pulse generator status
  - Remaining battery life
  - Capacitor formation and charge time
  - (Rarely) software update and correction
- Lead integrity
  - Real-time telemetry with provocative maneuvers
  - Evidence of failure on stored electrogram
  - X-ray assessment
  - Pacing threshold
  - R wave and P wave
  - Pacing impedance
  - High-voltage lead impedance
- Patient-specific programming and therapy
  - Adequate defibrillation threshold
  - Appropriate ventricular tachycardia programming (antitachycardia pacing, cardioversion)
  - Review of stored episodes

of medical status and for providing or arranging for additional medical evaluation as needed. Moreover, significant changes in cardiovascular status, such as myocardial infarction near the sensing lead, can directly affect device function. Knowledge of the patient's medical status may also guide management of arrhythmias (e.g., whether to add beta-blocking agents or reprogram a defibrillator to manage atrial fibrillation with rapid ventricular response).

Pulse Generator Assessment

With the current generation of implantable defibrillators, solid state pulse generator electronics have become highly reliable, and the main purpose of pulse generator assessment is to ensure that an adequate charge remains in the battery. Moreover, when pulse generator defects do occur, they can sometimes be manifested by premature battery depletion or be detected by other telemetered data. Telemetry failure itself may be a marker of significant malfunction or battery depletion.

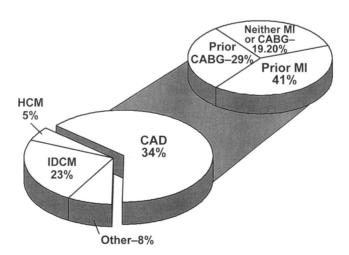

Fig. 13–21. Heart disease in implantable defibrillator recipients at the Mayo Clinic. CABG, coronary artery bypass graft; CAD, coronary artery disease; HCM, hypertrophic cardiomyopathy; IDCM, idiopathic dilated cardiomyopathy; MI, myocardial infarction. (Modified from Trusty et al.[11] By permission of Futura Publishing Company.)

Battery Status

The single most common indication for device replacement is battery depletion. Early devices used lithium vanadium pentoxide batteries, which maintained a constant voltage throughout their lifetimes when under a low current load. Therefore, battery status was indirectly assessed by charging the capacitor and recording the charge time. Most new ICDs use lithium silver vanadium oxide chemistry, in which the unloaded voltage provides a reasonable estimate of remaining battery life. Battery voltages gradually decline from beginning of life (BOL), to middle of life (MOL), to appearance of the elective replacement indicator (ERI), and to end of life (EOL). Guidant programmers show a gas gauge figure with labels BOL, ERI, and so on, graphically depicting the remaining useful battery life when the device is interrogated (Fig. 13–22 A). Other manufacturers display the actual device voltage in tabular format, often with reference values for ERI and EOL (Fig. 13–22 B).

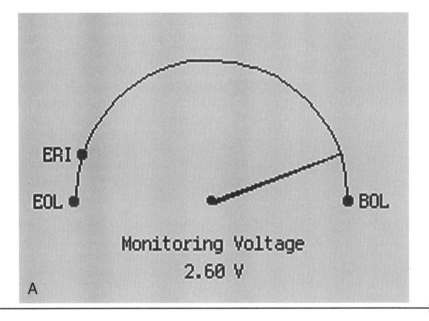

Fig. 13–22. Elective replacement indicators. A, The Guidant programmer has a "battery gauge" display that graphically depicts remaining battery life based on the monitoring (unloaded) battery voltage. BOL, beginning of life; ERI, elective replacement indicator; EOL, end of life. B, Device interrogation printouts provide the information in numerical tabular form and give the charge time. "Monitoring voltage" is the unloaded voltage used to assess longevity, whereas "charging voltage" is the lowest voltage recording during capacitor charge, used to determine EOL (further details in text). The pacemaker parameter summary is also shown. C, Medtronic status report. Battery voltage and reference values are provided at the top left; below is the capacitor information. "Last Capacitor Formation" is the most recent charge held for at least 10 minutes on the capacitor (starting with an energy of less than 1 J). "Last Charge" may not meet this criterion and is often the most recent capacitor charge for therapy delivery. On the right is the lead information. "Lead Impedance" shows the pacing impedance (assessing the conductors used by the pacing circuit). "Defibrillation (HVB)" shows the impedance of a low-energy (imperceptible) pulse delivered from the lead tip to the distal coil and measured between the coils. This value is normally lower than the impedance of an actual shock (typically from 11 to 20 Ω but varying depending on lead configuration), so that it should be compared with previous HVB measurements. "Last High Voltage Therapy" shows the actual impedance, energy, and waveform of the last shock delivered. Pacing parameters are summarized on a separate page (not shown).

```
Guidant                                          VENTAK PRIZM DR
                                                 29-MAR-00 12:18
Institution
Model      185:      RAM Version     2901 Programmer        007473
Serial     302076        1.2         2844 Software             1.1
                    Measured Data Report

┌─────────────────────────────────────────────────────────────────┐
│ Battery Status                                                    │
└─────────────────────────────────────────────────────────────────┘

Last Interrogation                  29-MAR-00 12:15

Last Delivered Shock                29-MAR-00 12:10
  Energy                                   31 J
  Charge Time                            10.5 sec
  Shock Impedance                          44 Ω

Auto Capacitor Re-form                     90 days
Last Capacitor Re-form              29-MAR-00 11:09
  Charge Time                            11.3 sec

Cumulative Charge Time              01:14 m:s
Time Since Implant                      0 months
Battery Status                         BOL
  Monitoring                           3.24 V
  Charging                             2.37 V
```

┌───┐
│ Intrinsic Amplitude Test   │
└───┘

Atrial	Date/Time	Ventricular	Date/Time
3.4 mV N/R	29-MAR-00 11:47	19.8 mV N/R	29-MAR-00 11:47

┌───┐
│ Lead Impedance Test   │
└───┘

Atrial	Date/Time	Ventricular	Date/Time
500 Ω N/R	29-MAR-00 11:47	642 Ω N/R	29-MAR-00 11:47

Shock	Date/Time
44 Ω N/R	29-MAR-00 11:47

┌───┐
│ Pace Threshold Test   │
└───┘

Atrial	Date/Time
0.6 V @ 0.5 ms N/R N/R N/R	29-MAR-00 11:47

Ventricular	Date/Time
0.6 V @ 0.5 ms N/R N/R N/R	29-MAR-00 11:48

B End of Report

ICD Model: Gem 7227   Sep 16, 1999 16:39:43
Serial Number: PIP105976H   9962 Software Version 2.0
                                                 Copyright (c) Medtronic, Inc. 1997
Status Report   Page 1

Last Interrogation: Sep 16, 1999 18:26:29

Battery Voltage
(ERI=2.55 V EOL=2.40 V)

Sep 16, 1999 18:14:03
Voltage   3.03 V

Last Capacitor Formation*

Sep 16, 1999 16:30:24
Charge Time   9.54 sec
Energy   0.0 - 35.0 J

Last Charge

Sep 16, 1999 18:12:07
Charge Time   7.19 sec
Energy   0.1 - 35.0 J

Lead Impedance
Sep 16, 1999 17:48:46
V. Pacing   349 ohms
Defibrillation (HVB)   16 ohms

Last High Voltage Therapy
Sep 16, 1999 18:12:08
Measured Impedance   36 ohms
Delivered Energy   35.3 J
Waveform   Biphasic
Pathway   AX>B

Device Status
Charge Circuit is OK.

C *Minimum Auto Cap Formation Interval is 6 months.

The ERI voltage varies from manufacturer to manufacturer and even from model to model from the same manufacturer (Table 13–3). The ERI voltage is a function of the power delivery of a particular battery, the current drain from the monitoring circuitry, and the capacitors used by the device. Thus, the ICD clinic

Table 13–3.
Device Replacement Indicators for Selected Defibrillators*

Manufacturer	Device	Elective replacement indicator	End of life
Guidant	Ventak P2/P3 (models 1620, 1625, 1630, 1635)	4.99–4.7 V	4.7–4.24 V
	Ventak PRx II/III (models 1715, 1720, 1721, 1725)	4.99–4.7 V	4.7–4.24 V
	Ventak Mini family (models 164x, 174x, 176x, 178x,179x)	2.45–2.3 V, or second charge time ≥ 18 sec (≥ 20 sec for Ventak Mini IV)	2.3 V or less, or second charge time ≥ 25 sec (≥ 30 sec for Ventak Mini IV)
	Ventak AV family (models 181x, 182x, 183x)	4.90–4.4 V, or second charge time ≥ 18 sec	4.4 V or less, or second charge time ≥ 30 sec
	Ventak VR (models 1774, 1775)	4.90–4.40 V, or second charge time ≥ 20 sec	4.40 V or less, or second charge time ≥ 45 sec
Medtronic	7216A	Battery voltage < 5.11 V, or two charge times ≥ 11 sec	Battery voltage ≤ 4.19 V
	7201, 7217	Battery voltage ≤ 4.97 V, or two charge times ≥ 11 sec	Battery voltage ≤ 4.74 V
	7202, 7218, 7219, 7220	Battery voltage ≤ 4.91 V, or two charge times ≥ 14.5 sec	Battery voltage ≤ 4.57 V
	7221	Battery voltage ≤ 4.91 V, or charge times ≥ 60 sec	Battery voltage ≤ 4.57 V
	Micro Jewel 7223 Cx	Battery voltage ≤ 4.91 V	Battery voltage ≤ 4.57 V or second charge time ≥ 60 sec
	GEM 7227	Battery voltage ≤ 2.55 V	Battery voltage ≤ 2.40 V
	GEM DR 7271	Battery voltage ≤ 4.91 V	Battery voltage ≤ 4.57 V
Ventritex	Profile M.D (model V186HV3)	2.55–2.50 V	2.50–2.40 V
	Augstrom M.D (model V190HV3)	2.55–2.50 V	2.50–2.40 V
	Augstrom II (model V180HV3)	2.55–2.50 V	2.50–2.40 V
	Contour M.D (model V175)	2.55–2.50 V	2.50–2.40 V
	Contour II (model V185)	2.55–2.50 V	2.50–2.40 V
	Contour (model V145)	2.50–2.40 V	2.50–2.40 V

*Replacement voltages vary from manufacturer to manufacturer and among individual devices from the same manufacturer, so that replacement voltage for a specific defibrillator must be confirmed.

must have a readily available list of device-specific ERI voltages. Additionally, the monitoring voltage may be depressed immediately after a capacitor charge, so that this measurement is best made more than 30 minutes after device discharge or capacitor formation.[12]

Once a battery is depleted to the ERI voltage, the time remaining until device malfunction varies, depending on the model, the degree of antibradycardia pacing, and the number of shocks delivered. Typically, plans for elective pulse generator replacement should be made within 3 months. To be certain that the ERI voltage is detected, patients are seen more often in the pacemaker clinic as the voltage gets lower. Newer generation Medtronic devices include a programmable patient alert feature that generates an audible tone for a number of device conditions, including battery depletion to the ERI voltage. Similarly, Guidant devices have a programmable "beep on ERI" feature. Patients are instructed to visit the clinic whenever they hear a tone from the device.

In contrast to the ERI voltage, which is measured in the unloaded state, the EOL voltage is the minimum loaded voltage, recorded while the battery is maximally stressed. This usually occurs during capacitor charge. If interrogation shows that the voltage has declined to EOL at any time, this response signifies that during a capacitor charge or other heavy current draw, the battery voltage dipped below acceptable levels. A device should be replaced before EOL is reached, and immediate device replacement should be considered if an EOL voltage is seen, as subsequent function may be unreliable.

Capacitor Status

Defibrillators require the use of capacitors to accumulate and store charge before a shock is delivered, because a battery is unable to deliver the high level of voltage and current needed over such a short interval. Implantable devices use electrolytic capacitors, since these have a high energy density and consequent small size. However, electrolytic capacitors develop relatively large leakage currents over time, which can be reduced by recharging ("reforming") the capacitors. With early ICDs, patients had to be seen in the clinic every few months for capacitor reforming. All new devices offer either programmable or automatic capacitor reforming. In devices with programmable charge times, the charge frequency can depend on the specific device, the age of the device, or the most recent charge time (so that capacitor formation frequency is increased if the charge time becomes too long). "Smart" reforming devices recognize a full energy charge as a capacitor-reforming event. Generally, failure to reform capacitors with sufficient frequency can result in significant delays for the *first* shock during therapy delivery; subsequent therapies in the same episode are not affected, because the capacitor is reformed after the first charge. Excessively frequent capacitor formation does not harm the device or its functionality, although battery depletion may be accelerated. With many newer devices, capacitor formation is as important for the battery as for the capacitor. If the battery is not "pulsed" periodically, internal resistance develops, which can lead to a voltage delay (and delayed capacitor charge) when the capacitor is charged to deliver a shock therapy.

For the clinician, the most pertinent capacitor information is the charge time, which is actually a measure of both battery and capacitor function; it is provided on device interrogation (Fig. 13–22 *B* and 13–22 *C*). Some manufacturers have used charge time to indicate pulse generator EOL. Although acceptable charge time can vary from device to device, a full capacitor charge generally should not exceed 15 to 20 seconds. Charge times associated with device ERI and EOL are listed in Table 13–3.

Software Revisions

Increasingly, implantable devices contain microprocessors, with programmable instructions (software) held in device memory, which determine function. Device functionality, including the addition of features such as new pacing algorithms, can be noninvasively loaded into the device by telemetry (done only for clinical studies, to date). Rarely, device malfunction may be due to a "software bug." For example, in some Guidant Ventak AV models (II, II DR, and III DR), a malfunction developed that could result in lack of pacing for 24 hours. These devices routinely perform an internal battery test every 24 hours. If this test occurs within 30 msec of a ventricular paced event, ventricular output is disabled for 24 hours (until the next check), although the marker channel continues to show a ventricular pacing marker (Fig. 13–23). A software patch was inserted into programmers, so that simply interrogating an affected device injects new software into the permanent memory of the ICD, eliminating the problem. The ability to modify, correct, or improve device function by noninvasively altering the contents of its permanent memory may permit even greater flexibility in the future.

Assessing Lead Function

Evaluation of pacing, sensing, and pacing impedance is similar to that of pacemakers, discussed in previous sections of this chapter. Like some pacemakers, newer defibrillators will soon incorporate automatic pacing threshold assessment features. In pacemakers, post-pacing polarization—present on most pacing leads—can obscure local evoked response, requiring special lead construction or current-utilizing algorithms. In defibrillators, however, determining capture from an evoked response (i.e., local myocardial depolarization in response to a pacing stimulus) is simplified by the absent or minimal polarization potential found on the far-field electrograms[13] (Fig. 13–24) (far-field and near-field electrograms are discussed below). The remainder of this section discusses assessment of lead function beyond pacing, sensing, and pacing impedance evaluation, focusing on issues unique to defibrillators.

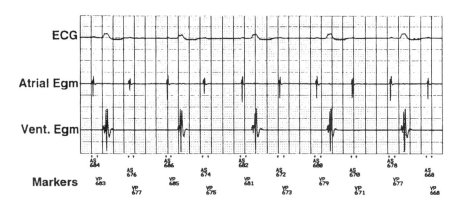

Fig. 13–23. Lack of ventricular output due to software error. Note that surface leads demonstrate absence of pacing artifact despite the suggestion of ventricular pacing by the interpretive markers. Noninvasive software injection corrects this malfunction permanently. Details in text. ECG, electrocardiogram; Egm, electrogram. (From Coppess MA, Miller JM, Zipes DP, Groh WJ: Software error resulting in malfunction of an implantable cardioverter defibrillator. J Cardiovasc Electrophysiol 10:871–873, 1999. By permission of Futura Publishing Company.)

Capture

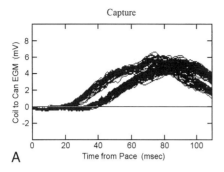

Non Capture

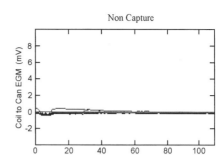

A

B

Fig. 13–24. Evoked response to assess capture. Since in defibrillators with true bipolar leads the coil and can are not used during pacing, polarization voltages are absent, permitting determination of whether a pacing pulse captures the ventricle. *A*, Composite tracing with multiple individual captured beats superimposed to show the evoked response in a 100-msec window following the pacing pulse. This evoked response is easily detected and could be used by future devices to automatically determine pacing capture and pacing thresholds. *B*, Composite tracing with multiple individual pacing pulses that failed to capture shows the absence of an evoked response. (Modified from Splett et al.[13] By permission of Futura Publishing Company.)

The defibrillator lead faces the harsh environment of the human body, undergoes mechanical stress at implantation and during its lifetime, and is the element of the defibrillation system most prone to failure. Lead design, implant location, and pulse generator location can influence the risk of lead failure.

Epicardial Systems

Lead failure rates are particularly high with epicardial systems. Although new epicardial systems are rarely used because nonthoracotomy systems are widely available, many patients still have these systems. As seen in Figure 13–25, up to 28% of epicardial patches with Medtronic models 6897 and 6927 fail at 4 years of follow-up. Moreover, we found that 58% of epicardial lead malfunctions were asymptomatic, diagnosed by failed defibrillation, lack of pacing output, lead abnormalities at routine pulse generator replacement, or radiographic evidence of fracture.[14] Because epicardial systems have mechanically separate defibrillation and pace-sense leads, lack an electrical method of assessing the defibrillation

patches other than by delivering a shock, and suffer from high rates of failure, we recommend annual ventricular fibrillation inductions to ensure appropriate system function.[15] Additionally, since 62% to 68% of fractures are found with careful radiographic review of the entire system (Fig. 13–26), radiographs should be checked every 6 months.[14] Complete recommendations for follow-up are discussed below. Importantly, subcutaneous patches have a construction design similar to that of epicardial patches and carry a 2.5% to 7.5% risk of malfunction, so that these systems may also require more careful follow-up. Although subcutaneous leads were used in 48% of monophasic endovascular systems, with the availability of biphasic waveforms they are required in only 3.7% of systems.[11]

Transvenous Systems

Pulse Generator Location. The remainder of this section deals with the now widely used totally endovascular biphasic systems. As with epicardial systems, pulse generator location and lead construction can importantly affect lead reliability.

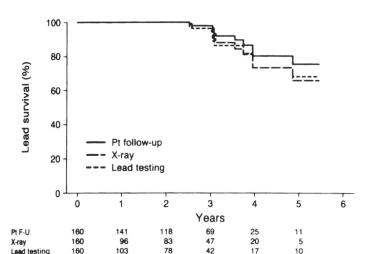

Pt F-U	160	141	118	69	25	11
X-ray	160	96	83	47	20	5
Lead testing	160	103	78	42	17	10

Fig. 13–25. Long-term epicardial lead survival free from malfunction. Each curve uses a different end point. "Patient follow-up" curve assumes leads are functioning in surviving patients at follow-up if there is no documented malfunction. "X-ray" curve determines lead survival as the interval from implantation to the most recent radiograph demonstrating an intact system. "Lead testing" curve (the most rigorous assessment) measures survival as the time from implantation to the last electrical test documenting normal lead function or as the interval from implantation to lead failure. The ordinate shows cumulative lead survival free from fracture, and the abscissa depicts follow-up in years. Note that the epicardial lead failure rate is 28% at 4 years. This suggests that epicardial systems require careful surveillance. Further details in text. (Modified from Brady et al.[14] By permission of the American College of Cardiology.)

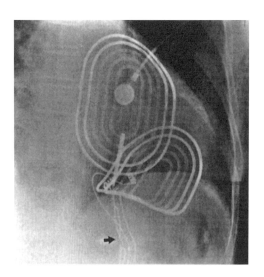 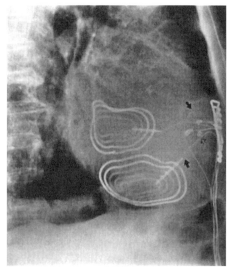

Fig. 13–26. Chest radiographs demonstrating conductor fractures in an epicardial lead system. *Left,* Subtle fracture (*arrow*) of midlead body of model 6897 patch is seen on posteroanterior view. *Right,* Lateral radiograph shows lead fractures close to anterior and inferior Medtronic model 6897 patches (*solid arrows*) and a fractured helix displaced from adjacent Medtronic model 6917 pace/sense lead (*open arrow*). (Modified from Brady et al.[14] By permission of the American College of Cardiology.)

Although abdominal placement is not widely used for transvenous biphasic systems, a number of such systems have been implanted, particularly with earlier, larger pulse generators or in small patients, who may not tolerate pectoral placement. In a long-term study of lead failure that included 379 patients, at 4 years of follow-up we found that the rate of lead failure was 12% for pectoral systems and 40% for abdominal systems[16] (Fig. 13–27). Lead failure was defined as an ICD system malfunction requiring surgical lead revision for correction. If an abdominal system fails, the abdominal pocket should be abandoned and a pectoral system implanted. We found that if a new lead was placed after lead failure with continued use of the abdominal pocket, the rate of recurrent failure within 6 months was 60% (Fig. 13–28). Failure in abdominal systems most likely is due to the greater lead length, tunneling required for lead insertion, and mechanical trauma of the lead against the pulse generator shell in the abdominal pocket. The high recurrence rate suggests that once failure is ev-

ident, the factors that led to abdominal system malfunction remain.

Lead Design. Lead design can also affect the risk of lead failure in transvenous systems. We found that 43% of failures were due to evident conductor or insulation defects (the remainder represented late dislodgment or an inability to appropriately pace or sense without manifest lead defect). All failures due to a clear conductor or insulation defect occurred in coaxial leads. In contrast to multiluminal leads, coaxial leads use concentric conductors with insulating layers between each coiled "cylinder" (Fig. 13–29). Because of their higher failure rate, systems with coaxial leads should also have closer follow-up; a reasonable schedule includes clinic evaluations every 3 months and consideration of annual defibrillation testing. Although the outer conductor in coaxial leads is the high-voltage defibrillation coil, available data show that when these leads fail, the possible manifestations are pace-sense abnormalities,

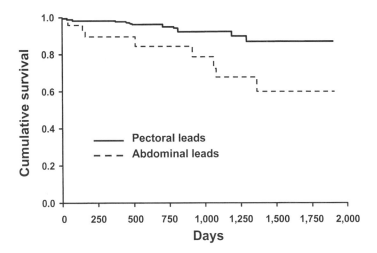

Fig. 13–27. Long-term freedom from malfunction of totally endovascular (transvenous) pectoral and abdominal lead systems. The ordinate shows cumulative survival and the abscissa time in days. At 48 months, the lead failure rate is significantly higher in systems with abdominally placed pulse generators (40%) than in pectoral systems (12%; $P = 0.01$). This finding suggests that abdominal systems require careful surveillance. (Modified from Friedman et al.[15] By permission of Futura Publishing Company.)

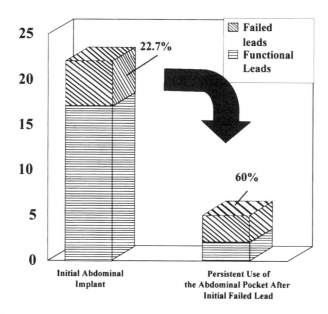

Fig. 13–28. Comparison of initial and recurrent lead failure for totally endovascular (transvenous) leads connected to an abdominally placed pulse generator. On the ordinate is the number of leads, with diagonal hatches in each bar indicating failed leads. The bar on the left shows the group with follow-up from the time of initial cardioverter-defibrillator implantation; 22.7% of the leads failed during this period. The bar on the right shows the outcome for five patients in whom a surgical procedure was performed to correct initial lead failure, with continued use of the abdominal pocket. In this group, three patients (60%) experienced recurrent lead failure within 6 months of the reoperation. This result suggests that after initial failure of an abdominal lead, a pectoral system should be used, because the factors that led to initial failure remain present.

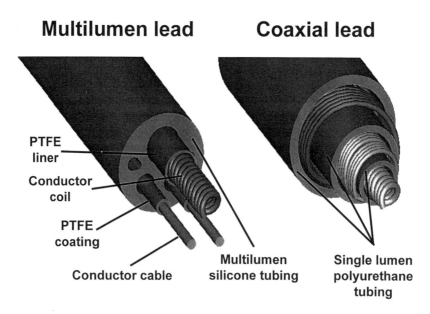

Fig. 13–29. Multilumen lead design (*left*) and coaxial lead design (*right*). Polytetrafluoroethylene (PTFE) is an insulation element. (Modified from Friedman et al.[15] By permission of Futura Publishing Company.)

inappropriate shocks (in 60%), electrogram evidence of electrical noise or oversensing (in 70%), and x-ray evidence of fracture (in 50%), so that the need for inductions and shock delivery is less well defined. Nonetheless, isolated defibrillation lead failures have been observed, and we prefer the more conservative approach (annual inductions) in these patients because of the increased risk of system malfunction and the potential for silent isolated outer conductor defect.

Diagnostic Tests for Assessing Lead Function. Of the diagnostic information available for assessing lead integrity—stored electrograms, inappropriate shocks, system radiography, and pacing parameter assessment (Table 13–2)—stored electrogram data were the most frequent indicators of lead malfunction in our series, consistent with their utility in other series[17–20] (Fig. 13–30). This occurs because the defibrillator's sensing function provides essentially continuous monitoring. Even though lead malfunction may be intermittent, if at any time enough electrical noise is created by failure to trigger detection of a "tachyarrhythmia" episode, it is recorded as a stored event (in most new devices) or will declare itself as an

inappropriate therapy (Fig. 13–31). Furthermore, in our series, there were no lead failures in multiluminal pectoral biphasic systems in which the only manifestation of malfunction was apparent at defibrillation threshold testing. In other words, even failures that adversely affected defibrillation or resulted in an abnormal high-voltage lead impedance were also detectable by another diagnostic test.[21] Thus, in contrast to failure in older epicardial and coaxial lead systems, defibrillation lead failure in biphasic systems becomes evident even without defibrillation testing. Therefore, in these newer systems, defibrillation testing is not needed to assess lead integrity.

Additionally, Medtronic recently introduced low-energy (imperceptible to the patient) test pulses of the high-voltage lead circuit. They can assess lead integrity daily and generate an audible tone when potential lead malfunction is detected.[22,23] Although low-energy pulses cannot detect all defibrillation lead failures (Fig. 13–32), they will further decrease the potential risk of "silent" defibrillation lead malfunction. Because in rare instances lead failure can be detected only by high-energy shock, delivering a maximum-energy shock during testing may be useful to confirm lead integrity. (Note: A

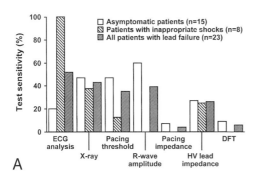
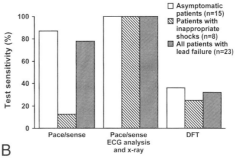

Fig. 13–30. Sensitivity of available diagnostic tests for the diagnosis of lead malfunction in biphasic transvenous implantable defibrillators in 379 patients with follow-up of 20 ± 16 months. *A*, Sensitivity of each test applied in isolation. *B*, Sensitivity of combined tests. In no case was defibrillation threshold (DFT) testing required to diagnose lead failure. ECG, electrocardiographic; HV, high-voltage.

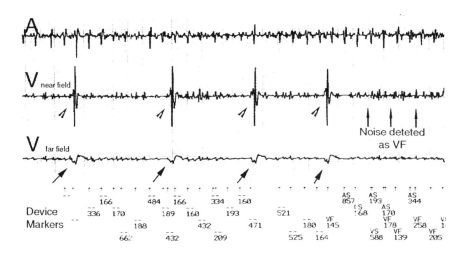

Fig. 13–31. Electrogram of noise caused by lead failure, leading to an inappropriate shock in a dual-chamber defibrillator. Shown from top to bottom are the atrial electrogram (during atrial fibrillation), the near-field ventricular electrogram, the far-field ventricular electrogram, and device markers. *Arrowheads* and *arrows* point to the actual QRS complexes. Noise occurs throughout the ventricular recordings, but on the far right the noise becomes large enough to be sensed by the defibrillator (note the "VF" markers at bottom far right of strip). The sensed noise is detected as ventricular fibrillation (VF), resulting in shock delivery. Stored electrograms make actual diagnosis possible. AS, atrial sensing; VS, ventricular sensing.

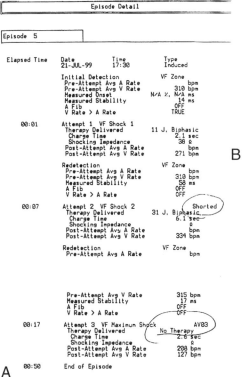

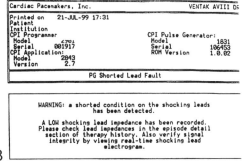

Fig. 13–32. Latent insulation defect that became manifest only after maximum-energy shock. Testing was performed at the time of pulse generator replacement, with use of chronic leads. During a previous test (not shown), a 17-J shock successfully terminated ventricular fibrillation (VF) with an impedance of 38 Ω. *A,* The first shock delivered, 11 J, failed but was associated with a normal impedance of 38 Ω. VF was appropriately redetected, and a maximum output shock ("Attempt 2," 31 J) resulted in a low impedance short circuit ("Shorted"). External rescue was successful (recorded by the device as "Attempt 3"). Direct inspection of the lead revealed a small insulation defect, which clinically became manifest only with high-energy shocks, leading to arcing between the lead and the active can in the pectoral pocket. *B,* A device warning printed after interrogation indicates the lead fault.

more detailed discussion, including the actual findings on stored electrograms suggestive of lead failure, can be found in Chapter 9.)

Radiography. Radiographic examination of the implantable defibrillator detected lead malfunction in 43% of nonthoracotomy systems and 68% of epicardial systems in our series.[14,21,24] Findings of authors have differed on the usefulness of chest and abdominal radiographs for detecting lead malfunction.[14,15,25] Nonetheless, because system radiography is simple, inexpensive, and noninvasive, it should be used routinely for periodic evaluation of system integrity.

In epicardial leads, no one fracture site predominates, and the entire lead system must be visualized.[14] In transvenous systems, particular attention should be paid to the region between the clavicle and the first rib, where anatomical constraints predispose to crush injury (Fig. 13–33). Also important to note is that the construction of many Endotak series leads produced an apparent radiographic fracture at the distal end of the proximal coil.

This "pseudofracture" of the Endotak lead (Fig. 13–34) should not be confused with an actual conductor defect. System radiography is discussed in greater detail in Chapter 11.

Assessing Patient-Specific Function

Defibrillation Threshold Testing

In addition to assessing lead integrity, the rationale for routine arrhythmia induction is to assess continuing defibrillation efficacy. The well-documented rise in the defibrillation threshold (DFT) over time in monophasic systems has been eliminated with the introduction of biphasic active can systems.[26–28] However, although the population DFT remains stable with biphasic systems, individual patients may have a critical increase in the DFT requiring system revision, and in previous reports (with fewer than 40 patients), these increases were not predictable.[28] However, we recently studied the long-term DFT in 262 patients with a mean follow-up of 32 ± 17 months.[24] As in the previous report, we found a 10-J increase

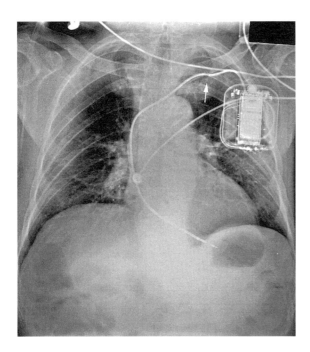

Fig. 13–33. Chest radiograph of lead with subclavian crush injury. Lead damage is at the site indicated by the *arrow*. (Modified from Friedman et al.[15] By permission of Futura Publishing Company.)

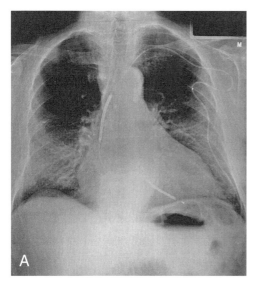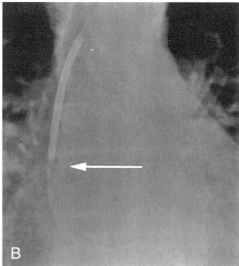

Fig. 13–34. "Pseudofracture" of an Endotak lead. *A,* In a chest radiograph of a normal Endotak lead, lead construction results in a radiographically apparent fracture at the distal end of the proximal coil without any true lead defect. This appearance should not be confused for a true fracture. *B,* Note lucency at *arrow.* This lucency is seen in Endotak leads in series 0060 and 0070.

in DFT in 13% of patients. However, all patients with a critical increase in DFT had an implantation DFT of 15 J or higher.[24] None of the 174 patients with an initial DFT of less than 15 J had a critical rise in DFT. Thus, although agreement is not universal, the preponderance of evidence and the largest series show that only a subset of patients—those with previously borderline defibrillation function—require routine DFT testing to detect increased DFTs at follow-up.[24,26,27,29] Note that these findings apply only to *routine* testing for screening. A number of specific clinical circumstances may suggest a need for additional arrhythmia induction; these are summarized in Table 13–4.

Ventricular Tachycardia Testing

Induction of ventricular tachycardia has long been regarded as useful for assessing the effectiveness of antitachycardia pacing (ATP) and for excluding arrhythmia acceleration. However, recent studies have questioned this approach and have suggested that empirical thera-

pies may be as effective as those guided by electrophysiologic study (EPS). In a study by Schaumann et al.,[30] the overall episode success rate for EPS-guided ATP was 95%, compared with 90% for empirical ATP. Importantly, for an individual patient, the success of ATP with guided therapy was no different from that with empirical therapy (82%, EPS-guided; 85%, empirical; P = NS). Additionally, the rates of arrhythmia acceleration were similar (2.5%, EPS-guided; 5%, empirical). We tend not to routinely induce ventricular tachycardia unless there is a clinical indication, such as to change programmed parameters because of clinical episodes of arrhythmias or inappropriate therapy.[29]

Stored and Real-time Electrogram Review

At routine follow-up, it is important to review real-time as well as stored electrograms. The real-time electrograms and markers can give important information on mechanical lead integrity and sensing function.[31] All third- and later-generation

Table 13–4.
Clinical Circumstances Suggesting the Need for Defibrillator
Evaluation and Consideration of Arrhythmia Induction

Clinical situation	Considerations
• Recurrent shocks, therapies	Lead failure; inappropriate therapies for atrial arrhythmias; recurrent or refractory ventricular arrhythmias
• New antiarrhythmic drugs (affect defibrillation threshold or ventricular tachycardia rate, or both)	Antiarrhythmic drugs can alter ventricular tachycardia rate, requiring reprogramming; can also affect defibrillation threshold
• Significant change in clinical status: myocardial infarction, deteriorating cardiac function	Can affect sensing (if infarction involves tissue near sensing lead); require new medications; rarely, affect defibrillation threshold
• Reprogramming to a lower sensitivity (e.g., for T-wave oversensing)	Might result in underdetection of ventricular fibrillation
• Other events: pneumonectomy, patch crinkle, and so forth	Can affect defibrillation threshold

ICDs can display both near-field and far-field electrograms (Fig. 13–35). Far-field electrograms are typically recorded between the defibrillation coil and the pulse generator shell. Thus, they are produced by widely spaced bipoles with electrodes having a large surface area, and recordings can be from more distant myocardium. The far-field electrogram more closely resembles the surface ECG, often demon-strates p waves (when they are present), and is useful for providing morphologic information about the QRS complex.

The morphologic information provided by far-field electrograms can be useful for differentiating supraventricular from ventricular tachycardias when stored electrograms are reviewed (Fig. 13–36). Differentiating supraventricular tachycardia from ventricular tachycardia

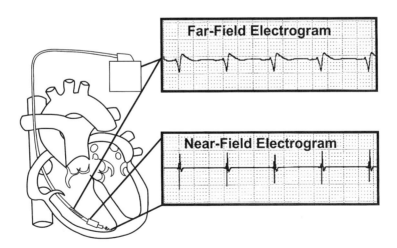

Fig. 13–35. Far-field and near-field electrograms. The far-field electrogram, recorded between the distal coil and the defibrillator can, provides morphologic information (e.g., narrow or wide complex), and p waves are often seen (as in this example). The near-field electrogram has a high slew (slope) and is useful for determination of intracardiac heart rate, but it provides limited morphologic information.

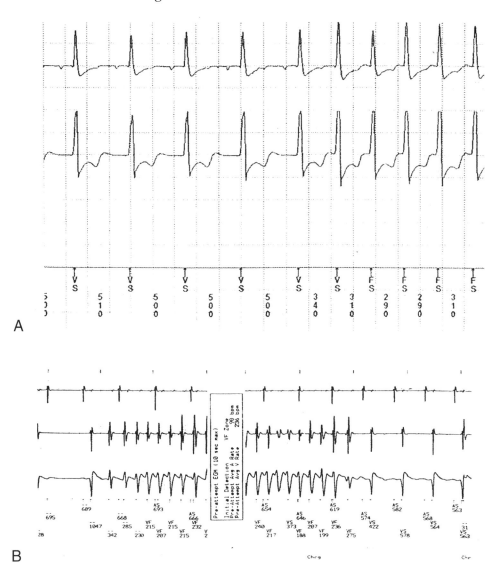

Fig. 13–36. Utility of electrograms for differentiating supraventricular tachycardia from ventricular tachycardia. *A,* Atrial fibrillation in ventricular fibrillation (VF) zone. Electrograms (top two tracings) and markers (bottom) are shown. Sinus rhythm (labeled "VS") is interrupted by atrial fibrillation (note lack of change in QRS morphology and increased heart rate), which is sensed by the device in the VF zone ("FS" markers). This could lead to inappropriate shock for atrial fibrillation; the electrograms permit actual rhythm diagnosis, so that reprogramming or rate control therapy can be used to correct the problem. *B,* Stored electrogram of a tachyarrhythmia episode in a patient with a dual-chamber implantable cardioverter-defibrillator. Shown, from top to bottom, are the atrial electrogram, ventricular near-field electrogram, ventricular far-field electrogram, and marker channel. Note that the first complex (above "689") has the same morphology as the last four complexes on the tracing, which are all sinus beats. The change in the far-field electrogram morphology suggests a ventricular origin for the arrhythmia, confirmed by atrial electrograms, which make it clear that the ventricular rate is greater than the atrial rate. This excludes the possibility of an aberrant supraventricular tachycardia. Note that after marker "VF 217," dropout of sensing due to electrogram diminution results in sensing of the next event outside the tachycardia zone ("VS 373"). The episode terminates spontaneously. (*B,* From Friedman et al.[15] By permission of Futura Publishing Company.)

is clearly important, because the approach to therapy can be quite different; this is discussed in greater depth in Chapter 9. Recording real-time far-field electrograms during sinus rhythm with the patient in various positions can also be useful to provide a comparison with the stored electrograms. Additionally, comparing near-field and far-field electrograms can at times determine which conductor is affected when lead fracture is present. In ICDs in which far-field electrograms are recorded between the shocking electrograms, noise present only in the far-field recordings identifies a defect involving the shocking lead but sparing the sensing leads (Fig. 13–37).

Near-field electrograms are recorded between the distal tip and the ring in true bipolar systems and between the tip and the distal coil in integrated systems (Fig. 13–35) (see Chapter 4). The more tightly spaced bipole causes a more discrete deflection to be generated by local myocardial activation (Fig. 13–35), which is superior for determining the ventricular rate but provides less morphologic information. Since the near-field electrogram is what the defibrillator "sees" for rhythm detection, it is usually the most useful electrographic source for troubleshooting device malfunction when oversensing or inappropriate shocks occur. A diminished near-field R wave, far-field (e.g., diaphragmatic) noise apparent on the near-field electrogram, and make-break electrical noise can all adversely affect device function (Fig. 13–31).

Episode logs provide summary information on the type of episode (supraventricular or ventricular), time and date of episodes, therapies delivered, and whether therapies were successful. Episode log review can provide useful information on

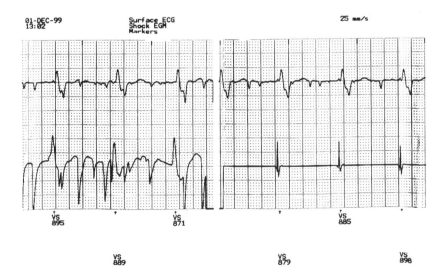

Fig. 13–37. Real-time recording during device testing. An abandoned lead is making contact with the proximal coil in this integrated bipolar lead. *Left,* Surface electrocardiogram (ECG), top, and shock electrogram (EGM), bottom. Note the marked electrical noise on the bottom tracing (Shock EGM). This contact noise is also seen on the surface recording, most likely because of an uncapped abandoned lead present at the time of this recording. *Right,* Surface ECG, top, and rate-sensing EGM (recorded between the tip and distal coil), bottom. Note the persistence of noise on the surface ECG and complete absence of noise on the rate-sensing electrogram. The clean signal on the rate-sensing electrogram at a time when noise is still present excludes association of the tip or distal coil with the noise; thus, the problem lies with the proximal coil. Lead repositioning eliminated the problem.

a change in frequency of episodes (which might suggest deteriorating cardiac status) and the effectiveness of painless ATP therapies (Fig. 13–38). Correlation between episode timing and a missed dose of medication may suggest the cause of a flurry of episodes (Fig. 13–38).

During a routine follow-up examination, provocative maneuvers should be performed (deep breathing, arm motion, sit up) during continuous telemetering and recording of near-field and far-field signals. These maneuvers may unmask lead or sensing problems (Fig. 13–39). An abnormal response to these

maneuvers may require device reprogramming or surgical revision. For discussion in greater detail, see Chapter 9.

Device-Device Interactions

Because current-generation ICDs are capable of fully functional antibradycardia therapy, implantation of separate pacemaker and defibrillator pulse generators has become rare. However, patients with separate systems require continuing follow-up, and occasionally a patient with a fully functional older generation pace-

```
TACHY EPISODE LOG REPORT ------------------------------- Page    1 of

Episode Data Interrogated: Mar 25, 2000 19:00:56
Episode Data Last Cleared:  Mar 23, 2000 11:35:38


   ID     DATE      TIME    TYPE AVG CYCLE   LAST Rx   SUCCESS DURATION
  -----  ------  --------- ---- --------- ---------- ------- --------
   43    Mar 25 15:15:59  VF    290 ms   VF  Rx 1     Yes    14 sec
   42    Mar 25 15:10:20  VF    290 ms   VF  Rx 1     Yes    11 sec
   41    Mar 25 15:03:07  VF    290 ms   (No Rx Delivered)   16 sec
   40    Mar 25 12:52:45  VF    300 ms   (No Rx Delivered)   13 sec
   39    Mar 25 12:45:09  VF    300 ms   (No Rx Delivered)   16 sec
   38    Mar 25 12:17:17  VF    290 ms   (No Rx Delivered)   19 sec
```

A   Medtronic 7221   SN   PFK204583H Rev 9891A302   Mar 25, 2000 19:25

```
VENTRICULAR EPISODE SUMMARY REPORT ------------------ Page  1 of  2

Date Interrogated: Mar 22, 2000 10:03:53
Date Last Cleared: Feb 14, 2000 08:35:38

ID    DATE    TIME    TYPE RRMEDIAN LAST THERAPY SUCCESS DURATION
---- ------ -------- ---- -------- ------------ ------- --------
00148 Mar 18 09:53:53  VT+  420 ms    VT Rx1     Yes    00:00:27
00146 Mar 18 04:33:50  VT+  410 ms    VT Rx1     Yes    00:01:34
00144 Mar 18 04:30:37  VT+  400 ms    VT Rx6     Yes    00:02:32
00142 Mar 18 04:27:45  VT+  410 ms    VT Rx4     Yes    00:02:16
00140 Mar 17 06:57:02  VT+  410 ms    VT Rx1     Yes    00:03:02
00138 Mar 17 06:55:18  VT+  420 ms    VT Rx1     Yes    00:01:14
00136 Mar 17 06:54:11  VT+  410 ms    VT Rx1     Yes    00:00:12
00135 Mar 17 06:53:52  VT+  410 ms    VT Rx1     Yes    00:00:09
00133 Mar 16 06:52:16  VT   410 ms    VT Rx4     Yes    00:03:31
00132 Mar 16 05:51:36  VT   410 ms    VT Rx1     Yes    00:00:28
00131 Mar 16 05:51:16  VT   420 ms    VT Rx1     Yes    00:00:16
00130 Mar 16 03:22:16  VT   420 ms    VT Rx1     Yes    00:01:06
00129 Mar 16 03:21:15  VT   420 ms    VT Rx1     Yes    00:00:19
00128 Mar 11 06:19:00  VT   410 ms    VT Rx1     Yes    00:00:15
00127 Mar 11 05:23:45  VT   410 ms    VT Rx1     Yes    00:00:16
00126 Mar 11 05:22:37  VT   410 ms    VT Rx1     Yes    00:00:32
00125 Mar 11 05:22:09  VT   410 ms    VT Rx1     Yes    00:00:22
```

```
VENTRICULAR EPISODE SUMMARY REPORT ----------- Page  2 of  2

ID    DATE    TIME    TYPE RRMEDIAN LAST THERAPY SUCCESS DURATION
---- ------ -------- ---- -------- ------------ ------- --------
00124 Mar 11 02:25:16  VT   410 ms    VT Rx1     Yes    00:00:22
00123 Mar 10 05:56:09  VT   400 ms    VT Rx1     Yes    00:00:31
00122 Mar 10 05:55:25  VT   400 ms    VT Rx1     Yes    00:00:41
00121 Mar 10 05:54:38  VT   400 ms    VT Rx1     Yes    00:00:15
00120 Mar 10 05:54:10  VT   400 ms    VT Rx1     Yes    00:00:17
00119 Mar 10 05:53:22  VT   410 ms    VT Rx1     Yes    00:00:15
00118 Mar 10 05:52:21  VT   410 ms    VT Rx1     Yes    00:00:16
00117 Mar 10 05:51:50  VT   390 ms    VT Rx1     Yes    00:00:16
```

B   Medtronic 7250   SN PID100034R Rev 9891A222   Mar 22, 2000 10:04   Medtronic 7250   SN PID100034R Rev 9891A222   Mar 22, 2000 10:04

Fig. 13–38. Event logs to guide diagnosis and assess the effectiveness of therapy. *A*, The patient forgot to take his antiarrhythmic medication in the morning of March 25 and then remembered to take it around 1:30 P.M. Note the development of frequent short episodes around noon (starting with episode ID 38 at 12:17). Since the episodes subsided at 3:15, the flurry may have been due to the missed dose. The patient was asymptomatic until two shocks were delivered (for episodes 42 and 43). *B*, The episode log for a patient with refractory ventricular tachycardia (VT) illustrates a high frequency of VT, which is predominantly successfully treated with antitachycardia pacing (VT R×1). Episodes 133, 142, and 144 were associated with shocks (note that the last therapies were VT R×4 and VT R×6), prompting the patient to seek evaluation.

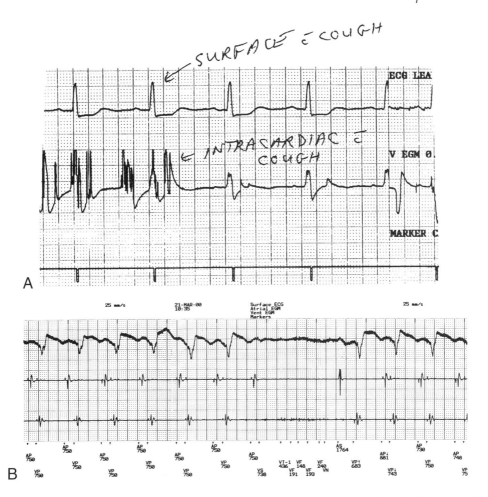

Fig. 13–39. Provocative maneuvers during real-time telemetry to detect lead malfunction. *A,* Recording of surface electrocardiogram (ECG) (top) and far-field electrogram (EGM) (middle), with a marker channel (bottom). During cough, electrical make-break contact noise is seen, confirming a fracture of the conductor to the shocking coil. Note that the marker channel demonstrates normal sensing of the QRS complexes, suggesting that the sensing conductor within the lead remains intact. *B,* Deep breathing during real-time recording. Shown from top to bottom are surface ECG, atrial EGM, ventricular near-field EGM, and markers. The patient has sinus bradycardia and high-grade atrioventricular block. Note that with deep inspiration, diaphragmatic noise is sensed as ventricular tachycardia/ventricular fibrillation (starting at marker VT-1, 436). This transiently inhibits pacing, leading to a pause. The patient had received a shock during deep-breathing exercises. Reprogramming to diminish ventricular sensitivity eliminated the problem.

maker or defibrillator requires additional device therapy and subsequently undergoes implantation of a second system.

Numerous interactions between pacemakers and ICDs can occur, and testing protocols have been developed to detect those interactions.[32–38] Since up to 50% of patients may have significant pacemaker-ICD interactions that can be avoided if properly identified, testing is warranted. Among the more common interactions described are inhibition of ventricular fibrillation detection by the pacemaker pacing artifacts (Fig. 3–40), in-

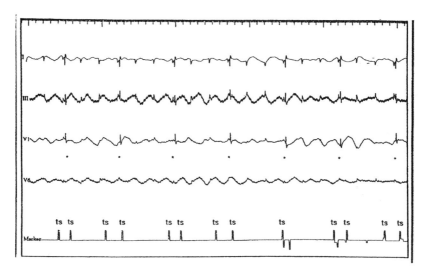

Fig. 13–40. Inhibition of the detection of implantable cardioverter-defibrillator ventricular fibrillation (VF) by artifacts generated by a concomitant pacemaker, found at the time of testing for device-device interactions. Asterisks denote pacemaker spikes. Because of the large amplitude of the pacing spike relative to the continuing VF, autoadjusting sensitivity becomes less sensitive (as if an R wave had been detected), and the VF is not appropriately sensed. (Modified from Friedman et al.[15] By permission of Futura Publishing Company.)

appropriate detection of tachycardia by the defibrillator because of overdetection of pacemaker stimulus artifacts, and various postshock phenomena.[37] Most of these interactions can be avoided if meticulous testing is done at implantation and follow-up. Our recommended testing is summarized in Table 13–5.[37]

Specific Situations Suggesting Further Evaluation or Arrhythmia Induction

As noted above, a number of clinical situations may suggest the need for further ICD testing (Table 13–4). The diagnosis and correction of frequent ICD therapies (symptomatic or asymptomatic) are discussed in Chapter 9). Other situations are discussed below.

Medications. The interaction of medications and defibrillators requires special mention in follow-up, because medications may be modified by other physicians without full appreciation of the interaction with ICDs. Medications, and particularly membrane-active antiarrhythmic drugs, can affect pacing function, defibrillation function, and the underlying arrhythmias. The effects of medications on defibrillator function are summarized in Table 13–6. Addition of medication can affect pacing thresholds, and these should be rechecked. Class IC agents have use dependency, so that their effects are amplified at higher heart rates; thus, ATP may have more of an effect than standard antibradycardia pacing. Most third- and later-generation devices permit independent programming of ATP outputs, and these should generally be set for values greater than those of the standard pacing therapies. A fuller discussion of the effects of medication on pacing function is found in Chapter 1.

The most prominent effect of antiarrhythmic drugs in patients with ICDs is the slowing of ventricular tachyarrhythmias. Ventricular tachycardia may slow

Table 13–5.
Recommended Testing to Screen for Implantable
Cardioverter-Defibrillator (ICD) and Pacemaker (PM) Interactions

Assess	PM	ICD	Comments
ICD sensing of PM artifact	• Pace at low rate • Maximum output, A and V channels • Long AV delay	• Record electrogram	Unacceptable values (may impair VF detection): • Stimulus artifact > 2 mV • Stimulus artifact: evoked electrogram ratio > 1:3 If unacceptable values found: • Reposition ICD sensing lead if possible (optimal) • Decrease pacing output and reassess
ICD detection of VF during asynchronous pacing outputs	• VOO or DOO (asynchronous) mode • High rate (90–120) • Long AV delay (≥ 200 msec)	• Induce VF • Record electrogram	• Assess worst case scenario for VF detection • Best to repeat at least once • Consider testing with PM programmed to power-on-reset values (in case ICD shock generates power on reset)
Pacemaker sensing of arrhythmia	• Parameters set to values for planned future use • Continuously record PPM telemetry	• Record electrograms	• Induce VF • Note PM response (asynchronous pacing?) • Noise reversion or arrhythmia non-sensing
Postshock interactions			Review all tracings from above and analyze for postshock phenomena: • Loss of capture • Oversensing

AV, atrioventricular; VF, ventricular fibrillation.
Data from Glickson et al.[37]

Table 13–6.
Interactions of Medications and Implantable Cardioverter-Defibrillators (ICDs)

ICD function	Potential medication effect
Sensing Detection	• Diminished slew rate could affect detection (rare) • Ventricular tachycardia rate slowed below detection cutoff rate • QRS widening can alter some detection criteria
Pacing	• Increase pacing threshold • Increase threshold at rapid pacing rates, as in antitachycardia pacing (use dependency, particularly class IC agents) • Induce bradycardia or atrioventricular block necessitating antibradycardia pacing
Defibrillation	• Proarrhythmia with increased shock frequency • Increase or decrease defibrillation threshold (detailed in Chapter 2)

below the cutoff rate and remain unde-tected. Increasing or decreasing the defib-rillation threshold can also alter the effec-tiveness of fibrillation termination. Thus, initiation of antiarrhythmic therapy is usu-ally best followed by ICD testing, includ-ing arrhythmia induction. The effects of medication on defibrillation function are discussed in greater detail in Chapter 1.

Decreasing Sensitivity to Prevent Over-sensing of Non-QRS Signals. At times, either from T-wave oversensing or from myopotential oversensing, the defibrilla-tor is made less sensitive (discussed in greater detail in Chapter 9). Although this may correct pacing or detection problems, the possibility of underdetection of small-amplitude electrograms during ventricu-lar fibrillation exists. This is particularly true after a failed shock, since lead polar-ization potentials as well as cell mem-brane electroporation result in diminished postshock electrograms. In Endotak series 0060 leads (in which the distance from the distal coil to the lead tip is small), the re-sult has occasionally been impaired rede-tection.[39,40] Although this phenomenon is less prominent in newer lead systems with greater space between the tip and the distal coil, assessment of ventricular fibril-lation detection, particularly after a failed shock, should be considered whenever sensitivity is diminished.

Putting It All Together: Evidence-based Implantable Defibrillator Follow-up

Clearly, the risks of system malfunc-tion or of patient-specific changes (such as an increase in DFT) that may compromise device function are not uniform but de-pend on multiple predictable risk factors, including lead type, pulse generator loca-tion, and a concomitant pacing system, among other factors. Thus, patients can be risk-stratified on the basis of the likeli-hood of system malfunction and follow-up tailored accordingly (Table 13–7).[15] Pa-tients with biphasic, active can, pectoral systems with multiluminal leads (i.e., not coaxial) and an implantation DFT of less than 15 J are at low risk for system com-plications. Furthermore, if complications do occur, they are well detected with vig-ilant outpatient clinic follow-up (by elec-trogram review, radiography, pacing pa-rameter, and painless high-voltage lead assessment, when available) without the need for arrhythmia induction. Since lead failures seem to increase over time and data are less robust after 3 to 4 years of follow-up, we increase the frequency of clinic visits after 3 years. In contrast to the low-risk group, patients who have systems with one or more risk factors un-dergo more frequent clinic visits (every 3 months) and annual inductions of ar-rhythmia (Table 13–7). Published reports that have recommended routine arrhyth-mia inductions have included patients who would be classified in the high-risk group.[19,25,41,42]

Patient Concerns

It is impossible to predict all con-cerns that might be raised by the patient with a permanent pacemaker. However, several specific issues are invariably raised, and they should be included in the information, whether written or oral, provided to the patient.

Electromagnetic Interference

Although patients do not use the term "electromagnetic interference" (EMI), they ask whether anything in the environment interferes with pacemakers. The reader is referred to Chapter 12 for a complete dis-cussion. Here, a few specific recurrent pa-tient concerns merit repeating.

Microwave ovens are not a concern at

Table 13–7.
Recommended Follow-up Based on Risk of System Complications of Malfunction

	Low risk	High risk
Group definition	All of the following characteristics present: DFT < 15 J Pectoral pulse generator Active can Endovascular (transvenous) leads	Any of the following present: DFT ≥ 15 J Abdominal pulse generator Cold can Epicardial leads Separate sensing lead PM and ICD: 2 devices Subcutaneous lead Coaxial lead
Recommended routine clinic follow-up	Every 6 months after implantation; every 3 months starting at 3 years	Every 3 months
Recommended routine arrhythmia inductions and DFT testing	At pulse generator change out only	Annual
Routine radiographic examination of entire system, from pulse generator to distal lead	Every 6 months	Every 6 months

DFT, defibrillation threshold; ICD, implantable cardioverter-defibrillator; PM, pacemaker.

this time despite the signs that remain posted near some microwave ovens in public places. Patients should be told that there were concerns with older pacemakers that were not as well shielded and older microwaves that were not as well sealed. Interference is no longer a problem.

Cellular telephones should not be a concern for the patient with a pacemaker. As discussed in Chapter 12, the patient should avoid holding the activated ("on") phone near the pacemaker or ICD. Ideally, the patient should use the phone at the ear contralateral to the pacemaker or ICD.[43]

Electronic article surveillance equipment has been a controversial issue in recent years. Although interference with pacemakers and ICDs is possible, some simple advice for the patient with an implantable device should suffice.[44–47] Patients should be aware of the location of surveillance equipment and avoid lingering within or near any antitheft device.

The phrase "don't linger, don't lean" has been popularized to summarize this advice. Legislation is pending that will require public places that use electronic article surveillance equipment to post signs indicating the location of the equipment.

Somewhat surprisingly, questions regarding welding equipment are not uncommon. For the non-pacemaker-dependent patient, the use of most hobby welding equipment should not be a problem. Patients should be questioned about the strength of the welding equipment they use. Previous work has demonstrated that alternating current hobby welding equipment in the range of 100 to 150 A should not cause a problem.[48] Industrial strength welding, that is, alternating current of 200 to 500 A, definitely has the potential for clinically significant EMI. Patients with pacemakers or ICDs who work with or close to such equipment should be individually assessed, especially if they are pacemaker-dependent. With ICDs, in theory, oversensing of the EMI could result in a false-positive interpretation that delivers a shock to the patient.

Specific work environments that contain equipment capable of producing EMI require individual assessment. Work environments with degaussing equipment, such as the television industry, induction ovens, and industrial welding, are of particular concern.[48] If a patient's livelihood depends on working in such an environment, the issues must be considered carefully; the patient should not be glibly told that return to this job is not possible. Testing procedures can be performed to determine whether the work environment is indeed hostile. For the non-pacemaker-dependent patient, the risk posed by EMI is obviously less significant. It may be possible to assess nondependent patients by ambulatory monitoring or patient-triggered event records.[49]

Medical Advisories and Recalls

Dealing with medical advisories and recalls from the manufacturer or the Food and Drug Administration (FDA) and reporting device failures are responsibilities of the physician or the institution, or both, providing follow-up care.[50]

The FDA categorizes recalls into three classes:

- Class I—Situations in which there is a reasonable probability that the use of, or exposure to, a violative product will cause serious adverse health consequences or death
- Class II—Situations in which the use of, or exposure to, a violative product may cause temporary or medically reversible adverse health consequences or in which the probability of serious adverse health consequences is remote
- Class III—Situations in which the use of, or exposure to, a violative

product is not likely to cause adverse health consequences

Safety advisories or safety alerts are sometimes issued and are, in general, less significant than class III recalls.

When informed of a recall or advisory, the physician or institution involved in follow-up of the patient with a pacemaker or ICD is responsible for making certain that the patient is aware of the potential problem and that appropriate steps are taken. Necessary action depends on the type of problem identified. Action may range from pulse generator or lead replacement to lead extraction, intensified follow-up, or patient notification only. Patient notification and advice should be documented in the medical chart.

Pacemaker clinic personnel should be available to discuss the alert or advisory with the patient after notification. They should also be knowledgeable about the specific problem and be able to explain the problem in a way the patient can understand.[51]

Under the Safe Medical Devices Act of 1990 (Public Law 101-629) and the Medical Device Amendments of 1992, hospitals, ambulatory surgical facilities, nursing homes, and outpatient treatment facilities that are not physicians' offices must report to the FDA or the manufacturer any death, serious illness, or serious injury caused or contributed to by a medical device. Such incidents should be reported within 10 working days of the event. Patient deaths must be reported to the FDA, and serious illness and injury must be reported only to the manufacturer. (If the manufacturer is unknown, the report should be made to the FDA.)

Lifestyle and Personal Concerns

Return to driving has traditionally been less of an issue with pacemakers than with ICDs. Both the North American Society of Pacing and Electrophysiology and the Canadian Cardiovascular Society have established guidelines for return to driving after pacemaker implantation.[52,53] These are summarized in Table 13–8. Regulations for return to driving differ from state to state.

We advise patients not to drive for 2 weeks after pacemaker implantation or revision of the ventricular lead, explaining that it is a medicolegal concern. Although rules vary among various countries and even states within the United States, general principles have been adopted by both American and European expert panels. Patients with ICDs are prohibited from any commercial driving. Personal driving is permissible but only after a prohibition of 6 months for patients who have clinical syncope or ICD discharge with significant symptoms.

Another relatively minor but driving-related issue is whether a seat belt interferes with the pacemaker. The seat belt may be over the pacemaker site for the driver with a left pectoral implant or a passenger with a right-sided implant. Seat belts are not an issue unless they cause some irritation at the implantation site in the early weeks after implantation. If irritation is a concern, the patient can place some padding over the pacing site or around the seat belt in the vicinity of the pacemaker. This should *not* be an excuse not to wear a seat belt.

Limitation of physical activities after pacemaker implantation must be addressed. For the adult patient, we recommend that ipsilateral arm movement be limited to 90° abduction for 3 to 4 weeks. Admittedly, this may be overcautious. The lead is secured to the pectoral muscle near the venous insertion site, and it is unlikely that more vigorous arm movements would dislodge the lead. However, some guidelines should be given, and this approach has been successful for us, with most adult patients seeming to follow the advice without difficulty.

Table 13–8.
Guidelines for Driving After Pacemaker Implantation

Condition	Noncommercial*	Commercial*
No symptoms No pacemaker	A	A
Syncope or near-syncope No pacemaker	C	C
Not pacemaker-dependent[†] Pacemaker	A	A
Pacemaker-dependent[†] Pacemaker	B, 1 wk	B, 4 wk

A, no driving restrictions; B, driving permitted after controlled arrhythmia is documented for a specified period and an adequate pacemaker follow-up regimen is followed; C, driving completely prohibited.

*Guidelines from the Canadian Cardiovascular Consensus Conference differ only in that all patients for private driving are restricted for 1 week after pacemaker implantation, must not have evidence of cerebral ischemia, and must have a pacemaker that is performing normally with normal sensing and capture. For commercial driving, the same guidelines apply except that the waiting period to drive is 4 weeks and the pacemaker output pulse must be at least 3 times the measured stimulation threshold.[53]

†For these purposes, "pacemaker-dependent" is applied to patients who have lost consciousness in the past due to bradyarrhythmias. The term may also be applied to patients immediately after atrioventricular junction ablation and to any other patient in whom sudden pacemaker failure is likely to result in alteration of consciousness.

From Epstein et al.[52] By permission of American Heart Association.

We also recommend that patients limit lifting to no more than 10 pounds with the ipsilateral arm for the first 2 weeks after implantation.

Pediatric patients are less likely to follow any activity guidelines. For the very small child, it is not unreasonable to have the child wear a loose sling on the ipsilateral arm as a reminder to limit arm motion.

Issues of return to work and disability arise. Once again, the advice should be individualized. Patients who have jobs that do not involve heavy physical exertion can return to work shortly after the procedure. It is unusual for the patient to experience postoperative pain significant enough to require more than ibuprofen or acetaminophen and to limit the ability to perform the job. Patients who have jobs that involve heavy physical exertion in which performance depends on upper body strength may need to wait longer to return to work.

Sports activities are important to many patients, young and old. Patients are told that they can return to most sports activities. For the younger patient, most competitive sports are all right with the exception of contact sports having a significant potential for injury. Specifically, football, wrestling, and boxing carry some risk. Patients should be informed of the risk and be given counseling to weigh the ratio of risk to benefit. The predominant concern with contact sports is direct trauma to the lead at or near the connector block. In other athletic activities, the concern is repetitive upper arm movement that might predispose the patient to a subclavian crush injury. There are case reports of lead injury with weightlifting. Again, the issues should be discussed with the patient and the importance of the activity weighed against the risk.

Golf and swimming are two of the most common athletic activities for the average patient with a pacemaker. We suggest waiting 4 weeks after implantation before returning to golfing. Swimming can be resumed as soon as the incision is healed, but the recommendation is to limit some strokes for 4 weeks to stay within the abduction guidelines already discussed.

Hunting and marksmanship also seem to be relatively frequent activities for our patient population. The pacemaker should be implanted on the side contralateral to that from which the patient shoots. We allow patients to return to these activities at any time so long as they stay within the shoulder movement guidelines outlined.

Activity restrictions for ICD recipients are in many ways similar to those for pacemaker recipients. Patients with slow ventricular tachycardia and young or active patients should undergo exercise testing to determine their peak heart rate with activity so that inappropriate detection of physiologic tachycardia as an arrhythmia can be avoided. ICD recipients are currently ineligible for competitive sports; however, noncompetitive athletics and physical activity are generally encouraged.

Concerns about resumption of sexual activities are frequent. Patients are often reluctant to ask questions about resuming sexual activities, and ideally the information should be offered. Patients are told that they may resume sexual activities whenever they like so long as they observe the shoulder motion guidelines.

Similar to the seat belt issue previously discussed, some women are concerned about irritation to the device site by their brassiere strap. Our patients are advised either not to wear a brassiere until the incision is well healed or nontender or to place extra padding around the strap.

Many unanticipated concerns arise. Initial education about the pacemaker and how it works is the best way to pre-empt the patient's apprehension.

Conclusion

Appropriate follow-up of pacemakers and implantable defibrillators is required to ensure continuing integrity of the system and to detect failures before they become clinically manifest. This requires a thorough understanding of both device function and interpretation of the extensive telemetered data provided by newer systems. However, with the incorporation of routine device self-assessment (including lead impedances and pacing thresholds), devices may soon be able to effectively advise patients when follow-up is required. Additionally, with continued maturation of device technology and emerging automated self-assessment, summaries highlighting potential problems, and one-button "quick checks," the emphasis at follow-up visits will shift from device evaluation to patient assessment, and the provider's role will change from technician-troubleshooter to practitioner of medicine.

References

1. Furman S, Parker B, Escher DJ: Transtelephone pacemaker clinic. J Thorac Cardiovasc Surg 61:827–834, 1971
2. Furman S, Escher DJ: Transtelephone pacemaker monitoring: five years later. Ann Thorac Surg 20:326–338, 1975
3. MED-MANUAL, MED-GUIDE ¶27,201, Coverage Issue Manual §50–1 Cardiac Pacemaker Evaluation Services [Effective date: October 1, 1984]
4. VonFeldt L, Neubauer SA, Hayes DL: Is transtelephonic monitoring a useful method to detect pacing system abnormalities? (Abstract.) Pacing Clin Electrophysiol 15:544, 1992
5. Hayes DL, Hyberger LK, Lloyd MA: Should the Medicare trans-telephonic pacemaker follow-up schedule be altered? (Abstract.) Pacing Clin Electrophysiol 20:1153, 1997
6. Mond HG: The Cardiac Pacemaker: Function and Malfunction. New York, Grune & Stratton, 1983, p 178
7. Roy PR, Sowton E: Clinical experience with the Elema Vario pacemaker. Br Med J 4:637–640, 1974
8. Goldschlager N, Ludmer P, Creamer C: Follow-up of the paced outpatient. *In* Clinical Cardiac Pacing. Edited by KA Ellenbogen, GN Kay, BL Wilkoff. Philadelphia, WB Saunders Company, 1995, pp 780–808
9. Parsonnet V, Neglia D, Bernstein AD: The frequency of pacemaker-system problems, etiologies, and corrective interventions (abstract). Pacing Clin Electrophysiol 15:510, 1992
10. Levine PA, Sanders R, Markowitz HT: Pacemaker diagnostics: measured data, event marker, electrogram, and event counter telemetry. *In* Clinical Cardiac Pacing. Edited by KA Ellenbogen, GN Kay, BL Wilkoff. Philadelphia, WB Saunders Company, 1995, pp 639–655
11. Trusty JM, Hayes DL, Stanton MS, Friedman PA: Factors affecting the frequency of subcutaneous lead usage in implantable defibrillators. Pacing Clin Electrophysiol 23:842–846, 2000
12. Adams TP: Patient followup systems. *In* Implantable Cardioverter Defibrillator Therapy: The Engineering-Clinical Interface. Edited by MW Kroll, MH Lehmann. Norwell, MA, Kluwer Academic Publishers, 1996, pp 421–434
13. Splett V, Trusty JM, Hammill SC, Friedman PA: Determination of pacing capture in implantable defibrillators. Evoked response detection using RV coil to can vector. Pacing Clin Electrophysiol (in press)
14. Brady PA, Friedman PA, Trusty JM, Grice S, Hammill SC, Stanton MS: High failure rate for an epicardial implantable cardioverter-defibrillator lead: implications for long-term follow-up of patients with an implantable cardioverter-defibrillator. J Am Coll Cardiol 31:616–622, 1998
15. Friedman PA, Glickson M, Stanton MS: Defibrillator challenges for the new millennium: the marriage of device and patient—making and maintaining a good match. J Cardiovasc Electrophysiol 11:697–709, 2000
16. Luria DM, Chugh SS, Lexvold NY, Hammill SC, Shen WK, Friedman PA: High rate of long-term endovascular lead failure with abdominally placed implantable defibrillators (abstract). Circulation 100 Suppl I:I-568, 1999
17. Schwartzman D, Nallamothu N, Callans DJ, Preminger MW, Gottlieb CD, Marchlinski FE: Postoperative lead-related complications in patients with nonthoracotomy

defibrillation lead systems. J Am Coll Cardiol 26:776–786, 1995

18. Mann DE, Kelly PA, Damle RS, Reiter MJ: Undersensing during ventricular tachyarrhythmias in a third-generation implantable cardioverter defibrillator: diagnosis using stored electrograms and correction with programming. Pacing Clin Electrophysiol 17:1525–1530, 1994

19. Lawton JS, Ellenbogen KA, Wood MA, Stambler BS, Herre JM, Nath S, Bernstein RC, DiMarco JP, Haines DE, Szentpetery S, Baker LD, Damiano RJ Jr: Sensing lead-related complications in patients with transvenous implantable cardioverter-defibrillators. Am J Cardiol 78:647–651, 1996

20. Auricchio A, Hartung W, Geller C, Klein H: Clinical relevance of stored electrograms for implantable cardioverter-defibrillator (ICD) troubleshooting and understanding of mechanisms for ventricular tachyarrhythmias. Am J Cardiol 78:33–41, 1996

21. Luria D, Rasmussen MJ, Hammill SC, Friedman PA: Frequency and mode of detection of nonthoracotomy implantable defibrillator lead failure (abstract). Pacing Clin Electrophysiol 22:705, 1999

22. O'Hara GE, Rashtian MY, Lemke B, Philippon F, Gilbert M, Brown AB, Cuijpers A, Koehler J, Soucy B, and the 7271 Gem DR Worldwide Investigators: Patient alert: clinical experience with a new patient monitoring system in a dual chamber defibrillator (abstract). Pacing Clin Electrophysiol 22:709, 1999

23. Philippon F, Johnson BW, Waldecker B, O'Hara GE, Gilbert M, Brown AB, Ayeni F, Soucy B: Painless lead impedance in a dual chamber defibrillator (abstract). Pacing Clin Electrophysiol 22:825, 1999

24. Luria D, Glikson M, Hammill S, Friedman P: Stability of long-term defibrillation thresholds in patients with nonthoracotomy implantable defibrillators. Cardiac Arrhythmias 1999. Proceedings of the 6th International Workshop on Cardiac Arrhythmias, Springer, 1999:40

25. Korte T, Jung W, Spehl S, Wolpert C, Moosdorf R, Manz M, Luderitz B: Incidence of ICD lead related complications during long-term follow-up: comparison of epicardial and endocardial electrode systems. Pacing Clin Electrophysiol 18:2053–2061, 1995

26. Olsovsky MR, Pelini MA, Shorofsky SR, Gold MR: Temporal stability of defibrillation thresholds with an active pectoral lead system. J Cardiovasc Electrophysiol 9:240–244, 1998

27. Gold MR, Kavesh NG, Peters RW, Shorofsky SR: Biphasic waveforms prevent the chronic rise of defibrillation thresholds with a transvenous lead system. J Am Coll Cardiol 30:233–236, 1997

28. Tokano T, Pelosi F, Flemming M, Horwood L, Souza JJ, Zivin A, Knight BP, Goyal R, Man KC, Morady F, Strickberger SA: Long-term evaluation of the ventricular defibrillation energy requirement. J Cardiovasc Electrophysiol 9:916–920, 1998

29. Glikson M, Luria D, Friedman PA, Trusty JM, Benderly M, Hammill SC, Stanton MS: Are routine arrhythmia inductions necessary in patients with pectoral implantable cardioverter defibrillators? J Cardiovasc Electrophysiol 11:127–135, 2000

30. Schaumann A, von zur Muhlen F, Herse B, Gonska BD, Kreuzer H: Empirical versus tested antitachycardia pacing in implantable cardioverter defibrillators: a prospective study including 200 patients. Circulation 97:66–74, 1998

31. Friedman PA, Stanton MS: The pacer-cardioverter-defibrillator: function and clinical experience. J Cardiovasc Electrophysiol 6:48–68, 1995

32. Clemo HF, Ellenbogen KA, Belz MK, Wood MA, Stambler BS: Safety of pacemaker implantation in patients with transvenous (nonthoracotomy) implantable cardioverter defibrillators. Pacing Clin Electrophysiol 17:2285–2291, 1994

33. Cohen AI, Wish MH, Fletcher RD, Miller FC, McCormick D, Shuck J, Shapira N, Delnegro AA: The use and interaction of permanent pacemakers and the automatic implantable cardioverter defibrillator. Pacing Clin Electrophysiol 11:704–711, 1988

34. Brooks R, Garan H, McGovern BA, Ruskin JN: Implantation of transvenous nonthoracotomy cardioverter-defibrillator systems in patients with permanent endocardial pacemakers. Am Heart J 129:45–53, 1995

35. Epstein AE, Wilkoff BL: Pacemaker-defibrillator interactions. In Clinical Cardiac Pacing. Edited by KA Ellenbogen, GN Kay, BL Wilkoff. Philadelphia, WB Saunders Company, 1995, pp 757–769

36. Geiger MJ, O'Neill P, Sharma A, Skadsen A, Zimerman L, Greenfield RA, Newby KH, Wharton JM, Kent V, Natale A: Interactions between transvenous nonthoracotomy cardioverter defibrillator systems and permanent transvenous endocardial pacemakers. Pacing Clin Electrophysiol 20:624–630, 1997

37. Glikson M, Trusty JM, Grice SK, Hayes DL, Hammill SC, Stanton MS: A stepwise testing protocol for modern implantable cardioverter-defibrillator systems to prevent pacemaker-implantable cardioverter-defibrillator interactions. Am J Cardiol 83: 360–366, 1999

38. Glikson M, Trusty JM, Grice SK, Hayes DL, Hammill SC, Stanton MS: Importance of pacemaker noise reversion as a potential mechanism of pacemaker-ICD interactions. Pacing Clin Electrophysiol 21: 1111–1121, 1998

39. Brady PA, Friedman PA, Stanton MS: Effect of failed defibrillation shocks on electrogram amplitude in a nonintegrated transvenous defibrillation lead system. Am J Cardiol 76:580–584, 1995

40. Jung W, Manz M, Moosdorf R, Luderitz B: Failure of an implantable cardioverter-defibrillator to redetect ventricular fibrillation in patients with a nonthoracotomy lead system. Circulation 86:1217–1222, 1992

41. Higgins SL, Rich DH, Haygood JR, Barone J, Greer SL, Meyer DB: ICD restudy: results and potential benefit from routine predischarge and 2-month evaluation. Pacing Clin Electrophysiol 21:410–417, 1998

42. Mattke S, Muller D, Markewitz A, Kaulbach H, Schmockel M, Dorwarth U, Hoffmann E, Steinbeck G: Failures of epicardial and transvenous leads for implantable cardioverter defibrillators. Am Heart J 130:1040–1044, 1995

43. Hayes DL, Wang PJ, Reynolds DW, Estes M III, Griffith JL, Steffens RA, Carlo GL, Findlay GK, Johnson CM: Interference with cardiac pacemakers by cellular telephones. N Engl J Med 336:1473–1479, 1997

44. Groh WJ, Boschee SA, Engelstein ED, Miles WM, Burton ME, Foster PR, Crevey BJ, Zipes DP: Interactions between electronic article surveillance systems and implantable cardioverter-defibrillators. Circulation 100:387–392, 1999

45. McIvor ME, Reddinger J, Floden E, Sheppard RC: Study of Pacemaker and Implantable Cardioverter Defibrillator Triggering by Electronic Article Surveillance Devices (SPICED TEAS). Pacing Clin Electrophysiol 21:1847–1861, 1998

46. Santucci PA, Haw J, Trohman RG, Pinski SL: Interference with an implantable defibrillator by an electronic antitheft-surveillance device. N Engl J Med 339:1371–1374, 1998

47. Burlington DB: Important information on anti-theft and metal detector systems and pacemakers, ICDs, and spinal cord stimulators (9–28-98). Safety alerts, public health advisories, and notices from Center for Devices and Radiological Health, Federal Drug Administration. Retrieved January 14, 2000, from the World Wide Web: http://www.fda.gov/cdrh/safety.html

48. Marco D, Eisinger G, Hayes DL: Testing of work environments for electromagnetic interference. Pacing Clin Electrophysiol 15:2016–2022, 1992

49. Machado C, Johnson D, Thacker JR, Duncan JL: Pacemaker patient-triggered event recording: accuracy, utility, and cost for the pacemaker follow-up clinic. Pacing Clin Electrophysiol 19:1813- 1818, 1996

50. Shein MJ, Brinker JA: Pacing: FDA and the regulatory environment. *In* Clinical Cardiac Pacing. Edited by KA Ellenbogen, GN Kay, BL Wilkoff. Philadelphia, WB Saunders Company, 1995, pp 809–820

51. Lloyd MA, Hyberger LK, Flavin DK, Hayes DL: Pacemaker lead advisories: patient perceptions and management (abstract). Pacing Clin Electrophysiol 20: 1212, 1997

52. Epstein AE, Miles WM, Benditt DG, Camm AJ, Darling EJ, Friedman PL, Garson A Jr, Harvey JC, Kidwell GA, Klein GJ, Levine PA, Marchlinski FE, Prystowsky EN, Wilkoff BL: Personal and public safety issues related to arrhythmias that may affect consciousness: implications for regulation and physician recommendations. A medical/scientific statement from the American Heart Association and the North American Society of Pacing and Electrophysiology. Circulation 94:1147–1166, 1996

53. CCS Consensus Conference Task Force: Assessment of the cardiac patient for fitness to drive. Can J Cardiol 8:406–412, 1992

Index

Page numbers in italics indicate figures; page numbers followed by *t* indicate tables.